WOMEN AND ADDICTION

WOMEN AND ADDICTION
A Comprehensive Handbook

Edited by
KATHLEEN T. BRADY
SUDIE E. BACK
SHELLY F. GREENFIELD

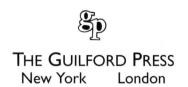

THE GUILFORD PRESS
New York   London

© 2009 The Guilford Press
A Division of Guilford Publications, Inc.
72 Spring Street, New York, NY 10012
www.guilford.com

Printed in the United States of America

This book is printed on acid-free paper.

Last digit is print number: 9 8 7 6 5 4 3 2 1

The editors have checked with sources believed to be reliable in their efforts to provide
information that is complete and generally in accord with the standards of practice that
are accepted at the time of publication. However, in view of the possibility of human
error or changes in medical sciences, neither the editors nor publisher, nor any other
party who has been involved in the preparation or publication of this work warrants
that the information contained herein is in every respect accurate or complete, and they
are not responsible for any errors or omissions or the results obtained from the use of
such information. Readers are encouraged to confirm the information contained in this
book with other sources.

Library of Congress Cataloging-in-Publication Data

Women and addiction : a comprehensive handbook / edited by Kathleen T. Brady,
Sudie E. Back, and Shelly F. Greenfield.
   p. cm.
  Includes bibliographical references and index.
  ISBN 978-1-60623-107-4 (hardcover : alk. paper)
  1. Women drug addicts. 2. Women—Substance abuse. I. Brady, Kathleen, 1952–
II. Back, Sudie E. III. Greenfield, Shelly F.
  HV4229.W65 2009
  616.860082—dc22

                                              2008056153

To my parents, Cecelia and Joseph V. Brady,
who inspired my lifelong interest in understanding
and helping women with addictive disorders
—KATHLEEN T. BRADY

With thanks to my parents, Harry and Bonnie Back,
for teaching me that anything is possible;
my grandmothers, Dilys Back and Elizabeth Harley,
for being such formidable women in my life;
and my husband, Stephen Caskie, for his love and support
—SUDIE E. BACK

Many thanks to Allan, Danny, and Jacob
for their ongoing love and support
—SHELLY F. GREENFIELD

About the Editors

Kathleen T. Brady, MD, PhD, is a board-certified psychiatrist specializing in addiction psychiatry. As Professor of Psychiatry at the Medical University of South Carolina, Dr. Brady is Director of the Clinical Neuroscience Division, Director of the Women's Research Center, Director of the General Clinical Research Center, and Associate Dean for Clinical and Translational Research. She received her doctorate in pharmacology from Virginia Commonwealth University and her medical degree from the Medical University of South Carolina, where she completed a residency in psychiatry and an addiction psychiatry fellowship. Dr. Brady's research interests are in the areas of drug and alcohol abuse/addiction and comorbid conditions such as posttraumatic stress disorder and other anxiety disorders. She has served as Principal Investigator, Co-Principal Investigator, and a mentor on numerous research projects and has received numerous awards for her research, teaching, and clinical work. Dr. Brady has been listed in *Best Doctors in America* since 1998. Her current research involves the investigation of stress response in individuals with substance use and co-occurring psychiatric disorders.

Sudie E. Back, PhD, a clinical psychologist, is Associate Professor of Psychiatry and Associate Director of the Drug Abuse Research Training program for psychiatry residents at the Medical University of South Carolina. Dr. Back received her doctorate in clinical psychology from the University of Georgia and completed her internship at Yale University School of Medicine, Department of Psychiatry. She serves as Principal Investigator or Co-Investigator on numerous federally funded research projects. Her current research involves prescription opioid dependence, the integrated psychosocial treatment of substance use disorders and posttraumatic stress disorder, and gender. The ultimate aim of this line of research is to improve the treatment of individuals with substance use disorders. Dr. Back is the current recipient of a National Institute on Drug Abuse (NIDA)-funded career award to investigate prescription opioid dependence and is the past recipient of an NIDA-funded National Research Service Award that investigated cocaine dependence and gender differences. She also maintains a small clinical practice at the Medical University of South Carolina.

Shelly F. Greenfield, MD, MPH, is Associate Professor of Psychiatry at Harvard Medical School and Chief Academic Officer and Director of Clinical and Health Services Research and Education, Division of Alcohol and Drug Abuse, McLean Hospital, Belmont, Massachusetts. Dr. Greenfield serves as Principal Investigator and Co-Investigator on federally funded research focusing on treatment for substance use disorders, gender differences in substance disorders, and health services for substance disorders. She is a past recipient of an NIDA-funded career award; a current recipient of an NIDA career award in patient-oriented research; Principal Investigator of an NIDA-funded grant to investigate the efficacy of a new manual-based group therapy for women with substance use disorders; Co-Investigator of a study to evaluate the effectiveness of integrating alcohol treatment into routine tuberculosis care in Tomsk Oblast, Russia; Co-Principal Investigator of the Northern New England node of the NIDA Clinical Trials Network; and chair of the NIDA Clinical Trial Network's Gender Special Interest Group. She is also Director of the Harvard Medical School/Partners Addiction Psychiatry Fellowship, a member of the Board of Directors of the American Academy of Addiction Psychiatry, and Editor-in-Chief of the *Harvard Review of Psychiatry*, and she serves on the Addiction Psychiatry Committee of the American Board of Psychiatry and Neurology. Dr. Greenfield is the recipient of the 2008 Massachusetts Psychiatric Society Research Award and the 2008 Jack H. Mendelson Memorial Research Award for multidisciplinary research on biological and behavioral bases of substance abuse.

Contributors

Sudie E. Back, PhD, Department of Psychiatry and Behavioral Sciences, Clinical Neuroscience Division, Medical University of South Carolina, Charleston, South Carolina

Chaya Bhuvaneswar, MD, MA, MPH, Department of Psychiatry, University of Pennsylvania, Philadelphia, Pennsylvania

Kathleen T. Brady, MD, PhD, Department of Psychiatry and Behavioral Sciences, Clinical Neuroscience Division, Medical University of South Carolina, Charleston, South Carolina

Rebecca W. Brendel, MD, JD, Law and Psychiatry Service, Massachusetts General Hospital, Harvard Medical School, Boston, Massachusetts

E. Sherwood Brown, MD, PhD, Psychoneuroendocrine Research Program, Department of Psychiatry, University of Texas Southwestern Medical Center, Dallas, Texas

Lisa A. Burckell, PhD, Department of Psychology, Stony Brook University, Stony Brook, New York

Grace Chang, MD, MPH, Department of Psychiatry, Brigham and Women's Hospital, Harvard Medical School, Boston, Massachusetts

Lisa R. Cohen, PhD, Department of Psychiatry, College of Physicians and Surgeons of Columbia University, and New York State Psychiatric Institute, New York, New York

Pamela Collins, BA, Department of Psychology, Dalhousie University, Halifax, Nova Scotia, Canada

Latoya C. Conner, PhD, Department of Educational Foundations and Counseling, Hunter College of The City University of New York, New York

Kelly P. Cosgrove, PhD, Department of Psychiatry, Yale University School of Medicine, and VA Connecticut Healthcare System, West Haven, Connecticut

C. Lindsay DeVane, PharmD, Department of Psychiatry and Behavioral Sciences, Clinical Neuroscience Division, Medical University of South Carolina, Charleston, South Carolina

Amanda Elton, BS, Department of Psychiatry and Behavioral Sciences, Emory University School of Medicine, Atlanta, Georgia

Suzette M. Evans, PhD, Department of Psychiatry, College of Physicians and Surgeons of Columbia University, and New York State Psychiatric Institute, New York, New York

William Fals-Stewart, PhD, School of Nursing, Addiction and Family Research Group, University of Rochester, Rochester, New York

Helen Fox, PhD, Department of Psychiatry, Yale University School of Medicine, and Substance Abuse Center, Connecticut Mental Health Center, New Haven, Connecticut

Dubravka Gavric, BA, Department of Psychology, Dalhousie University, Halifax, Nova Scotia, Canada

Risë B. Goldstein, PhD, MPH, Laboratory of Epidemiology and Biometry, Division of Intramural Clinical and Biological Research, National Institute on Alcohol Abuse and Alcoholism, National Institutes of Health, Bethesda, Maryland

Susan M. Gordon, PhD, Seabrook House, Seabrook, New Jersey

Kevin M. Gray, MD, Youth Psychiatry Division, Institute of Psychiatry, Medical University of South Carolina, Charleston, South Carolina

Shelly F. Greenfield, MD, MPH, Department of Psychiatry, Harvard Medical School, and Alcohol and Drug Abuse Treatment Program, McLean Hospital, Harvard Medical School, Belmont, Massachusetts

Christine E. Grella, PhD, Integrated Substance Abuse Programs, the University of California, Los Angeles, Los Angeles, California

Karen Hartwell, MD, Department of Psychiatry and Behavioral Sciences, Clinical Neuroscience Division, Medical University of South Carolina, Charleston, South Carolina

Denise Hien, PhD, Department of Clinical Psychology, The City University of New York, and College of Physicians and Surgeons of Columbia University, New York, New York

Thomas W. Irwin, PhD, The McLean Center at Fernside, Princeton, Massachusetts

Amanda Kalaydjian, PhD, Section on Developmental Genetic Epidemiology, National Institute of Mental Health, Bethesda, Maryland

Clinton D. Kilts, PhD, Department of Psychiatry and Behavioral Sciences, Emory University School of Medicine, Atlanta, Georgia

Michelle L. Kelley, PhD, Department of Psychology, Old Dominion University, Norfolk, Virginia

Wendy K. K. Lam, PhD, University of Rochester School of Nursing, Rochester, New York

Charlene E. Le Fauve, PhD, Co-Occurring and Homeless Activities Branch, Substance Abuse and Mental Health Services Administration, Center for Substance Abuse Treatment, Division of State and Community Assistance, Rockville, Maryland

Ching-ju Lu, MPH, Department of Psychiatry, University of Florida, Gainesville, Florida

Wendy J. Lynch, PhD, Department of Psychiatry, University of Virginia, Charlottesville, Virginia

Carolyn M. Mazure, PhD, Department of Psychiatry, Yale University School of Medicine, New Haven, Connecticut

Alexandra McCaffrey, BA, Cognitive Neuroimaging Laboratory, Brain Imaging Center, McLean Hospital, Harvard Medical School, Belmont, Massachusetts

Shelley McMain, PhD, Borderline Personality Disorder Clinic, Centre for Addiction and Mental Health, Toronto, Ontario, Canada

Aimee L. McRae-Clark, PharmD, BCPP, Department of Psychiatry and Behavioral Sciences, Clinical Neuroscience Division, Medical University of South Carolina, Charleston, South Carolina

Nancy K. Mello, PhD, Alcohol and Drug Abuse Research Center, Department of Psychiatry, McLean Hospital, Harvard Medical School, Belmont, Massachusetts

Kathleen Ries Merikangas, PhD, Section on Developmental Genetic Epidemiology, National Institute of Mental Health, Bethesda, Maryland

Jennifer L. Newman, PhD, Alcohol and Drug Abuse Research Center, Department of Psychiatry, McLean Hospital, Harvard Medical School, Belmont, Massachusetts

Kim-Chi Nguyen, BS, BA, Psychoneuroendocrine Research Program, Department of Psychiatry, University of Texas Southwestern Medical Center, Dallas, Texas

Rebecca Payne, MD, Department of Psychiatry and Behavioral Sciences, Clinical Neuroscience Division, Medical University of South Carolina, Charleston, South Carolina

Kenneth A. Perkins, PhD, Department of Psychiatry, Western Psychiatric Institute and Clinic, University of Pittsburgh Medical Center, Pittsburgh, Pennsylvania

Helen M. Pettinati, PhD, Department of Psychiatry, Treatment Research Center, University of Pennsylvania, Philadelphia, Pennsylvania

Teresa A. Pigott, MD, Department of Psychiatry, University of Florida, Gainesville, Florida

Sandrine Pirard, MD, PhD, Department of Psychiatry, McLean Hospital, Harvard Medical School, Belmont, Massachusetts

Jennifer G. Plebani, PhD, Department of Psychiatry, Treatment Research Center, University of Pennsylvania, Philadelphia, Pennsylvania

Marc N. Potenza, MD, PhD, Department of Psychiatry, Yale University School of Medicine, New Haven, Connecticut

Kimber L. Price, PhD, MSCR, Department of Psychiatry and Behavioral Sciences, Clinical Neuroscience Division, Medical University of South Carolina, Charleston, South Carolina

Stephanie Collins Reed, PhD, Department of Psychiatry, College of Physicians and Surgeons of Columbia University, and New York State Psychiatric Institute, New York, New York

Simona Sava, MD, PhD, Department of Radiology, Children's Hospital Boston, Waltham, Massachusetts

Rajita Sinha, PhD, Department of Psychiatry, Yale University School of Medicine, New Haven, Connecticut

Matthew F. Soulier, MD, Division of Psychiatry and the Law, University of California, Davis, Sacramento, California

Sherry H. Stewart, PhD, Department of Psychology, Dalhousie University, Halifax, Nova Scotia, Canada

Scott A. Teitelbaum, MD, Department of Psychiatry, and McKnight Brain Institute, University of Florida, Gainesville, Florida

Himanshu P. Upadhyaya, MBBS, Department of Psychiatry and Behavioral Sciences, Clinical Neuroscience Division, Medical University of South Carolina, Charleston, South Carolina

Angela E. Waldrop, PhD, University of California, San Francisco, San Francisco VA Medical Center, San Francisco, California

Maryann H. Walker, PhD, Department of Psychiatry, University of Florida, Gainesville, Florida

Barbara C. Wallace, PhD, Research Group on Disparities in Health, Department of Health and Behavior Studies, Teachers College, Columbia University, New York, New York

Deborah A. Yurgelun-Todd, PhD, The Brain Institute, University of Utah, Salt Lake City, and Cognitive Neuroimaging Laboratory, Brain Imaging Center, McLean Hospital, Harvard Medical School, Belmont, Massachusetts

Monica L. Zilberman MD, PhD, Institute of Psychiatry, University of São Paulo, São Paulo, Brazil

Preface

Until the early 1990s, there was scant research on women with alcohol and drug use disorders. Prior to 1990, the coexisting belief that men and women were equivalent except for their reproductive capacity and secondary sex characteristics was embedded in much of clinical research. In this context, the substance abuse literature was based primarily on male samples, and studies utilizing mixed-gender samples generally had too few women to examine gender differences meaningfully. In clinical trials, women were often excluded from research because of their childbearing potential. As a result, much of what we previously knew about addiction was based on men, as the investigators and study participants were predominantly men, and the treatments were most often designed by and tested in men. Prior to 1990, the implications of most addiction research and treatment outcomes were that findings derived from male samples would apply equally well to female samples.

In the early 1990s, things began to change at the level of the national research agenda. In 1990, the U.S. Government Accounting Office reported continuing underinclusion of women in biomedical research. In 1993, U.S. government guidelines highlighted the importance of expanding research to include women of childbearing potential, and the National Institutes of Health's (NIH) Office of Research on Women's Health was established in order to track the inclusion of women in NIH-funded research and to set priorities for women's health research at NIH. In 1994, NIH published its guidelines on the inclusion of women and took another step by mandating that women be recruited into clinical investigations sponsored by NIH, unless investigators could provide a strong and viable justification for recruiting only men.

Since that time, awareness of the importance of gender differences has grown in the addiction field, and the last 15 years have brought a rapid acceleration both in studies of gender differences in substance use disorders, and studies focusing specifically on women and addiction. Among the most reproducible findings has been that of heightened vulnerability among women to the adverse medical and social consequences of substance abuse. More broadly, ongoing research continues to document genetic, neurobiological, physiological, psychiatric, and other psychosocial differences between women and men that influence the etiology, epidemiology, clinical presentation, psychiatric comorbidity, course of illness, and treatment outcome of substance use disorders.

This book seeks to highlight current research in these areas and to synthesize the findings of recent studies of gender differences in substance use disorders, with a focus on women and addiction. In addition, the chapters identify remaining gaps in our knowledge base and obstacles still left to overcome. The work represented here is intended as a foundation for understanding the importance of substance use disorders in women's lives, and how sex and gender likely moderate all aspects of the addiction process.

We have divided the book into seven sections that focus on an overview of the field, biological issues in women's addiction, co-occurring psychiatric disorders, treatment outcome, women and specific substances of abuse, special populations, and social and policy issues as they affect women with substance use disorders. In Part I, Monica L. Zilberman synthesizes the literature on women and addiction across the lifespan. The second chapter in this part gives a context for the research in this field by summarizing research design and methodology in studies of women and addiction. In this chapter, Stephanie Collins Reed and Suzette M. Evans also discuss future research designs and methodologies that can be utilized to examine gender differences.

In Part II, biological issues that affect women's addiction are covered. Jennifer L. Newman and Nancy K. Mello summarize the recent literature on neuroactive gonadal steroid hormones and drug addiction in women, and Helen Fox and Rajita Sinha present human and animal investigations on the role of stress and the neuroendocrine response in women's addiction. Amanda Kalaydjian and Kathleen Ries Merikangas focus on sex differences in the transmission of substance use disorders. Their discussion is followed by a chapter in which Teresa A. Pigott, Maryann H. Walker, Scott A. Teitelbaum, and Ching-ju Lu review the recent findings of studies examining gender and the neurotransmitter systems in addiction. C. Lindsay DeVane integrates the findings on sex differences in pharmacokinetics and pharmacodynamics. Gender differences in neuroimaging are the focus of the final two chapters in this section. The first of these, by Simona Sava, Alexandra McCaffrey, and Deborah A. Yurgelun-Todd, reports on the findings in the field of gender, cognition, and addiction, and in the final chapter, Amanda Elton and Clinton D. Kilts summarize the roles of sex differences in the drug addiction process through a close examination of recent findings from neuroimaging studies.

The chapters in Part III explore gender differences in rates and impact of co-occurring psychiatric disorders among women and men with substance use disorders. This section begins with Risë B. Goldstein's summary of the data from the National Epidemiologic Survey on Alcohol and Related Conditions on co-occurring substance use and mood and anxiety disorders in women. The next six chapters of this section focus on the findings related to specific co-occurring psychiatric disorders among women with substance use disorders. Helen M. Pettinati and Jennifer G. Plebani update the evidence on depression and substance use disorders in women. Kathleen T. Brady and Karen Hartwell review the field of gender, anxiety, and substance abuse, and Lisa R. Cohen and Susan M. Gordon examine co-occurring eating and substance use disorders among women. Denise Hien synthesizes the literature on trauma, posttraumatic stress disorder, and addiction in women, including new evidence from several multisite trials in this area. Part III concludes with chapters from Kim-Chi Nguyen and E. Sherwood Brown on psychotic disorders in women with substance abuse, as well as an integration of research findings by Lisa A. Burckell and Shelley McMain on concurrent personality and substance use disorders in women.

Part IV reviews treatment outcomes for women with substance use disorders, and consists of three chapters. In the first of these chapters, Shelly F. Greenfield and Sandrine Pirard present an overview and synthesis of treatment outcome findings for gender-specific treatment of women with substance use disorders. Christine E. Grella's chapter covers the important area of treatment seeking and utilization among women with substance use disorders. Finally, William Fals-Stewart, Wendy K. K. Lam, and Michelle L. Kelley review partner-involved treatment for women with substance use disorders.

The five chapters in Part V focus on the role specific substances play in women's addiction. Sherry H. Stewart, Dubravka Gavric, and Pamela Collins synthesize a large literature on women, girls, and alcohol use, and Kenneth A. Perkins outlines the results of studies examining gender differences and the treatment of nicotine dependence in women. Sudie E. Back and Rebecca Payne review the emerging field of gender and prescription opioid addiction, and Aimee L. McRae-Clark and Kimber L. Price summarize the issues and opportunities for research and treatment of women with marijuana dependence. Part V concludes with a synthesis by Wendy J. Lynch, Marc N. Potenza, Kelly P. Cosgrove, and Carolyn M. Mazure on a translational perspective on sex differences in vulnerability to addiction.

Part VI is devoted to special populations and is comprised of four chapters. Himanshu P. Upadhyaya and Kevin M. Gray present findings on the role of gender in adolescent substance use and abuse, and Chaya Bhuvaneswar and Grace Chang summarize new findings on the epidemiology, presentation, and treatment of substance use in pregnancy. Latoya C. Conner, Charlene E. Le Fauve, and Barbara C. Wallace cover the broad and critical field of ethnic and cultural correlates of addiction among diverse populations of women. Finally, Thomas W. Irwin discusses current clinical and research findings on substance use disorders among sexual-minority women.

Part VII reviews the social and policy issues relevant to women and addiction. First, Angela E. Waldrop details the public health and clinical crisis of violence and victimization among women with substance use disorders. Rebecca W. Brendel and Matthew F. Soulier provide a comprehensive overview of the legal issues surrounding women and addiction.

More than 90% of studies investigating gender differences in substance abuse treatment have been published since 1990, and of these, nearly 40% have been published since 2000. We anticipate that there will be a continued acceleration in research findings in the area of gender differences in the etiology, course, and treatment of substance use disorders and that these findings will enhance our understanding of the process of addiction in women. We believe that such understanding will ultimately lead to enhanced prevention, detection, and treatment of substance use disorders in women. As the first decade of the 21st century comes to a close, it is our hope that this book will synthesize what we know now and will provide a launch point for clinicians and investigators to move forward this critical public health and clinical field of women and addiction.

ACKNOWLEDGMENTS

Kathleen T. Brady would like to acknowledge Grant No. K24 DA00435 from the National Institute on Drug Abuse and Grant No. P50 DA0165 from the National Institute of Arthritis and Musculoskeletal and Skin Diseases and the Office of Research on Women's Health. Sudie E. Back would like to acknowledge Grant No. K23 DA021228 from the National Institute on Drug Abuse. Shelly F. Greenfield would like to acknowledge Grant No. K24 DA019855 from the National Institute on Drug Abuse.

Contents

VI. SPECIAL POPULATIONS

VII. SOCIAL AND POLICY ISSUES

PART I

OVERVIEW

CHAPTER 1

Substance Abuse across the Lifespan in Women

Monica L. Zilberman, MD, PhD

In the last decades, a considerable body of knowledge regarding differential gender issues in substance abuse has evolved. Researchers have focused on topics such as prevention, treatment, harm reduction, and public policies across genders. This chapter aims to review and summarize how a woman's life cycle stage influences her substance use and risk for developing abuse or dependence.

EPIDEMIOLOGY

In 2005, the Monitoring the Future survey, that evaluates substance use of 14- to 18-year-old students enrolled in 8th to 12th grades, found that, when data from the five grades were pooled, male students presented higher rates of heavy drinking and illicit drug use than female students. However, this did not hold true among the 8th graders in the last years. Also, at 10th grade, girls presented higher last-30-days prevalence rates of drinking. As for cigarette smoking, similar rates have been observed across genders, but at 8th grade girls presented higher 30-day prevalence rates of use than boys. It was observed that gender differences (with boys presenting higher rates of use) emerged as students grow older, whereas for younger students (8th grade) a pattern of gender convergence or higher rates of use for girls was evidenced at least for some drugs (Johnston, O'Malley, Bachman, & Schulenberg, 2007).

Combined data from the 2002, 2003, and 2004 National Surveys on Drug Use and Health (NSDUH) conducted annually in the United States also provides evidence for gender convergence among youths ages 12–17 for misuse of psychoactive prescription medications. Past year rates for girls were 9.9% (8.2% for boys; Colliver, Kroutil, Dai, & Gfroerer, 2006).

In the general population, alcohol dependence or abuse is more frequent for men than for women. However, among men and women ages 12 or older that are heavy drinkers (e.g., those drinking five or more drinks on the same occasion on each of five or more days in the 30-day period prior to the survey), similar rates of past year alcohol dependence or abuse were found (Substance Abuse and Mental Health Services Administration [SAMHSA], 2007a).

Younger women are a matter of particular concern given their increased likelihood of smoking while pregnant compared to older pregnant women. Roughly one-quarter of pregnant women ages 15–17 and 18–25 reported past-month smoking compared to 10% of those ages 26–44 (SAMHSA, 2007b). Recent data from NSDUH conducted from 2004 to 2006 estimate that annually almost 10% of women of childbearing age (18–49 years) needed treatment for a substance-use problem. Of these, 85% did not receive or perceive their need for treatment. The most frequently cited reasons for not receiving treatment were not being ready to stop using substances (36%), lack of funding (34%), and social stigma (29%; SAMHSA, 2007c).

ADOLESCENCE: DEPRESSION, TRAUMA, AND EATING DISORDERS

Several studies point out that psychological factors play a distinct role in substance use and abuse across genders. The seminal Oakland Growth Study identified that for girls, but not for boys, feelings of low self-esteem and coping difficulties at junior high and high school levels predicted future problem drinking (Jones, 1968, 1971). In the following decade, Fillmore, Bacon, and Hyman (1979) conducted a 27-year follow-up study of drinking among college students in the United States, reporting considerable gender differences in predictive factors for future problem drinking. For college women, drinking to relieve shyness, to get high, and to get along better on dates were all predictors of future problem drinking, whereas for men, the best predictor of future problem drinking was having "incipient problems." In a U.S. national survey published in 1997, 1,099 women were asked about sexual experiences occurring before age 18, and it was found that those women who reported childhood sexual abuse were significantly more likely to report recent alcohol use, intoxication, drinking-related problems, and alcohol dependence symptoms; lifetime use of prescribed psychoactive drugs and illicit drugs; depression and anxiety; pain that prevented intercourse; and consensual sexual intercourse before age 15, suggesting that women's experience of sexual abuse in childhood may be an important risk factor for later substance abuse, psychopathology, and sexual dysfunction (Wilsnack, Vogeltanz, Klassen, & Harris, 1997). More recently, the National Center on Addiction and Substance Abuse ([CASA]; 2003) released a comprehensive study of girls and young women in the United States confirming that feelings of depression, hopelessness, sadness, and suicidal ideation are a great deal more frequent in high school girls than boys and these same feelings are significantly associated with a heightened risk for not only drinking but also for other drug use for girls.

These findings suggest that prevention strategies at high school and college levels should focus on those girls and young women who display emotional distress and those who drink to enhance self-esteem and ability to function. Providers of health and mental services for girls and young women can play an important role in prevention by helping them avoid self-medicating with alcohol or drugs of abuse.

Drinking also influences young women's aggressive behavior differently from men. Results from the National Longitudinal Survey of Youth of 808 drinkers ages 17–21 in 1994, 1996, and 1998 revealed a stronger relationship between heavy episodic drinking and fights after drinking for females than for males. Particularly, those young women who dropped out of high school were significantly more likely to fight after drinking compared with college students (Wells, Speechley, Koval, & Graham, 2007).

Reasons for substance-use initiation differ in young females and males. Substance use is often perceived by young women as a coping mechanism in dealing with shyness, anxiety, and/or depression. Curiosity is the main reason for substance use initiation for boys. Also, more girls now are focused on body image and thinness, and cigarette smoking and stimulants use may be one strategy in accomplishing these ideals. Standard treatment and prevention strategies may be difficult to apply in these young women, requiring additional effort and gender-specific content in helping them maintain a good relationship with their bodies (Blume, Zilberman, & Tavares, 2005).

ADULTHOOD

Menstrual Cycle and Fertility

Many of the effects of substance use on women's sexuality and fertility, as well as use of substances in the perinatal period, have been elucidated. The relationship between drinking and the menstrual cycle was reviewed by Mumenthaler, Taylor, O'Hara, and Yesavage (1999). They concluded that the menstrual cycle is unlikely to have a significant influence over alcohol pharmacokinetics. Conversely, although at low levels alcohol seems to have little effect on female sex hormones, there is evidence that acute alcohol intoxication is associated with increased plasma levels of testosterone in women. This is due to an increased rate of conversion of androstenedione to testosterone in the liver caused by alcohol even in healthy women who drink episodically (Sarkola, Fukunaga, Makisala, & Peter Eriksson, 2000). This may be the basis for a variety of fertility problems such as ovulation inhibition, decreased gonadal mass, infertility, and other sexual dysfunctions often observed in women who drink heavily women (Blume & Zilberman, 2004). In men, alcohol intoxication produces a transient reduction in testosterone levels (Frias, Torres, Miranda, Ruiz, & Ortega, 2002).

The effects of drinking on sexuality involve a complex interaction of socially determined expectations and pharmacological effects. A commonly held societal belief is that women who are drinking crave sex and become promiscuous. This stereotype encourages men to seek sexual intercourse with women who show intoxication. A 1981 national survey of 917 women showed that a large proportion of women drinkers reported that drinking lessens their sexual inhibitions and helps them feel close to others, 22% reported feeling more sexually assertive, but only 8% reported becoming less selective in partner choice. However, 60% reported having been the target of other drinkers' sexual aggression. Women who were heavier drinkers higher rates of sexual dysfunction such as lack of sexual interest, difficulties reaching orgasm, and vaginismus (Klassen & Wilsnack, 1986).

Another interesting finding is the dissociation observed in women between subjective feelings of sexual arousal and physiological responses after drinking. Physiological measures demonstrate that alcohol consumption actually reduces sexual arousal in women, although they subjectively reported feeling more aroused (Wilson & Lawson, 1976). The same dissociation was observed regarding their ability to reach orgasm, which was depressed by alcohol in a dose-response relationship (Malatesta, Pollack, Crotty, & Peacock, 1982).

Likewise, some women rely on the use of drugs for their presumed aphrodisiac properties. The literature, instead, reveals that, apart from the subjective effects, substance use negatively affects the sexual response (Johnson, Phelps, & Cottler, 2004). For instance, although the acute effect of cocaine is as a stimulant, its chronic use causes sexual dysfunction mainly due to hyperprolactinemia, but is also linked to increased levels of luteinizing hormone (Mello & Mendelson, 1997). Cocaine use is associated with negative effects over the menstrual cycle, producing amenorrhea, luteal phase dysfunction, galactorrhea, and infertility (Mendelson, Sholar, Siegel, & Mello, 2001).

Opioids at high doses inhibit the hypothalamus–pituitary–gonadal axis and increase prolactin levels that, in turn, interfere with sexual response and fertility (Cofrancesco et al., 2006). Cigarette smoking has been associated with a number of menstrual abnormalities, fertility problems, and early menopause in women, related to nicotine inhibitory effect over luteinizing hormone and prolactin release (Fuxe, Andersson, Eneroth, Härfstrand, & Agnati, 1989). Acute cannabis use during the luteal phase of the menstrual cycle is also associated with decreased prolactin and luteinizing hormone levels, whereas chronic cannabis use does not alter hormone levels (Block, Farinpour, & Schlechte, 1991), suggesting that cannabis effects on women's hormones may not be persistent.

Pregnancy and Breastfeeding

Substance use during the perinatal period poses significant risks for women and their offspring. Antenatal alcohol exposure has a broad range of adverse effects on placental development and function including placental dysfunction, decreased size, impaired blood flow and nutrient transport, endocrine changes, increased rates of stillbirth and abruption, umbilical cord vasoconstriction, and low birth weight (Burd, Roberts, Olson, & Odendaal, 2007). Fetal alcohol syndrome (FAS) is one of the most common developmental disabilities in the United States. FAS occurs at a rate of 0.5–2.0 per 1000 live births, making it one of the three most frequent causes of birth defects associated with mental retardation. The syndrome includes prenatal and postnatal growth retardation and central nervous system abnormalities. A characteristic facial dysmorphism, composed of short palpebral fissures, epicanthic folds, and maxillary hypoplasia, may be present. Other signs may include birth defects such as microcephaly, altered palmar creases, and heart abnormalities. The full-blown FAS is seen in the offspring of approximately one third of women who are alcoholics drinking the equivalent of 10 standard drinks daily, but other fetal alcohol effects such as spontaneous abortion, reduced birth weight, and behavior changes have been associated with lower levels of alcohol intake (Warren et al., 2001). Binge drinking is an important risk factor, but studies of genetic associations have focused on the alcohol dehydrogenase 1B gene, suggesting a protective effect for genotypes containing ADH1B2 or ADH1B3, associated with faster alcohol metabolism, while the ADH1B1 homozygous genotype would be involved with slower metabolism and FAS susceptibility (Green & Stoler, 2007). There are controversial data regarding potential adverse effects of low to moderate alcohol levels during pregnancy. A recent systematic review observed no conclusive evidence regarding the matter but observed that methodological weaknesses in the studies reviewed precluded assumptions about the safety of light drinking during pregnancy. In addition, countries vary broadly in definitions of low-risk drinking (Henderson, Gray, & Brocklehurst, 2007). Therefore, the recommendation for women who are pregnant or attempting to become pregnant is to refrain from drinking.

There is a need for more data on drinking patterns during the breastfeeding period. Results from the 1993–1994 Food and Drug Administration Infant Feeding Practices Study I, a longitudinal study of infant–mother pairs that included 772 breastfeeding women and 776 controls, found no significant differences in self-reported alcohol consumption at 3 months postpartum among breastfeeding and non-breastfeeding women (approximately 38%). However, data about levels of infant exposure and consequences are lacking for the most part (Breslow, Falk, Fein, & Grummer-Strawn, 2007). A study uncovered a significant (albeit relatively small) difference in motor development at one year of age between infants breastfed by mothers who drank during lactation and infants of mothers who were abstinent (Little,

Anderson, Ervin, Worthington-Roberts, & Clarren, 1989). This finding was not replicated in a more recent study conducted by the same group of investigators (Little, Northstone, Golding, & ALSPAC Study Team, 2002).

Data from pregnant women participating in the four-site Maternal Lifestyle Study estimated that 5–10% of pregnant women in North America use cocaine during pregnancy (Lester et al., 2001). Only 2% of these women reported cocaine use only. Hence, it is difficult to isolate the specific pharmacological effects of cocaine on pregnancy and offspring due to polydrug use. Perinatal complications associated with cocaine use include sexually transmitted diseases, abruptio placentae, meconium staining, premature rupture of membranes, and low birth weight (Bauer et al., 2002).

A recent review highlighted findings about the effects of prenatal cocaine exposure on offspring's mental health. These effects tend to be nonpersistent and are largely mediated by psychosocial factors, such as malnutrition, increased maternal age, and other drug use including alcohol and tobacco, in such a way that most associations between child development and intrauterine cocaine exposure disappear when psychosocial factors are taken into account (Williams & Ross, 2007). However, longer follow-up studies are still needed, as cognitive demands tend to be higher in adolescence. For instance, recent studies in children and adolescents with in utero cocaine exposure uncovered reduced cerebral blood flow (Rao et al., 2007) and slower growth rate (Richardson, Goldschmidt, & Larkby, 2007), even when psychosocial factors are taken into account. Unlike antenatal cocaine exposure, there is a lack of information regarding recommendations for breastfeeding mothers who were cocaine users, although case studies record detection of cocaine in breast milk in levels that could lead to symptoms such as seizures, tachycardia, and irritability in the newborn (Sarkar, Djulus, & Koren, 2005).

Being highly lipophylic, tetrahydrocannabinol may be sequestrated in fat tissue for weeks in chronic users. Hence, even if the user quits cannabis use after finding out about pregnancy, tetrahydrocannabinol will still be slowly released from fat tissue into the bloodstream, freely crossing the placental barrier and exerting its potentially deleterious effects on pregnancy and offspring. These effects are caused by cannabis-induced decreased uteroplacental perfusion, preterm delivery, and intrauterine growth retardation with low birth weight. Regarding regular antenatal exposure to cannabis, data support a subtle neurodevelopmental effect upon later functioning that includes specific cognitive deficits, particularly in visuospatial working memory (Smith, Fried, Hogan, & Cameron, 2006), and also hyperactivity, impulsivity, attention deficit, depressive symptomatology, and substance use disorders (Sundram, 2006). Environmental factors and use of other substances may have additive effects with cannabis use during pregnancy and in many cases may be even stronger factors in determining perinatal morbidity. Antenatal cannabis exposure effects tend to increase with heavier use. There is no study evaluating the impact of cannabis exposure in early as opposed to late pregnancy, and the literature lacks data about potential effects of cannabis use during breastfeeding.

Intravenous opiate use during pregnancy is associated with problems linked to injection risks, such as HIV and hepatitis and increased neonatal morbidity associated with various environmental factors, such as lack of prenatal care, poverty, and malnutrition (Bauer et al., 2002). Prenatal opiate exposure in the last trimester of pregnancy elicits a well-described neonatal withdrawal syndrome (NWS) affecting central nervous, autonomic, and gastrointestinal systems, characterized by weight loss, feeding difficulties, sleep abnormalities, and seizures. Although methadone maintenance is the treatment of choice for pregnant women who are opioid dependent in the United States, most neonates who are methadone exposed develop NWS of enough severity to require treatment (Chiriboga, 2003). In a sample of pregnant women who were opioid maintained, the largest proportion of neonates requiring treatment for NWS was found in the morphine-maintained group (82%), followed by the methadone-maintained group (60%). The smallest percentage of clinically significant NWS was found among women who were buprenorphine maintained (21%; Ebner et al., 2007). Maternal and neonate factors that may affect vulnerability to NWS in infants born to mothers who are methadone maintained are not completely understood. Population data show that 27% of babies born to pregnant women who are methadone maintained present NWS. These mothers had more previous pregnancies and were more likely to be heavy cigarette smokers (Burns & Mattick, 2007). Available evidence indicates that the administration of opiates to the neonate with significant NWS appears to reduce time to regain birth weight but may increase the duration of hospital stay. This approach seems to be more effective than the use of sedatives, clonidine, or benzodiazepines (Osborn, Jeffery, & Cole, 2005). Maternal methadone dose does not predict the need for neonate treatment. A study comparing breastfeeding women who were methadone maintained and women who were formula feeding showed that fewer breastfed neonates required additional pharmacotherapy for NWS (Jansson et al., 2008). Hence breastfeeding has been suggested as an appropriate treatment strategy for managing the symptoms of withdrawal in infants who were methadone exposed. Women still unstable in their recoveries or prone to relapse and those infected with HIV should not breastfeed. Hepatitis C per se is not a contraindication, unless nipples are cracked or bleeding (Jansson, Velez, & Harrow, 2004). Methadone stabilization at the lowest possible dose, adjusted for the increased body mass, is the recommended treatment for pregnant women with opiate dependence in the United States. Comparatively little data exist on buprenorphine treatment during pregnancy. Most data on buprenorphine comes from European countries (Auriacombe, Fatséas, Dubernet, Daulouède, & Tignol, 2004). A recent prospective study of 259 pregnant women maintained on methadone or high-dose buprenorphine showed that approximately 12% had premature delivery and 70% of neonates displayed a NWS with similar perinatal outcome for women and their infants across groups (Lejeune, Simmat-Durand, Gourarier, & Aubisson, 2006). Similar to what happens with cocaine, the mental, motor, and behavioral consequences of prenatal opiate exposure on infants up to age 3, as measured by the Maternal Lifestyle Study, were associated mostly with low birth weight and reflect environmental risks such as lack of adequate prenatal care, malnutrition, cigarette smoking, and polydrug use, rather than with direct effects of opiates (Messinger et al., 2004).

Nicotine use is the most important preventable risk factor for an unsuccessful pregnancy outcome, even surpassing poverty in many countries (Cnattingius, 2004). Exposure to tobacco constituents can affect placental development directly (by negatively influencing cytotrophoblast proliferation and differentiation) or indirectly by reducing blood flow (Zdravkovic, Genbacev, McMaster, & Fisher, 2005). Various effects of tobacco on pregnancy are derived from oxytocin stimulation and include still birth, preterm birth, placental abruption, fetal growth restriction with low birth weight and height, obstetric complications (such as spontaneous abortions, ectopic pregnancies, and placenta previa) and neonatal mortality (Cnattingius, 2004). Maternal smoking, either prenatal or after birth, is currently the most frequent and preventable risk factor for sudden infant death syndrome, and this relationship appears to be dose dependent. This is possibly due to arousal impairments in association with changes in control of autonomic cardiac function (Horne, Franco, Adamson, Grosswasser, & Kahn, 2004). Long-term physical and behavioral consequences of prenatal exposure to maternal smoking have also been reported, such as impaired lung function and delinquency, independent of other confounding variables (Zilberman & Blume, 2004). Regarding breastfeeding, there is evidence that, given its clear benefits in counterbalancing morbidity in neonates of smoking mothers and the potential additive effects of pre- and postnatal maternal smoking and second-hand paternal smoking, breast milk nutrition should be encouraged for infants born to parents who smoke (Dorea, 2007).

Women who use substances that become pregnant suffer severe disapproval for exposing their future babies to drugs. There is evidence, however, that many women stop using drugs during this period. For example, from 1993–1999, the odds of quitting smoking during pregnancy raised 51% (Colman & Joyce, 2003). Among those who do not quit, the quantity and frequency of drug use are often considerably reduced, demonstrating that these women are indeed concerned about their offspring (Bottorff et al., 2006). A nonjudgmental approach is essential in attracting more pregnant women to treatment. Preliminary evidence suggests good results for therapeutic interventions for this population (Windsor, 2003). The additional challenge is to help them remain abstinence in the postpartum period. A particular cause for concern is the fact that most women who quit smoking during pregnancy eventually return to using tobacco within 6 months after delivery (Solomon et al., 2007).

AGING: MENOPAUSE

Over the next two decades, a huge increase in the rates of drinking among older women is expected due to the gender convergence of prevalence rates of alcohol use in adolescents observed in recent cohorts. At this stage of the life cycle, women are confronted with additional challenges, biological and social in nature, including menopause, motor limitations, osteoporosis, retirement, and "empty nest." Vulnerability to alcohol is augmented in older women, although there is limited evidence that drinking of one standard drink per day might confer some protection against heart disease and osteoporosis. Heavy drinking, however, increases osteoporosis risk, and there is evidence that bone damage provoked by early heavy drinking may be irreversible (Sampson, 2002). Additionally, drinking has been linked to increased rates of breast cancer (Key et al., 2006; MacMahon, 2006). Furthermore, the risk of combined effects of alcohol with prescription drugs should not be overlooked. Alcohol also increases risks for trauma, hypertension, cardiac arrythmias, gastrointestinal problems, neurocognitive deficits, and depressive/anxiety symptomatology (Register, Cline, & Shively, 2002). Many older women who drink alcoholic beverages also take medications that may interact negatively with alcohol. Age-related changes in the absorption, distribution, and metabolism of alcohol and medications may partly explain these negative interactions (Epstein, Fischer-Elber, & Al-Otaiba, 2007). Some medications have disulfiram-like reactions when taken together with alcohol. Additionally alcohol may interfere with the effectiveness of some medications. Practitioners and patients need to be aware of these potential risks of combined alcohol and medication use. Approximately 10% of older women misuse prescribed medications (Johnell, Fastbom, Rosén, & Leimanis, 2007). Substance abuse in older women is usually a consequence of social isolation and psychiatric comorbidity. Particular attention should be given to the abusive potential of sedative and opioid medications among older people (Simoni-Wastila & Yang, 2006).

There have been findings from epidemiological studies suggesting that light-to-moderate drinking is associated with reduced risk of atherosclerosis (by altering cholesterol metabolism and reducing blood clotting and platelet function). This may be the basis for its protective effect for cardiovascular and Alzheimer's diseases. Moderate drinking is also associated with increased bone mineral density and consequent decreased fracture risk in older women. The problem is to safely define the limits of light-to-moderate drinking given great individual vulnerability to alcohol particularly among women (Mancinelli, Binetti, & Ceccanti, 2006).

Only recently specific treatment programming for this age bracket has attracted attention. In designing treatment strategies, cognitive limitations and social isolation need to be taken into consideration. Support groups are particularly helpful, and themes such as widowhood and role loss should be addressed (Epstein et al., 2007).

KEY POINTS

- A pattern of gender convergence or higher rates of substance use has been evidenced among younger women at least for some drugs (including cigarette smoking and prescribed medications).
- Emotional problems and psychiatric comorbidity are more prevalent in women compared to men and are important risk factors for substance use in women.
- Women are particularly vulnerable to the physical effects of different substances, being at greater risk of developing health-related problems.
- Substance use among women poses particular programming and treatment issues given women's specificities in different phase of their life cycle such as fertility, pregnancy, breastfeeding, menopause, and aging.
- There is a critical need for the development of prevention strategies aimed at retarding substance-use initiation among girls. Also, media campaigns designed to reduce the stigma attached to substance use among women are required to alert and help women with substance-use problems.

REFERENCES

Asterisks denote recommended readings.

Auriacombe, M., Fatséas, M., Dubernet, J., Daulouède, J. P., & Tignol, J. (2004). French field experience with buprenorphine. *American Journal of Addictions*, 13(Suppl. 1), S17–S28.

Bauer, C. R., Shankaran, S., Bada, H. S., Lester, B., Wright, L. L., Krause-Steinrauf, H., et al. (2002). The Maternal Lifestyle Study: Drug exposure during pregnancy and short-term maternal outcomes. *American Journal of Obstetrics and Gynecology*, 186, 487–495. (*)

Block, R. I., Farinpour, R., & Schlechte, J. A. (1991). Effects of chronic marijuana use on testosterone, luteinizing hormone, follicle stimulating hormone, prolactin and cortisol in men and women. *Drug and Alcohol Dependence*, 28(2), 121–128.

Blume, S. B., & Zilberman, M. L. (2004). Women: Clinical aspects. In J. Lowinson, P. Ruiz, R. B. Millman, & J. G. Langrod (Eds.), *Substance abuse: A comprehensive textbook* (4th ed., pp. 1049–1064). Philadelphia: Lippincott Williams & Wilkins.

Blume, S. B., Zilberman, M. L., & Tavares, H. (2005). Substance use, abuse, and dependence in adolescent girls. In S. Romans & M. V. Seeman (Eds.), *Women's mental health: A life cycle approach* (pp. 133–145). Philadelphia: Lippincott Williams & Wilkins.

Bottorff, J. L., Kalaw, C., Johnson, J. L., Stewart, M., Greaves, L., & Carey, J. (2006). Couple dynamics during women's tobacco reduction in pregnancy and postpartum. *Nicotine and Tobacco Research*, 8(4), 499–509.

Breslow, R. A., Falk, D. E., Fein, S. B., & Grummer-Strawn, L. M. (2007). Alcohol consumption among breastfeeding women. *Breastfeeding Medicine*, 2, 152–157.

Burd, L., Roberts, D., Olson, M., & Odendaal, H. (2007). Ethanol and the placenta: A review. *Journal of Maternal–Fetal & Neonatal Medicine*, 20, 361–375.

Burns, L., & Mattick, R. P. (2007). Using population data to examine the prevalence and correlates of neonatal abstinence syndrome. *Drug and Alcohol Review*, 26(5), 487–492.

Chiriboga, C. A. (2003). Fetal alcohol and drug effects. *Neurologist*, 9(6), 267–279.

Cnattingius, S. (2004). The epidemiology of smoking during pregnancy: Smoking prevalence, maternal characteristics, and pregnancy outcomes. *Nicotine and Tobacco Research*, 6(Suppl. 2), S125–140. (*)

Cofrancesco, J., Jr., Shah, N., Ghanem, K. G., Dobs, A. S., Klein, R. S., Mayer, K., et al. (2006). The effects of illicit drug use and HIV infection on sex hormone levels in women. *Gynecological Endocrinology*, 22(5), 244–251.

Colliver, J. D., Kroutil, L. A., Dai, L., & Gfroerer, J. C. (2006). *Misuse of prescription drugs: Data from the 2002, 2003, and 2004 National Surveys on Drug Use and Health* (DHHS Publication No. SMA 06-4192, Analytic Series A-28). Rockville, MD: Substance Abuse and Mental Health Services Administration, Office of Applied Studies.

Colman, G. J., & Joyce, T. (2003). Trends in smoking before, during, and after pregnancy in ten states. *American Journal of Preventive Medicine*, 24(1), 29–35.

Dorea, J. G. (2007). Maternal smoking and infant feeding: Breastfeeding is better and safer. *Maternal and Child Health Journal*, 11, 287–291.

Ebner, N., Rohrmeister, K., Winklbaur, B., Baewert, A., Jagsch, R., Peternell, A., et al. (2007). Management of neonatal abstinence syndrome in neonates born to opioid maintained women. *Drug and Alcohol Dependence*, 87(2/3), 131–138.

Epstein, E. E., Fischer-Elber, K., & Al-Otaiba, Z. (2007). Women, aging, and alcohol use disorders. *Journal of Women & Aging*, 19, 31–48. (*)

Fillmore, K. M., Bacon, S. D., & Hyman, M. (1979). *The 27 year longitudinal panel study of drinking by students in college. Report 1979 to National Institute of Alcoholism and Alcohol Abuse* (Contract No: ADM 281–76-0015). Washington DC: . (*)

Frias, J., Torres, J. M., Miranda, M. T., Ruiz, E., & Ortega, E. (2002). Effects of acute alcohol intoxication on pituitary–gonadal axis hormones, pituitary–adrenal axis hormones, beta-endorphin and prolactin in human adults of both sexes. *Alcohol and Alcoholism*, 37, 169–173.

Fuxe, K., Andersson, K., Eneroth, P., Härfstrand, A., & Agnati, L. F. (1989). Neuroendocrine actions of nicotine and of exposure to cigarette smoke: Medical implications. *Psychoneuroendocrinology*, 14(1/2), 19–41.

Green, R. F., & Stoler, J. M. (2007). Alcohol dehydrogenase 1B genotype and fetal alcohol syndrome: A HuGE minireview. *American Journal of Obstetrics and Gynecology*, 197, 12–25.

Henderson, J., Gray, R., & Brocklehurst, P. (2007). Systematic review of effects of low–moderate prenatal alcohol exposure on pregnancy outcome. *British Journal of Obstetrics and Gynecology*, 114, 243–252.

Horne, R. S., Franco, P., Adamson, T. M., Groswasser, J., & Kahn, A. (2004). Influences of maternal cigarette smoking on infant arousability. *Early Human Development*, 79, 49–58.

Jansson, L. M., Choo, R., Velez, M. L., Harrow, C., Schroeder, J. R., Shakleya, D. M., et al. (2008). Methadone maintenance and breastfeeding in the neonatal period. *Pediatrics*, 121(1), 106–114.

Jansson, L. M., Velez, M., & Harrow, C. (2004). Methadone maintenance and lactation: A review of the literature and current management guidelines. *Journal of Human Lactation*, 20, 62–71.

Johnell, K., Fastbom, J., Rosén, M., & Leimanis, A. (2007). Inappropriate drug use in the elderly: A nationwide register-based study. *Annals of Pharmacotherapy*, 41(7), 1243–1248.

Johnson, S. D., Phelps, D. L., & Cottler, L. B. (2004). The association of sexual dysfunction and substance use among a community epidemiological sample. *Archives of Sexual Behavior*, 33(1), 55–63.

Johnston, L. D., O'Malley, P. M., Bachman, J. G., & Schulenberg, J. E. (2007). *Monitoring the Future national results on adolescent drug use: Overview of key findings, 2006* (NIH Publication No. 07-6202). Bethesda, MD: National Institute on Drug Abuse.

Jones, M. C. (1968). Personality correlates and antecedents of drinking patterns in adult males. *Journal of Consulting and Clinical Psychology*, 32, 2–12.

Jones, M. C. (1971). Personality antecedents and correlates of drinking patterns in women. *Journal of Consulting and Clinical Psychology*, 36, 61–69.

Key, J., Hodgson, S., Omar, R. Z., Jensen, T. K., Thompson, S. G., Boobis, A. R., et al. (2006). Meta-analysis of studies of alcohol and breast cancer with consideration of the methodological issues. *Cancer Causes & Control*, 17(6), 759–770.

Klassen, A. D., & Wilsnack, S. C. (1986). Sexual experience and drinking among women in a U.S. national survey. *Archives of Sexual Behavior, 15,* 363–392. (*)

Lejeune, C., Simmat-Durand, L., Gourarier, L., & Aubisson, S. (2006). Prospective multicenter observational study of 260 infants born to 259 opiate-dependent mothers on methadone or high-dose buprenophine substitution. *Drug and Alcohol Dependence, 82,* 250–257.

Lester, B. M., ElSohly, M., Wright, L. L., Smeriglio, V. L., Verter, J., Bauer, C. R., et al. (2001). The Maternal Lifestyle Study: Drug use by meconium toxicology and maternal self-report. *Pediatrics, 107*(2), 309–317.

Little, R. E., Anderson, K. W., Ervin, C. H., Worthington-Roberts, B., & Clarren, S. K. (1989). Maternal alcohol use during breast-feeding and infant mental and motor development at one year. *New England Journal of Medicine, 321,* 425–430.

Little, R. E., Northstone, K., Golding, J., & ALSPAC Study Team. (2002). Alcohol, breastfeeding, and development at 18 months. *Pediatrics, 109*(5), E72–2.

MacMahon, B. (2006). Epidemiology and the causes of breast cancer. *International Journal of Cancer, 118*(10), 2373–2378.

Malatesta, V. J., Pollack, R. H., Crotty, T. D., & Peacock, L. J. (1982). Acute alcohol intoxication and female orgasmic response. *Journal of Sex Research, 18*(1), 1–17.

Mancinelli, R., Binetti, R., & Ceccanti, M. (2006). Female drinking, environmental and biological markers. *Annali dell'Istituto superiore di sanita, 42*(1), 31–38.

Mello, N. K., & Mendelson, J. H. (1997). Cocaine's effects on neuroendocrine systems: Clinical and preclinical studies. *Pharmacology, Biochemistry, and Behavior, 57*(3), 571–599.

Mendelson, J. H., Sholar, M. B., Siegel, A. J., & Mello, N. K. (2001). Effects of cocaine on luteinizing hormone in women during the follicular and luteal phases of the menstrual cycle and in men. *Journal of Pharmacology and Experimental Therapeutics, 296,* 972–979.

Messinger, D. S., Bauer, C. R., Das, A., Seifer, R., Lester, B. M., Lagasse, L. L., et al. (2004). The Maternal Lifestyle Study: Cognitive, motor, and behavioral outcomes of cocaine-exposed and opiate-exposed infants through three years of age. *Pediatrics, 113,* 1677–1685.

Mumenthaler, M. S., Taylor, J. L., O'Hara, R., & Yesavage, J. A. (1999). Gender differences in moderate drinking effects. *Alcohol Research & Health, 23,* 55–64.

National Center on Addiction and Substance Abuse at Columbia University. (2003). *The formative years: Pathways to substance abuse among girls and young women ages 8–22.* Available at *www.casacolumbia.org.* (*)

Osborn, D. A., Jeffery, H. E., & Cole, M. J. (2005, July 20). Sedatives for opiate withdrawal in newborn infants. *Cochrane Database of Systematic Reviews* (3), CD002059.

Rao, H., Wang, J., Giannetta, J., Korczykowski, M., Shera, D., Avants, B. B., et al. (2007). Altered resting cerebral blood flow in adolescents with in utero cocaine exposure revealed by perfusion functional MRI. *Pediatrics, 120*(5), e1245–1254.

Register, T. C., Cline, J. M., & Shively, C. A. (2002). Health issues in postmenopausal women who drink. *Alcohol Research & Health, 26*(4), 299–307. (*)

Richardson, G. A., Goldschmidt, L., & Larkby, C. (2007). Effects of prenatal cocaine exposure on growth: A longitudinal analysis. *Pediatrics, 120*(4), e1017–1027.

Sampson, H. W. (2002). Alcohol and other factors affecting osteoporosis risk in women. *Alcohol Research & Health, 26,* 292–298.

Sarkar, M., Djulus, J., & Koren, G. (2005). When a cocaine-using mother wishes to breastfeed: Proposed guidelines. *Therapeutic Drug Monitoring, 27,* 1–2.

Sarkola, T., Fukunaga, T., Makisalo, H., & Peter Eriksson, C. J. (2000). Acute effect of alcohol on androgens in premenopausal women. *Alcohol and Alcoholism, 35,* 84–90.

Simoni-Wastila, L., & Yang, H. K. (2006). Psychoactive drug abuse in older adults. *American Journal of Geriatric Pharmacotherapy, 4*(4), 380–394.

Smith, A. M., Fried, P. A., Hogan, M. J., & Cameron, I. (2006). Effects of prenatal marijuana on visuospatial working memory: An fMRI study in young adults. *Neurotoxicology and Teratology, 28*(2), 286–295.

Solomon, L. J., Higgins, S. T., Heil, S. H., Badger, G. J., Thomas, C. S., & Bernstein, I. M. (2007). Predictors of postpartum relapse to smoking. *Drug and Alcohol Dependence, 90*(2/3), 224–227.

Substance Abuse and Mental Health Services Administration, Office of Applied Studies. (2007a). *The NSDUH report: Cigarette use among pregnant women and recent mothers.* Rockville, MD: Author.

Substance Abuse and Mental Health Services Administration, Office of Applied Studies. (2007b). *The NSDUH report: Gender differences in alcohol use and alcohol dependence or abuse: 2004 and 2005.* Rockville, MD: Author.

Substance Abuse and Mental Health Services Administration, Office of Applied Studies. (2007c). *The NSDUH report: Substance use treatment among women of childrearing age.* Rockville, MD: Author.

Sundram, S. (2006). Cannabis and neurodevelopment: Implications for psychiatric disorders. *Human Psychopharmacology, 21,* 245–254.

Warren, K. R., Calhoun, F. J., May, P. A., Viljoen, D. L., Li, T. K., Tanaka, H., et al. (2001). Fetal alcohol syndrome: An international perspective. *Alcoholism, Clinical and Experimental Research, 25*(5 Suppl. ISBRA), 202S–206S.

Wells, S., Speechley, M., Koval, J. J., & Graham, K. (2007). Gender differences in the relationship between heavy episodic drinking, social roles, and alcohol-related aggression in a U.S. sample of late adolescent and young adult drinkers. *American Journal of Drug and Alcohol Abuse, 33,* 21–29.

Williams, J. H., & Ross, L. (2007). Consequences of prenatal toxin exposure for mental health in children and adolescents: A systematic review. *European Child & Adolescent Psychiatry, 16,* 243–253.

Wilsnack, S. C., Vogeltanz, N. D., Klassen, A. D., & Harris, T. R. (1997). Childhood sexual abuse and women's substance abuse: National survey findings. *Journal of Studies on Alcohol, 58,* 264–271.

Wilson, G. T., & Lawson, D. M. (1976). Effects of alcohol on sexual arousal in women. *Journal of Abnorm Psychology, 85*(5), 489–497.

Windsor, R. (2003). Smoking cessation or reduction in pregnancy treatment methods: A meta-evaluation of the impact of dissemination. *The American Journal of the Medical Sciences, 326*(4), 216–222.

Zdravkovic, T., Genbacev, O., McMaster, M. T., & Fisher, S. J. (2005). The adverse effects of maternal smoking on the human placenta: A review. *Placenta, 26*(Suppl. A), S81–S86.

Zilberman, M. L., & Blume, S. B. (2004). Women and drugs. In J. Lowinson, P. Ruiz, R. B. Millman, & J. G. Langrod (Eds.), *Substance abuse: A comprehensive textbook* (4th ed., pp. 1064–1075). Philadelphia: Lippincott Williams & Wilkins.

CHAPTER 2

Research Design and Methodology in Studies of Women and Addiction

Stephanie Collins Reed, PhD
Suzette M. Evans, PhD

Sex is a factor often overlooked with respect to preclinical human drug abuse research, despite the fact that women make up 30% of substance abuse treatment admissions (Substance Abuse and Mental Health Services Administration [SAMHSA], 2007). Until about 15 years ago, most studies with drugs of abuse did not include women, in part because of the risk of pregnancy. However, as pregnant women with substance use disorders (SUDs) and women with SUDs and HIV/AIDS became increasingly prevalent, National Institutes of Health mandated that research studies not only include women, but also focus on women. In response, there has been a growing focus on male/female differences in drug abuse and sex differences research (Wetherington, 2007).

Although there is a growing literature indicating sex differences in response to drugs of abuse, the studies have been somewhat inconsistent. This may be due to certain risk factors or comorbidities that differ by gender and impact response to drugs of abuse and treatments. These sex differences, as well as issues related specifically to women (e.g., the menstrual cycle) need to be taken into consideration in designing studies to examine women or sex differences. This chapter focuses primarily on the methodological issues that need to be considered when designing or conducting human laboratory research, particularly studies that involve the administration of drugs of abuse. Careful attention to these issues provides important information that can then be utilized in improving our understanding and treatment of SUDs in men and women.

STUDY ISSUES

Women's Issues

Menstrual Cycle

One obvious difference between men and women is the menstrual cycle. The human female typically has a 28-day menstrual cycle. During the first half of the menstrual cycle, progesterone levels are minimal and estradiol levels rise gradually, peaking just before ovulation. The luteal phase begins after ovulation, and progesterone levels increase, peaking 3–8 days after ovulation and declining several days prior to menses. During the luteal phase, estradiol levels remain at levels similar to, or slightly higher, than those observed in the early to midfollicular phase. The menstrual cycle can be further divided into five hormonally distinct phases: menstrual or early follicular, mid- to late follicular, ovulatory, midluteal, and late luteal.

Ideally, when conducting research in women, the menstrual cycle should be prospectively tracked throughout a research or treatment study for two major reasons. First, there is growing evidence that women respond differently to drugs (particularly stimulants) across the menstrual cycle (see "Role of the Menstrual Cycle"). Second, the majority of women do not accurately track their menstrual cycle, making retrospective self-reports highly unreliable. An easy method for tracking is a standardized form for daily self-report, such as the Daily Ratings Form (Evans, Haney, Levin, Foltin, & Fischman, 1998). This form tracks changes in mood across the menstrual cycle, documents the onset and duration of menstruation, and can be modified to obtain prospective information on daily alcohol use, cigarette use, and other drug use. It can also be used to assess clinically meaningful premenstrual mood changes. If more accurate information is required, periodic blood samples to determine the actual levels of estradiol and progesterone and to confirm ovulation will clearly delineate the menstrual cycle phases. If testing during the luteal phase is essential, then urinary ovulations kits should be used to determine the time of ovulation for scheduling purposes. Laboratory studies specifically interested in the role of the menstrual cycle should ideally use a within-subject design, rather than a between-subject design, due to the inherent variability across individuals and the small sample sizes typically employed (Han & Evans, 2005). In summary, prospectively tracking the menstrual cycle is something that all studies involving premenopausal women should include because the menstrual cycle can affect a number of variables, including response to drugs of abuse and potential treatment medications.

Oral Contraceptives

In 2005, the prevalence of oral contraceptive (OC) use in the United States ranged from approximately 20–40% of the female population (Bensyl, Iuliano, Carter, Santelli, & Gilbert, 2005); however, we could find no data on the prevalence of OC use in women with SUDs. OCs can alter the metabolism of medication and substances of abuse. For example, nicotine metabolism was faster in women taking certain OCs compared to those who were not and compared to men (Benowitz, Lessov-Schlaggar, Swan, & Jacob, 2006). Conversely, OCs can decrease the metabolism of caffeine (see D. J. Back & Orme, 1990, for review).

Although relatively few studies have administered drugs of abuse to women taking OCs, available evidence suggests that OCs do not substantially alter the response (e.g., Kouri, Lundahl, Borden, McNeil, & Lukas, 2002). However, a recent study showed that the administration of estradiol enhanced the discriminative stimulus effects and some subjective effects of *d*-amphetamine compared to placebo in women who were in the placebo phase of their OCs (Lile, Kendall, Babalonis, Martin, & Kelly, 2007). Because data on the impact of OCs on drug response are limited, the prudent approach is to control for OC use in studies and to document the specific type (i.e., monophonic, biphasic, triphasic) and brand of OC. Ideally, studies that administer drugs and include women should strive to recruit homogeneous groups by either including only normally cycling women or women on the same type of OC.

Pre- and Postmenopausal Women

Unfortunately, there is little, if any research on differential effects of substances of abuse in premenopausal and postmenopausal women. However, there is evidence that women with

SUDs go through menopause earlier than women without SUDs (e.g., Kinney, Kline, & Levin, 2006) and that estradiol levels are disrupted in women with alcohol use disorders (Gavaler, Deal, VanThiel, Arria, & Allan, 1993).

With respect to smoking cessation treatment, premenopausal women drop out of treatment earlier than postmenopausal women (Copeland, Martin, Geiselman, Rash, & Kendzor, 2006). This is partially related to a greater concern about weight gain in younger women, but premenopausal women may also experience more withdrawal symptoms, particularly during the late luteal phase of the menstrual cycle (see "Role of the Menstrual Cycle"). In addition, premenopausal women may be less likely to stay in treatment due to their other responsibilities, such as child care. Among postmenopausal women, hormone replacement therapy may decrease withdrawal and craving and improve treatment retention (Allen, Hatsukami, Christianson, & Nelson, 2004). Thus, the responses to drugs or treatments for women may differ across the life span. Clearly more research needs to be conducted to address the special needs of perimenopausal and postmenopausal women.

Risk Factors Prevalent in Women

Depression

Overall, the prevalence of depression is higher in women than men (SAMSHA, 2006), and there is a high rate of depression in individuals with SUDs, particularly women (Sinha & Rounsaville, 2002). Psychiatric comorbidity can influence study results in important ways. For example, among cigarette smokers with a history of depression, positive mood induced by a script was increased more after nicotine administration in female smokers compared to male smokers (Spring et al., 2007), suggesting that nicotine may be beneficial to mood, particularly in women.

Studies focused on gender differences should carefully assess lifetime and current depressive disorders. The most commonly used instruments to identify depression are the Beck Depression Inventory (BDI) and the Hamilton Depression Scale (HAM-D). The BDI, a 21-item self-report questionnaire (Beck, Steer, & Brown, 1996), is a good screening instrument for depressive symptoms, but should always be followed up with a structured clinical interview to determine lifetime or current *DSM-IV* criteria for depression. To assess changes in depression symptomatology during a study, the self-report BDI and/or the clinician-administered HAM-D (Hamilton, 1960) can be conducted every 1–2 weeks.

Eating Disorders

Eating disorders are far more common in women as compared to men (e.g., Afifi, 2007), with the period of adolescence (Kearney-Cooke, 1999) to college age (Cullari, Rohrer, & Bahm, 1998) being the most vulnerable times for the development of eating disorders. Although there are limited data on sex differences in anorexia, the prevalence of bulimia nervosa (BN) is estimated to be 9 to 10 times greater in women than in men (e.g., Crowther, Wolf, & Sherwood, 1992).

Having an eating disorder is associated with alcohol and drug use (e.g., Bulik et al., 2004), particularly in women (Landheim, Bakken, & Valum, 2003). The prevalence of BN is about ten times greater (20%) in women with alcohol and substance-use disorders (e.g., Specker, Westermeyer, & Thuras, 2000), as compared to the general population (Bushnell, Wells, Hornblow, Oakley-Browne, & Joyce, 1990). Similarly, the prevalence of alcohol dependence is greater in patients with BN (e.g., 23%; meta-analysis by Holderness, Brooks-Gunn, & Warren, 1994) than in the general population (6%; SAMHSA, 2003). Stimulant use is also greater in patients with BN than controls (e.g., Wiederman & Pryor, 1996). The eating disorder typically precedes drug and alcohol problems (e.g., Hudson, Pope, Yergelun-Todd, Jonas, & Frenkenburg, 1987). Thus, it is necessary to explore eating disorders in women with substance abuse problems. There are several self-reports to determine BN, such as the Eating Disorders Examination Questionnaire (Fairburn & Beglin, 1994), the self-rating scale for bulimia (the "BITE"; Henderson & Freeman, 1987) and the eating disorder inventory (Garner, Olmstead, & Polivy, 1983). However, a structured clinical interview is needed to determine if an individual meets lifetime or current *DSM-IV* criteria for an eating disorder.

Premenstrual Dysphoric Disorder

Although the majority of premenopausal women experience some level of premenstrual symptoms (Dickerson, Mazyek, & Hunter, 2003), only 8% of women suffer from premenstrual symptoms that interfere with normal functioning and are diagnosed with premenstrual dysphoric disorder (PMDD; Bhatia & Bhatia, 2002). PMDD can affect mood, cognition, and appetite (e.g., Evans, 1998; Evans, Foltin, & Fischman, 1999), as well as response to pain (Straneva et al., 2002), and is characterized primarily by a cluster of mood symptoms, especially depression, tension, anxiety, irritability, and fatigue (American Psychiatric Association [APA], 1994). The Premenstrual Assessment Form (Halbreich, Endicott, & Schacht, 1982), which is a retrospective self-report questionnaire regarding changes in mood, behavior, and physical symptoms for the previous three menstrual cycles, is a good screening tool for PMDD. However, to accurately determine the presence or absence of PMDD, women should prospectively monitor symptoms for at least two consecutive symptomatic menstrual cycles (American Psychiatric Association, 1994) using self–reports such as the Daily Ratings Form (Evans et al., 1998), the Daily Symptom Report (Freeman, DeRubeis, & Rickels, 1996), the Daily Record of Severity of Problems (Endicott, Nee, & Harrison, 2006), or another form of diary each evening. Although tracking for two menstrual cycles can be time-consuming, it is essential to prospectively monitor symptoms, particularly when doing menstrual cycle-based research.

Few studies have directly examined the response to drugs and alcohol in women with PMDD (e.g., Marks, Hair, Klock, Ginsburg, & Pomerleau, 1994), and most studies have relied on prospective self-reports, with inconsistent results. For instance, among light and moderate drinkers with PMDD, there was no evidence that alcohol consumption varied as a function of menstrual cycle phase (e.g., Evans et al., 1999). However, another study found that women with PMDD reported more alcohol use, cigarette smoking, and nonprescription drug use during menses than other phases of the menstrual phase (Marks et al., 1994). Therefore, fluctuations in drug use and/or response across the menstrual cycle in women with PMDD needs further clarification.

Other Risk Factors That May Affect Women Differently from Men

Family History of Alcoholism

Males and females are at an increased risk to develop alcohol-use disorders if they have parents who are alcoholics (e.g., Merikangas, 1990). Moreover, having a family history of alcoholism (FHP) is more common among women who are alcoholics than either men who are alcoholics or women who are not alcoholics (Gomberg, 1993). Several studies have shown that individuals with FHP show less impairment after alcohol administration than individuals who do not have a family history of alcoholism (FHN; e.g., Schuckit et al., 2000), although this effect may be less robust in women with FHP (Evans & Levin, 2003).

Several studies have suggested that environmental factors play a greater role among females with FHP (e.g., Pickens et al., 1991). Consistent with this, Heath et al. (1999) reported that reduced alcohol sensitivity predicted increased genetic risk for men, but not for women.

Although individuals with FHP are also at increased risk for drug abuse (e.g., McCaul, Turkkan, Svikis, Bigelow, & Cromwell, 1990), only a few studies have examined the effects of drugs other than alcohol, with the majority testing benzodiazepines. Two of the benzodiazepine studies were conducted in women with FHP (Ciraulo et al., 1996; Evans, Levin, & Fischman, 2000), but no studies have directly compared men and women with FHP. Only one study examined the effects of cocaine in males with FHP and found no differences between males with FHP and FHN (Kouri, Raga, McNeil, & Lukas, 2000). Thus, much more research needs to be conducted in males and females with FHP, with alcohol and other drugs.

When conducting studies that involve the administration of drugs of abuse, particularly alcohol, it is important to carefully assess the presence or absence of family history of alcohol and substance abuse. The best way to ensure accurate information on family history is to conduct a structured family interview with first-degree relatives, such as the structured diagnostic instrument used in The Collaborative Study on the Genetics of Alcoholism (COGA; Rice et al., 1995). Although this may appear impractical, time-consuming, and expensive, it is feasible (Evans & Levin, 2003). We have been using this procedure in our studies for the past 12 years and have been unable to confirm a participant's self-report of a paternal family history of alcoholism in 5% of female participants and 10% of male participants. Consequently, if we had included these individuals based on the self-report of the participant, our results may have been compromised.

Trauma

STRESS

Preclinical and clinical laboratory studies indicate that exposure to stressors and hypothalamic–pituitary–adrenal (HPA) axis activation, which increases cortisol and other stress-related hormones, increases drug craving (e.g., see Sinha, 2001, for review). Women are more likely to abuse substances subsequent to trauma exposure than men (e.g., Kendler et al., 2000). McKee, Maciejewski, Falba, and Mazure (2003) found that stressful life events had a greater negative effect on ability to quit smoking for women compared to men. These studies suggest that women may be more vulnerable to the impact of stress on substance use as compared to men.

Stress has also been shown to disrupt a woman's menstrual cycle (Edozien, 2006); 33% of women who were incarcerated reported menstrual irregularity associated with a history of SUDs or childhood sexual abuse (CSA) (Allsworth et al., 2007). Women also have differential responses to stress across the menstrual cycle. For example, there is an increased response to stress (Kajantie & Phillips, 2006, for review) and higher stress hormone levels (adrenocorticotropic hormone [ACTH] and cortisol; Kirschbaum, Kudielka, Gaab, Schommer, & Hellhammer, 1999) in the luteal phase compared to the follicular phase.

Induction of stress in the laboratory is usually done using a psychological stressor or a physical stressor. The most commonly used psychological stressors are the Trier Social Stress Test (TSST; e.g., Kirschbaum, Pirke, & Hellhammer, 1993) and imagery scripts (e.g., Sinha, Catapano, & O'Malley, 1999). The TSST consists of a public speaking task and a mental arithmetic task. Stress imagery scripts have participants describe and imagine a recent personally stressful experience. A common physical stressor is the Cold Pressor Test (CPT; e.g.,

Zacny et al., 1996). Subjective response can be measured by self-report questionnaires, such as the Perceived Stress Scale (Cohen, Kamarck, & Mermelstein, 1983) and the State Anxiety Inventory (Spielberger, Gorsuch, & Lushene, 1970). Stress response can also be measured by cardiovascular (i.e., heart rate) and endocrine (cortisol, ACTH) measures, which increase in response to stress exposure.

To date, much of the data assessing response to stress among substance abusers has focused on cocaine. Males who are cocaine dependent showed a greater physiological response at baseline and after exposure to stress imagery than females (Fox et al., 2006). Similarly, men who are cocaine dependent had a greater physiological response to a Mental Arithmetic Task and the CPT, but women who are cocaine dependent had a greater subjective anxiety response to these two stressors (S. E. Back, Brady, Jackson, Salstrom, & Zinzow, 2005). This suggests that women who are cocaine dependent may be more vulnerable to the subjective effects of stress compared to men who are cocaine dependent. Two studies that examined sex differences in response to the physical stressor, the CPT, in response to opioids found that women had greater pain tolerance (Pud et al., 2006) and reduced self-report of pain (al'Absi et al., 2004) in response to opioids than men. In one study that examined sex differences in stress response after alcohol consumption, cardiovascular effects were decreased in women with FHP in response to a speech stressor, whereas this was not observed in men with FHP (Sinha, Robinson, & O'Malley, 1998). Based on the limited existing data, women who abuse drugs have a differential response to stress than men who abuse drugs, thus there is a need to better understand if stress is a trigger for drug use or relapse and how this may affect men and women differently. Further, studies have shown that women with childhood abuse (Bremner et al., 2003) or bulimia (Bekker & Boselie, 2002) have a different physiological and psychological response to stress compared to control women. Therefore, when assessing response to laboratory stressors, a comprehensive battery of subjective, physiological, and hormonal responses should be measured, and ideally more than one type of stressor should be conducted.

CHILDHOOD SEXUAL ABUSE

Although CSA occurs in females and males (Walker, Carey, Mohr, Stein, & Seedat, 2004), in the United States, the prevalence of CSA is 3 to 5 times greater in females (e.g., Harrison, Fulkerson, & Beebe, 1997). Further, there appear to be differences between male and female CSA victims in terms of their subsequent disorders, including substance abuse (e.g., Walker et al., 2004). The prevalence rates of CSA in women in the general population range from 10–60% (e.g., MacMillan et al., 2001); are associated with a number of adult psychiatric disorders including depression, bulimia, and alcohol and substance abuse disorders (e.g., Kendler et al., 2000); and these associations appear to be stronger for women than for men (Widom, Marmorstein, & White, 2006). Clinical studies have shown high rates of CSA (20–80%) among women seeking treatment for alcohol or drug abuse (e.g., Simpson & Miller, 2002). Similarly, the rates of alcohol and drug abuse are higher among women with CSA (e.g., Corstorphine, Waller, Lawson, & Ganis, 2007) than the general population. Thus, in substance abusers, it is important to determine whether there is a history of sexual abuse (or other forms of abuse) or childhood trauma because individuals with CSA may be less responsive to treatment and need targeted treatment for the CSA. When conducting research in women, questionnaires should be included, such as the Early Trauma Inventory (Bremner, Vermetten, & Mazure, 2000) or the Childhood Trauma Questionnaire (Bernstein et al., 2003) to determine childhood histories of trauma even in those who do not have posttraumatic stress disorder (PTSD).

POSTTRAUMATIC STRESS DISORDER

Traumatic events occurring in one's lifetime are associated with high levels of emotional and physiological distress that can lead to PTSD (e.g., Regehr, Goldberg, Glancy, & Knott, 2002). Women, in particular, may be more vulnerable to the development of PTSD (Breslau, Davis, Andreski, Peterson, & Schultz, 1997). PTSD has also been linked to SUDs (e.g., Brady, Myrick, & McElroy, 1998), with one study reporting that 21–43% of individuals with PTSD also abuse drugs (Jacobsen, Southwick, & Kosten, 2001). In women, PTSD more commonly precedes the development of SUDs as compared to men (e.g., Johnson & Rn, 2006). As such, careful assessment of PTSD is important in studies of SUDs in women.

Impulsivity

"Impulsivity comprises a heterogeneous cluster of lower-order traits that includes terms such as impulsivity, sensation seeking, risk-taking, novelty seeking, boldness, adventuresomeness, boredom susceptibility, unreliability, and unorderliness" (Depue & Collins, 1999, p. 495). Not surprisingly, individuals with SUDs (e.g., Petry, 2001) exhibit more impulsive behavior than normal controls. Sensation seeking has also been associated with risky behaviors, including drug use (e.g., Zuckerman & Kuhlman, 2000) and sexual risk taking (Donohew et al., 2000). The relationship between SUDs and impulsivity is unclear and probably variable. For example, an individual who is intoxicated may be more likely to engage in impulsive behaviors, such as unprotected sex. Conversely, an individual who behaves impulsively may be more likely to use drugs and engage in excessive drinking.

Impulsivity is currently assessed by a range of self-report questionnaires and behavioral measures. Self-report questionnaires include (1) the Impulsivity Questionnaire (Eysenck, Pearson, Easting, & Allsopp, 1985), (2) the Barratt Impulsiveness Scale (Patton, Stanford, & Barratt, 1995), and (3) the Zuckerman Sensation-Seeking Scale (Zuckerman, Eysenck, & Eysenck, 1978). Behavioral measures include (1) the Immediate Memory Task/Delayed Memory Task (e.g., Dougherty, 1999), which measures attention and rapid-response impulsivity, (2) the Go–Stop Task (Dougherty, Mathias, & Marsh, 2003), which measures behavioral inhibition, (3) the Delay Discounting Task (e.g., Kirby & Marakovic, 1996) and the Iowa Gambling Task (Bechara, Damasio, Damasio, & Anderson, 1994), which measure decision making; and (4) the Balloon Analogue Risk Task (Lejuez et al., 2002), which measures risk taking. Not all of these measures produce the same profile of effects, either across different groups of people or when different drugs are administered. Therefore, it is important to assess a range of impulsivity measures.

With respect to sex differences, most studies conducted in normal non-SUD populations indicate that men are more impulsive than women (e.g., Zuckerman, 1996). Although no sex differences in impulsivity were observed in cigarette smokers (Lejuez et al., 2003) or drinkers (Goudriaan, Grekin, & Sher, 2007), Petry, Kirby, and Kranzler (2002) found that females with FHP were more impulsive (had higher discount rates) than females with FHN, a relationship not observed for males. Among cocaine abusers, one study found that females were more impulsive than males, and impulsivity was a risk factor in the relationship between gender and crack/cocaine dependence and lifetime heaviest use (Lejuez, Boprnovalova, Reynolds, Daughters, & Curtin, 2007), whereas no sex differences on two measures of impulsivity were observed in abstinent cocaine users in treatment (Bornovalova, Lejuez, Daughters, Zachary Rosenthal, & Lynch, 2005).

Self-reported impulsivity has been shown to predict worse treatment retention in heroin-dependent cocaine abusers (see Poling, Kosten, & Sofuoglu, 2007, for review), however, sex differences were not specifically examined in these studies. Although it is still unclear whether sex differences play a role in the relationship between impulsivity and SUDs, data suggest that impulsivity may have an important role in treatment. Thus, baseline measures of impulsivity, as well as changes in impulsivity during treatment, should be addressed in study design.

Specific Considerations When Assessing the Effects of Drugs

Pharmacokinetics/Body Weight

Metabolism of some drugs may differ between men and women (Beierle, Meibohm, & Derendorf, 1999). Nicotine, for example, is metabolized faster in women than in men (Benowitz et al., 2006). There are also important differences in alcohol pharmacokinetics, in part due to differences in body composition. Because men have a lower body fat content than women, with the same dose of alcohol (assuming other factors are controlled for, including drinking level, family history of alcoholism, etc.), men will have lower breath alcohol levels and less of a behavioral response to alcohol than women (see Han & Evans, 2005 for review), although the elimination rate of alcohol is generally faster in women (Ammon, Schäfer, Hofmann, & Kutz, 1996). Sex differences in alcohol metabolism and distribution can be minimized by adjusting for body weight (e.g., Breslin, Kapur, Sobell, & Cappell, 1997) and calculating doses based on estimated total body water (e.g., Kushner, Schoeller, Fjeld, & Danford, 1992). However, there is minimal evidence that the pharmacokinetics of cocaine differ between men and women or across the menstrual cycle for intravenous cocaine (Mendelson et al., 1999), intranasal cocaine (Collins, Evans, Foltin, & Haney, 2007) or smoked cocaine (e.g., Evans & Foltin, 2006). Regardless, because women generally weigh less than men, investigators should try to dose based on body weight or body composition, particularly for alcohol or intravenous drugs.

Route of Administration

Although studies of intranasal cocaine have shown minimal differences as a function of sex or menstrual cycle phase (e.g., Collins et al., 2007), sex differences have been reported in response to smoked cocaine (e.g., Evans & Foltin, 2006) particularly when the menstrual cycle was controlled for. Similarly, sex differences in response to nicotine also depend on the method of nicotine administration (see Perkins, 1999, for review). For example, nicotine spray (Perkins et al., 1996) and gum (Killen, Fortmann, Newman, & Varady, 1990) are self-administered more in men than in women, but women report greater positive subjective ratings after tobacco smoking than men (e.g., Perkins et al., 1994).

Although a number of studies have assessed the effects of orally administered alcohol in men and women, the sex differences have been modest and inconsistent. In one study alcohol reduced tension in women but increased arousal in men (Sutker, Allain, Brantley, & Randall, 1982). In another study, ratings of anxiety were decreased to a similar extent in men and women (de Boer, Schippers, & van der Staak, 1993). The only study that compared the subjective effects of intravenous alcohol in men and women found no sex differences in response to a low dose of alcohol (Nyberg, Wahlström, Bäckström, & Poromaa, 2004). Thus, the effects of alcohol may differ depending on the route of administration, however more research is needed.

Unfortunately, relatively few studies with other drugs of abuse have evaluated different routes of administration in men and women. With respect to cannabinoids, there is limited evidence that men are more sensitive to the positive subjective effects of smoked marijuana (Penetar et al., 2005) and oral delta-9-tetrahydrocannabinol (THC; Haney, 2007) than women. More research is clearly needed in this area, but available evidence suggests that men and women should be tested when examining drug effects by differing routes of administration because there may be sex differences that depend on the route or method of administration.

Role of the Menstrual Cycle

Recently, a number of studies have examined the effects of drugs across the menstrual cycle in humans (see Terner & de Wit, 2006, for review). The majority of research in this area has focused on the effects of stimulants (cocaine, amphetamine, nicotine) and alcohol. The most consistent finding to date is that the effects of d-amphetamine and cocaine vary across the menstrual cycle in women, and this may account for the sex differences observed in response to these stimulants. Specifically, the subjective effects of d-amphetamine (e.g., Justice & de Wit, 1999) or cocaine (e.g., Sofuoglu, Dudish-Poulsen, Nelson, Pentel, & Hatsukami, 1999) are greater during the follicular phase when progesterone levels are minimal, compared to the luteal phase when progesterone levels are elevated. Further, the response to stimulants in women during the follicular phase is similar to that observed in men (e.g., White, Justice, & de Wit, 2002) and oral progesterone dampens the effects of cocaine during the follicular phase (e.g., Evans & Foltin, 2006), further suggesting that hormonal fluctuations across the menstrual cycle alter the response to stimulants (see Evans, 2007, for review). However, for cocaine, these menstrual cycle differences appear to depend on the route of administration because several studies have failed to observe changes across the menstrual cycle following intranasal cocaine (e.g., Kouri et al., 2002).

Similarly, studies with nicotine have shown that nicotine craving and nicotine withdrawal vary across the menstrual cycle. It has been reported that nicotine craving (Franklin et al., 2004), cigarettes smoked per day (Snively, Ahijevych, Bernhard, & Wewers, 2000), nicotine withdrawal (e.g., Perkins, 2001), and desire to smoke were increased during the late luteal phase, particularly in women who experienced premenstrual symptoms (Allen, Hatsukami, Bade, & Center, 1999). With respect to cigarette smoking, one study reported that women smoked more during menses (Marks, Hair, Klock, Ginsburg, & Pomerleau, 1994), while other studies showed that smoking (Pomerleau, Cole, Lumley, Marks, & Pomerleau, 1994) and the effects of intranasal nicotine spray did not vary across the menstrual cycle (Marks, Pomerleau, & Pomerleau, 1999).

In contrast to stimulants, alcohol appears to produce minimal differences across the menstrual cycle, including subjective effects (e.g., Nyberg et al., 2004a), performance effects (Holdstock & de Wit, 2000), or peak blood-alcohol concentrations (Corrêa & Oga, 2004). Changes in self-reported alcohol intake across the menstrual cycle have been variable across studies (e.g., Pastor & Evans, 2003). However, one study that assessed alcohol consumption while women resided as inpatients found that alcohol consumption increased during the luteal phase in those women who experienced premenstrual symptoms (Mello, Mendelson, & Lex, 1990). Therefore, changes in alcohol consumption across the menstrual cycle in women may depend on their drinking level and premenstrual symptom levels.

In contrast to stimulants and alcohol, the number of studies that have assessed changes in response to opioids across the menstrual cycle is limited and virtually nonexistent for marijuana. One study (Gear et al., 1996) reported no menstrual cycle phase differences in analgesia effects after a kappa-opiate for postoperative pain. Another study found that higher doses were needed for anesthesia during the follicular phase (Erden et al., 2005), yet another study reported greater opioid use in the luteal phase to treat postoperative pain (Sener et al., 2005). Taken together, there is growing evidence that the response to some drugs of abuse, particularly stimulants, vary as a function of menstrual cycle phase. Given the paucity of data with other drugs of abuse, until it has been clearly established that the response to a drug does not vary across the menstrual cycle, studies need to control for this important variable (see "Oral Contraceptives").

Recruitment and Retention

A major hurdle in conducting human substance-abuse research is recruitment and retention, and this appears to be even more difficult in women than in men. In our own experience, men are more willing to participate in laboratory studies involving the administration of drugs of abuse. Similarly, among individuals seeking treatment, although women may enter treatment earlier than men (Brady & Randall, 1999), overall, they are less likely to enter treatment at all (Greenfield et al., 2007). The recruitment of women can be even more difficult if studies have to control for the menstrual cycle or have to be conducted at specific phases of the menstrual cycle. Further, women often have child care responsibilities, making it challenging for them to schedule and keep appointments or participate in long-term inpatient studies, so shorter studies or outpatient studies may be better suited to female drug abusers. In addition, based on our own experience recruiting cocaine abusers for laboratory studies, women are excluded for medical or psychiatric reasons more often than men. Further, in outpatient studies that require cocaine abusers to be drug free, women are less able to refrain from drug use than men. Therefore, recruiting women into either laboratory research or treatment studies requires more intensive efforts and the development of specific strategies, such as advertising in publications or locations that women are likely to see, including hair and nail salons, laundromats, women's health clinics, and so on. Also, a good strategy is to ask women already involved to tell their friends about the research opportunities.

FUTURE DIRECTIONS

Sex differences related to drug abuse may be due to various factors such as stress response (e.g., Kirschbaum et al., 1999), age of first use (e.g., Brady & Randall, 1999), environment (e.g., Brady & Randall, 1999), subjective effects (e.g., Evans & Foltin, 2006), hormone levels (e.g., Mendelson, Sholar, Siegel, & Mello, 2001), menstrual cycle effects (e.g., Evans, Haney, & Foltin, 2002), other Axis I or II disorders, or even impulsive behavior, as discussed throughout this chapter. Thus, it is necessary to take these factors into consideration when conducting research in women, and importantly, when examining future treatment options for female substance abusers.

The most important methodological suggestion for research, particularly when the goal is to assess response to drugs of abuse and differences between men and women, is to carefully collect as much information as possible on all research participants, including a full clinical interview to assess current and lifetime Axis I disorders. Other factors that will affect and potentially confound results include obtaining information on family history of alcoholism and substance abuse, history of various traumas, and information on impulsivity. Further, in studies that look at women or sex differences and include premenopausal women it is important to carefully monitor the menstrual cycle and/or control for oral contraceptive use, as these factors have been shown to affect research study outcomes in women who are drug abusers and may have an affect on treatment.

To improve upon the existing literature examining women or sex differences it is necessary to continue to include women in research studies and to focus on enhancing the recruitment and retention of women in research studies. More importantly, it is necessary to improve treatments for women by specifically tailoring treatment programs and medications for women to provide more effective and sensitive treatments that will result in better retention and treatment outcomes.

KEY POINTS

- Include women in all research studies.
- Carefully monitor the menstrual cycle in women.
- Control for oral contraceptive use in women.
- Collect as much information as possible on all research participants, especially about current and previous levels of drug use and Axis I disorders.
- Consider factors that aren't typically captured in a structured clinical interview, but that would affect response to drugs and treatment outcome. These may include a family history of drug and alcohol abuse, impulsive tendencies, and a history of stress or trauma (including childhood abuse).
- Tailor treatment programs to sex-specific issues to increase chances of a successful treatment outcome.

ACKNOWLEDGMENTS

We would like to thank the National Institute on Drug Abuse for their support on Grant Nos. KO1 DA022282, RO1 DA021242, RO1 DA009114, and RO1 DA08105.

REFERENCES

Asterisks denote recommended readings.

Afifi, M. (2007). Gender differences in mental health. *Singapore Medical Journal*, 48, 385–391. (*)

al'Absi, M., Wittmers, L. E., Ellestad, D., Nordehn, G., Kim, S. W., Kirschbaum, C., et al. (2004). Sex differences in pain and hypothalamic–pituitary–adrenocortical responses to opioid blockade. *Psychosomatic Medicine*, 66, 198–206.

Allen, S. S., Hatsukami, D. K., Bade, T., & Center, B. (2004). Transdermal nicotine use in postmenopausal women: Does the treatment efficacy differ in women using and not using hormone replacement therapy? *Nicotine and Tobacco Research*, 6, 777–788.

Allen, S. S., Hatsukami, D. K., Christianson, D., & Nelson, D. (1999). Withdrawal and premenstrual symptomatology during the menstrual cycle in short-term smoking abstinence: Effects of menstrual cycle on smoking abstinence. *Nicotine and Tobacco Research*, 1, 129–142.

Allsworth, J. E., Clarke, J., Peipert, J. F., Hebert, M. R., Cooper, A., & Boardman, L. A. (2007). The influence of stress on the menstrual cycle among newly incarcerated women. *Womens Health Issues*, 17, 202–209.

American Psychiatric Association. (1994). *Diagnostic and statistical manual of mental disorders* (4th ed.). Washington, DC: Author.

Ammon, E., Schäfer, C., Hofmann, U., & Klotz, U. (1996). Disposition and first-pass metabolism of ethanol in humans: Is it gastric or hepatic and does it depend on gender? *Clinical Pharmacology and Therapeutics*, 59, 503–513.

Back, D. J., & Orme, M. L. (1990). Pharmacokinetic drug interactions with oral contraceptives. *Clinical Pharmacokinetics*, 18, 472–484.

Back, S. E., Brady, K. T., Jackson, J. L., Salstrom, S., & Zinzow, H. (2005). Gender differences in stress reactivity among cocaine-dependent individuals. *Psychopharmacology*, *180*, 169–176.

Bechara, A., Damasio, A. R., Damasio, H., & Anderson, S. W. (1994). Insensitivity to future consequences following damage to human prefrontal cortex. *Cognition*, *50*, 7–15.

Beck, A. T., Steer, R. A., & Brown, G. K. (1996). *BDI-II Beck Depression Inventory manual* (2nd ed.). San Antonio, TX: Psychological Corp.

Beierle, I., Meibohm, B., & Derendorf, H. (1999). Gender differences in pharmacokinetics and pharmacodynamics. *International Journal of Clinical Pharmacology and Therapeutics*, *37*, 529–547.

Bekker, M. H. J., & Boselie, K. A. H. M. (2002). Gender and stress: Is gender role stress? A reexamination of the relationship between feminine gender role stress and eating disorders. *Stress and Health*, *18*, 141–149.

Benowitz, N. L., Lessov-Schlaggar, C. N., Swan, G. E., & Jacob, P., 3rd. (2006). Female sex and oral contraceptive use accelerate nicotine metabolism. *Clinical Pharmacology and Therapeutics*, *79*, 480–488.

Bensyl, D. M., Iuliano, D. A., Carter, M., Santelli, J., & Gilbert, B. C. (2005). Contraceptive use—United States and territories, Behavioral Risk Factor Surveillance System, 2002. *Morbidity and Mortality Weekly Report. Surveillance Summary*, *54*, 1–72.

Bernstein, D. P., Stein, J. A., Newcomb, M. D., Walker, E., Pogge, D., Ahluvalia, T., et al. (2003). Development and validation of a brief screening version of the Childhood Trauma Questionnaire. *Child Abuse and Neglect*, *27*, 169–190.

Bhatia, S. C., & Bhatia, S. K. (2002). Diagnosis and treatment of premenstrual dysphoric disorder. *American Family Physician*, *66*, 1239–1248.

Bornovalova, M. A., Lejuez, C. W., Daughters, S. B., Zachary Rosenthal, M., & Lynch, T. R. (2005). Impulsivity as a common process across borderline personality and substance use disorders. *Clinical Psychology Review*, *25*, 790–812.

Brady, K. T., Myrick, H., & McElroy, S. (1998). The relationship between substance use disorders, impulse control disorders, and pathological aggression. *American Journal on Addictions*, *7*, 221–230.

Brady, K. T., & Randall, C. L. (1999). Gender differences in substance use disorders. *Psychiatric Clinics of North America*, *22*, 241–252. (*)

Bremner, J. D., Vermetten, E., & Mazure, C. M. (2000). Development and preliminary psychometric properties of an instrument for the measurement of childhood trauma: The Early Trauma Inventory. *Depression and Anxiety*, *12*, 1–12.

Bremner, J. D., Vythilingam, M., Vermetten, E., Adil, A., Khan, S., Nazeer, A., et al. (2003). Cortisol response to a cognitive stress challenge in posttraumatic stress disorder (PTSD) related to childhood abuse. *Psychoneuroendocrinology*, *28*, 733–750.

Breslau, N., Davis, G. C., Andreski, P., Peterson, E. L., & Schultz, L. R. (1997). Sex differences in posttraumatic stress disorder. *Archives of General Psychiatry*, *54*, 1044–1048.

Breslin, F. C., Kapur, B. M., Sobell, M. B., & Cappell, H. (1997). Gender and alcohol dosing: A procedure for producing comparable breath alcohol curves for men and women. *Alcoholism, Clinical and Experimental Research*, *21*, 928–930.

Bulik, C. M., Klump, K. L., Thornton, L., Kaplan, A. S., Devlin, B., Fichter, M. M., et al. (2004). Alcohol use disorder comorbidity in eating disorders: A multicenter study. *Journal of Clinical Psychiatry*, *65*, 1000–1006.

Bushnell, J. A., Wells, J. E., Hornblow, A. E., Oakley-Browne, M. A., & Joyce, P. (1990). Prevalence of three bulimia syndromes in the general population. *Psychological Medicine*, *20*, 671–680.

Ciraulo, D. A., Sarid-Segal, O., Knapp, C., Ciraulo, A. M., Greenblatt, D. J., & Shader, R. I. (1996). Liability to alprazolam abuse in daughters of alcoholics. *American Journal of Psychiatry*, *153*, 956–958.

Cohen, S., Kamarck, T., & Mermelstein, R. (1983). A global measure of perceived stress. *Journal of Health and Social Behavior*, *24*, 385–396.

Collins, S. L., Evans, S. M., Foltin, R. W., & Haney, M. (2007). Intranasal cocaine in humans: Effects of sex and menstrual cycle. *Pharmacology, Biochemistry, and Behavior*, *86*, 117–124.

Copeland, A. L., Martin, P. D., Geiselman, P. J., Rash, C. J., & Kendzor, D. E. (2006). Predictors of pretreatment attrition from smoking cessation among pre- and postmenopausal, weight-concerned women. *Eating Behaviors, 7,* 243–251.

Corrêa, C. L., & Oga, S. (2004). Effects of the menstrual cycle of white women on ethanol toxicokinetics. *Journal of Studies on Alcohol, 65,* 227–231.

Corstorphine, E., Waller, G., Lawson, R., & Ganis, C. (2007). Trauma and multi-impulsivity in the eating disorders. *Eating Behaviors, 8,* 23–30.

Crowther, J. H., Wolf, E. M., & Sherwood, N. (1992). Epidemiology of bulimia nervosa. In M. Crowther, D. L. Tennenbaum, S. E. Hobfoll, & M. A. P. Stephens (Eds.), *The etiology of bulimia nervosa: The individual and familial context* (pp. 1–26). Washington, DC: Taylor & Francis.

Cullari, S., Rohrer, J. M., & Bahm, C. (1998). Body-image perceptions across sex and age groups. *Perceptual and Motor Skills, 87,* 839–847.

de Boer, M. C., Schippers, G. M., & van der Staak, C. P. (1993). Alcohol and social anxiety in women and men: Pharmacological and expectancy effects. *Addictive Behaviors, 18,* 117–126.

Depue, R. A., & Collins, P. F. (1999). Neurobiology of the structure of personality: Dopamine, facilitation of incentive motivation, and extraversion. *Behavioral and Brain Sciences, 22,* 491–569.

Dickerson, L. M., Mazyck, P. J., & Hunter, M. H. (2003). Premenstrual syndrome. *American Family Physician, 67,* 1743–1752.

Donohew, L., Zimmerman, R. S., Cupp, P. S., Novak, S., Colon, S., & Abell, R. (2000). Sensation seeking, impulsive decision-making, and risky sex: Implications for risk-taking and design of interventions. *Personality and Individual Differences, 28,* 1079–1091.

Dougherty, D. M. (1999). *IMT/DMT Immediate Memory Task and Delayed Memory Task: A research tool for studying attention and memory processes* (Version 1.3) (Computer software manual). Houston: University of Texas Health Science Center at Houston, Neurobehavioral Research Laboratory and Clinic.

Dougherty, D. M., Mathias, C. W., & Marsh, D. M. (2003). Laboratory measures of impulsivity. In E. F. Coccaro (Ed.), *Aggression: Psychiatric assessment and treatment* (pp. 247–265). New York: Marcel Dekker.

Edozien, L. C. (2006). Mind over matter: Psychological factors and the menstrual cycle. *Current Opinions in Obstetrics & Gynecology, 18,* 452–456.

Endicott, J., Nee, J., & Harrison, W. (2006). Daily Record of Severity of Problems (DRSP): Reliability and validity. *Archives of Womens Mental Health, 9,* 41–49.

Erden, V., Yangin, Z., Erkalp, K., Delatioglu, H., Bahceci, F., & Seyhan, A. (2005). Increased progesterone production during the luteal phase of menstruation may decrease anesthetic requirement. *Anesthesia and Analgesia, 101,* 1007–1011.

Evans, S. M. (2007). The role of estradiol and progesterone in modulating the subjective effects of stimulants in humans. *Experimental and Clinical Psychopharmacology, 15,* 418–426.

Evans, S. M., & Foltin, R. W. (2006). Exogenous progesterone attenuates the subjective effects of smoked cocaine in women, but not in men. *Neuropsychopharmacology, 31,* 659–674.

Evans, S. M., Foltin, R. W., & Fischman, M. W. (1999). Food "cravings" and the acute effects of alprazolam on food intake in women with premenstrual dysphoric disorder. *Appetite, 32,* 331–349.

Evans, S. M., Haney, M., & Foltin, R. W. (2002). The effects of smoked cocaine during the follicular and luteal phases of the menstrual cycle in women. *Psychopharmacology, 159,* 397–406.

Evans, S. M., Haney, M., Levin, F. R., Foltin, R. W., & Fischman, M. W. (1998). Mood and performance changes in women with premenstrual dysphoric disorder: Acute effects of alprazolam. *Neuropsychopharmacology, 19,* 499–516.

Evans, S. M., & Levin, F. R. (2003). Response to alcohol in females with a paternal history of alcoholism. *Psychopharmacology, 169,* 10–20.

Evans, S. M., Levin, F. R., & Fischman, M. W. (2000). Increased sensitivity to alprazolam in females with a paternal history of alcoholism. *Psychopharmacology, 150,* 150–162.

Eysenck, S. B. G., Pearson, P. R., Easting, G., & Allsopp, J. F. (1985). Age norms for impulsiveness, venturesomeness and empathy in adults. *Personality and Individual Differences, 6,* 613–619.

Fairburn, C. G., & Beglin, S. J. (1994). Assessment of eating disorders: Interview or self-report questionnaire? *The International Journal of Eating Disorders, 16,* 363–370.

Fox, H. C., Garcia, M., Jr., Kemp, K., Milivojevic, V., Kreek, M. J., & Sinha, R. (2006). Gender differences in cardiovascular and corticoadrenal response to stress and drug cues in cocaine dependent individuals. *Psychopharmacology, 185,* 348–357.

Franklin, T. R., Napier, K., Ehrman, R., Gariti, P., O'Brien, C. P., & Childress, A. R. (2004). Retrospective study: Influence of menstrual cycle on cue-induced cigarette craving. *Nicotine and Tobacco Research, 6,* 171–175.

Freeman, E. W., DeRubeis, R. J., & Rickels, K. (1996). Reliability and validity of a daily diary for premenstrual syndrome. *Psychiatry Research, 65,* 97–106.

Garner, D. M., Olmsted, M. P., & Polivy, J. (1983). Development and validation of a multidimensional eating disorder inventory for anorexia nervosa and bulimia. *International Journal of Eating Disorders, 2,* 15–34.

Gavaler, J. S., Deal, S. R., Van Thiel, D. H., Arria, A., & Allan, M. J. (1993). Alcohol and estrogen levels in postmenopausal women: The spectrum of effect. *Alcoholism, Clinical and Experimental Research, 17,* 786–790.

Gear, R. W., Gordon, N. C., Heller, P. H., Paul, S., Miaskowski, C., & Levine, J. D. (1996). Gender difference in analgesic response to the kappa-opioid pentazocine. *Neuroscience Letters, 205,* 207–209.

Gomberg, E. S. (1993). Women and alcohol: Use and abuse. *Journal of Nervous and Mental Disease, 181,* 211–219.

Goudriaan, A. E., Grekin, E. R., & Sher, K. J. (2007). Decision making and binge drinking: A longitudinal study. *Alcoholism, Clinical and Experimental Research, 31,* 928–938.

Greenfield, S. F., Brooks, A. J., Gordon, S. M., Green, C. A., Kropp, F., McHugh, R. K., et al. (2007). Substance abuse treatment entry, retention, and outcome in women: A review of the literature. *Drug and Alcohol Dependence, 86,* 1–21. (*)

Halbreich, U., Endicott, J., & Schacht, S. (1982). Premenstrual syndromes: A new instrument for their assessment. *Journal of Psychiatric Treatment and Evaluation, 4,* 161–164.

Hamilton, M. (1960). A rating scale for depression. *Journal of Neurology, Neurosurgery, and Psychiatry, 3,* 56–62.

Han, S. C., & Evans, S. M. (2005). Sex and drugs: Do women differ from men in their subjective response to drugs of abuse? In M. Earlywine (Ed.), *Mind-altering drugs, the science of subjective experience* (pp. 183–216). New York: Oxford University Press.

Haney, M. (2007). Opioid antagonism of cannabinoid effects: Differences between marijuana smokers and nonmarijuana smokers. *Neuropsychopharmacology, 32,* 1391–1403.

Harrison, P. A., Fulkerson, J. A., & Beebe, T. J. (1997). Multiple substance use among adolescent physical and sexual abuse victims. *Child Abuse and Neglect, 21,* 529–539.

Heath, A. C., Madden, P. A., Bucholz, K. K., Dinwiddie, S. H., Slutske, W. S., Bierut, L. J., et al. (1999). Genetic differences in alcohol sensitivity and the inheritance of alcoholism risk. *Psychological Medicine, 29,* 1069–1081.

Henderson, M., & Freeman, C. P. (1987). A self-rating scale for bulimia. The "BITE." *British Journal of Psychiatry, 150,* 18–24.

Holderness, C. C., Brooks-Gunn, J., & Warren, M. P. (1994). Co-morbidity of eating disorders and substance abuse: Review of the literature. *International Journal of Eating Disorders, 16,* 1–34.

Holdstock, L., & de Wit, H. (2000). Effects of ethanol at four phases of the menstrual cycle. *Psychopharmacology, 150,* 374–382.

Hudson, J. I., Pope, H. G., Yurgelun-Todd, D., Jonas, J. M., & Frenkenburg, F. R. (1987). A controlled study of lifetime prevalence of affective and other psychiatric disorders in bulimic outpatients. *American Journal of Psychiatry, 144,* 1283–1287.

Jacobsen, L. K., Southwick, S. M., & Kosten, T. R. (2001). Substance use disorders in patients with posttraumatic stress disorder: A review of the literature. *American Journal of Psychiatry, 158,* 1184–1190.

Johnson, K. L., & Rn, C. R. (2006). The hypothalamic–pituitary–adrenal axis in critical illness. *AACN Clinical Issues, 17,* 39–49.

Justice, A. J., & de Wit, H. (1999). Acute effects of *d*-amphetamine during the follicular and luteal phases of the menstrual cycle in women. *Psychopharmacology, 145,* 67–75.

Kajantie, E., & Phillips, D. I. (2006). The effects of sex and hormonal status on the physiological response to acute psychosocial stress. *Psychoneuroendocrinology, 31,* 151–178.

Kearney-Cooke, A. (1999). Gender differences and self-esteem. *Journal of Gender Specific Medicine, 2,* 46–52.

Kendler, K. S., Bulik, C. M., Silberg, J., Hettema, J. M., Myers, J., & Prescott, C. A. (2000). Childhood sexual abuse and adult psychiatric and substance use disorders in women: An epidemiological and cotwin control analysis. *Archives of General Psychiatry, 57,* 953–959.

Killen, J. D., Fortmann, S. P., Newman, B., & Varady, A. (1990). Evaluation of a treatment approach combining nicotine gum with self-guided behavioral treatments for smoking relapse prevention. *Journal of Consulting and Clinical Psychology, 58,* 85–92.

Kinney, A., Kline, J., & Levin, B. (2006). Alcohol, caffeine and smoking in relation to age at menopause. *Maturitas, 54,* 27–38.

Kirby, K. N., & Marakovic, N. N. (1996). Delay-discounting probabilistic rewards: Rates decrease as amounts increase. *Psychonomic Bulletin and Review, 3,* 100–104.

Kirschbaum, C., Kudielka, B. M., Gaab, J., Schommer, N. C., & Hellhammer, D. H. (1999). Impact of gender, menstrual cycle phase, and oral contraceptives on the activity of the hypothalamus–pituitary–adrenal axis. *Psychosomatic Medicine, 61,* 154–162.

Kirschbaum, C., Pirke, M.-M., & Hellhammer, D. H. (1993). The "Trier Social Stress Test"—A tool for investigating psychobiological stress responses in a laboratory setting. *Neuropsychobiology, 28,* 76–81.

Kouri, E. M., Lundahl, L. H., Borden, K. N., McNeil, J. F., & Lukas, S. E. (2002). Effects of oral contraceptives on acute cocaine response in female volunteers. *Pharmacology, Biochemistry, and Behavior, 74,* 173–180.

Kouri, E. M., Raga, J. M., McNeil, J. F., & Lukas, S. E. (2000). Impact of family history of alcoholism on cocaine-induced subjective effects and pharmacokinetic profile. *Psychopharmacology, 152,* 268–274.

Kushner, R. F., Schoeller, D. A., Fjeld, C. R., & Danford, L. (1992). Is the impedence index (ht2/R) significant in predicting total body water? *American Journal of Clinical Nutrition, 6,* 835–839.

Landheim, A. S., Bakken, K., & Vaglum, P. (2003). Gender differences in the prevalence of symptom disorders and personality disorders among poly-substance abusers and pure alcoholics. Substance abusers treated in two counties in Norway. *European Addiction Research, 9,* 8–17.

Lejuez, C. W., Aklin, W. M., Jones, H. A., Richards, J. B., Strong, D. R., Kahler, C. W., et al. (2003). The Balloon Analogue Risk Task (BART) differentiates smokers and nonsmokers. *Experimental and Clinical Psychopharmacology, 11,* 26–33.

Lejuez, C. W., Bornovalova, M. A., Reynolds, E. K., Daughters, S. B., & Curtin, J. J. (2007). Risk factors in the relationship between gender and crack/cocaine. *Experimental and Clinical Psychopharmacology, 15,* 165–175.

Lejuez, C. W., Read, J. P., Kahler, C. W., Richards, J. B., Ramsey, S. E., Stuart, G. L., et al. (2002). Evaluation of a behavioral measure of risk taking: The Balloon Analogue Risk Task (BART). *Journal of Experimental Psychology Applied, 8,* 75–84.

Lile, J. A., Kendall, S. L., Babalonis, S., Martin, C. A., & Kelly, T. H. (2007). Evaluation of estradiol administration on the discriminative-stimulus and subject-rated effects of *d*-amphetamine in healthy pre-menopausal women. *Pharmacology, Biochemistry, and Behavior, 87,* 258–266.

MacMillan, H. L., Fleming, J. E., Streiner, D. L., Lin, E., Boyle, M. H., Jamieson, E., et al. (2001). Childhood abuse and lifetime psychopathology in a community sample. *American Journal of Psychiatry, 158,* 1878–1883.

Marks, J. L., Hair, C. S., Klock, S. C., Ginsburg, B. E., & Pomerleau, C. S. (1994). Effects of menstrual phase on intake of nicotine, caffeine, and alcohol and nonprescribed drugs in women with late luteal phase dysphoric disorder. *Journal of Substance Abuse, 6,* 235–243.

Marks, J. L., Pomerleau, C. S., & Pomerleau, O. F. (1999). Effects of menstrual phase on reactivity to nicotine. *Addictive Behaviors, 24,* 127–134.

McCaul, M. E., Turkkan, J. S., Svikis, D. S., Bigelow, G. E., & Cromwell, C. C. (1990). Alcohol and drug use by college males as a function of family alcoholism history. *Alcoholism, Clinical and Experimental Research, 14,* 467–471.

McKee, S. A., Maciejewski, P. K., Falba, T., & Mazure, C. M. (2003). Sex differences in the effects of stressful life vents on changes in smoking status. *Addiction*, *98*, 847–855.

Mello, N. K., Mendelson, J. H., & Lex, B. W. (1990). Alcohol use and premenstrual symptoms in social drinkers. *Psychopharmacology*, *101*, 448–455.

Mendelson, J. H., Mello, N. K., Sholar, M. B., Siegel, A. J., Kaufman, M. J., Levin, J. M., et al. (1999). Cocaine pharmacokinetics in men and in women during the follicular and luteal phases of the menstrual cycle. *Neuropsychopharmacology*, *21*, 294–303.

Mendelson, J. H., Sholar, M. B., Siegel, A. J., & Mello N. K. (2001). Effects of cocaine on luteinizing hormone in women during the follicular and luteal phases of the menstrual cycle and in men. *Journal of Pharmacology and Experimental Therapeutics*, *296*, 972–979.

Merikangas, K. R. (1990). The genetic epidemiology of alcoholism. *Psychological Medicine*, *20*, 11–22.

Nyberg, S., Wahlström, G., Bäckström, T., & Poromaa, I. S. (2004a). Altered sensitivity to alcohol in the late luteal phase among patients with premenstrual dysphoric disorder. *Psychoneuroendocrinology*, *29*, 767–777.

Nyberg, S., Wahlström, G., Bäckström, T., & Sundström Poromaa, I. (2004b). No difference in responsiveness to a low dose of alcohol between healthy women and men. *Pharmacology, Biochemistry, and Behavior*, *78*, 603–610.

Pastor, A. D., & Evans, S. M. (2003). Alcohol outcome expectancies and risk for alcohol use problems in women with and without a family history of alcoholism. *Drug and Alcohol Dependence*, *70*, 201–214.

Patton, J. H., Stanford, M. S., & Barratt, E. S. (1995). Factor structure of the Barratt Impulsiveness Scale. *Journal of Clinical Psychology*, *51*, 768–774.

Penetar, D. M., Kouri, E. M., Gross, M. M., McCarthy, E. M., Rhee, C. K., Peters, E. N., et al. (2005). Transdermal nicotine alters some of marihuana's effects in male and female volunteers. *Drug and Alcohol Dependence*, *79*, 211–223.

Perkins, K. A. (1999). Nicotine discrimination in men and women. *Pharmacology, Biochemistry, and Behavior*, *64*, 295–299.

Perkins, K. A. (2001). Smoking cessation in women. Special considerations. *CNS Drugs*, *15*(5), 391–411.

Perkins, K. A., Grobe, J. E., D'Amico, D., Fonte, C., Wilson, A. S., & Stiller, R. L. (1996). Low-dose nicotine nasal spray use and effects during initial smoking cessation. *Experimental and Clinical Psychopharmacology*, *4*, 157–165.

Perkins, K. A., Sexton, J., Reynolds, W. A., Grobe, J. E., Fonte, C., & Stiller, R. L. (1994). Comparison of acute subjective and heart rate effects of nicotine intake via tobacco smoking versus nasal spray. *Pharmacology, Biochemistry, and Behavior*, *47*, 295–299.

Petry, N. M. (2001). Delay discounting of money and alcohol in actively using alcoholics, currently abstinent alcoholics, and controls. *Psychopharmocology*, *154*, 243–250.

Petry, N. M., Kirby, K. N., & Kranzler, H. R. (2002). Effects of gender and family history of alcohol dependence on a behavioral task of impulsivity in healthy subjects. *Journal of Studies on Alcohol*, *63*, 83–91.

Pickens, R. W., Svikis, D. S., McGue, M., Lykken, D. T., Heston, L. L., & Clayton, P. J. (1991). Heterogeneity in the inheritance of alcoholism. A study of male and female twins. *Archives of General Psychiatry*, *48*, 19–28.

Poling, J., Kosten, T. R., & Sofuoglu, M. (2007). Treatment outcome predictors for cocaine dependence. *American Journal of Drug and Alcohol Abuse*, *33*, 191–206.

Pomerleau, C. S., Cole, P. A., Lumley, M. A., Marks, J. L., & Pomerleau, O. F. (1994). Effects of menstrual phase on nicotine, alcohol, and caffeine intake in smokers. *Journal of Substance Abuse*, *6*, 227–234.

Pud, D., Yarnitsky, D., Sprecher, E., Rogowski, Z., Adler, R., & Eisenberg, E. (2006). Can personality traits and gender predict the response to morphine? An experimental cold pain study. *European Journal of Pain*, *10*, 103–112.

Regehr, C., Goldberg, G., Glancy, G. D., & Knott, T. (2002). Posttraumatic symptoms and disability in paramedics. *Canadian Journal of Psychiatry*, *47*, 953–958.

Rice, J. P., Reich, T., Bucholz, A. K., Neuman, R. J., Fishman, R., Rochberg, N., et al. (1995). Comparison of direct interview and family history diagnoses of alcohol dependence. *Alcoholism, Clinical
and Experimental Research*, 19, 1018–1023.

Schuckit, M. A., Smith, T. L., Kalmijn, J., Tsuang, J., Hesselbrock, V., & Bucholz, K. (2000). Response
to alcohol in daughters of alcoholics: A pilot study and a comparison with sons of alcoholics.
Alcohol and Alcoholism, 35, 242–248.

Sener, E. B., Kocamanoglu, S., Cetinkaya, M. B., Ustun, E., Bildik, E., & Tur, A. (2005). Effects of menstrual cycle on postoperative analgesic requirements, agitation, incidence of nausea and vomiting
after gynecological laparoscopy. *Gynecological and Obstetric Investigation*, 59, 49–53.

Simpson, T. L., & Miller, W. R. (2002). Concomitance between childhood sexual and physical abuse
and substance use problems: A review. *Clinical Psychology Review*, 22, 27–77.

Sinha, R. (2001). How does stress increase risk of drug abuse and relapse? *Psychopharmacology*, 158,
343–359. (*)

Sinha, R., Catapano, D., & O'Malley, S. (1999). Stress-induced craving and stress response in cocaine
dependent individuals. *Psychopharmacology*, 142, 343–351.

Sinha, R., Robinson, J., & O'Malley, S. (1998). Stress response dampening: Effects of gender and family history of alcoholism and anxiety disorders. *Psychopharmacology*, 137, 311–320.

Sinha, R., & Rounsaville, B. J. (2002). Sex differences in depressed substance abusers. *Journal of Clinical Psychiatry*, 63, 616–627.

Snively, T. A., Ahijevych, K. L., Bernhard, L. A., & Wewers, M. E. (2000). Smoking behavior, dysphoric
states and the menstrual cycle: Results from single smoking sessions and the natural environment.
Psychoneuroendocrinology, 25, 677–691.

Sofuoglu, M., Dudish-Poulsen, S., Nelson, D., Pentel, P. R., & Hatsukami, D. K. (1999). Sex and menstrual cycle differences in the subjective effects from smoked cocaine in humans. *Experimental and
Clinical Psychopharmacology*, 7, 274–283.

Specker, S., Westermeyer, J., & Thuras, P. (2000). Course and severity of substance abuse in women
with comorbid eating disorder. *Substance Abuse*, 21, 137–147.

Spielberger, C. D., Gorsuch, R. L., & Lushene, R. E. (1970). *STAI Manual for the State–Trait Anxiety
Inventory ("Self-Evaluation Questionnaire")*. Palo Alto, CA: Consulting Psychologists Press.

Spring, B., Cook, J. W., Appelhans, B., Maloney, A., Richmond, M., Vaughn, J., et al. (2007) Nicotine
effects on affective response in depression-prone smokers. *Psychopharmacology*, 196, 461–471.

Straneva, P. A., Maixner, W., Light, K. C., Pedersen, C. A., Costello, N. L., & Girdler, S. S. (2002).
Menstrual cycle, beta-endorphins, and pain sensitivity in premenstrual dysphoric disorder. *Health
Psychology*, 21, 358–367.

Substance Abuse and Mental Health Services Administration. (2003). *Results from the 2002 National
Survey on Drug Use and Health*. Rockville, MD: Substance Abuse and Mental Health Services
Administration, Office of Applied Studies.

Substance Abuse and Mental Health Services Administration. (2006). *Results from the 2005 National
Survey on Drug Use and Health*. Rockville, MD: Substance Abuse and Mental Health Services
Administration, Office of Applied Studies.

Substance Abuse and Mental Health Services Administration. (2007). *Results from the 2006 National
Survey on Drug Use and Health*. Rockville, MD: Substance Abuse and Mental Health Services
Administration, Office of Applied Studies.

Sutker, P. B., Allain, A. N., Brantley, P. J., & Randall, C. L. (1982). Acute alcohol intoxication, negative
affect, and autonomic arousal in women and men. *Addictive Behaviors*, 7, 17–25.

Terner, J. M., & de Wit, H. (2006). Menstrual cycle phase and responses to drugs of abuse in humans.
Drug and Alcohol Dependence, 84, 1–13. (*)

Walker, J. L., Carey, P. D., Mohr, N., Stein, D. J., & Seedat, S. (2004). Gender differences in the prevalence of childhood sexual abuse and in the development of pediatric PTSD. *Archives of Womens
Mental Health*, 7, 111–121.

Wetherington, C. L. (2007). Sex-gender differences in drug abuse: A shift in the burden of proof?
Experimental and Clinical Psychopharmacology, 15, 411–417.

White, T. L., Justice, A. J., & de Wit, H. (2002). Differential subjective effects of D-amphetamine by gender, hormone levels and menstrual cycle phase. *Pharmacology, Biochemistry, and Behavior*, 73, 729–741.

Widom, C. S., Marmorstein, N. R., & White, H. R. (2006). Childhood victimization and illicit drug use in middle adulthood. *Psychology of Addictive Behavior*, 20, 394–403.

Wiederman, M. W., & Pryor, T. (1996). Substance use among women with eating disorders. *International Journal of Eating Disorders*, 20, 163–168.

Zacny, J. P., Coalson, D. W., Young, C. J., Klafta, J. M., Lichtor, J. L., Rupani, G., et al. (1996). Propofol at conscious sedation doses produces mild analgesia to cold pressor-induced pain in healthy volunteers. *Journal of Clinical Anesthesia*, 8, 469–474.

Zuckerman, M. (1996). The psychobiological model for impulsive unsocialized sensation seeking: A comparative approach. *Neuropsychobiology*, 34, 125–129.

Zuckerman, M., Eysenck, S., & Eysenck, H. J. (1978). Sensation seeking in England and America: Cross-cultural, age and sex comparisons. *Journal of Consulting and Clinical Psychology*, 46, 139–149.

Zuckerman, M., & Kuhlman, D. M. (2000). Personality and risk-taking: Common biosocial factors. *Journal of Personality*, 68, 999–1029.

PART II

BIOLOGICAL ISSUES

CHAPTER 3

Neuroactive Gonadal Steroid Hormones and Drug Addiction in Women

Jennifer L. Newman, PhD
Nancy K. Mello, PhD

There is accumulating evidence that the hormonal milieu may influence alcohol and drug addiction in women. The changing levels of anterior pituitary and gonadal hormones that define the menstrual cycle appear to influence mood as well as responsivity to drugs of abuse. Preclinical studies in female rodents and in nonhuman primates also suggest that the neuroactive gonadal steroid hormones affect the reinforcing and discriminative stimulus properties of drugs under many conditions. The gonadal steroid hormones may also contribute to sex/gender differences in drug addiction. The scientific importance of studying sex/gender differences in susceptibility to the addictive disorders, and to disease states generally, is increasingly appreciated (Becker et al., 2008; Institute of Medicine [IOM], 2001; Wetherington, 2007). Although a number of brain regions are sexually dimorphic (Becker et al., 2008; Cahill, 2006), the extent to which this may translate into sex differences in susceptibility to drug addiction remains to be determined.

Research on the interactions between the neuroactive gonadal steroid hormones, sex and drug abuse provides an exciting new perspective on the neurobiology of drug addiction. The gonadal steroid hormones (estradiol, testosterone, and progesterone) are classified as "neuroactive" because each may have excitatory and inhibitory effects on the brain (Rupprecht, 2003; Rupprecht & Holsboer, 1999a, 1999b). Moreover, the neuroactive steroid hormones can directly alter dopamine release under many conditions (Becker, 1999; Becker, Molenda, & Hummer, 2001; Becker et al., 2008; Cabrera, Bregonzia, Laconi, & Mampel, 2002; Castner, Xia, & Becker, 1993; Pasqualini, Olivier, Guibert, Frain, & Leviel, 1995, 1996; Thilbin, Finn, Ross, & Stenfors, 1999) and dopamine appears to mediate the abuse-related effects of many drugs (Koob, 1992; Kuhar, Ritz, & Boja, 1991; Ritz, Lamb, Goldberg, & Kuhar, 1987; Woolverton & Johnson, 1992).

An emerging literature suggests that the neuroactive steroid hormones may influence the saliency of drug effects, as well as alterations in mood. These findings in turn suggest that the neuroactive gonadal steroid hormones may come to play an important role in the treatment of some psychiatric disorders such as depression and anxiety (Rupprecht, 2003; Rupprecht & Holsboer, 1999a, 1999b) as well as drug abuse (Gasior, Carter, & Witkin, 1999; Zinder & Dar, 1999). It is increasingly recognized that the neuroactive steroid hormones have a broad range of neurobehavioral effects in addition to their role in reproductive function. Exploration of this new dimension in the interactions between the hormonal milieu and the abuse-related effects of drugs has been possible, in part, because of a series of changes in federal regulations developed in recognition of the importance of studying disease processes in women. A brief history of these regulatory changes and their effect on clinical research is described below.

FEDERAL MANDATES FOR STUDIES OF DRUG ABUSE PROBLEMS IN WOMEN AND SEX/GENDER COMPARISONS

Until the early 1990s, women's health problems received relatively little research attention, and it was generally assumed that data obtained in men were generalizable to women. A gradual increased awareness of the need for more balanced attention to women's health issues led to explicit policy statements from the Public Health Service (PHS, 1985), the National Institutes of Health (NIH) (Healy, 1991; NIH, 1990), the Food and Drug Administration (FDA) (Centers for Disease Control [CDC], 1993; Merkatz, Temple, Soble, Feiden, & Kessler, 1993) and from congressional leaders (Schroeder, 1990). In 1990, NIH and the Alcohol, Drug Abuse and Mental Health Administration (ADAMHA) announced a revised policy, designed to increase health-related research on women, by requiring investigators to justify the exclusion of women from research study populations. In 1990, the NIH created the Office of Research on Women's Health (ORWH) to provide a focus on women's health issues (Pinn, 2004, 2006). ORWH has increased awareness of the importance of understanding the role of sex and gender factors in health and disease (Pinn, 2003, 2005a, 2005b; Stone, Pinn, Rudick, Lawrence, & Carlyn, 2006) and has initiated new interdisciplinary training and research programs. These evolving changes in federal policy have facilitated research on the role of sex/gender factors in the addictive disorders. The National Institute on Drug Abuse (NIDA) has consistently supported research on drug abuse in women, as well as the analysis of possible sex/gender differences in the origins and consequences of drug abuse. NIDA first summarized its several program announcements in a pamphlet titled *Research Opportunities on Women's Health and Gender Differences* in 1998, and this has remained a continuing programmatic interest (Wetherington, 2007).

FDA POLICY ON MEDICATION TRIALS IN WOMEN

In 1993, FDA policy also changed to emphasize the importance of examining possible sex/ gender and hormonal influences on drug pharmacokinetics and pharmacodynamics. The FDA published *Guidelines for the Study and Evaluation of Gender Differences in the Clinical Evaluation of Drugs* (CDC, 1993; Merkatz et al., 1993). The FDA stated that studies of the safety and effectiveness of new pharmacotherapies must be conducted in women as well as in men. The *FDA Medical Bulletin* (CDC, 1993) stated:

> The hormonal environment may influence both pharmacokinetics and pharmacodynamic parameters of drugs. Four factors can be identified that might lead to hormonally mediated gender differences in drug effects: (1) variations in levels of gonadotropins and circulating steroidal hormones, notably estradiol and progesterone, during the menstrual cycle; (2) differences in the hormonal milieu between pre menopausal and post menopausal women, including the use of exogenous hormonal replacement therapy; (3) the effects of different hormonal levels during pregnancy and the metabolic consequences of pregnancy itself; and

(4) the effects of steroidal contraceptives on the metabolism of drugs taken concomitantly and, conversely, the effects of other drugs on the efficacy of contraceptives. (p. 2)

This was a landmark policy change. Before 1993, there were many concerns about including women in research on medications. Paramount among these concerns was the possibility of compromising pregnancy. The current availability of many tests to detect pregnancy makes it safe to study nonpregnant women and to exclude women who are pregnant.

SEX DIFFERENCES IN ADDICTION

The existence of sex differences in the pharmacological and mood-altering effects of abused drugs is now widely accepted, and this difference is influenced by social and biological factors. Epidemiological data indicate that more men than women abuse drugs (Substance Abuse and Mental Health Services Administration [SAMHSA], 2007), and it has been suggested that the higher rate of male drug abusers is due to the earlier age of exposure to and greater opportunity to try drugs (Van Etten, Neumark, & Anthony, 1999). There are also sex differences in drug use that differ by group and type of drug. Among adults who smoke, males tend to exceed females; however, among a younger demographic, girls ages 12–17 are more likely to have smoked cigarettes than their male counterparts (SAMHSA, 2007). Clearly, social factors are involved in the initiation of, and exposure to, drug abuse; however, biological factors also contribute (Mello & Mendelson, 2002, 2009). Although much remains to be learned about the role of the neuroactive gonadal steroid hormones in the physiological, neuropharmacological, and psychological effects of drugs, it is likely that these are an important factor in sex differences in drug abuse. The contribution of the neuroactive gonadal steroid hormones to drug abuse and addiction in women is the focus of this review.

NEUROACTIVE GONADAL STEROID HORMONES

Gonadal steroid hormones have many roles in the development and organization of the mammalian brain. In males, androgens are the primary gonadal hormones and are produced in the testes. In females, the ovaries produce estrogens (estradiol, estriol, and estrone) and progestins (progesterone), as well as testosterone, which is the precursor for estrogen. The testes also synthesize estrogen from testosterone. Although the primary role of the gonadal steroid hormones is to regulate reproduction and related behaviors, their effects extend well beyond the reproductive function. For example, estrogen appears to have neuroprotective effects, as well as effects on learning and memory. Historically, the actions of steroid hormones have been thought to be primarily genomic mechanisms involved in the regulation of gene expression and protein synthesis within the cell nucleus. More recently, attention has been focused on the nongenomic mechanisms by which neuroactive steroids function (Falkenstein, Tillmann, Christ, Feuring, & Wehling, 2000). Nongenomic effects of steroids are identified as rapidly occurring effects mediated by ligand-gated ion channels or membrane-bound receptors coupled to intracellular second messenger systems (McEwen, 1991; Rupprecht, 2003; Rupprecht & Holsboer, 1999a, 1999b).

The hypothalamic–pituitary–gonadal (HPG) axis controls gonadotropin and gonadal steroid hormone release through a complex feedback mechanism. The hypothalamus, located at the base of the thalamus, serves as an interface between the endocrine system and the nervous system. The hypothalamus secretes gonadotropin-releasing peptide hormone (GnRH) into the pituitary, by way of a closed-circuit portal system. GnRH stimulates the synthesis and release of tropic hormones from the anterior pituitary, which act on target tissues and endocrine glands, including the gonads. Throughout the menstrual cycle, luteinizing hormone (LH) and follicle stimulating hormone (FSH) stimulate the synthesis of the ovarian steroids, estrogen, and progesterone. Secretion of estrogen and progesterone leads to decreases in LH and FSH, through negative feedback regulation. Follicular, ovulatory, and luteal phases of the menstrual cycle are defined by fluctuations of the ovarian steroid hormones, as well as the cyclic changes in gonadotropins that stimulate and inhibit their release.

Gonadal steroid hormones are inextricably involved in mediating neurobehavioral processes related to the reward system, including naturally rewarding activities such as feeding and reproduction. In an evolutionary context, these behaviors ensure survival and perpetuation of a species. However, recent observations indicate that gonadal steroid hormones are involved in other reward-seeking behaviors incompatible with survival, including drug abuse and addiction. According to one theory, addictive substances disrupt the homeostasis of the natural reward system (Robinson & Berridge, 2000) leading to dysfunction of normal reward processing. The ovarian steroid hormones, estrogen and progesterone, interact with a number of neurotransmitter systems and affect various aspects of neurological function mediating the reinforcing effects of abused drugs (Frye, 2007; McEwen, 2002). For example, estradiol regulates dopamine neurotransmission (Becker, 1999, 2000; Thompson & Moss, 1994). It has been suggested that estrogen and progesterone produce opposing effects on dopamine release (Fernandez-Ruiz, de Miguel, Hernandez, & Ramos, 1990), on dopamine binding (Bazzett & Becker, 1994), and on the behavioral effects of abused drugs including the indirect dopamine agonist, cocaine (Carroll, Lynch, Roth, Morgan, & Cosgrove, 2004; Jackson, Robinson, & Becker, 2006; Larson, Anker, Gliddon, Fons, & Carroll, 2007).

Metabolites of progesterone are neuroactive and appear to influence the behavioral effects of drugs. The neuroactive metabolites of progesterone, such as pregnanolone, allopregnanolone, and allotetrahydrodeoxycorticosterone (THDOC) are modulators of the gamma-aminobutyric acid–A (GABA-A) receptor and N-methyl-D-aspartate (NMDA) subtype of the glutamate receptor. These neuroactive steroids produce many behavioral effects and have sedative–hypnotic, anxiolytic, and anticonvulsant effects similar to alcohol, benzodiazepines, and barbiturates that potently modulate GABA neurotransmission (for a detailed description of the behavioral effects of neuroactive steroids, see Reddy, 2003). Recent studies have shown that the neuroactive steroids modulate the behavioral effects of drugs related to their abuse. For example, THDOC and allopregnanolone produced discriminative stimulus effects similar to that of alcohol, diazepam, and pentobarbital in rats (Ator, Grant, Purdy, Paul, & Griffiths, 1993), and allopregnanolone produced alcohol-like discriminative stimulus effects in monkeys (Grant, Azarov, Bowen, Mirkis, & Purdy, 1996). Allopregnanolone itself may produce positive subjective effects (Finn, Phillips, Okorn, Chester, & Cunningham, 1997). The neuroactive metabolites also fluctuate as a function of the menstrual cycle and therefore are likely to contribute to the changes of neuropharmacological effects of drugs of abuse across the cycle. Potentially relevant to the neuropharmacology of addiction, neuroactive steroids appear to be involved in the modulation of stress, anxiety, and depression often associated with premenstrual dysphoric disorders (Grant et al., 1996; Hardoy et al., 2006; N-Whilback, Sundström-Poromaa, & Bäckström, 2006; Pluchino et al., 2006).

Another class of neuroactive steroids is the negative allosteric modulators of the GABA-A receptor, that includes pregnenolone sulfate and dehydroepiandrosterone (DHEA). These negative allosteric modulators exert inhibitory effects on GABA neurotransmission and enhance NMDA receptor function and thus produce excitatory, proconvulsant, and angiogenic effects. DHEA has been shown to reduce cocaine self-administration and reduce cocaine-seeking behavior in a model of relapse in rats (Doron et al., 2006; Maayan et al., 2006). Acute treatment with cocaine and nicotine increases DHEA levels in humans (Doron et al., 2006; Maayan et al., 2006; Mendelson, Goletiani, Sholar, Siegel, & Mello, 2008; Mendelson et al., 2002; Mendelson, Sholar, Goletiani, Siegel, & Mello, 2005) and in rats (Maayan et al., 2006) and it has been suggested that high endogenous levels of DHEA may facilitate abstinence in males who abuse cocaine (Wilkins et al., 2005).

PRECLINICAL RESEARCH IN EXPERIMENTAL ANIMALS

Sex dimorphisms in drug abuse and addiction are mediated by biological factors as well as social and cultural influences. Although investigation of the effects of hormones on addiction in humans is of critical importance, the use of nonhuman animal subjects allows for a more precise examination of the neuroendocrine contributions underlying these differences by circumventing the psychosocial factors to which human subjects are exposed. Additionally, many research questions cannot be addressed in humans due to ethical constraints (see Weerts, Fantegrossi, & Goodwin, 2007 for review).

The behavioral and neuropharmacological effects of drugs have been studied in preclinical animal models, primarily in rodents. The reproductive cycle of the rodent differs in several ways from the menstrual cycle in humans and nonhuman primates. The rodent estrous cycle lasts for 4 or 5 days (Freeman, 1994) whereas the menstrual cycle lasts for about 28 days (Hotchkiss & Knobil, 1994). The four phases of the rodent estrous cycle are proestrus, estrus, metestrus, and diestrus (Freeman, 1994). The proestrus phase is characterized by peak levels of estrogen and a second surge of progesterone; the estrus phase is characterized by rapidly decreasing levels of estrogen and progesterone; metestrus by low estrogen and rising progesterone levels; and diestrus characterized by increasing estrogen and decreasing progesterone levels. The endogenous fluctuation of hormones in rodents is difficult to examine because of the rapidly changing hormones and the short duration of the estrous cycle. An effective method for directly studying the role of gonadal hormones in laboratory animals is by gonadectomy and subsequent hormone replacement. Castration or ovariectomy involves surgical removal of the testes or ovaries, respectively, thus eliminating the major source of endogenous sex hormone production. Subsequently, the hormones can be replaced by injection of estradiol, progesterone, and testosterone to simulate physiologically relevant levels of these hormones in an experimentally controlled manner.

The duration of the menstrual cycle and patterns of neuroendocrine release in the nonhuman primate is similar to that of humans (Hotchkiss & Knobil, 1994; Knobil, 1980; Knobil & Hotchkiss, 1988). The primate menstrual cycle consists of four phases: menses (days 1–5), the follicular phase (days 6–11), the periovulatory phase (12–14), ovulation, and the luteal phase (days 16–28). The duration of each phase tends to vary across individuals, and the follicular phase is the most variable. The follicular phase is characterized by low levels of estrogen, progesterone, LH and FSH. In the early follicular phase, a follicle is selected and achieves dominance in the late follicular phase. Estrogen levels increase at the end of the follicular phase and stimulate a surge in LH and FSH that culminates in ovulation, and a rapid decrease in LH and FSH. After ovulation, the site of the dominant follicle becomes densely vascularized and forms the corpus luteum, the source of progesterone. Progesterone increases to high levels for 5 to 7 days, then decreases over several days before menses. Estrogen levels also increase and decrease in parallel with progesterone. If pregnancy does not occur, the corpus luteum regresses during the luteal phase. If ovulation does not occur, hormones remain at a low level until the next menses. In anovulatory menstrual cycle, once regression of the corpus luteum is complete, FSH levels rise and the process of selecting a new follicle begins. Accurate verification of menstrual cycle phase requires hormone measures or vaginal cytology in rats. Hormone replacement in gonadectomized subjects, and hormone treatment in intact subjects are two approaches often used to characterize the effects of hormones on behavior.

The relationship between hormones and behavior, including hormone-mediated changes in mood and the effects of abused substances, are complex. Estrogen and progesterone receptors are found widely throughout the central nervous system (CNS). Estrogen has been shown to have a neuroprotective role as it reduces cocaine-induced toxicity in rats (Rapp, Kourounakis, & Selye, 1979). Importantly, estradiol and progesterone affect dopamine, GABA, and glutamate neurotransmission, which are intimately involved in mediating the effects of many abused drugs (Becker, 2000; Cyr, Ghribi, & Di Paolo, 2000; DeMaria, Livingstone, & Freeman, 2000; Luine, Grattan, & Selmanoff, 1997).

THE INFLUENCE OF NEUROACTIVE GONADAL STEROID HORMONES ON THE EFFECTS OF DRUGS OF ABUSE

Recent advancements in brain imaging techniques permit observation of sex differences in reward-related brain activity. Positron emission tomography (PET) has revealed that striatal presynaptic dopamine synthesis is greater in postmenopausal women than in men of similar age (Laakso et al., 2002). Brain regions activated by the reinforcing effects of drugs also differ between men and women. For example, a PET study that examined amphetamine-stimulated dopamine release found that striatal dopamine release and positive subjective effects in response to d-amphetamine were greater in men than in women (Munro et al., 2006). Additionally, no differences in dopamine release or subjective effects between the follicular and luteal phases were found; however only one day of one cycle was examined in each of the women (Munro et al., 2006). Others have reported changes in brain function and neurochemistry that are altered across phases of the menstrual cycle, probably reflecting fluctuations in ovarian hormones, estrogen and progesterone. Functional magnetic resonance imaging (fMRI) showed that women during their midfollicular phase (days 4–8 following menses onset) showed greater activation of the orbitofrontal cortex and amygdala in response to anticipated monetary reward than during the luteal phase (6–10 days following LH surge) (Dreher et al., 2007). A correlation analysis between gonadal steroid hormone levels (measured to verify menstrual cycle phase) found that dorsolateral prefrontal cortical activity was positively correlated with estrogen levels (Dreher et al., 2007). These findings suggest a role for gonadal steroid hormones in activating reward-related brain activity. Similarly, in nonhuman primates, dopamine D_2 receptor availability, a substrate known to mediate the reinforcing effects of drugs, is greater in the luteal phase than the follicular phase of the menstrual cycle (Czoty et al., 2008). In rats, dopamine activity also fluctuates according to the phase of estrous cycle (Thompson & Moss, 1997).

SEX AND HORMONAL INFLUENCES ON DRUG AND ALCOHOL ABUSE AND DEPENDENCE

Alcohol

Alcohol abuse and alcoholism is often associated with heavy cigarette smoking as well as use of illicit substances. During 2006, an estimated 17 million people reported heavy drinking, defined as five or more drinks per occasion on 5 or more days during the past month (SAMHSA, 2007). An estimated 2.5 million persons were treated for alcohol abuse and dependence during 2006 (SAMHSA, 2007). Alcohol dependence generally affects more men than women, but the rate at which alcohol abuse escalates to alcohol dependence may be greater in women than men in adulthood (Brady & Randall, 1999). Age also influences apparent sex differences. Among young adults (ages 18–25), men tend to consume more alcohol than women; however, among adolescents (ages 12–17), an equivalent number of males (16.3%) and females (17.0%) regularly consumed alcohol (SAMHSA, 2007). Importantly, adolescence represents a transitional phase as gonadal steroid hormone levels rapidly increase and the greatest physiological differentiation between males and females (outside of prenatal development) is observed. Early onset of puberty in girls has been associated with earlier smoking and alcohol drinking (Wilson et al., 1994).

A number of biological factors may influence sex differences in the effects of alcohol. Women may have higher blood alcohol levels than men after equivalent amounts of alcohol due to lower body weight and lower levels of alcohol dehydrogenase and aldehyde dehydrogenase, enzymes necessary for the breakdown of alcohol (Chrostek, Jelski, Szmitkowski, & Puchalski, 2003; Frezza et al., 1990). Some pharmacological effects of alcohol have been shown to vary as a function of the menstrual cycle in females. For example, there was a significant correlation between anxiety and blood alcohol levels during the luteal phase of the menstrual cycle (Logue, Linnoila, Wallman, & Erwin, 1981). Retrospective reports also suggest that alcohol consumption is greater during the luteal phase, and this increase may be associated with premenstrual dysphoria (Harvey & Beckman, 1985; Mello, Mendelson, & Lex, 1990). However in controlled clinical laboratory studies, the effects of menstrual cycle phase and alcohol's subjective and pharmacokinetic effects have been inconsistent. Several studies reported that the positive subjective effects (Brick, Nathan, Westrick, Frankenstein, & Shapiro, 1986; Freitag & Adesso, 1993; Holdstock & de Wit, 2000) and the pharmacokinetic effects of alcohol do not vary as a function of phase of the menstrual cycle (Brick et al., 1986; Freitag & Adesso, 1993; Holdstock & de Wit, 2000; Mumenthaler, Taylor, O'Hara, Fisch, & Yesavage, 1999). However, there are also reports of higher blood alcohol levels (B. M. Jones & Jones, 1976) and more rapid elimination rates in women during the midluteal phase compared to early follicular phases (Sutker, Goist, Allain, & Bugg, 1987; Sutker, Goist, & King, 1987). In one study, alcohol elimination and disappearance rates were significantly lower in women taking oral contraceptives than in women not taking contraceptives (M. K. Jones & Jones, 1984); however, others did not detect significant differences in alcohol pharmacokinetics in women taking oral contraceptives (King & Hunter, 2005). Importantly, methodological differences between studies can lead to contradictory findings (Lammers, Mainzer, & Breteler, 1995). Definitions of phases are often inconsistent, and often there is no verification of menstrual cycle phase by measurement of hormonal status.

Studies using laboratory animals generally correspond to the findings in human participants. For example, studies in rhesus monkeys have found that intravenous alcohol self-administration was not significantly altered in the follicular or luteal phases of the menstrual cycle regardless of dose, though it was significantly lower during menstruation (Mello, Bree, & Mendelson, 1986). Peak blood alcohol levels were also not affected by menstrual cycle phase in monkeys (Mello, Bree, Skupny, & Mendelson, 1984). There is considerable evidence suggesting that the neuroactive steroids modulate alcohol's behavioral effects (Purdy et al., 2005). Treatment with the neuroactive steroid and progesterone metabolite, allopregnanolone, increases alcohol self-administration in rats (Janak & Gill, 2003; Janak, Redfern, & Samson, 1998). Allopregnanolone shares discriminative stimulus effects with alcohol in rats and female monkeys (Ator et al., 1993; Grant et al., 1996), and female monkeys are more sensitive to the discriminative stimulus effects of alcohol and allopregnanolone during the luteal phase of the menstrual cycle (Grant, Azarov, Shively, & Purdy, 1997). Female rats tend to have higher rates of alcohol self-administration than male rats, and this is associated with greater increases in extracellular dopamine (Blanchard, Steindorf, Wang, & Glick, 1993).

Nicotine

Cigarette smoking is a major public health concern that is associated with significantly debilitating conditions and lethality due to cardiopulmonary diseases, stroke, and cancer. Tobacco related-diseases account for over 400,000 deaths each year (CDC, 2004) and are the major preventable causes of death and disease in the United States. Lung cancer has become the leading cause of cancer deaths in women, and cigarette smoking is the primary cause of lung cancer in women (CDC, 2001; Patel, Bach, & Kris, 2004). Some diseases, such as chronic obstructive pulmonary disease (COPD), are becoming more prevalent in women smokers than in men (Han et al., 2007). The risk of certain types of ovarian cancer is amplified in women who smoke (Jordan, Whiteman, Purdie, Green, & Webb, 2006), and the risk for myocardial infarct is greater in women who smoke and take contraceptive medications containing hormones (Burkman, 1999). Over the past 5 years, consistently more adolescent girls than boys (ages 12–17) smoked cigarettes (SAMHSA, 2007).

Nicotine is the principle dependence-producing substance in tobacco products. Nicotine is absorbed through the skin, oral and nasal mucosa, and the lungs. Smoking produces central pharmacological effects within 7 seconds of inhalation (O'Brien, 2006). Nicotine is self-administered intravenously by experimental animals (Corrigall & Coen, 1989; Donny et al., 1999; Goldberg, Spealman, & Goldberg, 1981; Henningfield & Goldberg, 1983; Le Foll, Wertheim, & Goldberg, 2007; Spealman & Goldberg, 1982), and by humans in a clinical laboratory setting (Harvey et al., 2004; Henningfield & Goldberg, 1983; Henningfield, Miyasato, & Jasinski, 1983; Sofuoglu, Yoo, Hill, & Mooney, 2008). Nicotine is an agonist at nicotinic acetylcholine receptors, which are located in the central and peripheral nervous system. In addition to its cholinergic mechanism of action, nicotine indirectly inhibits or enhances the release of neurotransmitters (glutamate, dopamine, and norepinephrine) thought to be involved in mediating nicotine reinforcement (Di Chiara, 2000; Rauhut, Mullins, Dwoskin, & Bardo, 2002; Wang, Chen, Steketee, & Sharp, 2007; Zakharova, Danysz, & Bespalov, 2005). Nicotine acetylcholine receptors are found in brain regions involved in mediating the reinforcing effects of drugs, such as the mesolimbic circuit, and nicotine stimulates dopamine release (Di Chiara, 2000).

Sex Differences in Nicotine's Effects

Men and women appear to respond differently to the reinforcing effects of cigarette smoking (Pauly, 2008; Perkins et al., 2006; Pomerleau, Pomerleau, & Garcia, 1991). Recent brain-imaging studies have confirmed sex differences in response to nicotine. For example, women and men showed reactivity in different brain areas in response to smoking-related cues as measured by fMRI (McClernon, Kozink, & Rose, 2007). This finding is consistent with earlier reports that men and women react differently to the pharmacological and nonpharmacological effects of nicotine (Perkins et al., 2001). However, preclinical studies of sex differences in the pharmacological effects of nicotine have often been inconclusive. Female rats were more responsive than males to the antinociceptive effects of nicotine in one study (Craft & Milholland, 1998), and less sensitive to nicotine's antinociceptive effects in another study

(Damaj, 2001). Female rats show greater behavioral sensitivity to repeated administration of nicotine compared to male rats and ovariectomized rats (Booze et al., 1999).

Male and female rodents also respond differently to nicotine's reinforcing effects. Consistent sex differences in nicotine self-administration by rodents on a progressive ratio schedule of reinforcement have been reported. Under the progressive ratio schedule, the response requirement for an infusion of nicotine increased until the rats ceased responding. The ratio at which the rat stopped responding was defined as the break point. Using this approach, females reached higher break points and began nicotine self-administration more rapidly than males (Donny et al., 2000). However, female rats also showed a general increase in nonreinforced lever responding, suggesting that the differences in nicotine self-administration may have reflected an overall increase in motor behavior. Females did not have greater plasma and brain nicotine levels or more brain nicotine receptors than males (Donny et al., 2000). This finding is inconsistent with an earlier study showing female rats had higher brain levels of nicotine than male rats following administration of the same nicotine dose (Rosecrans, 1972). Evidence from human and animal studies suggest that females are more sensitive to the nonpharmacological effects of smoking-related cues, whereas men are more affected by the direct pharmacological effects (Perkins, Donny, & Caggiula, 1999; Perkins et al., 2001). For example, in female rats, pairing a visual stimulus with self-administered infusions of nicotine led to greater increases in responding for nicotine than in males (Chaudhri et al., 2005).

Role of Gonadal Hormones in Mediating Nicotine's Effects

Sex differences in nicotine self-administration are mediated, at least in part, by the differences in the hormonal milieu in males and females. The effects of endogenous ovarian hormones on smoking have been examined in women across phases of the menstrual cycle. Women smoke more during the luteal phase, when progesterone levels are elevated (Craig, Parrott, & Coomber, 1992; DeBon, Klesges, & Klesges, 1995; Marks, Hair, Klock, Ginsburg, & Pomerleau, 1994; Mello, Mendelson, & Palmieri, 1987) and during menses, when estrogen and progesterone are low, than during other phases of the menstrual cycle (DeBon et al., 1995). One study did not detect an effect of menstrual cycle phase on withdrawal symptomatology, however, women reported an increased desire to smoke to alleviate premenstrual discomfort (Allen, Hatsukami, Christianson, & Nelson, 1999). When presented with smoking-related cues, women reported less craving for cigarettes during the follicular phase than women in the luteal phase or men (Franklin et al., 2004). Less preclinical research on endogenous hormonal fluctuations and nicotine's effects has been conducted. No effect of estrous cycle on nicotine self-administration in rats (Donny et al., 2000) or on nicotine's locomotor stimulatory effects have been reported (Kuo et al., 1999). Exogenously administered estrogen has been shown to increase nicotine-induced dopamine release in striatal tissue of ovariectomized rats, but not in castrated males (Dluzen & Anderson, 1997). Progesterone and 17ß-estradiol each block nicotine receptors *in vitro* and *in vivo* as evidenced by attenuation of nicotine-induced analgesia in mice (Damaj, 2001).

Sex differences in nicotine's effects may also reflect pharmacokinetic factors. For example, plasma nicotine levels are significantly greater in female rats than in males, and ovariectomy reverses these effects (Harrod, Booze, & Mactutus, 2007). Similarly, the same dose of nicotine may produce higher brain levels of nicotine in female rats than in male rats (Rosecrans, 1972). Hormone contraceptives and pregnancy each appear to increase the rate of nicotine metabolism (Benowitz, Lessov-Schlaggar, Swan, & Jacob, 2006; Dempsey, Jacob, & Benowitz, 2002). These findings are consistent with evidence that circulating ovarian hormones contribute to the pharmacokinetic differences in nicotine metabolism. The liver enzyme cyto-chrome P450 2A6 is activated by endogenous estrogen and has been identified as a potential mechanism underlying the greater rate of nicotine metabolism in *in vitro* preparations (Higashi et al., 2007), however, the *in vivo* evidence in humans is contradictory (Hukkanen, Gourlay, Kenkare, & Benowitz, 2005). A recent study examining the reinforcing effects and pharmacokinetics of nicotine in pregnant rats found that nicotine self-administration was lower and elimination slower in late pregnancy, however, steroid hormones were not measured (Lesage, Keyler, Burroughs, & Pentel, 2007).

Although sex differences in the reinforcing and behavioral effects of nicotine may be influenced by sex differences in nicotine metabolism and elimination, there is evidence to suggest that pharmacodynamic differences also contribute. For example, nicotine receptor binding was significantly higher in male rats compared to female rats (Koylu, Demigoren, London, & Pogum, 1997), but the phase of estrous cycle was not reported. Other studies have shown that dopamine transporter proteins increase, and dopamine D_3 subtype of receptors decrease in the nucleus accumbens in response to experimenter-administered nicotine in female rats (Harrod et al., 2004). Further research is necessary to delineate the pharmacokinetic (processes of absorption, distribution, metabolism, and elimination) and pharmacodynamic (drug's mechanism of action) mediated sex differences in response to nicotine's effects.

Smoking Cessation and Withdrawal

Accumulating evidence suggests that withdrawal symptoms and craving for nicotine is greatest during the luteal phase of the menstrual cycle when progesterone levels are high. Studies examining the effects of menstrual cycle on cessation and abstinence have produced varying results, but these disparate findings probably reflect the measurements utilized. Nicotine withdrawal signs and symptoms have been examined across the menstrual cycle in humans. Such studies typically use physiological markers such as cortisol, blood pressure, and heart rate, as well as self-report measures. One important consideration in interpreting self-report data is that many withdrawal symptoms overlap with symptoms associated with premenstrual dysphoria, including depression, increased appetite, decreased energy, and irritability (Allen, Hatsukami, Christianson, & Nelson, 1996; Carpenter, Upadhyaya, LaRowe, Saladin, & Brady, 2006; DeBon et al., 1995). Women had more severe withdrawal symptoms after quitting in their luteal phase than the women who quit during their follicular phase; however, estradiol and progesterone levels were not measured in this study (Perkins et al., 2000). Findings from several recent studies indicate that women who attempt smoking cessation in the follicular phase tend to remain abstinent longer than women who attempt to quit smoking during the luteal phase (Carpenter, Saladin, Leinbach, Larowe, & Upadhyaya, 2008; Franklin et al., 2008).

Nonpharmacological factors also mediate nicotine's reinforcing effects and its potential for producing and maintaining dependence. Environmental cues associated with nicotine's reinforcing effects can serve as powerful determinants of self-reported craving and relapse during periods of abstinence. Exposure to smoking-related cues can potentially initiate relapse in smokers trying to abstain (Shiffman, Paty, Gnys, Kessel, & Hickcox, 1996), and the reaction to such cues is predictive of the success of the cessation attempt. The effect of smoking-related cues varies as a function of desire to smoke and current withdrawal severity (Payne, McClernon, & Dobbins, 2007). One study suggests that females report a greater level of craving when exposed to smoking-related cues than males (Field & Duka, 2004). Presentation of cues, scripted and real, evokes a significant change in confidence to abstain from smoking (Niaura et al., 1998). Studies using imaging techniques have elegantly demonstrated that specific brain areas become active when smokers are presented with smoking-related cues (Brody et al., 2002; Franklin et al., 2007).

Gonadal steroid hormones may mediate reactivity to nicotine-associated environmental cues. Women report less craving when presented with smoking-related cues in the follicular phase of their cycle than women in the luteal phase and men (Franklin et al., 2004). These studies support the involvement of environmental variables in the reinforcement of nicotine in females. However, more research is needed to determine the contribution of gonadal steroid hormones to regulation of nonpharmacological stimulus effects in nicotine-seeking behaviors. Circulating ovarian hormones can affect the pharmacological effects of nicotine in women and, importantly, may suggest improved treatments of smoking cessation in female smokers.

Stimulants: Cocaine and Amphetamine

Cocaine abuse is a major public health problem and has many deleterious effects on health (Mendelson & Mello, 2008). In 2006, an estimated 2.4 million persons ages 12 and older were current cocaine users (SAMHSA, 2007). Cocaine continues to be the most frequently cited illicit drug in emergency room visits (Drug Abuse Warning Network [DAWN], 2007). There has been considerable research on cocaine's effects on the endocrine system, and more recently, the contribution of the endocrine system to the effects of cocaine (see Carroll et al., 2004; Evans, 2007; Lynch, Roth, & Carroll, 2002; Mello & Mendelson, 2002; Mendelson et al., 2008). The remainder of this section summarizes some recent research on stimulants, sex, and menstrual cycle phase.

To date, research on stimulants has provided the most evidence for sex differences and menstrual cycle effects. Stimulant drugs such as cocaine, d-amphetamine, and methamphetamine, each increase brain dopamine levels. Cocaine binds to the dopamine, serotonin, and norepinephrine transporters and thus blocks reuptake of these monoamines into the presynaptic neurons. Although serotonin and norepinephrine are important modulators of these drugs, dopamine is the primary transmitter involved in mediating the reinforcing effects (Kuhar et al., 1991; Ritz et al., 1987).

A number of clinical studies have examined the influence of sex differences and the menstrual cycle on the physiological and subjective effects of stimulants. The positive subjective and reinforcing effects of stimulants generally appear to be greater during the follicular phase of the menstrual cycle, when levels of estrogen and progesterone are low, compared to the luteal phase when estrogen and progesterone levels are high (Evans, 2007). Men reported higher positive subjective ratings after smoking cocaine than women as a group, but women in the luteal phase reported lower ratings of "feel high" than women in the follicular phase and men (Sofuoglu, Dudish-Poulsen, Nelson, Pentel, & Hatsukami, 1999). No sex differences in plasma cocaine levels or in heart rate and blood pressure were detected among the three groups (Sofuoglu et al., 1999). In another study, smoked cocaine produced similar subjective effects across men and women, but higher peak cocaine plasma levels and a more sustained increase in heart rate among women (Evans, Haney, Fischman, & Foltin, 1999). However, the women received functionally higher doses of cocaine than the men because of differences in body weight (Evans et al., 1999). One study examined the effects of cocaine in the same women across both the follicular and midluteal phases of their menstrual cycle and found the women reported a greater increase in the positive subject-rated effects of cocaine during their follicular phase (Evans, Haney, & Foltin, 2002). A PET imaging study found that men reported greater positive subjective effects and greater striatal dopamine release in response to amphetamine than women during the follicular or the luteal phase of the menstrual cycle, but no menstrual cycle phase differences were detected in women (Munro et al., 2006).

Cocaine's pharmacokinetics appear to be the same in men and women and in male and female rodents and nonhuman primates. There were no significant differences in cocaine's peak plasma levels, elimination half-life, area under the curve, cardiovascular effects, or subjective effects between men and women when cocaine was given intravenously (Mendelson et al., 1999). When women were compared across phases of the menstrual cycle, women in the follicular phase reached peak cocaine plasma levels significantly more rapidly than men or women in the luteal phase. Although the difference of 2.7 minutes to reach peak cocaine levels was statistically significant, it was deemed to have little "biological significance" (Mendelson et al., 1999). Consistent with previously reported data (Mello, Mendelson, Kelly, & Bowen, 2000), a study of cocaine's pharmacokinetics in rhesus monkeys did not find any differences in cocaine plasma levels across four menstrual cycle phases (menses, midfollicular, periovulatory, and midluteal) (Evans & Foltin, 2006b). The lack of menstrual cycle phase effects on cocaine plasma levels were consistent with data reported previously (Mello et al., 2000). Finally, no sex differences in cocaine's pharmacokinetics were detected in rats (Bowman et al., 1999).

Like cocaine, *d*-amphetamine produces greater positive subjective effects during the follicular phase than in the luteal phase. Self-report ratings of "high," "energetic," and "euphoric" after oral *d*-amphetamine compared to placebo were higher during the follicular phase than during the luteal phase in the same women studied as their own control (Justice & de Wit, 1999). Salivary estrogen levels were positively correlated with reports of "elation," "vigor," and "positive mood" after *d*-amphetamine, whereas progesterone levels were negatively correlated with "friendliness" (White, Justice, & de Wit, 2002). However, subjective effects of *d*-amphetamine during the early follicular phase, when estradiol was low, were not appreciably different than during the late stages of the follicular phase when estradiol levels were higher (Justice & de Wit, 2000a). Exogenous estradiol administered in the early follicular phase produced estradiol levels 10 times that observed in the early follicular phase, but did not alter *d*-amphetamine's subjective effects relative to estrogen placebo (Justice & de Wit, 2000b). In contrast, estradiol has also been shown to enhance the discriminative stimulus effects and some positive subjective effects of *d*-amphetamine (Lile, Kendall, Babalonis, Martin, & Kelly, 2007).

Sex differences in the behavioral effects of stimulants are consistently supported by research in laboratory animals. In nonhuman primates, female cynomolgus monkeys reached significantly greater break points for intravenous infusion of cocaine than males on a progressive ratio schedule of reinforcement (Mello, Knudson, & Mendelson, 2007). This finding was consistent with previous reports using a similar procedure in rats (Roberts, Bennett, & Vickers, 1989). Adult female rats acquired self-administration of low cocaine doses (0.2 mg/kg) more rapidly than males (Lynch & Carroll, 1999), and adolescent female rats acquired self-administration at high cocaine doses (0.75 mg/kg) more readily than adolescent males. Female rats also acquired methamphetamine self-administration more rapidly (Roth & Carroll, 2004) and were more sensitive to the locomotor activating effects of methamphetamine than male rats (Schindler, Bross, & Thorndike, 2002). In a laboratory model of relapse using cocaine-priming injections, females showed a greater degree of reinstatement (i.e., pressed more on the lever previously associated with cocaine) than males, despite similar levels of prior cocaine self-administration and extinction (Lynch & Carroll, 2000). In other behavioral procedures, cocaine consistently produced greater effects in females than males. For example, cocaine produced greater stimulation of locomotor activity in female rats than in males (Craft & Stratmann, 1996; Sell, Scalzitti, Thomas, & Cunningham, 2000; van Haaren

& Meyer, 1991). Female rats also showed greater behavioral sensitization to repeated cocaine injections, and this effect was attenuated by ovariectomy (Sircar & Kim, 1999). Treating the ovariectomized rats with estradiol restored the ability of cocaine to produce behavioral sensitization (Sircar & Kim, 1999).

The effects of the estrous cycle on cocaine self-administration in rats has been studied extensively (see Carroll et al., 2004; Lynch et al., 2002; Mello & Mendelson, 2002, 2009, for review). One of the first studies found that female rats reached higher break points for cocaine infusions during estrus when estrogen and progesterone were falling (Roberts et al., 1989). The effect of estrous cycle was only evident when response requirements were high, but not under a continuous reinforcement schedule, when each response produced an infusion. Another study demonstrated female rats in the estrus phase of the estrous cycle self-administered higher doses of cocaine than metestrus/diestrus or proestrus phases (Lynch, Arizzi, & Carroll, 2000). It has been suggested that estrogen is an important mediator of positive and reinforcing effects of the stimulants (Carroll et al., 2004). Cocaine and estradiol produce increases in extracellular dopamine in rats (Becker et al., 2001; Becker & Rudick, 1999; Hemby, Co, Koves, Smith, & Dworkin, 1997). Ovariectomized rats treated with estradiol acquired cocaine self-administration more readily than untreated ovariectomized rats (Hu, Crombag, Robinson, & Becker, 2004; Lynch, Roth, Mickelberg, & Carroll, 2001). Furthermore, treatment with the antiestrogen, tamoxifen, in gonadally intact female rats reduced acquisition of cocaine self-administration (Lynch et al., 2001). However, the effect of ovariectomy may be limited to acquisition of cocaine self-administration. Ovariectomy did not affect cocaine self-administration in rats previously trained to self-administer cocaine (Caine et al., 2004). Moreover, in rhesus monkeys, estradiol administration over a broad dose range, did not alter cocaine self-administration at reinforcing doses (Mello et al., 2007).

Estradiol appears to have a facilitatory role in the reinforcing effects of stimulants under some conditions, whereas progesterone has an inhibitory effect. Women who were cocaine dependent in their midluteal phase, when progesterone levels were highest, reported less stress and cocaine cue–induced craving than women in the late follicular phase when estrogen levels were higher than progesterone (Evans, 2007). This finding in humans is consistent with a finding in rats demonstrating that reinstatement of cocaine seeking is lowest during proestrus, when levels of progesterone are at their highest, and highest during estrus when progesterone levels were low (Feltenstein & See, 2007). The inhibitory role of progesterone is supported by findings indicating heightened positive effects of stimulants during the follicular phase relative to the luteal phase, but also from studies examining exogenous administration of progesterone. Progesterone administered to women during the follicular phase, attenuated the positive subjective effects of cocaine and cocaine-induced increases in diastolic blood pressure and heart rate (Evans & Foltin, 2006a; Sofuoglu, Mitchell, & Kosten, 2004). The findings obtained in human participants are similar to findings from studies using laboratory animals. Pretreatment with progesterone reduces acquisition of cocaine self-administration in estrogen-primed female rats (Jackson et al., 2006), cocaine-induced conditioned place preference (Russo et al., 2008), and reinstatement of cocaine-seeking behavior during of period of extinction (abstinence) (Anker, Larson, Gliddon, & Carroll, 2007). In an escalation procedure, rats were allowed extended access to cocaine, and when rats were returned to an abbreviated self-administration period, drug self-administration levels were higher than before the extended cocaine access period. When ovariectomized rats were treated with estrogen, escalation of cocaine self-administration was similar to intact rats; however, escalation was inhibited after treatment with progesterone (Larson et al., 2007). Ovariectomy reduced cocaine self-administration in female rats, and this effect was reversed when estradiol was exogenously administered (Lynch et al., 2001), and reduced when progesterone was co-administered (Jackson et al., 2006). One study conducted with rhesus monkeys has shown that progesterone decreased cocaine self-administration and shifts the cocaine dose–effect curve downwards (Mello & Mendelson, 2009). Progesterone may act as a functional antagonist of estrogen's ability to enhance cocaine's effects, and progesterone is generally more effective in reducing stimulant effects in women than in men.

Progesterone and its metabolites modulate several neurotransmitter systems, and therefore may alter stimulant effects through a nonsteroid receptor mechanism. Progesterone's effects may be due in large part to the neuroactive steroid metabolites of progesterone, such as allopregnanolone and pregnanolone. Allopregnanolone is a GABA-A positive modulator (McEwen, 1991; Rupprecht & Holsboer, 1999a, 1999b), and this class of drugs suppress cocaine's effects under some but not all conditions (Barrett, Negus, Mello, & Caine, 2005; Negus, Mello, & Fivel, 2000). Pregnanolone decreases the discriminative stimulus effects of cocaine in rats (Quinton, Gerak, Moerschbaecher, & Winsauer, 2006). Sedative, anesthetic, and anxiolytic effects of progesterone and its metabolites have also been observed (Ator et al., 1993; Majewska, Harrison, Schwartz, Barker, & Paul, 1986; Rupprecht & Holsboer, 1999a; Selye, 1941). Currently there is growing interest in the role of GABA modulators for treatment of cocaine dependence (Kalivas, 2007).

Opioids

Opioid abuse involving heroin and the nonmedical use of prescription drugs continues to increase among men, but not among women (SAMHSA, 2007). An estimated 91,000 people used heroin for the first time in 2006 (SAMHSA, 2007). Treatment was provided to approximately 466,000 heroin abusers and 547,000 persons dependent on opioids. In addition, an estimated 5.2 million people engaged in the nonmedical use of pain relievers in 2006. Compared to alcohol, nicotine, cocaine, and amphetamine, there has been considerably less research on sex differences or menstrual cycle effects on the behavioral, pain-alleviating, and abuse-related effects of opioids. Opioids also differ from most abused drugs insofar as endogenous opioid peptides regulate the HPG axis and inhibit release of luteinizing-hormone-releasing-hormone (LHRH) that stimulates LH and FSH (Yen, 1999a, 1999b). An opioid antagonist, naltrexone, antagonizes endogenous opioid inhibition and stimulates LH release. This has been useful for the treatment of infertility disorders (see Mello & Mendelson, 2009, for review). In men, opioids suppress testosterone and LH (Mendelson, Mendelson, & Patch, 1975; Mendelson, Meyer, Ellingboe, Mirin, & McDougle, 1975). The opioids with the greatest abuse and dependence producing potential are those that bind with high efficacy to the mu-opioid receptor. Kappa and delta opioids do not appear to have similar abuse potential. Mu-receptor agonists include heroin and morphine, in addition to many opioid analgesic medications. Laudanum, a tincture of opium, was frequently prescribed to women for gynecological problems and neurasthenia in the late 1800s and early 1900s (Kandall, 1998).

Today, the nonmedical use of prescription drugs appears to be increasing (SAMHSA, 2007). One multivariate study examined previously collected self-report data on the use of psychoactive prescription medications, including opioid analgesics, and found that women were more likely to take medications containing opioids than men (Simoni-Wastila, 2000; Simoni-Wastila, Ritter, & Strickler, 2004). One retrospective study found the females were more sensitive than males to some subjective effects of morphine such as "dry mouth," "sluggish," and "coasting" (Zacny, 2001). Controlled laboratory studies in humans usually report that women are more sensitive to cold pressor pain than men (Zacny & Beckman, 2004), however, women may adapt to repeated painful stimuli more effective than men (Kowalczyk et al., 2006). However, no significant differences in pain threshold or tolerance for pain were detected as a function of menstrual cycle phase (Kowalczyk et al., 2006).

Sex differences in response to opioid analgesics have also been reported (Fillingim & Gear, 2004; Gear, Miaskowski, et al., 1996; Gear et al., 1999). For example, one controlled laboratory study found that women were more sensitive to the analgesic effects of morphine than men, but the onset and offset of the effects were slower in women (Sarton, Romberg, & Dahan, 2003). Kappa opioid agonists appear to be more potent as analgesics in women than in men (Gear, Gordon, et al., 1996; Gear et al., 1999). However, analgesic responsivity to the kappa opioid agonist, pentazocine, did not vary across different phases of the menstrual cycle (Gear, Gordon, et al., 1996). To date, research on analgesic responses across the menstrual cycle has provided inconsistent results. The disparate findings could be due to differences in type of pain measured (e.g., spinally vs. supraspinally mediated pain), and lack of methodological consistency in measuring pain and determining menstrual cycle phase. Menstrual cycle effects on pain perception add to the complexity of determining analgesic response to opioid medications. One meta-analysis review of 16 experiments concluded that pain perception varies with menstrual cycle phase; and, generally, pain thresholds appear to be highest during the follicular phase and lower during periovulatory, luteal, and premenstrual phases (Riley, Robinson, Wise, & Price, 1999). Consistent with the meta-analysis, a recent study found that women in the luteal phase had lower pain threshold and that this correlated with serum progesterone levels (Stening et al., 2007).

In contrast, preclinical research generally indicates that males are more sensitive than females to the analgesic effects of mu-opioid agonists. This has been demonstrated in rhesus monkeys (males compared to ovariectomized females) (Negus & Mello, 1999) and rats (Cicero, Nock, & Meyer, 1997). Furthermore, treating ovariectomized female monkeys with ovarian steroid hormones produced little effect on mu-opioid-mediated analgesia (Negus & Mello, 1999, 2002). Male rats may also be more susceptible to the physical dependence producing effects of opioids. One study showed that after 5 days of treatment with the same dose of morphine, naloxone, a mu-opioid antagonist, precipitated more severe withdrawal signs in males than females (Craft, Stratmann, Bartok, Walpole, & King, 1999). It has been suggested that sex differences in response to opioids may reflect organizational effects of gonadal steroid hormones in development, particularly that of testosterone, rather than the activational effects in adulthood (Cicero, Nock, O'Connor, & Meyer, 2002). Morphine generally produces a biphasic effect on locomotor activity in rodents, with initial suppression followed by hyperactivity, and suppression of locomotor activity was greater in males than females after a high acute dose of morphine (Craft, Clark, Hart, & Pinckney, 2006). Proestrus females were more sensitive to morphine-induced increases in locomotor activity, than at other phases of the estrous cycle. Ovariectomy enhanced morphine-induced increases in locomotor activity, and estradiol attenuated this effect (Craft et al., 2006).

In contrast to locomotor activity and withdrawal sign severity, the reinforcing saliency of opioids appear to be greater in female rodents than in males. Female rats intravenously self-administer greater amounts of heroin and morphine than male rats (Cicero, Aylward, & Meyer, 2003; Lynch & Carroll, 1999). Moreover, female rats reach significantly higher progressive ratio break points for heroin and morphine infusions than male rats (Cicero et al., 2003). Similarly, female rats also acquire heroin self-administration at a faster rate than male rats (Lynch & Carroll, 1999). However, other investigators have not detected sex differences or hormone treatment effects in rats acquiring heroin self-administration (Stewart, Woodside, & Shaham, 1996). Consistent with sex differences in the reinforcing effects of opioids, female rats are more sensitive to the discriminative stimulus effects of morphine than male rats (Craft, Kalivas, & Stratmann, 1996; but see Craft, Morgan, & Bernal, 1998). However, in gonadectomized animals, hormone replacement did not alter morphine's discriminative stimulus effects (Craft, Heideman, & Bartok, 1999). Two studies have shown that morphine plasma and brain levels do not differ between male and female rats (Cicero et al., 1997; Craft et al., 1996), suggesting that sex differences in opioid pharmacokinetics do not account for the sex differences observed in behavior.

Examinations of hormone treatment on heroin self-administration have yielded equivocal results. Ovariectomized rats treated with estradiol acquired heroin self-administration more rapidly and self-administered more heroin infusions than ovariectomized, untreated rats in one study (Roth, Casimir, & Carroll, 2002), but no significant effects of estradiol and progesterone replacement in ovariectomized rats on acquisition of heroin self-administration were detected in another study (Stewart et al., 1996). However, neither of these studies examined the plasma levels of hormones to determine whether physiologically relevant levels had been reached. Differences in heroin self-administration across the estrous cycle were not detected in female rats (Cicero et al., 2003).

Female rats have higher densities of mu-opioid receptors in some brain areas, and there is evidence to suggest that estrogen has modulatory effects on mu-opioid receptor levels (Brown, Psai, & Etgen, 1996; Hammer, Zhou, & Cheung, 1994; Quinones-Jenab, Jenab, Ogawa, Inturrisi, & Pfaff, 1997). A recent PET imaging study demonstrated that, in presence of a painful stimulus, women had higher mu-opioid binding potential than men, and that treatment with estradiol during the early follicular phase produced an increase in mu-opioid receptor binding potential (Smith et al., 2006). Although there is some evidence to suggest that females may be more sensitive than males to some effects of opioids, controlled laboratory studies in humans are needed.

Marijuana

Marijuana remains the most abused illicit substance in the United States. An estimated 4.2 million abused marijuana during 2006, and 14.8 million persons reported using marijuana during the past month. At least 3.1 million persons reported using marijuana on a daily or almost daily basis (SAMHSA, 2007). Treatment data indicate that 1.2 million persons received treatment for marijuana abuse (SAMHSA, 2007). Generally, less than one-half of marijuana users are female, although among adolescents, the numbers of male and female marijuana users were nearly equal.

Delta-9-tetrahydrocannabinol (delta9-THC) is the main psychoactive ingredient in marijuana. Currently, two cannabinoid receptors, CB-1 and CB-2, have been identified (Pertwee, 1997). One endogenous ligand, anandamide, has been characterized (Devane et al., 1992). The pharmacological effects of marijuana or its active constituent have been examined in humans, but the nature of possible sex differences is unclear. There appear to be no pharmacokinetic differences of intravenous or oral delta9-THC in men and women and no differences in subjective effects were reported (Wall, Sadler, Brine, Taylor, & Perez-Reyes, 1983). Although less tachycardia was produced by a second dose of delta9-THC in females than in males, no differences in subjective effects were detected (Cocchetto, Owens, Perez-Reyes, DiGuiseppi, & Miller, 1981). Each of these early studies had a relatively small sample size (three males, three females). Only two studies have examined the effects of menstrual cycle phase on marijuana's subjective effects. One study examined the effects of delta9-THC in 28 women during the follicular, ovulatory, and luteal phases in a placebo-controlled laboratory setting (Lex, Mendelson, Bavli, Harvey, & Mello, 1984). No significant differences in heart rate or subjective effects were observed across the cycle after smoking one cigarette containing 1.8% delta9-THC. The other study evaluated daily marijuana use for three menstrual cycles in 30 women (Griffin, Mendelson, Mello, & Lex, 1986). Self-reports of marijuana smoking also did not reveal an effect of menstrual cycle phase. When given the opportunity to earn marijuana cigarettes in a inpatient setting, women as a group did not smoke more marijuana during the premenstruum (3 days preceding menses) than at other phases of the cycle. However, those women that increased marijuana smoking also reported increased premenstrual dysphoria (i.e., depression, anxiety, irritability, mood lability, and impaired social functioning) compared to the other women who did not increase marijuana smoking (Mello & Mendelson, 1985). These data suggested that these women increased marijuana smoking to counter the adverse effects associated with premenstrual dysphoria. Marijuana smoking did not appear to disrupt the menstrual cycle in these women, however a decrease in LH was observed (Mendelson & Mello, 1999).

To date, relatively few preclinical studies have examined the potential sex differences or ovarian hormone effects on the reinforcing effects of marijuana or synthetic cannabinoids. However, gonadal steroid hormones appear to contribute to the pharmacodynamics of cannabinoids. One study reported that female rats acquired self-administration of WIN 55,212-2, a synthetic cannabinoid agonist, more rapidly than male rats (Fattore et al., 2007). Moreover, ovariectomy reduced the rate of acquisition, suggesting that the ovarian steroid hormones influenced the reinforcing effects of WIN 55,212-2. Other behavioral studies indicate that female rats are generally more sensitive to cannabinoid-induced antinociception, locomotor decreasing effects, and catalepsy (Tseng & Craft, 2001). In ovariectomized rats, estradiol augmented the antinociceptive effects of delta9-THC (Craft, Ulibarri, Leitl, & Sumner, 2008). Female rats accumulate greater concentrations of delta9-THC, and its active metabolite 11-hydroxy-delta9-THC in the brain than male rats, and this may be due to differences in pharmacokinetics (Tseng, Harding, & Craft, 2004). Moreover, CB_1 receptor density within the medial hypothalamus and binding affinity within the limbic forebrain fluctuated with the estrous cycle in females, such that CB_1 receptor density and binding affinity in these areas were highest during diestrus and low during estrus (Rodriguez de Fonseca, Cebeira, Ramos, Martin, & Fernandez-Ruiz, 1994). CB_1 receptor transcription was lower in the anterior pituitary of females than in males (Gonzalez et al., 2000). Gonadectomy reduced CB_1 transcription levels in males and increased it in females. These effects of gonadectomy were reversed by estradiol replacement in females, but dihydrotestosterone replacement in males was without effect (Gonzalez et al., 2000). Furthermore, anandamide and CB_1 receptor transcription levels within the anterior pituitary and hypothalamus varied with the estrous cycle in female rats (Gonzalez et al., 2000). Taken together, these findings suggest that the gonadal steroid hormones may have some role in regulating the endogenous cannabinoid system.

IMPLICATIONS FOR ADDICTION TREATMENT

The influence of the neuroactive steroid hormones on drug abuse varies as a function of the species, the endpoint measures, and the drug studied. There is now considerable evidence of sex differences in use patterns and reactions to abused drugs measured in clinical laboratory studies. Except for marijuana, sex differences have been observed on several endpoint measures for alcohol, nicotine, cocaine, and opioids. Women and female rodents are often more responsive to the abuse-related or analgesic effects of drugs than males. However, it has been more difficult to detect menstrual cycle phase differences in response to drugs. Although menstrual cycle phase effects have been reported, the phase of the menstrual cycle associated with the greatest drug effect has not been consistent across drugs. For example, the follicular phase is usually associated with the greatest responsivity to stimulants, such as cocaine, whereas the effects of alcohol and nicotine are often most salient during the luteal phase. Interpretation of studies in which drug use was greatest during luteal phase is often complicated by reports of concurrently premenstrual dysphoria. Unfortunately, parallel clinical studies of menstrual cycle phase effects using a similar methodology have not been conducted across drugs.

The most compelling evidence that neuroactive gonadal steroid hormones affect the abuse-related effects of drugs comes from preclinical studies in rodents. It has been shown that ovariectomy usually decreases responsivity to drugs, and replacement of estradiol restores drug-seeking behavior in several paradigms. Also female rats are often most responsive to the reinforcing effects of drugs, such as cocaine, during the estrus phase of the estrous cycle. However, the unit dose of drug available for self-administration appears to be one critical determinant of estrous-cycle phase effects. When a highly reinforcing dose of a drug is available for self-administration, the effects of estradiol and/or estrous cycle phase are less consistent than when low doses of a drug are studied.

Another approach to evaluating the role of the neuroactive steroid hormones in drug abuse is to administer a hormone, rather than attempting to correlate endogenous hormonal fluctuations with drug effects. Recent clinical and preclinical data indicate that administration of progesterone may decrease the positive subjective effects and the reinforcing effects of cocaine in women. In clinical studies, cocaine usually produces more positive subjective ratings and reinforcing effects during the follicular phase, when progesterone levels are low. Evidence from clinical, placebo-controlled studies in humans (Evans & Foltin, 2006a; Sofuoglu et al., 2004; Sofuoglu et al., 2007), and studies using laboratory animals (Anker et al., 2007; Mello & Mendelson, 2009), suggests that progesterone treatment may be a viable treatment option for female stimulant abusers. The potential use of neuroactive steroids for the treatment of the anxiety, depression, and panic disorder is an exciting new development in psychiatry (Rupprecht, 2003; Rupprecht & Holsboer, 1999a, 1999b). Moreover there is support for the concept that the neuroactive steroid hormones may be useful for the treatment of drug abuse (Gasior et al., 1999; Zinder & Dar, 1999). Further exploration of the interactions between drugs of abuse and the neuroactive gonadal steroid hormones will be important for increasing our understanding of the basic neurobiology of drug abuse.

KEY POINTS

- There is now considerable evidence of sex differences in use patterns and reactions to alcohol, nicotine, cocaine, and opioids measured in clinical laboratory studies.
- Women, female rodents, and nonhuman primates are often more responsive to the abuse-related or analgesic effects of drugs than males.
- Menstrual-cycle phase differences in response to drugs have been reported, but the phase of the menstrual cycle associated with the greatest drug effect has not been consistent across drugs.
- Recent clinical and preclinical data indicate that administration of progesterone may decrease the positive subjective effects and the reinforcing effects of cocaine in women.
- The potential use of neuroactive steroids for the treatment of anxiety, depression, panic disorder, and drug abuse is an exciting new development in psychiatry.
- Research on the interactions between the neuroactive gonadal steroid hormones, sex, and drug abuse provides an exciting new perspective on the neurobiology of drug addiction.

ACKNOWLEDGMENTS

Preparation of this review was prepared with support from Grants Nos. K05-DA00101, P01-DA14528, and R01-DA14670 from the National Institute on Drug Abuse, National Institutes of Health. We are grateful to Rita Head for preparation of the manuscript and to Inge Knudson for her many contributions to the literature reviews.

REFERENCES

Asterisks denote recommended readings.

Allen, S. S., Hatsukami, D., Christianson, D., & Nelson, D. (1996). Symptomatology and energy intake during the menstrual cycle in smoking women. *Journal of Substance Abuse*, 8, 303–319.

Allen, S. S., Hatsukami, D. K., Christianson, D., & Nelson, D. (1999). Withdrawal and premenstrual symptomatology during the menstrual cycle in short-term smoking abstinence: Effects of menstrual cycle on smoking abstinence. *Nicotine and Tobacco Research*, 1, 129–142.

Anker, J. J., Larson, E. B., Gliddon, L. A., & Carroll, M. E. (2007). Effects of progesterone on the reinstatement of cocaine-seeking behavior in female rats. *Experimental and Clinical Psychopharmacology*, 15, 472–480.

Ator, N. A., Grant, K. A., Purdy, R. H., Paul, S. M., & Griffiths, R. R. (1993). Drug discrimination analysis of endogenous neuroactive steroids in rats. *European Journal of Pharmacology*, 241, 237-243.

Barrett, A. C., Negus, S. S., Mello, N. K., & Caine, S. B. (2005). Effect of GABA agonists and GABA-A receptor modulators on cocaine- and food-maintained responding and cocaine discrimination in rats. *Journal of Pharmacology and Experimental Therapeutics*, 315, 858–871.

Bazzett, T. J., & Becker, J. B. (1994). Sex differences in the rapid and acute effects of estrogen on striatal D2 dopamine receptor binding. *Brain Research*, 637, 163–172.

Becker, J. B. (1999). Gender differences in dopaminergic function in striatum and nucleus accumbens. *Pharmacology, Biochemistry, and Behavior*, 64, 803–812.

Becker, J. B. (2000). Oestrogen effects on dopaminergic function in striatum. *Novartis Foundation Symposium*, 230, 134–145; discussion 145–154.

Becker, J. B., Berkley, K. J., Geary, N., Hampson, E., Herman, J. P., & Young, E. A. (2008). *Sex differences in the brain from genes to behavior*. New York: Oxford University Press. (*)

Becker, J. B., Molenda, H., & Hummer, D. L. (2001). Gender differences in the behavioral responses to cocaine and amphetamine. Implications for mechanisms mediating gender differences in drug abuse. *Annals of the New York Academy of Science*, 937, 172–187.

Becker, J. B., & Rudick, C. N. (1999). Rapid effects of estrogen or progesterone on the amphetamine-induced increase in striatal dopamine are enhanced by estrogen priming: A microdialysis study. *Pharmacology, Biochemistry, and Behavior*, 64, 53–57.

Benowitz, N. L., Lessov-Schlaggar, C. N., Swan, G. E., & Jacob, P., 3rd. (2006). Female sex and oral contraceptive use accelerate nicotine metabolism. *Clinical Pharmacology and Therapeutics*, 79, 480–488.

Blanchard, B. A., Steindorf, S., Wang, S., & Glick, S. D. (1993). Sex differences in ethanol-induced dopamine release in nucleus accumbens and in ethanol consumption in rats. *Alcoholism, Clinical and Experimental Research*, 17, 968–973.

Booze, R. M., Welch, M. A., Wood, M. L., Billings, K. A., Apple, S. R., & Mactutus, C. F. (1999). Behavioral sensitization following repeated intravenous nicotine administration: Gender differences and gonadal hormones. *Pharmacology, Biochemistry, and Behavior*, 64, 827–839.

Bowman, B. P., Vaughan, S. R., Walker, Q. D., Davis, S. L., Little, P. J., Scheffler, N. M., et al. (1999). Effects of sex and gonadectomy of cocaine metabolism in the rat. *Journal of Pharmacology and Experimental Therapeutics*, 290, 1316–1323.

Brady, K. T., & Randall, C. L. (1999). Gender differences in substance use disorders. *Psychiatric Clinics of North America, 22,* 241–252.

Brick, J., Nathan, P. E., Westrick, E., Frankenstein, W., & Shapiro, A. (1986). The effect of menstrual cycle on blood alcohol levels and behavior. *Journal of Studies on Alcohol, 47,* 472–477.

Brody, A. L., Mandelkern, M. A., London, E. D., Childress, A. R., Lee, G. S., Bota, R. G., et al. (2002). Brain metabolic changes during cigarette craving. *Archives of General Psychiatry, 59,* 1162–1172.

Brown, L. L., Pasi, S., & Etgen, A. M. (1996). Estrogen regulation of mu opioid receptor density in hypothalamic premammillary nuclei. *Brain Research, 742,* 347–351.

Burkman, R. T. (1999). Oral contraceptives: An update. *Drugs Today (Barcelona, Spain), 35,* 857–866.

Cabrera, R. J., Bregonzio, D., Laconi, M., & Mampel, A. (2002). Allopregnanolone increase in striatal N-methyl-D-aspartic acid evoked [3H] dopamine release is estrogen and progesterone dependent. *Cell and Molecular Neurobiology, 22,* 445–454.

Cahill, L. (2006). Why sex matters for neuroscience. *Nature Reviews Neuroscience, 7,* 477–484.

Caine, S. B., Bowen, C. A., Yu, G., Zuzga, D., Negus, S. S., & Mello, N. K. (2004). Effect of gonadectomy and gonadal hormone replacement on cocaine self-administration in female and male rats. *Neuropsychopharmacology, 29,* 929–942.

Carpenter, M. J., Saladin, M. E., Leinbach, A. S., Larowe, S. D., & Upadhyaya, H. P. (2008). Menstrual phase effects on smoking cessation: A pilot feasibility study. *Journal of Women's Health (Larchmt), 17,* 293–301.

Carpenter, M. J., Upadhyaya, H. P., LaRowe, S. D., Saladin, M. E., & Brady, K. T. (2006). Menstrual cycle phase effects on nicotine withdrawal and cigarette craving: A review. *Nicotine and Tobacco Research, 8,* 627–638.

Carroll, M. E., Lynch, W. J., Roth, M. E., Morgan, A. D., & Cosgrove, K. P. (2004). Sex and estrogen influence drug abuse. *Trends in Pharmacological Sciences, 25,* 273–279. (*)

Castner, S. A., Xiao, L., & Becker, J. B. (1993). Sex differences in striatal dopamine: In vivo microdialysis and behavioral studies. *Brain Research, 610,* 127–134.

Centers for Disease Control. (1993). Guidelines for the study and evaluation of gender differences in the clinical evaluation of drugs. *FDA Medical Bulletin, 23,* 2–4.

Centers for Disease Control. (2001). *Women and smoking. Surgeon general's report on smoking and tobacco use.* Washington, DC: Public Health Service.

Centers for Disease Control. (2004) Adult cigarette smoking in the United States: Current estimates National Center for Chronic Disease Prevention and Health Promotion. *Tobacco Information and Prevention Source (TIPS), 15,* 20–58.

Chaudhri, N., Caggiula, A. R., Donny, E. C., Booth, S., Gharib, M. A., Craven, L. A., et al. (2005). Sex differences in the contribution of nicotine and nonpharmacological stimuli to nicotine self-administration in rats. *Psychopharmacology (Berl), 180,* 258–266.

Chrostek, L., Jelski, W., Szmitkowski, M., & Puchalski, Z. (2003). Gender-related differences in hepatic activity of alcohol dehydrogenase isoenzymes and aldehyde dehydrogenase in humans. *Journal of Clinical Lab Analysis, 17,* 93–96.

Cicero, T. J., Aylward, S. C., & Meyer, E. R. (2003). Gender differences in the intravenous self-administration of mu opiate agonists. *Pharmacology, Biochemistry, and Behavior, 74,* 541–549.

Cicero, T. J., Nock, B., & Meyer, E. R. (1997). Sex-related differences in morphine's antinociceptive activity: Relationship to serum and brain morphine concentrations. *Journal of Pharmacology and Experimental Therapeutics, 282,* 939–944.

Cicero, T. J., Nock, B., O'Connor, L., & Meyer, E. R. (2002). Role of steroids in sex differences in morphine-induced analgesia: Activational and organizational effects. *Journal of Pharmacology and Experimental Therapeutics, 300,* 695–701.

Cocchetto, D. M., Owens, S. M., Perez-Reyes, M., DiGuiseppi, S., & Miller, L. L. (1981). Relationship between plasma delta-9-tetrahydrocannabinol concentration and pharmacologic effects in man. *Psychopharmacology (Berl), 75,* 158–164.

Corrigall, W. A., & Coen, K. M. (1989). Nicotine maintains robust self-administration in rats on a limited-access schedule. *Psychopharmacology (Berl), 99,* 473–478.

Craft, R. M., Clark, J. L., Hart, S. P., & Pinckney, M. K. (2006). Sex differences in locomotor effects of morphine in the rat. *Pharmacology, Biochemistry, and Behavior, 85,* 850–858.

Craft, R. M., Heideman, L. M., & Bartok, R. E. (1999). Effect of gonadectomy on discriminative stimulus effects of morphine in female versus male rats. *Drug and Alcohol Dependence, 53,* 95–109.

Craft, R. M., Kalivas, P. W., & Stratmann, J. A. (1996). Sex differences in discriminative stimulus effects of morphine in the rat. *Behavioral Pharmacology, 7,* 764–778.

Craft, R. M., & Milholland, R. B. (1998). Sex differences in cocaine- and nicotine-induced antinociception in the rat. *Brain Research, 809,* 137–140.

Craft, R. M., Morgan, C. L., & Bernal, S. A. (1998). Reinforcement frequency, but not gender, determines sensitivity to discriminative stimulus effects of morphine. *Behavioral Pharmacology, 9,* 357–362.

Craft, R. M., & Stratmann, J. A. (1996). Discriminative stimulus effects of cocaine in female versus male rats. *Drug and Alcohol Dependence, 42,* 27–37.

Craft, R. M., Stratmann, J. A., Bartok, R. E., Walpole, T. I., & King, S. J. (1999). Sex differences in development of morphine tolerance and dependence in the rat. *Psychopharmacology (Berl), 143,* 1–7.

Craft, R. M., Ulibarri, C., Leitl, M. D., & Sumner, J. E. (2008). Dose- and time-dependent estradiol modulation of morphine antinociception in adult female rats. *European Journal of Pain, 12,* 472–479.

Craig, D., Parrott, A., & Coomber, J. A. (1992). Smoking cessation in women: Effects of the menstrual cycle. *International Journal of the Addictions, 27,* 697–706.

Cyr, M., Ghribi, O., & Di Paolo, T. (2000). Regional and selective effects of oestradiol and progesterone on NMDA and AMPA receptors in the rat brain. *Journal of Neuroendocrinology, 12,* 445–452.

Czoty, P. W., Riddick, N. V., Gage, H. D., Sandridge, M., Nader, S. H., Garg, S., et al. (2008). Effect of menstrual cycle phase on dopamine d2 receptor availability in female cynomolgus monkeys. *Neuropsychopharmacology.* Available at *http://dx.doi.org/10.1038/^pp.2008.3.*

Damaj, M. I. (2001). Influence of gender and sex hormones on nicotine acute pharmacological effects in mice. *Journal of Pharmacology and Experimental Therapeutics, 296,* 132–140.

DeBon, M., Klesges, R. C., & Klesges, L. M. (1995). Symptomatology across the menstrual cycle in smoking and nonsmoking women. *Addictive Behaviors, 20,* 335–343.

DeMaria, J. E., Livingstone, J. D., & Freeman, M. E. (2000). Ovarian steroids influence the activity of neuroendocrine dopaminergic neurons. *Brain Research, 879,* 139–147.

Dempsey, D., Jacob, P., 3rd, & Benowitz, N. L. (2002). Accelerated metabolism of nicotine and cotinine in pregnant smokers. *Journal of Pharmacology and Experimental Therapeutics, 301,* 594–598.

Devane, W. A., Hanus, L., Breuer, A., Pertwee, R. G., Stevenson, L. A., Griffin, G., et al. (1992). Isolation and structure of a brain constituent that binds to the cannabinoid receptor. *Science, 258,* 1946–1949.

Di Chiara, G. (2000). Role of dopamine in the behavioural actions of nicotine related to addiction. *European Journal of Pharmacology, 393,* 295–314.

Dluzen, D. E., & Anderson, L. I. (1997). Estrogen differentially modulates nicotine-evoked dopamine release from the striatum of male and female rats. *Neuroscience Letters, 230,* 140–142.

Donny, E. C., Caggiula, A. R., Mielke, M. M., Booth, S., Gharib, M. A., Hoffman, A., et al. (1999). Nicotine self-administration in rats on a progressive ratio schedule of reinforcement. *Psychopharmacology (Berl), 147,* 135–142.

Donny, E. C., Caggiula, A. R., Rowell, P. P., Gharib, M. A., Maldovan, V., Booth, S., et al. (2000). Nicotine self-administration in rats: Estrous cycle effects, sex differences and nicotinic receptor binding. *Psychopharmacology (Berl), 151,* 392–405.

Doron, R., Fridman, L., Gispan-Herman, I., Maayan, R., Weizman, A., & Yadid, G. (2006). DHEA, a neurosteroid, decreases cocaine self-administration and reinstatement of cocaine-seeking behavior in rats. *Neuropsychopharmacology, 31,* 2231–2236.

Dreher, J. C., Schmidt, P. J., Kohn, P., Furman, D., Rubinow, D., & Berman, K. F. (2007). Menstrual cycle phase modulates reward-related neural function in women. *Proceedings of the National Academy of Sciences USA, 104,* 2465–2470.

Drug Abuse Warning Network. (2007). *Drug Abuse Warning Network, 2005: National estimates of drug-related emergency department visits.* Rockville, MD: Substance Abuse and Mental Health Services Administration, Office of Applied Studies, National Clearinghouse for Alcohol and Drug Information (NCADI).

Evans, S. M. (2007). The role of estradiol and progesterone in modulating the subjective effects of stimulants in humans. *Experimental and Clinical Psychopharmacology, 15,* 418–426.

Evans, S. M., & Foltin, R. W. (2006a). Exogenous progesterone attenuates the subjective effects of smoked cocaine in women, but not in men. *Neuropsychopharmacology, 31,* 659–674.

Evans, S. M., & Foltin, R. W. (2006b). Pharmacokinetics of repeated doses of intravenous cocaine across the menstrual cycle in rhesus monkeys. *Pharmacology, Biochemistry, and Behavior, 83,* 56–66.

Evans, S. M., Haney, M., Fischman, M. W., & Foltin, R. W. (1999). Limited sex differences in response to "binge" smoked cocaine use in humans. *Neuropsychopharmacology, 21,* 445–454.

Evans, S. M., Haney, M., & Foltin, R. W. (2002). The effects of smoked cocaine during the follicular and luteal phases of the menstrual cycle in women. *Psychopharmacology (Berl), 159,* 397–406.

Falkenstein, E., Tillmann, H. C., Christ, M., Feuring, M., & Wehling, M. (2000). Multiple actions of steroid hormones—A focus on rapid, nongenomic effects. *Pharmacological Reviews, 52,* 513–556.

Fattore, L., Spano, M. S., Altea, S., Angius, F., Fadda, P., & Fratta, W. (2007). Cannabinoid self-administration in rats: Sex differences and the influence of ovarian function. *British Journal of Pharmacology, 152,* 795–804.

Feltenstein, M. W., & See, R. E. (2007). Plasma progesterone levels and cocaine-seeking in freely cycling female rats across the estrous cycle. *Drug and Alcohol Dependence, 89,* 183–189.

Fernandez-Ruiz, J. J., de Miguel, R., Hernandez, M. L., & Ramos, J. A. (1990). Time-course of the effects of ovarian steroids on the activity of limbic and striatal dopaminergic neurons in female rat brain. *Pharmacology, Biochemistry, and Behavior, 36,* 603–606.

Field, M., & Duka, T. (2004). Cue reactivity in smokers: The effects of perceived cigarette availability and gender. *Pharmacology, Biochemistry, and Behavior, 78,* 647–652.

Fillingim, R. B., & Gear, R. W. (2004). Sex differences in opioid analgesia: Clinical and experimental findings. *European Journal of Pain, 8,* 413–425.

Finn, D. A., Phillips, T. J., Okorn, D. M., Chester, J. A., & Cunningham, C. L. (1997). Rewarding effect of the neuroactive steroid 3 alpha-hydroxy-5 alpha-pregnan-20-one in mice. *Pharmacology, Biochemistry, and Behavior, 56,* 261–264.

Franklin, T. R., Ehrman, R., Lynch, K. G., Harper, D., Sciortino, N., O'Brien, C. P., et al. (2008). Menstrual cycle phase at quit date predicts smoking status in an NRT treatment trial: A retrospective analysis. *Journal of Women's Health (Larchmt), 17,* 287–292.

Franklin, T. R., Napier, K., Ehrman, R., Gariti, P., O'Brien, C. P., & Childress, A. R. (2004). Retrospective study: Influence of menstrual cycle on cue-induced cigarette craving. *Nicotine and Tobacco Research, 6,* 171–175.

Franklin, T. R., Wang, Z., Wang, J., Sciortino, N., Harper, D., Li, Y., et al. (2007). Limbic activation to cigarette smoking cues independent of nicotine withdrawal: A perfusion fMRI study. *Neuropsychopharmacology, 32,* 2301–2309.

Freeman, M. E. (1994). The neuroendocrine control of the ovarian cycle of the rat. In E. Knobil & J. D. Neill (Eds.), *The physiology of reproduction* (2nd ed., pp. 613–658). New York: Raven Press.

Freitag, W. J., & Adesso, V. J. (1993). Mood effects of alcohol and expectancies across the menstrual cycle. *Alcohol, 10,* 291–298.

Frezza, M., di Padova, C., Pozzato, G., Terpin, M., Baraona, E., & Lieber, C. S. (1990). High blood alcohol levels in women. The role of decreased gastric alcohol dehydrogenase activity and first-pass metabolism. *New England Journal of Medicine, 322,* 95–99.

Frye, C. A. (2007). Progestins influence motivation, reward, conditioning, stress, and/or response to drugs of abuse. *Pharmacology, Biochemistry, and Behavior, 86,* 209–219.

Gasior, M., Carter, R. B., & Witkin, J. M. (1999). Neuroactive steroids: Potential therapeutic use in neurological and psychiatric disorders. *Trends in Pharmacological Science, 20,* 107–112.

Gear, R. W., Gordon, N. C., Heller, P. H., Paul, S., Miaskowski, C., & Levine, J. D. (1996). Gender difference in analgesic response to the kappa-opioid pentazocine. *Neuroscience Letters*, *205*, 207–209.

Gear, R. W., Miaskowski, C., Gordon, N. C., Paul, S. M., Heller, P. H., & Levine, J. D. (1996). Kappa-opioids produce significantly greater analgesia in women than in men. *Nature Medicine*, *2*, 1248–1250.

Gear, R. W., Miaskowski, C., Gordon, N. C., Paul, S. M., Heller, P. H., & Levine, J. D. (1999). The kappa opioid nalbuphine produces gender- and dose-dependent analgesia and antianalgesia in patients with postoperative pain. *Pain*, *83*, 339–345.

Goldberg, S. R., Spealman, R. D., & Goldberg, D. M. (1981). Persistent behavior at high rates maintained by intravenous self-administration of nicotine. *Science*, *214*, 573–575.

Gonzalez, S., Bisogno, T., Wenger, T., Manzanares, J., Milone, A., Berrendero, F., et al. (2000). Sex steroid influence on cannabinoid CB(1) receptor mRNA and endocannabinoid levels in the anterior pituitary gland. *Biochemical and Biophysical Research Communications*, *270*, 260–266.

Grant, K. A., Azarov, A., Bowen, C. A., Mirkis, S., & Purdy, R. H. (1996). Ethanol-like discriminative stimulus effects of the neurosteroid 3 alpha-hydroxy-5 alpha-pregnan-20-one in female Macaca fascicularis monkeys. *Psychopharmacology (Berl)*, *124*, 340–346.

Grant, K. A., Azarov, A., Shively, C. A., & Purdy, R. H. (1997). Discriminative stimulus effects of ethanol and 3 alpha-hydroxy-5 alpha-pregnan-20-one in relation to menstrual cycle phase in cynomolgus monkeys (Macaca fascicularis). *Psychopharmacology (Berl)*, *130*, 59–68.

Griffin, M. L., Mendelson, J. H., Mello, N. K., & Lex, B. W. (1986). Marihuana use across the menstrual cycle. *Drug and Alcohol Dependence*, *18*, 213–224.

Hammer, R. P., Jr., Zhou, L., & Cheung, S. (1994). Gonadal steroid hormones and hypothalamic opioid circuitry. *Hormones and Behavior*, *28*, 431–437.

Han, M. K., Postma, D., Mannino, D. M., Giardino, N. D., Buist, S., Curtis, J. L., et al. (2007). Gender and chronic obstructive pulmonary disease: Why it matters. *American Journal of Respiratory and Critical Care Medicine*, *176*, 1179–1184.

Hardoy, M. C., Serra, M., Carta, M. G., Contu, P., Pisu, M. G., & Biggio, G. (2006). Increased neuroactive steroid concentrations in women with bipolar disorder or major depressive disorder. *Journal of Clinical Psychopharmacology*, *26*, 379–384.

Harrod, S. B., Booze, R. M., & Mactutus, C. F. (2007). Sex differences in nicotine levels following repeated intravenous injection in rats are attenuated by gonadectomy. *Pharmacology, Biochemistry, and Behavior*, *86*, 32–36.

Harrod, S. B., Mactutus, C. F., Bennett, K., Hasselrot, U., Wu, G., Welch, M., et al. (2004). Sex differences and repeated intravenous nicotine: Behavioral sensitization and dopamine receptors. *Pharmacology, Biochemistry, and Behavior*, *78*, 581–592.

Harvey, D. M., Yasar, S., Heishman, S. J., Panlilio, L. V., Henningfield, J. E., & Goldberg, S. R. (2004). Nicotine serves as an effective reinforcer of intravenous drug-taking behavior in human cigarette smokers. *Psychopharmacology (Berl)*, *175*, 134–142.

Harvey, S. M., & Beckman, L. J. (1985). Cyclic fluctuation in alcohol consumption among female social drinkers. *Alcoholism, Clinical and Experimental Research*, *9*, 465–467.

Healy, B. (1991). The yentl syndrome. *New England Journal of Medicine*, *325*, 274–276.

Hemby, S. E., Co, C., Koves, T. R., Smith, J. E., & Dworkin, S. I. (1997). Differences in extracellular dopamine concentrations in the nucleus accumbens during response-dependent and response-independent cocaine administration in the rat. *Psychopharmacology (Berl)*, *133*, 7–16.

Henningfield, J. E., & Goldberg, S. R. (1983). Nicotine as a reinforcer in human subjects and laboratory animals. *Pharmacology, Biochemistry, and Behavior*, *19*, 989–992.

Henningfield, J. E., Miyasato, K., & Jasinski, D. R. (1983). Cigarette smokers self-administer intravenous nicotine. *Pharmacology, Biochemistry, and Behavior*, *19*, 887–890.

Higashi, E., Fukami, T., Itoh, M., Kyo, S., Inoue, M., Yokoi, T., et al. (2007). Human CYP2A6 is induced by estrogen via estrogen receptor. *Drug Metabolism and Disposition*, *35*, 1935–1941.

Holdstock, L., & de Wit, H. (2000). Effects of ethanol at four phases of the menstrual cycle. *Psychopharmacology (Berl)*, *150*, 374–382.

Hotchkiss, J., & Knobil, E. (1994). The menstrual cycle and its neuroendocrine control. In E. Knobil

& J. D. Neill (Eds.), *The physiology of reproduction* (2nd ed., pp. 711–749). New York: Raven Press.

Hu, M., Crombag, H. S., Robinson, T. E., & Becker, J. B. (2004). Biological basis of sex differences in the propensity to self-administer cocaine. *Neuropsychopharmacology, 29,* 81–85.

Hukkanen, J., Gourlay, S. G., Kenkare, S., & Benowitz, N. L. (2005). Influence of menstrual cycle on cytochrome P450 2A6 activity and cardiovascular effects of nicotine. *Clinical Pharmacology and Therapeutics, 77,* 159–169.

Institute of Medicine. (2001). *Exploring the biological contributions to human health. Does sex matter?* Washington, DC: National Academy Press.

Jackson, L. R., Robinson, T. E., & Becker, J. B. (2006). Sex differences and hormonal influences on acquisition of cocaine self-administration in rats. *Neuropsychopharmacology, 31,* 129–138.

Janak, P. H., & Gill, T. (2003). Comparison of the effects of allopregnanolone with direct GABAergic agonists on ethanol self-administration with and without concurrently available sucrose. *Alcohol, 30,* 1–7.

Janak, P. H., Redfern, J. E., & Samson, H. H. (1998). The reinforcing effects of ethanol are altered by the endogenous neurosteroid, allopregnanolone. *Alcoholism, Clinical and Experimental Research, 22,* 1106–1112.

Jones, B. M., & Jones, M. K. (1976). Alcohol effects in women during the menstrual cycle. *Annals of the New York Academy of Science, 273,* 576–587.

Jones, M. K., & Jones, B. M. (1984). Ethanol metabolism in women taking oral contraceptives. *Alcoholism, Clinical and Experimental Research, 8,* 24–28.

Jordan, S. J., Whiteman, D. C., Purdie, D. M., Green, A. C., & Webb, P. M. (2006). Does smoking increase risk of ovarian cancer? A systematic review. *Gynecologic Oncology, 103,* 1122–1129.

Justice, A. J., & de Wit, H. (1999). Acute effects of *d*-amphetamine during the follicular and luteal phases of the menstrual cycle in women. *Psychopharmacology (Berl), 145,* 67–75.

Justice, A. J., & de Wit, H. (2000a). Acute effects of *d*-amphetamine during the early and late follicular phases of the menstrual cycle in women. *Pharmacology, Biochemistry, and Behavior, 66,* 509–515.

Justice, A. J., & de Wit, H. (2000b). Acute effects of estradiol pretreatment on the response to *d*-amphetamine in women. *Neuroendocrinology, 71,* 51–59.

Kalivas, P. W. (2007). Neurobiology of cocaine addiction: Implications for new pharmacotherapy. *American Journal of Addictions, 16,* 71–78.

Kandall, S. R. (1998). The history of drug abuse and women in the United States. In C. L. Wetherington & A. B. Roman (Eds.), *Drug addiction research and the health of women* (pp. 8–16). Rockville, MD: U.S. Department of Health and Human Services.

King, A. R., & Hunter, P. J. (2005). Alcohol elimination at low blood concentrations among women taking combined oral contraceptives. *Journal of Studies on Alcohol, 66,* 738–744.

Knobil, E. (1980). The neuroendocrine control of the menstrual cycle. *Recent Progress in Hormone Research, 36,* 53–88.

Knobil, E., & Hotchkiss, J. (1988). The menstrual cycle and its neuroendocrine control. In E. Knobil, J. Neill, L. Ewing, G. Greenwald, C. Markert, & D. Pfaff (Eds.), *The physiology of reproduction* (pp. 1971–1994). New York: Raven Press.

Koob, G. F. (1992). Drugs of abuse: Anatomy, pharmacology and function of reward pathways. *Trends in Pharmacological Sciences, 13,* 177–184.

Kowalczyk, W. J., Evans, S. M., Bisaga, A. M., Sullivan, M. A., & Comer, S. D. (2006). Sex differences and hormonal influences on response to cold pressor pain in humans. *Journal of Pain, 7,* 151–160.

Koylu, E., Demirgoren, S., London, E. D., & Pogun, S. (1997). Sex difference in up-regulation of nicotinic acetylcholine receptors in rat brain. *Life Sciences, 61,* 185–190.

Kuhar, M. J., Ritz, M. C., & Boja, J. W. (1991). The dopamine hypothesis of the reinforcing properties of cocaine. *Trends in Neurosciences, 14,* 299–302.

Kuo, D. Y., Lin, T. B., Huang, C. C., Duh, S. L., Liao, J. M., & Cheng, J. T. (1999). Nicotine-induced hyperlocomotion is not modified by the estrous cycle, ovariectomy and estradiol replacement at physiological level. *Chinese Journal of Physiology, 42,* 83–88.

Laakso, A., Vilkman, H., Bergman, J., Haaparanta, M., Solin, O., Syvalahti, E., et al. (2002). Sex differences in striatal presynaptic dopamine synthesis capacity in healthy subjects. *Biological Psychiatry*, *52*, 759–763.

Lammers, S. M., Mainzer, D. E., & Breteler, M. H. (1995). Do alcohol pharmacokinetics in women vary due to the menstrual cycle? *Addiction*, *90*, 23–30.

Larson, E. B., Anker, J. J., Gliddon, L. A., Fons, K. S., & Carroll, M. E. (2007). Effects of estrogen and progesterone on the escalation of cocaine self-administration in female rats during extended access. *Experimental and Clinical Psychopharmacology*, *15*, 461–471.

Le Foll, B., Wertheim, C., & Goldberg, S. R. (2007). High reinforcing efficacy of nicotine in non-human primates. *PLoS ONE*, *2*, e230.

Lesage, M. G., Keyler, D. E., Burroughs, D., & Pentel, P. R. (2007). Effects of pregnancy on nicotine self-administration and nicotine pharmacokinetics in rats. *Psychopharmacology (Berl)*, *194*, 413–421.

Lex, B. W., Mendelson, J. H., Bavli, S., Harvey, K., & Mello, N. K. (1984). Effects of acute marijuana smoking on pulse rate and mood states in women. *Psychopharmacology (Berl)*, *84*, 178–187.

Lile, J. A., Kendall, S. L., Babalonis, S., Martin, C. A., & Kelly, T. H. (2007). Evaluation of estradiol administration on the discriminative-stimulus and subject-rated effects of *d*-amphetamine in healthy pre-menopausal women. *Pharmacology, Biochemistry, and Behavior*, *87*, 258–266.

Logue, P. E., Linnoila, M., Wallman, L., & Erwin, C. W. (1981). Effects of ethanol and psychomotor tests on state anxiety: Interaction with menstrual cycle in women. *Perceptual and Motor Skills*, *52*, 643–648.

Luine, V. N., Grattan, D. R., & Selmanoff, M. (1997). Gonadal hormones alter hypothalamic GABA and glutamate levels. *Brain Research*, *747*, 165–168.

Lynch, W. J., Arizzi, M. N., & Carroll, M. E. (2000). Effects of sex and the estrous cycle on regulation of intravenously self-administered cocaine in rats. *Psychopharmacology (Berl)*, *152*, 132–139.

Lynch, W. J., & Carroll, M. E. (1999). Sex differences in the acquisition of intravenously self-administered cocaine and heroin in rats. *Psychopharmacology (Berl)*, *144*, 77–82.

Lynch, W. J., & Carroll, M. E. (2000). Reinstatement of cocaine self-administration in rats: Sex differences. *Psychopharmacology (Berl)*, *148*, 196–200.

Lynch, W. J., Roth, M. E., & Carroll, M. E. (2002). Biological basis of sex differences in drug abuse: Preclinical and clinical studies. *Psychopharmacology*, *164*, 121–137.

Lynch, W. J., Roth, M. E., Mickelberg, J. L., & Carroll, M. E. (2001). Role of estrogen in the acquisition of intravenously self-administered cocaine in female rats. *Pharmacology, Biochemistry, and Behavior*, *68*, 641–646.

Maayan, R., Lotan, S., Doron, R., Shabat-Simon, M., Gispan-Herman, I., Weizman, A., et al. (2006). Dehydroepiandrosterone (DHEA) attenuates cocaine-seeking behavior in the self-administration model in rats. *European Neuropsychopharmacology*, *16*, 329–339.

Majewska, M. D., Harrison, N. L., Schwartz, R. D., Barker, J. L., & Paul, S. M. (1986). Steroid hormone metabolites are barbiturate-like modulators of the GABA receptor. *Science*, *232*, 1004–1007.

Marks, J. L., Hair, C. S., Klock, S. C., Ginsburg, B. E., & Pomerleau, C. S. (1994). Effects of menstrual phase on intake of nicotine, caffeine, and alcohol and nonprescribed drugs in women with late luteal phase dysphoric disorder. *Journal of Substance Abuse*, *6*, 235–243.

McClernon, F. J., Kozink, R. V., & Rose, J. E. (2007). Individual differences in nicotine dependence, withdrawal symptoms, and sex predict transient fMRI-Bold responses to smoking cues. *Neuropsychopharmacology*, *33*, 2148–2157.

McEwen, B. (2002). Estrogen actions throughout the brain. *Recent Progress in Hormone Research*, *57*, 357–384.

McEwen, B. S. (1991). Non-genomic and genomic effects of steroids on neural activity. *Trends in Pharmacological Sciences*, *12*, 141–147.

Mello, N. K., Bree, M. P., & Mendelson, J. H. (1986). Alcohol and food self-administration by female Macaque monkeys as a function of menstrual cycle phase. *Physiology & Behavior*, *36*, 959–966.

Mello, N. K., Bree, M. P., Skupny, A. S., & Mendelson, J. H. (1984). Blood alcohol levels as a function of menstrual cycle phase in female macaque monkeys. *Alcohol*, *1*, 27–31.

Mello, N. K., Knudson, I. M., Kelly, M., & Mendelson, J. H. (2001). *Effects of progesterone and tes-*

tosterone on cocaine self-administration and cocaine discrimination by female rhesus monkeys. Manuscript under review.

Mello, N. K., Knudson, I. M., & Mendelson, J. H. (2007). Sex and menstrual cycle effects on progressive ratio measures of cocaine self-administration in cynomolgus monkeys. *Neuropsychopharmacology, 32,* 1956–1966.

Mello, N. K., & Mendelson, J. H. (1985). Operant acquisition of marihuana by women. *Journal of Pharmacology and Experimental Therapeutics, 235,* 162–171.

Mello, N. K., & Mendelson, J. H. (2002). Cocaine, hormones and behavior: Clinical and preclinical studies. In D. W. Pfaff, A. P. Arnold, A. M. Etgen, S. E. Fahrbach, & R. T. Rubin (Eds.), *Hormones, brain, and behavior* (pp. 665–745). New York: Academic Press.

Mello, N. K., & Mendelson, J. H. (2009). Cocaine, hormones and behavior: Clinical and preclinical studies. In D. W. Pfaff, A. P. Arnold, A. M. Etgen, S. E. Fahrbach, & R. T. Rubin (Eds.), *Hormones, brain and behavior* (2nd ed.). San Diego: Elsevier. (*)

Mello, N. K., Mendelson, J. H., Kelly, M., & Bowen, C. A. (2000). The effects of cocaine on basal and human chorionic gonadotropin-stimulated ovarian steroid hormones in female rhesus monkeys. *Journal of Pharmacology and Experimental Therapeutics, 294,* 1137–1145.

Mello, N. K., Mendelson, J. H., & Lex, B. W. (1990). Alcohol use and premenstrual symptoms in social drinkers. *Psychopharmacology (Berl), 101,* 448–455.

Mello, N. K., Mendelson, J. H., & Palmieri, S. L. (1987). Cigarette smoking by women: interactions with alcohol use. *Psychopharmacology (Berl), 93,* 8–15.

Mendelson, J. H., Goletiani, N., Sholar, M. B., Siegel, A. J., & Mello, N. K. (2008). Effects of smoking successive low- and high-nicotine cigarettes on hypothalamic–pituitary–adrenal axis hormones and mood in men. *Neuropsychopharmacology, 33,* 749–760.

Mendelson, J. H., & Mello, N. K. (1999). Marihuana effects on pituitary and gonadal hormones in women. In G. Nahas, K. Sutin, D. Harvey, & S. Agurell (Eds.), *Marijuana and medicine* (pp. 385–392). Totowa, NJ: Humana Press.

Mendelson, J. H., & Mello, N. K. (2008). Cocaine and other commonly abused drugs. In A. S. Fauci, D. L. Kasper, E. Braunwald, S. L. Hauser, D. L. Longo, J. L. Jameson, et al. (Eds.), *Harrison's principles of internal medicine, 17th edition* (pp. 2733–2736). New York: McGraw-Hill.

Mendelson, J. H., & Mello, N. K. (in press). Endocrine effects of opioid antagonists. In R. Dean, E. Bilsky, D. Gastfriend, & S. S. Negus (Eds.), *Opiate receptors and antagonists.* Totowa, NJ: Humana Press.

Mendelson, J. H., Mello, N. K., Sholar, M. B., Siegel, A. J., Kaufman, M. J., Levin, J. M., et al. (1999). Cocaine pharmacokinetics in men and in women during the follicular and luteal phases of the menstrual cycle. *Neuropsychopharmacology, 21,* 294–303.

Mendelson, J. H., Mello, N. K., Sholar, M. B., Siegel, A. J., Mutschler, N., & Halpern, J. (2002). Temporal concordance of cocaine effects on mood states and neuroendocrine hormones. *Psychoneuroendocrinology, 27,* 71–82.

Mendelson, J. H., Mendelson, J. E., & Patch, V. D. (1975). Plasma testosterone levels in heroin addiction and during methadone maintenance. *Journal of Pharmacology and Experimental Therapeutics, 192,* 211–217.

Mendelson, J. H., Meyer, R. E., Ellingboe, J., Mirin, S. M., & McDougle, M. (1975). Effects of heroin and methadone on plasma cortisol and testosterone. *Journal of Pharmacology and Experimental Therapeutics, 195,* 296–302.

Mendelson, J. H., Sholar, M. B., Goletiani, N., Siegel, A. J., & Mello, N. K. (2005). Effects of low- and high-nicotine cigarette smoking on mood states and the HPA axis in men. *Neuropsychopharmacology, 30,* 1751–1763.

Merkatz, R. B., Temple, R., Sobel, S., Feiden, K., & Kessler, D. A. (1993). Women in clinical trials of new drugs: A change in food and drug administration policy. *New England Journal of Medicine, 329,* 292–296.

Mumenthaler, M. S., Taylor, J. L., O'Hara, R., Fisch, H. U., & Yesavage, J. A. (1999). Effects of menstrual cycle and female sex steroids on ethanol pharmacokinetics. *Alcoholism, Clinical and Experimental Research, 23,* 250–255.

Munro, C. A., McCaul, M. E., Wong, D. F., Oswald, L. M., Zhou, Y., Brasic, J., et al. (2006). Sex differences in striatal dopamine release in healthy adults. *Biological Psychiatry*, *59*, 966–974.

National Center on Addiction and Substance Abuse at Columbia University. (2006). *Women under the influence*. Baltimore: Johns Hopkins University Press. (*)

Negus, S. S., & Mello, N. K. (1999). Opioid antinociception in ovariectomized monkeys: Comparison with antinociception in males and effects of estradiol replacement. *Journal of Pharmacology and Experimental Therapeutics*, *290*, 1132–1140.

Negus, S. S., & Mello, N. K. (2002). Effects of gonadal steroid hormone treatments on opioid antinociception in ovariectomized rhesus monkeys. *Psychopharmacology (Berl)*, *159*, 275–283.

Negus, S. S., Mello, N. K., & Fivel, P. A. (2000). Effects of GABA agonists and GABA-A receptor modulators on cocaine discrimination in rhesus monkeys. *Psychopharmacology (Berl)*, *152*, 398–407.

Niaura, R., Shadel, W. G., Abrams, D. B., Monti, P. M., Rohsenow, D. J., & Sirota, A. (1998). Individual differences in cue reactivity among smokers trying to quit: Effects of gender and cue type. *Addictive Behaviors*, *23*, 209–224.

National Institutes of Health. (1990). *NIH/ADAMHA policy concerning inclusion of women in study populations* (NIH Guide Grants Contracts P.T. 34. II: K.W. 1014002. 1014006). Bethesda, MD: Department of Health and Human Services.

N-Wihlback, A. C., Sundström-Poromaa, I., & Bäckström, T. (2006). Action by and sensitivity to neuroactive steroids in menstrual cycle related CNS disorders. *Psychopharmacology (Berl)*, *186*, 388–401.

O'Brien, C. P. (2006). Drug addiction and drug abuse. In L. Brunton, J. Lazo, & K. Parker (Eds.), *Goodman and Gilman's the pharmacological basis of therapeutics* (pp. 607–627). New York: McGraw-Hill.

Pasqualini, C., Olivier, V., Guibert, B., Frain, O., & Leviel, V. (1995). Acute stimulatory effect of estradiol on striatal dopamine synthesis. *Journal of Neurochemistry*, *65*, 1651–1657.

Pasqualini, C., Olivier, V., Guibert, B., Frain, O., & Leviel, V. (1996). Rapid stimulation of striatal dopamine synthesis by estradiol. *Cell and Molecular Neurobiology*, *16*, 411–415.

Patel, J. D., Bach, P. B., & Kris, M. G. (2004). Lung cancer in US women: A contemporary epidemic. *Journal of the American Medical Association*, *291*, 1763–1768.

Pauly, J. R. (2008). Gender differences in tobacco smoking dynamics and the neuropharmacological actions of nicotine. *Frontiers in Bioscience*, *13*, 505–516.

Payne, B. K., McClernon, F. J., & Dobbins, I. G. (2007). Automatic affective responses to smoking cues. *Experimental and Clinical Psychopharmacology*, *15*, 400–409.

Perkins, K. A., Donny, E., & Caggiula, A. R. (1999). Sex differences in nicotine effects and self-administration: Review of human and animal evidence. *Nicotine and Tobacco Research*, *1*, 301–315.

Perkins, K. A., Doyle, T., Ciccocioppo, M., Conklin, C., Sayette, M., & Caggiula, A. (2006). Sex differences in the influence of nicotine dose instructions on the reinforcing and self-reported rewarding effects of smoking. *Psychopharmacology (Berl)*, *184*, 600–607.

Perkins, K. A., Gerlach, D., Vender, J., Grobe, J., Meeker, J., & Hutchison, S. (2001). Sex differences in the subjective and reinforcing effects of visual and olfactory cigarette smoke stimuli. *Nicotine and Tobacco Research*, *3*, 141–150.

Perkins, K. A., Levine, M., Marcus, M., Shiffman, S., D'Amico, D., Miller, A., et al. (2000). Tobacco withdrawal in women and menstrual cycle phase. *Journal of Consulting and Clinical Psychology*, *68*, 176–180.

Pertwee, R. G. (1997). Pharmacology of cannabinoid CB1 and CB2 receptors. *Pharmacology & Therapeutics*, *74*, 129–180.

Pinn, V. W. (2003). Sex and gender factors in medical studies. Implications for health and clinical practice. *Journal of the American Medical Association*, *289*, 397–400.

Pinn, V. W. (2004). The view from the National Institutes of Health: A decade with the Office of Research on Women's Health. *Gender Medicine*, *1*, 5–7.

Pinn, V. W. (2005a). Interdisciplinary research on women's health and sex/gender factors. *Gender Medicine*, *2*, 121–123.

Pinn, V. W. (2005b). Research on women's health. *Journal of the American Medical Association*, *294*, 1407–1410.

Pinn, V. W. (2006). Women's health research and health leadership: Benchmarks of the continuum. *Journal of Dental Education*, *70*, 27–34.

Pluchino, N., Luisi, M., Lenzi, E., Centofanti, M., Begliuomini, S., Freschi, L., et al. (2006). Progesterone and progestins: Effects on brain, allopregnanolone and beta-endorphin. *Journal of Steroid Biochemistry and Molecular Biology*, *102*, 205–213.

Pomerleau, C. S., Pomerleau, O. F., & Garcia, A. W. (1991). Biobehavioral research on nicotine use in women. *British Journal of Addictions*, *86*, 527–531.

Public Health Service. (1985). *Public Health Service Task Force on Women's Health Issues Public Health Report*, pp. 74–106.

Purdy, R. H., Valenzuela, C. F., Janak, P. H., Finn, D. A., Biggio, G., & Backstrom, T. (2005). Neuroactive steroids and ethanol. *Alcoholism, Clinical and Experimental Research*, *29*, 1292–1298.

Quinones-Jenab, V., Jenab, S., Ogawa, S., Inturrisi, C., & Pfaff, D. W. (1997). Estrogen regulation of mu-opioid receptor mRNA in the forebrain of female rats. *Brain Research Molecular Brain Research*, *47*, 134–138.

Quinton, M. S., Gerak, L. R., Moerschbaecher, J. M., & Winsauer, P. J. (2006). Effects of pregnanolone in rats discriminating cocaine. *Pharmacology, Biochemistry, and Behavior*, *85*, 385–392.

Rapp, U., Kourounakis, P., & Selye, H. (1979). Effect of steroids and diethylstilbestrol on cocaine toxicity, plasma concentrations and urinary excretion. *Arzneimittelforschung*, *29*, 48–50.

Rauhut, A. S., Mullins, S. N., Dwoskin, L. P., & Bardo, M. T. (2002). Reboxetine: Attenuation of intravenous nicotine self-administration in rats. *Journal of Pharmacology and Experimental Therapeutics*, *303*, 664–672.

Reddy, D. S. (2003). Pharmacology of endogenous neuroactive steroids. *Critical Reviews in Neurobiology*, *15*, 197–234.

Riley, J. L., 3rd, Robinson, M. E., Wise, E. A., & Price, D. D. (1999). A meta-analytic review of pain perception across the menstrual cycle. *Pain*, *81*, 225–235.

Ritz, M. C., Lamb, R. J., Goldberg, S. R., & Kuhar, M. J. (1987). Cocaine receptors on dopamine transporters are related to self-administration of cocaine. *Science*, *237*, 1219–1223.

Roberts, D. C., Bennett, S. A., & Vickers, G. J. (1989). The estrous cycle affects cocaine self-administration on a progressive ratio schedule in rats. *Psychopharmacology (Berl)*, *98*, 408–411.

Robinson, T. E., & Berridge, K. C. (2000). The psychology and neurobiology of addiction: An incentive-sensitization view. *Addiction*, *95*(Suppl. 2), S91–S117.

Rodriguez de Fonseca, F., Cebeira, M., Ramos, J. A., Martin, M., & Fernandez-Ruiz, J. J. (1994). Cannabinoid receptors in rat brain areas: Sexual differences, fluctuations during estrous cycle and changes after gonadectomy and sex steroid replacement. *Life Sciences*, *54*, 159–170.

Rosecrans, J. A. (1972). Brain area nicotine levels in male and female rats with different levels of spontaneous activity. *Neuropharmacology*, *11*, 863–870.

Roth, M. E., & Carroll, M. E. (2004). Sex differences in the acquisition of IV methamphetamine self-administration and subsequent maintenance under a progressive ratio schedule in rats. *Psychopharmacology (Berl)*, *172*, 443–449.

Roth, M. E., Casimir, A. G., & Carroll, M. E. (2002). Influence of estrogen in the acquisition of intravenously self-administered heroin in female rats. *Pharmacology, Biochemistry, and Behavior*, *72*, 313–318.

Rupprecht, R. (2003). Neuroactive steroids: Mechanisms of action and neuropsychopharmacological properties. *Psychoneuroendocrinology*, *28*, 139–168.

Rupprecht, R., & Holsboer, F. (1999a). Neuropsychopharmacological properties of neuroactive steroids. *Steroids*, *64*, 83–91.

Rupprecht, R., & Holsboer, F. (1999b). Neuroactive steroids: Mechanisms of action and neuropsychopharmacological perspectives. *Trends in Neuroscience*, *22*, 410–416.

Russo, S. J., Sun, W. L., Minerly, A. C., Weierstall, K., Nazarian, A., Festa, E. D., et al. (2008). Progesterone attenuates cocaine-induced conditioned place preference in female rats. *Brain Research*, *1189*, 229–235.

Sarton, E., Romberg, R., & Dahan, A. (2003). Gender differences in morphine pharmacokinetics and dynamics. *Advances in Experimental Medicine and Biology, 523*, 71–80.

Schindler, C. W., Bross, J. G., & Thorndike, E. B. (2002). Gender differences in the behavioral effects of methamphetamine. *European Journal of Pharmacology, 442*, 231–235.

Schroeder, P. (1990). Pay attention to women's health. *Journal of NIH Research, 2*, 38.

Sell, S. L., Scalzitti, J. M., Thomas, M. L., & Cunningham, K. A. (2000). Influence of ovarian hormones and estrous cycle on the behavioral response to cocaine in female rats. *Journal of Pharmacology and Experimental Therapeutics, 293*, 879–886.

Selye, H. (1941). Anesthetic effects of steroid hormones. *Proceedings of the Society for Experimental Biology and Medicine, 46*, 116–121.

Shiffman, S., Paty, J. A., Gnys, M., Kassel, J. A., & Hickcox, M. (1996). First lapses to smoking: Within-subjects analysis of real-time reports. *Journal of Consulting and Clinical Psychology, 64*, 366–379.

Simoni-Wastila, L. (2000). The use of abusable prescription drugs: The role of gender. *Journal of Women's Health and Gender-Based Medicine, 9*, 289–297.

Simoni-Wastila, L., Ritter, G., & Strickler, G. (2004). Gender and other factors associated with the nonmedical use of abusable prescription drugs. *Substance Use & Misuse, 39*, 1–23.

Sircar, R., & Kim, D. (1999). Female gonadal hormones differentially modulate cocaine-induced behavioral sensitization in Fischer, Lewis, and Sprague-Dawley rats. *Journal of Pharmacology and Experimental Therapeutics, 289*, 54–65.

Smith, Y. R., Stohler, C. S., Nichols, T. E., Bueller, J. A., Koeppe, R. A., & Zubieta, J. K. (2006). Pronociceptive and antinociceptive effects of estradiol through endogenous opioid neurotransmission in women. *Journal of Neuroscience, 26*, 5777–5785.

Sofuoglu, M., Dudish-Poulsen, S., Nelson, D., Pentel, P. R., & Hatsukami, D. K. (1999). Sex and menstrual cycle differences in the subjective effects from smoked cocaine in humans. *Experimental and Clinical Psychopharmacology, 7*, 274–283.

Sofuoglu, M., Mitchell, E., & Kosten, T. R. (2004). Effects of progesterone treatment on cocaine responses in male and female cocaine users. *Pharmacology, Biochemistry, and Behavior, 78*, 699–705.

Sofuoglu, M., Poling, J., Gonzalez, G., Gonsai, K., Oliveto, A., & Kosten, T. R. (2007). Progesterone effects on cocaine use in male cocaine users maintained on methadone: A randomized, double-blind, pilot study. *Experimental and Clinical Psychopharmacology, 15*, 453–460.

Sofuoglu, M., Yoo, S., Hill, K. P., & Mooney, M. (2008). Self-administration of intravenous nicotine in male and female cigarette smokers. *Neuropsychopharmacology, 33*, 715–720.

Spealman, R. D., & Goldberg, S. R. (1982). Maintenance of schedule-controlled behavior by intravenous injections of nicotine in squirrel monkeys. *Journal of Pharmacology and Experimental Therapeutics, 223*, 402–408.

Stening, K., Eriksson, O., Wahren, L., Berg, G., Hammar, M., & Blomqvist, A. (2007). Pain sensations to the cold pressor test in normally menstruating women: Comparison with men and relation to menstrual phase and serum sex steroid levels. *American Journal of Physiology. Regulatory, Integrative and Comparative Physiology, 293*, R1711–R1716.

Stewart, J., Woodside, B., & Shaham, Y. (1996). Ovarian hormones do not affect the initiation and maintenance of intravenous self-administration of heroin in the female rat. *Psychobiology, 24*, 154–159.

Stone, J., Pinn, V. W., Rudick, J., Lawrence, M., & Carlyn, M. (2006). Evaluation of the first 10 years of the Office of Research on Women's Health at the National Institutes of Health: Selected findings. *Journal of Women's Health (Larchmt), 15*, 234–247.

Substance Abuse and Mental Health Services Administration. (2007). Overview of findings from the 2006 National Survey on Drug Use and Health. National Household Survey on Drug Abuse Series H-21). Rockville, MD: Author.

Sutker, P. B., Goist, K. C., Jr., Allain, A. N., & Bugg, F. (1987). Acute alcohol intoxication: Sex comparisons on pharmacokinetic and mood measures. *Alcoholism, Clinical and Experimental Research, 11*, 507–512.

Sutker, P. B., Goist, K. C., Jr., & King, A. R. (1987). Acute alcohol intoxication in women: Relationship to dose and menstrual cycle phase. *Alcoholism, Clinical and Experimental Research, 11,* 74–79.

Thilbin, I., Finn, A., Ross, S. B., & Stenfors, C. (1999). Increased dopaminergic and 5-hydroxytryptaminergic activities in male rat brain following long-term treatment with anabolic androgenic steroids. *British Journal of Pharmacology, 126,* 1301–1306.

Thompson, T. L., & Moss, R. L. (1994). Estrogen regulation of dopamine release in the nucleus accumbens: Genomic- and nongenomic-mediated effects. *Journal of Neurochemistry, 62,* 1750–1756.

Thompson, T. L., & Moss, R. L. (1997). Modulation of mesolimbic dopaminergic activity over the rat estrous cycle. *Neuroscience Letters, 229,* 145–148.

Tseng, A. H., & Craft, R. M. (2001). Sex differences in antinociceptive and motoric effects of cannabinoids. *European Journal of Pharmacology, 430,* 41–47.

Tseng, A. H., Harding, J. W., & Craft, R. M. (2004). Pharmacokinetic factors in sex differences in Delta 9-tetrahydrocannabinol-induced behavioral effects in rats. *Behavioral Brain Research, 154,* 77–83.

Van Etten, M. L., Neumark, Y. D., & Anthony, J. C. (1999). Male–female differences in the earliest stages of drug involvement. *Addiction, 94,* 1413–1419.

van Haaren, F., & Meyer, M. E. (1991). Sex differences in locomotor activity after acute and chronic cocaine administration. *Pharmacology, Biochemistry, and Behavior, 39,* 923–927.

Wall, M. E., Sadler, B. M., Brine, D., Taylor, H., & Perez-Reyes, M. (1983). Metabolism, disposition, and kinetics of delta-9-tetrahydrocannabinol in men and women. *Clinical Pharmacology and Therapeutics, 34,* 352–363.

Wang, F., Chen, H., Steketee, J. D., & Sharp, B. M. (2007). Upregulation of ionotropic glutamate receptor subunits within specific mesocorticolimbic regions during chronic nicotine self-administration. *Neuropsychopharmacology, 32,* 103–109.

Weerts, E. M., Fantegrossi, W. E., & Goodwin, A. K. (2007). The value of nonhuman primates in drug abuse research. *Experimental and Clinical Psychopharmacology, 15,* 309–327.

Wetherington, C. L. (2007). Sex-gender differences in drug abuse: A shift in the burden of proof? *Experimental and Clinical Psychopharmacology, 15,* 411–417.

White, T. L., Justice, A. J., & de Wit, H. (2002). Differential subjective effects of D-amphetamine by gender, hormone levels and menstrual cycle phase. *Pharmacology, Biochemistry, and Behavior, 73,* 729–741.

Wilkins, J. N., Majewska, M. D., Van Gorp, W., Li, S. H., Hinken, C., Plotkin, D., et al. (2005). DHEAS and POMS measures identify cocaine dependence treatment outcome. *Psychoneuroendocrinology, 30,* 18–28.

Wilson, D. M., Killen, J. D., Hayward, C., Robinson, T. N., Hammer, L. D., Kraemer, H. C., et al. (1994). Timing and rate of sexual maturation and the onset of cigarette and alcohol use among teenage girls. *Archives of Pediatric & Adolescent Medicine, 148,* 789–795.

Woolverton, W. L., & Johnson, K. M. (1992). Neurobiology of cocaine abuse. *Trends in Pharmacological Sciences, 13,* 193–200.

Yen, S. S. C. (1999a). The human menstrual cycle: Neuroendocrine regulation. In S. S. C. Yen, R. B. Jaffe, & R. L. Barbieri (Eds.), *Reproductive endocrinology: Physiology, pathophysiology, and clinical management* (4th ed., pp. 191–217). Philadelphia: W.B. Saunders.

Yen, S. S. C. (1999b). Chronic anovulation due to CNS–hypothalamic–pituitary dysfunction. In S. S. C. Yen, R. B. Jaffe, & R. L. Barbieri (Eds.), *Reproductive endocrinology: Physiology, pathophysiology, and clinical management* (4th ed., pp. 516–561). Philadelphia: W.B. Saunders.

Zacny, J. P. (2001). Morphine responses in humans: A retrospective analysis of sex differences. *Drug and Alcohol Dependence, 63,* 23–28.

Zacny, J. P., & Beckman, N. J. (2004). The effects of a cold-water stimulus on butorphanol effects in males and females. *Pharmacology, Biochemistry, and Behavior, 78,* 653–659.

Zakharova, E. S., Danysz, W., & Bespalov, A. Y. (2005). Drug discrimination analysis of NMDA receptor channel blockers as nicotinic receptor antagonists in rats. *Psychopharmacology (Berl), 179,* 128–135.

Zinder, O., & Dar, D. E. (1999). Neuroactive steroids: Their mechanism of action and their function in the stress response. *Acta Physiologica Scandinavia, 167,* 181–188.

CHAPTER 4

Stress, Neuroendocrine Response, and Addiction in Women

Helen Fox, PhD
Rajita Sinha, PhD

Until very recently, drug abuse has been viewed as a marginal issue for women and portrayed largely as a male problem. However, in the last decade, due to changing socioeconomic and sociocultural factors, results from national surveys have shown that 2.5 million women in the United States meet criteria for alcohol dependence (Grant et al., 2004), and increasing rates of heavy episodic drinking by younger women are becoming more apparent (Russell, Light, & Gruenewald, 2004). As a result, international research projects have begun to highlight the comparative vulnerability of women to abuse-related issues. Despite generally lower consumption levels, women reach higher blood concentration levels when consuming equivalent weight-adjusted amounts of alcohol and/or drugs (Lieber, 1997) and have drug-related death rates of 50–100% higher than those of males (Walter, Dvorak, Gutierrez, Zitterl, & Lesch, 2005). Moreover, risk-related sex differences that set women at a disadvantage for compulsive drug use have been identified at every phase of the addiction cycle, including initiation, maintenance, and outcome (Quinones-Jenab, 2006). For example, women report very different reasons, compared with men, for using alcohol (Piko, Wills, & Walker, 2007; Sonne, Back, Diaz Zuniga, Randall, & Brady, 2003) and are more likely to attribute their alcohol use to a traumatic event or stressor and self-medicate. Women also experience markedly different acute physiological and subjective effects of drugs and alcohol (McCance-Katz, Hart, Boyarsky, Kosten, & Jatlow, 2005; Sofuoglu, Dudish-Poulsen, Nelson, Pentel, & Hatsukami, 1999). Moreover, these responses are intrinsic to the maintenance of substance use. As such, the negative consequences of drinking in females often appear accelerated or "telescoped," particularly in relation to co-occurring psychopathology such as depression, panic disorders, phobia and eating pathology (Back, Brady, Jackson, Salstrom, & Zinzow, 2005; Sinha & Rounsaville, 2002).

Preclinical studies that have utilized models to mimic the transition to loss of control in drug-seeking behavior have also corroborated the fact that males and females differ in relation to addiction vulnerability. Research using laboratory rats has indicated that female rats show greater sensitization to the reinforcing effects of drugs, compared with male rats (see Lynch, 2006, for review). Female rats acquire cocaine, methamphetamine, nicotine, and heroin self-administration much more rapidly than male rats (Carroll, Sinha, Nich, Babuscio, & Rounsaville, 2002; Donny et al., 2000; Hu, Crombag, Robinson, & Becker, 2004; Lynch &

Carroll, 1999; Roth & Carroll, 2004). They also demonstrate significantly higher breaking points to progressive ratio schedules, compared with male rats, across a range of substances (Roth & Carroll, 2004) and acquire conditioned place preference (CPP) more quickly than male rats following exposure to cocaine (Russo et al., 2003). Furthermore, they show greater escalation and dysregulation in pattern and quantity of drug intake during extended-access regimens (Lynch, 2006; Lynch, Lynch, Arizzi, & Carroll, 2000).

Both clinical and preclinical research has identified a markedly more rapid and risk-oriented path to compulsive drug seeking in females. Furthermore, in view of the fact that women have typically been underrepresented in clinical trials and biobehavioral experimental research, in general, elucidating sex-specific variation in addiction etiology is not only timely but also integral to clarifying the influence of gender in compulsive drug use. While many biological and psychosocial factors may influence this sex-related disparity in the etiology, course, and consequences of addiction, the main objective of the current chapter is to focus specifically upon the impact of gender on neuroendocrine adaptations to stress and reward system function as a potential mediator for women's path to addiction. From a broad perspective, anecdotal data as well as clinical and laboratory-based findings have documented both stressors and drug-related environmental cues as being among the most important facilitators of drug reinstatement and/or drug seeking in both animals and humans (Sinha, 2001, for review). Moreover, clinical research has indicated that in the United States, women are markedly over represented with regard to rates of stress-related psychopathology, including anxiety and depression (see Blanchard, 1998, for review).

Findings from recent studies, including those from our own laboratory, have assessed gender variations in stress-system neuroadaptations, either by examining emotional and autonomic differences between addicted men and women in relation to stress and cue response, or by assessing the interactions of gonadal hormones and/or menstrual cycle (MC) phase on physiological and subjective responses to both acute drug consumption and stress. Initially, however, it may be important to understand why hormonal alterations in stress and reward systems are important to assess in addiction.

HORMONAL ALTERATIONS IN STRESS AND REWARD SYSTEMS

Although the perception of distress relies on specific factors such as the emotional state of the individual (coping strategies and cognitive appraisal) and social-environmental characteristics, the stress response or "stress cascade" typically elicits the activation of two major neuroendocrine systems in the face of homeostatic challenge: namely, the hypothalamic–pituitary–adrenal (HPA) axis and the sympathetic adrenal medullary (SAM) system. More importantly, in terms of addiction, the stress pathways stimulate or "prime" the reward circuits of the brain (Sinha, 2001). Glucocorticoid or stress hormones (e.g., cortisol) secreted via HPA activation in response to stress exposure, acute drug use, or residual and protracted withdrawal states, modify reward-related behaviors through stimulation of mesencephalic dopaminergic transmission (Piazza & Le Moal, 1997). According to the allostatic model of addiction, a sustained increase in the secretion of dopamine (DA) may culminate in a failure to maintain homeostatsis and result in a decrease in the function of normal reward-related neurocircuitry and persistence or sensitivity of the stress-related systems (Koob & Le Moal, 2005).

As such, both animal and human research has shown that neuroadaptations to these stress systems may underlie the pathophysiology of stimulant, opioid, alcohol, and nicotine addictions. Extensive preclinical research has refined stress-related animal reinstatement models, highlighting the importance of HPA adaptations in cocaine, heroin, alcohol, and nicotine seeking (for review, see Sarnyai, Shaham, & Heinrichs, 2001; Shalev, Grimm, & Shaham, 2002). Substantial preclinical evidence also shows that stress systems are stimulated by acute nicotine (Andersson, Eneroth, & Agnati, 1981; Balfour, 1989; Donny et al., 2000), cocaine (Shaham, Erb, & Stewart, 2000; Stewart, 2000), and alcohol administration (Gianoulakis, Krishnan, & Thavundayil, 1996). In rats and monkeys, sensitized stress-induced increases in glucocorticoids are associated with increased alcohol intake (Higley, Hasert, Suomi, & Linnoila, 1991; Prasad & Prasad, 1995), and levels of corticosterone are correlated with amount of amphetamine consumed at the initial presentation of the novelty-related stress (Piazza et al., 1991, 1993). Moreover, in adrenalectomized animals, in which corticosterone secretion is suppressed, a decrease in behavioral response to both amphetamine and morphine is documented (Deroche et al., 1995), as well as decreased alcohol consumption (Hansen, Fahlke, Söderpalm, & Hård, 1995; Lamblin & De Witte, 1996).

In humans, chronic smoking as well as cocaine and alcohol consumption have also been associated with enhanced stress-system activity. Acute alcohol intake and recent withdrawal from alcohol have been associated with elevated basal cortisol (Adinoff et al., 1991; Adinoff, Ruether, Krebaum, Iranmanesh, & Williams, 2003; Costa et al., 1996; Kutscher et al., 2002) and lower basal Adrenocorticotropic Hormone (ACTH) levels (Dai, Thavundayil, & Gianoulakis, 2002). Moreover, blunted ACTH and cortisol response to both pharmacological challenges and psychosocial stressors in chronic alcohol abusers have also been reported (Adinoff, Junghanns, Kiefer, & Krishnan-Sarin, 2005; Al'Absi, Bongard, & Lovallo, 2000; Costa et al., 1996; Errico, Parsons, King, & Lovallo, 1993; Inder et al., 1995; Junghanns et al., 2003; Lovallo, Dickensheets, Myers, Thomas, & Nixon, 2000; Wand & Dobs, 1991). Similarly, cigarette smoking has been shown to elevate circulating levels of both ACTH and cortisol in moderate smokers (Pomerleau & Pomerleau, 1990; Seyler, Fertig, Pomerleau, Hunt, & Parker, 1984), and blunted ACTH and cortisol response to stress has been reported in smokers in withdrawal (Al'Absi, Hatsukami, & Davis, 2005).

In relation to protracted abstinence, the stress and drug/alcohol cue-related craving state has also been associated with enhanced negative emotion and anxiety as well as changes in HPA axis and SAM systems in early-abstinent cocaine abusers (Fox et al., 2006; Sinha et al., 2003), comorbid cocaine and alcohol abusers (Fox et al., 2005), and alcohol abusers (Fox, Berquist, Hong, & Sinha, 2007; Sinha, Fuse, Aubin, & O'Malley, 2000; Sinha, Garcia, Kemp, Krystal, & O'Malley, 2005). Notably, enhanced stress-related plasma cortisol levels have been associated with relapse factors in those with cocaine abuse (Sinha, Garcia, Paliwal, Kreek, & Rounsaville, 2006), and suppressed levels associated with a shorter time to relapse in those with alcohol dependence (Adinoff et al., 2005; Breese et al., 2005) and males who smoke (Al'Absi, 2006). Taken together, these findings show that the reinforcing effects of psychoactive drugs such as cocaine, alcohol, and nicotine could be modulated by alterations in the major stress pathways. Moreover, adaptations in these HPA and SAM stress-system mechanisms may represent the transition from controlled to compulsive drug seeking in both laboratory animals and humans across a range of substances. Most importantly, these neuroadaptations are also sex-specific.

SEX DIFFERENCES IN ACUTE DRUG ADMINISTRATION AND STRESS SENSITIVITY

Relatively consistent neuroadaptations have been observed as a function of gender in both preclinical and clinical research. Gender differences have been shown predominantly in studies that have assessed sensitization either to acute drug administration, stress, or both. Such sex differences in the emotional, behavioral, and neurohormonal cross-sensitization of stress and the acute effects of many psychoactive drugs, including cocaine, alcohol, and nicotine (Deutch & Roth, 1990; Sorg & Stekette, 2002), suggest that gender variation in either may point to important indicators of the stress-induced compulsive drug-seeking state and relapse liability. In general, findings have indicated that female rats demonstrate increased behavioral sensitivity to both acute drug administration and different forms of stress. Female rats show greater HPA-axis response to alcohol (Ogilvie & Rivier, 1997) and greater locomotor activity following cocaine exposure, compared with male rats (Carroll, Anderson, & Morgan, 2007). They also show significantly increased locomotor activity, orofacial activity, increased ACTH and cortisol levels, and a decrease in D3 dopamine transporters in response to nicotine, compared with male rats (Faraday, Blakeman, & Grunberg, 2005; Harrod et al., 2004; Harrod, Booze, Welch, Browning, & Mactutus, 2005).

Sex differences in stress and reward-related HPA- and SAM-system function have also been documented. Female rats show significantly greater corticosterone and ACTH levels, compared with male rats, both at baseline (Atkinson & Waddell, 1997) and in response to stressors such as footshock and restraint stress (Handa, Bungess, Kerr, & O'Keefe, 1994; Rivier, 1999; Yoshimura et al., 2003). They also show longer activation of the HPA axis (Heinsbroek, van Haaren, Feenstra, Boon, & van de Poll, 1991) and demonstrate greater behavioral sensitivity (locomotor activity, vocalizations, and flinching) to stressors, compared with male rats (van Haaren & Meyer, 1991). In relation to catecholaminergic markers, norepinephrine (NE) response to controlled, compared with uncontrolled, stress is also greater in female compared with male rats, and footshock initiates greater neural activity in monoaminergic brain regions of female compared with male rats (Heinsbroek, van Haaren, Feenstra, van Galen, Boer, et al., 1990; Heinsbroek, van Haaren, van de Poll, & Steenbergen, 1991). Studies that have examined the effects of both stress and drug administration on behavioral sensitivity have shown that maternal separation facilitates behavioral sensitization to alcohol in female, but not male, rats (Kawakami, Quadros, Takahashi, & Sucheki, 2007). Similarly, following restraint stress and nicotine exposure, female rats show greater increases in horizontal activity and decreases in feeding and body weight than male rats (Faraday, O'Donoghue, & Grunberg, 2003, 2005).

In humans, gender variations in response to different types of stress challenge have also highlighted broad sex-based differences in neuroendocrine stress and reward function. However, some studies have emphasized the fact that gender variation may be specific to particular types of stress induction. Although HPA axis response to physiological exercise has not been shown to differ by gender (Kirschbaum, Wust, & Helhammer, 1992), men show a consistently higher HPA drive, compared with women, following psychosocial stressors, despite females reporting significantly higher levels of distress (Kudielka & Kirschbaum, 2005). The stressors have included public speaking, mental arithmetic (Kirschbaum et al. 1992; Kirschbaum, Kudielka, Gaab, Schommer, & Helhammer, 1999; Kudielka et al., 1998), examination stress (Frankenhaeuser et al., 1978), pain (Zimmer, Basler, Vedder, & Lautenbacher, 2003) and cognitive challenge (Seeman, Singer, Wilkinson, & McEwen, 2001). Higher levels of basal ACTH have been reported in males, compared with females, although no simultaneous differences in basal cortisol have been reported (Dorn et al., 1996; Horrocks et al., 1990; Roelfsema et al., 1993). Males have also demonstrated increased vascular reactivity to harassment, mirror drawing tasks, and mental arithmetic (Allen, Stoney, Owens, & Matthews, 1993; Earle, Linden, & Weinberg, 1999; Matthews, Gump, & Owens, 2001).

Given that there are intrinsic sex-specific variations in neuroendocrine stress and reward system function, and that chronic drug-use-related neuroadaptations in these systems are associated with relapse susceptibility, we may expect to observe gender differences in the emotional and physiological response to stress in substance abusers. Moreover, these gender-related response differences could potentially highlight important risk factors specific to relapse, co-occurring psychopathology, and treatment outcome in women.

GENDER DIFFERENCES IN STRESS RESPONSE IN SUBSTANCE ABUSERS

Several recent studies have assessed stress and drug-cue response within addicted populations and have highlighted important gender variations in autonomic and affective functioning. In our laboratory, we have used personalized, stressful, and cue-related imagery techniques in order to induce a distress state in groups of early-abstinent men and women with cocaine dependence (CD). All patients were treatment seeking and kept on a locked inpatient unit for 4 weeks of treatment and study participation. All of our laboratory studies were typically conducted following 3–4 weeks of inpatient stay and involved exposing all participants to a brief 5-minute guided imagery of individually calibrated stressful situations, personal drug/ alcohol-related situations, and neutral relaxing situations, presented in random order con-secutively over 3 days, with one imagery session presented per day. Subjective drug craving, and anxiety ratings, emotion rating scales, physiological measures, and HPA (cortisol, ACTH, prolactin) markers were collected at baseline, immediately following imagery, and at various recovery time points. This personalized stress paradigm allowed us, first, to elucidate some of the subjective, behavioral, physiological, and neuroendocrine markers of the stress and cue-related craving state during early, protracted withdrawal (Fox et al., 2005, 2006; Sinha et al., 2003, 2006) and, second, to assess potential gender differences in alterations in stress and reward pathways. Because the personalized stress paradigm permits individual calibration of levels of distress, the method has helped account for gender variation in relation to salience of stressors. Prior studies have shown that whereas achievement stress has been shown to have greater salience for men, women have been shown to be more reactive to social rejec-tion (Kajantie & Phillips, 2006; Stroud, Salovey, & Epel, 2002). In our samples, therefore, participants' stress-related scenarios were used only if they were scored higher than an 8 on a 10-point Likert scale for emotional distress calibrated by participants themselves. As an added validation of emotional stress, all stress scripts were similarly rated by two clinicians for degree of stressfulness on a 5-point scale ranging from 1 = *not at all* to 5 = *most stressful*.

COCAINE

Consistent with research in healthy volunteers, we found that 25 men with CD demonstrated a significantly higher ACTH, cortisol, and blood pressure drive, compared with 25 females with CD, following exposure to stress, drug cue, and neutral imagery (Fox et al., 2006). Although women with CD showed significantly lower levels of basal and response plasma cortisol compared with males with CD, they still demonstrated hyperarousal to stress in rela-tion to their response to the neutral condition. Furthermore, another recent study from our laboratory showed 12 women with CD to have significantly enhanced basal daily salivary cortisol levels at waking, compared with 10 healthy control women, across one complete menstrual cycle (Fox et al., 2008a). The study also demonstrated a basal upregulation of corticotropin-releasing factor (CRF) and the hypothalamic–pituitary–adrenal (HPA) axis (CRF–HPA axis) in women with CD.

Extended analyses from Fox et al. (2006) found that ACTH and cortisol were correlated in the 25 males with CD following both stress and drug cue, but not in females. This low ACTH and cortisol conformity may highlight a failure of the adrenal cortex to respond normally to ACTH stimulation when the HPA system is challenged under psychologically stressful conditions. Previous research has interpreted a lack of synchrony between ACTH and cortisol as a possible disturbance in the regulation of cortisol secretion and disruption in hormonal release patterns, which could increase vulnerability to neuroendocrine dysfunction (Galard et al., 1991; Roelfsema, Pincus, & Veldhuis, 1998). Further alterations in adrenal responsiveness were also highlighted in that females with CD did not demonstrate the hypersensitivity to ACTH in relation to the production of glucocorticoids typically observed in normal healthy females (Kajantie & Phillips, 2006). This finding was demonstrated by the fact that males with CD showed significantly higher basal levels of cortisol, compared with women with CD. In comparison, prior studies have tended to show higher levels of basal ACTH, but not cortisol, in males (Dorn et al., 1996; Horrocks et al., 1990; Roelfsema et al., 1993), suggesting that females, in general, may display a different setpoint to cortisol feedback.

Additional to these potential changes in ACTH sensitivity, other findings have also indicated that females with CD report significantly higher levels of negative affect, compared with males, despite demonstrating a lower stress and cue-induced HPA drive. For example, findings from one of our studies indicated that 26 women with CD who socially drank reported significantly higher levels of sadness and anxiety following exposure to stress, compared with 44 males with CD who drank socially (Fox, Hong, Siedlarz, & Sinha, 2008b). Enhanced subjective response to stress is also consistent with a prior study by Back and colleagues (2005), in which women with CD reported higher ratings of stress, nervousness, and pain, compared with men with CD, following exposure to both psychological (mental arithmetic task) and physiological (cold pressor task) stressors.

Whereas a significantly higher HPA drive in males with CD (Fox et al., 2006) may represent a direct risk factor for men, our findings also indicate that females with CD may show a potentially different stress-related dysregulation of the HPA system. Both the low conformity in stress and drug-cue-related ACTH and cortisol response in women with CD, as well as possible alterations in cortisol feedback (Fox et al., 2006), may highlight a failure of the adrenal cortex to respond normally to ACTH stimulation under challenging situations. Additionally, females with CD also display a more sensitized change in emotional setpoint, despite a lower HPA drive (i.e., they may experience greater emotional intensity at lower levels of HPA arousal than men, Fox et al., 2008b). This finding is consistent with findings in social drinkers (Chaplin, Hong, Berquist, & Sinha, 2007), as well as in research that has identified levels of depression to be associated with increased basal cortisol, more so in both drug-abusing and non-drug-abusing women, compared to men (Wisniewski et al., 2006; Young, 1995).

ALCOHOL

Using an identical imagery paradigm, we also compared a group of males and females with alcohol dependence (AD) across three imagery conditions (stress, alcohol cue and neutral/relaxing) and assessed emotional and behavioral responses at baseline, immediately following imagery exposure, and at various time points. Findings again highlighted gender-specific changes in both emotional and behavioral set points following exposure to stress and alcohol-cue-related imagery (Fox & Sinha, 2007). Similar to females with CD, 21 early-abstinent females with AD reported significantly higher ratings of stress-induced sadness, anxiety, anger, fear, and behavioral arousal, compared with 21 males with AD, and 21 males who engaged in social drinking (SD), and 21 females who engaged in SD (Fox & Sinha, 2007).

In relation to HPA axis markers, a recent study by Brady et al. (2006) demonstrated gender-related basal and response differences to the cold pressor task (CPT) in three groups of individuals (those with AD, posttraumatic stress disorder [PTSD], and comorbid AD and PTSD). Findings indicated that females showed significantly lower levels of ACTH, compared with males (across all three groups), and that females with either AD or PTSD showed greater ACTH blunting following stress exposure, compared with males diagnosed with similar drinking or PTSD criteria. This finding also corroborates earlier findings from a study by Gianoulakis, Dai, and Brown (2003) in which decreased ACTH levels were shown to be more pronounced in women ages 30–60, compared with men of a similar age group. This finding may indicate an important risk factor for women with AD in view of the fact that HPA-axis hyporeactivity to social stress, alcohol-cue exposure, and alcohol consumption have been associated with greater craving and a return to early drinking in people with AD (Adinoff et al., 2005; Breese et al., 2005; Junghanns et al., 2005; O'Malley, Krishnan-Sarin, Farren, Sinha, & Kreek, 2002), as well as deemed a risk marker for the development of substance use disorders in individuals with a positive family history for alcoholism (Sorocco, Lovallo, Vincent, & Collins, 2006).

NICOTINE

A recent study by Back, Waldrop, Saladin, Yeatts, Simpson, McRae, et al. (2008) has indicated that, similar to women with AD, stress-induced-HPA-axis response is dampened in females who smoke than males who smoke. The study involved exposing males and females who smoked and nonsmoking individuals to both the Triers Social Stress Test (TSST) and a corticotropin-releasing hormone (CRH) challenge. Females who smoked demonstrated significantly lower basal cortisol levels, compared with females who did not smoke, as well as a blunted cortisol response to both the physiological and psychosocial stressors, compared with females who did not smoke. Importantly, these variations in smoking-related adaptations were not observed between the males who smoked and did not smoke and may again reflect risk markers for the fact that women have markedly greater difficulty quitting smoking than men (Green, Lynn, & Montgomery, 2008; Ward, Haney, Fischman, & Foltin, 1997; Wileyto et al., 2005).

THE IMPACT OF SEX HORMONES ON STRESS RESPONSES

Researchers have attempted to understand the basis of these gender differences in stress response by examining the impact of gonadatrophic hormones on autonomic response to stress as well as subjective, physiological, and hormonal responses to acute drug administration. Drugs such as cocaine and *d*-amphetamine are known to stimulate the HPA-axis stress systems in rodents and humans (Sarnyai, Mello, Mendelson, Erös-Sarnyai, & Mercer, 1996), and there is cross-sensitization between response to stress and psychostimulant drugs. As such, assessing the influence of sex hormones on acute responses to stimulant drugs as well as on stress responses may additionally help clarify sexual dimorphism in stress-related behaviors that are intrinsic to the maintenance and reinforcing effects of stimulants.

Preclinical studies have indicated that sex steroids are intrinsically involved in the regulation of the HPA axis and sympathoadrenal activity and, as such, may play an important role in the rewarding effects of drugs. Specifically, estradiol may have an excitatory effect on the HPA axis in animals (see McCormick & Mathews, 2007, for review); female rats, for example, have been shown to have higher levels of ACTH and corticosterone and a higher ACTH response to stress during proestrus, which is marked by high estradiol levels (Atkinson & Waddell, 1997). In further support of this hypothesis, other studies have shown that estradiol and progesterone substitutions stimulate HPA-axis function in nonhuman primates (Norman, Smith, Pappas, & Hall, 1992), and mean daily levels of cortisol are significantly reduced following ovariectomy in rhesus macaques (Smith & Norman, 1987). Estrogen also modulates DA activity in the striatum and nucleus accumbens (Nacc; Becker, 1999) and has been shown to enhance behavioral sensitization to cocaine in female, but not male rats (Becker, Molenda, & Hummer, 2001).

In healthy human females, several studies have shown the HPA modulating effects of progesterone and estrogen. ACTH secretion has been shown to be increased during the luteal menstrual cycle (MC) phase (Roca, Schmidt, & Rubinow, 1999), and estrogen replacement has been shown to blunt ACTH, cortisol, NE, and blood pressure in postmenopausal women (Lindheim et al., 1994). Findings have also shown increased glucocorticoid response in the luteal, compared with the follicular, phase of the MC following stressors that included mental arithmetic, the CPT (Tersman, Collins, & Eneroth, 1991), and the TSST (Kirschbaum et al., 1995, 1999).

In drug-abusing populations, the impact of sex hormones on the stress and reward system has broadly included assessing the effects of a drug at different stages of the MC in women or assessing the effects of exogenous hormone levels on drug exposure at different stages of the MC. Some studies have also compared responses to hormone and drug exposure in both men and women. The majority of the research to date has indicated that the MC phase appears to have a significant impact on both the subjective and pharmacokinetic effects of stimulant drugs, including cocaine, amphetamine, and methamphetamine. Drugs such as alcohol, nicotine, marijuana, and benzodizipines have been shown to have a limited effect on the MC in both animals and humans (Terner & de Wit, 2006); however, reproductive problems such as early menopause, amenorrhea, and luteal phase dysfunction have been associated with chronic misuse of these drugs (Mello, 1988; Teoh, Lex, Mendelson, Mello, & Cochlin, 1992). As such, a more precise endocrine profile of MC disruption in nonstimulant drugs may still need to be elucidated.

In relation to stimulants, an initial study by Justice and De Wit (1999) reported that the positive subjective effects of d-amphetamine, such as "high," "euphoria," and "Like Drug," were potentiated during the follicular, compared to the midluteal, phase, when progesterone levels are typically low. Similar subjective effects of cocaine were also potentiated in the follicular, compared with midluteal, phase of women following smoked cocaine—although ratings were dependent upon dose (Evans, Haney, & Foltin, 2002). Follow-up research comparing women in both the early (low estradiol) and late (high estradiol) follicular phase of their MC found no significant differences in the subjective effects of d-amphetamine, suggesting less of a role for estradiol in potentiating the effects of amphetamines and a potentially greater role for progesterone in masking the acute effects (Evans, 2007; Justice & de Wit, 2000a). In support of this hypothesis, exogenous administration of estradiol was not shown to enhance either the subjective or pharmacokinetic effects of d-amphetamine in either normally cycling (Justice & de Wit, 2000b) or postmenopausal (Schleifer, Justice, & de Wit, 2002) women. In addition, subsequent studies comparing men with women in both the follicular and luteal phases of their cycle also demonstrated that the subjective effects of a drug were potentiated in women during the follicular phase, but comparable to men. Conversely, women in the luteal phase of their cycle were shown to report attenuated subjective effects of both *d*-amphetamine (White, Justice, & de Wit, 2002) and cocaine (Evans & Foltin, 2006; Sofuoglu et al., 1999), compared with men. In other research, exogenous progesterone had an attenuating effect on the subjective (Evans & Foltin, 2006; Sofuoglu, Babb, & Hatsukami, 2002) and physiological (Sofuoglu, Mitchell, & Kosten, 2004) effects of smoked cocaine. Although progesterone exerts an attenuating influence with regard to the subjective effects of stimulants, the precise sex-specific mechanisms underlying this process remain ambiguous. Whereas Sofuoglu et al. (2004) reported reduced DBP and feelings of "high," from cocaine in both women and men, Evans and Fortin (2006) reported attenuated effects of cocaine in women only.

Recent research from our own laboratory has further investigated the role of these sex hormones in relation to relapse vulnerability during the first month of abstinence, a period associated with increased distress. We assessed and compared daily levels of salivary cortisol, estradiol, and progesterone at waking in a group of 12 women with CD following admission to inpatient treatment, with a group of 10 healthy control women, across one complete 28-day MC. Weekly measures of negative emotion were also collected in all women and cocaine craving measures were collected only in the women with CD (Fox et al., 2008a). Findings indicated that levels of waking cortisol and progesterone, but not estradiol, were significantly higher in the women with CD, compared with the healthy control women. Significantly lower estradiol-to-progesterone ratios were also observed in women with CD, compared with healthy control women, largely as a result of high waking levels of progesterone. Women with CD also reported significantly higher overall negative emotion, compared with the healthy women. Although ratings of cocaine craving did not change in women with CD as a function of MC phase, craving did correlate positively with negative mood in the follicular and luteal phases.

Increased levels of salivary cortisol, progesterone, and negative affect observed in the women with CD are also consistent with our findings of enhanced stress-related sensitivity to negative emotion reported in women with CD, compared with men (Fox et al., 2008b). Moreover, increased levels of progesterone in early-abstinent females with CD may potentially represent compensatory adaptations to an enhanced HPA-driven distressed state and are consistent with the possibility that progesterone may reduce the positive effects of *d*-amphetamine and cocaine (Evans & Foltin, 2006; Sofuoglu et al., 2002, 2004).

In a follow-up study that aimed to assess the effects of the MC phase more systematically on stress and cue-related cocaine craving, we compared the responses of three groups of women with CD at various stages of their MC to stress, drug-cue, and neutral imagery exposure, using our standard procedures (Sinha et al., 2007). The groups included five women with high progesterone (P) levels to match the midluteal phase of the menstrual cycle (P = 11.8 ng/ml, *SD* = 2.9; estradiol [E] = 69.1 pg/ml, *SD* = 43.2), five women with low P levels to match the late follicular phase of the cycle (P = 0.44 ng/ml, *SD* = .21; E = 112.46 pg/ml, *SD* = 118.3), and nine women with moderate levels of P (P = 2.7 ng/ml, *SD* = 2.85; E = 60.19 pg/ml; *SD* = 66.9), corresponding to the early luteal phase of the cycle.

Findings indicated that the women with CD and high P levels reported significantly lower ratings of stress and cue-induced cocaine craving, cue-induced anxiety, and decreased cue-induced blood pressure, compared with the women with low P levels. This finding corroborated previous human studies that had also shown intramuscular P treatment to significantly attenuate epinephrine and heart rate responses to mental stress (Del Rio et al., 1998). Most importantly, findings demonstrated that increased progesterone levels were able to regulate selective aspects of the stress- and cue-induced craving state in midluteal women with CD.

IMPLICATIONS FOR RELAPSE
VULNERABILITY AND TREATMENT

The findings described in the previous sections indicate drug- and alcohol-related neuroadaptations in sex and stress hormone function that are likely to contribute to an increased risk of relapse in substance-abusing women.

1. Sex hormones may impact neuroadaptation in stress response and drug craving in several ways. (a) The positive effects of cocaine may be potentiated in women during the follicular phase of their cycle to the same levels as men (Evans & Foltin, 2006; Sofuoglu et al., 1999). Although follicular estradiol has been shown to play a lesser role in altering response to stimulants in humans, the equivalent hedonic experience in women compared with men may highlight the follicular phase as a period of increased allostatic susceptibility. This response is particularly likely in view of the fact that females with CD may potentially experience greater emotional intensity in reaction to HPA arousal (Chaplin et al., 2007; Young, 1995), as observed in our laboratory studies (Fox et al., 2008b; Fox & Sinha, 2007). Furthermore, mid-luteal phase progesterone levels may "mask" the positive effects of stimulants (Evans, 2007), as well as attenuate stress and cue-related craving, anxiety and blood pressure in early abstinent cocaine women (Sinha et al., 2007).

(b) While increased levels of P across the MC in women with CD may initially reflect an neuroadaptive response to enhanced stress-induced HPA function and negative affect, persistence of distress and repeated adaptations may lead to depleted P and allopregnanolone levels (Girdler & Klatzkin, 2007). This deletion could further predispose women to increased anxiety, negative emotion and lowered tolerance to stress, which in turn may increase vulnerability to relapse. The attenuating effects of progesterone may also suggest that the late-luteal (premenstrual) MC phase, which is characterized by endogenous progesterone withdrawal (Moran, Goldberg, & Smith, 1998), could represent a phase of increased vulnerability to stress and cue-related craving. These P-related mechanisms may serve to increase anxiety (Smith et al., 1998) and insensitivity to the potentiating effects of GABA modulatory drugs such as alcohol (Gulinello et al., 2001) in substance abusing women. It is notable that in our study we found that E2/P ratios in the late luteal phase of 12 women with CD were significantly associated with increased cocaine craving (Fox et al., 2008a).

2. Gender differences in emotional and endocrine stress response may heighten drug-seeking behavior in women by increasing risk of comorbid disorders. Increased reports of stress-related anxiety and negative affect have previously been observed in females who drink socially (Chaplin et al., 2007) and are also consistent with studies of subjective emotional experience in normal healthy women (Brebner, 2003; Fischer, Mosquera, van Vianen, & Manstead, 2004). As such, findings from our laboratory studies of woman who abuse cocaine and alcohol (Fox et al., 2006; Fox & Sinha, 2007) may largely reflect trends in anxiety and affective disorders in the general population (Brady & Sinha, 2005). However, in women who abuse drugs, enhanced emotional sensitivity to a stress-related craving state and differences in adrenal response may increase risk of relapse vulnerability as well as highlight discrepancies in risk for comorbid disorders between men and women.

Increased anxiety, anger, fear, and sadness reported by females with alcohol dependence (Fox & Sinha, 2007) have been significantly associated with stress-induced alcohol craving (Fox et al., 2007; Sinha et al., 2008), and increased stress-related anxiety and sadness have been significantly associated with stress-related cocaine craving in cocaine abusers (Fox et al., 2008b). Furthermore, meta-analyses of international longitudinal surveys have shown that emotionally driven internalizing disorders, such as depression, are predictive of drinking in women, but not men (Fillmore et al., 1997). Similarly, affective problems such as low self-esteem, guilt (Reed, 1985), stigmatization (Bepko, 1991), and social withdrawal (Turnbull & Gomberg, 1991) have all been highlighted as risk factors in alcohol- and drug-abusing women.

Findings from our laboratory studies are consistent with findings that women generally surpass men in the number of psychiatric problems related to their drug/alcohol use, despite men having significantly higher consumption levels and dependence problems (Kajantie & Phillips, 2006; Wilsnack, 1996). Moreover, National Comorbidity Surveys have reported greater prevalence of anxiety, depression, panic disorder, and phobia in female abusers of alcohol, compared with males (Kessler et al., 1997), and almost twice the prevalence of anxiety disorders have been reported in treatment-seeking women with CD, compared with men (Rounsville et al., 1991). As such, allostasis of stress-related HPA and SAM systems, increased emotional intensity, and the potential for comorbid affective disorders may interact as unique risk factors in women who abuse alcohol and drugs. Such compounded problems may, in turn, highlight the necessity for gender-specific treatment programs that emphasize the development of assertiveness and coping skills for affective disorders, guilt, and low self-esteem (Kauffman, Dore, & Nelson-Zlupko, 1995; Reed, 1985). Indeed, recent studies have shown that women-focused single-gender group treatment has improved long-term clinical outcomes in substance-abusing women (Greenfield, Trucco, McHugh, Lincoln, & Gallop, 2007).

3. Gender differences in emotional and endocrine stress response, as well as co-occurring psychopathology, may also highlight the need for more tailored pharmacological treatments for women. In relation to pharmacological implications, sex-specific differences in HPA dysregulation exemplify the need for the oversampling of women in treatment studies. In the nicotine literature, for example, various drugs for smoking cessation (e.g., mecamylamine and clonidine) have demonstrated an ability to enhance abstinence in women compared with men, particularly women with risk factors for treatment failure, such as recurrent major depression (Glassman et al., 1993; Perkins, 2001). Sex differences have also been documented in relation to the efficacy of disulfiram on cocaine abuse, wherein men have shown significantly better treatment outcome, possibly due to the fact that women may be more sensitized to the potentially anxiety-inducing alterations in DA- to -NE ratios often induced by disulfiram (Nich et al., 2004).

As men and women differ in relation to the nature and severity of co-occurring psychopathology and the manner in which they respond to stress and cues, it is also likely that the efficacy of pharmacological treatments will differ across gender, again emphasizing the importance of developing sex-specific pharmacological treatment therapies.

KEY POINTS

- Findings from several studies assessing neuroendocrine response to stress indicate that women with cocaine or alcohol dependence show increased emotional sensitivity to stress and cues compared with men, alongside sex-specific differences in HPA axis function.
- Stress- and reward-system alterations may be modulated by sex hormones and/or MC phase. Findings also suggest that women are less susceptible to stress and cue-related craving during the midluteal phase, when progesterone levels are typically high.
- These unique neuroadaptations in affect and autonomic function may impact relapse vulnerability, susceptibility to comorbid affective disorders, and treatment outcome.
- All of these factors may necessitate the need for gender-specific clinical, pharmacological, and psychological interventions to improve treatment outcomes in addiction.

REFERENCES

Asterisks denote recommended readings.

Adinoff, B., Junghanns, K., Kiefer, F., & Krishnan-Sarin, S. (2005). Suppression of the HPA axis stress-response: Implications for relapse. *Alcoholism: Clinical and Experimental Research, 29*(7), 1351–1355. (*)

Adinoff, B., Risher-Flowers, D., De Jong, J., Ravitz, B., Bone, G. H., Nutt, D. J., et al. (1991). Disturbances of hypothalamic–pituitary–adrenal axis functioning during ethanol withdrawal in six men. *American Journal of Psychiatry, 148*(8), 1023–1025.

Adinoff, B., Ruether, K., Krebaum, S., Iranmanesh, A., & Williams, M. J. (2003). Increased salivary cortisol concentrations during chronic alcohol intoxication in a naturalistic clinical sample of men. *Alcoholism: Clinical and Experimental Research, 27*(9), 1420–1427.

Al'Absi, M. (2006). Altered psychoendocrine responses to psychological stress and smoking relapse. *International Journal of Psychophysiology, 59,* 218–227.

Al'Absi, M., Bongard, S., & Lovallo, W. R. (2000). Effects of habitual anger expression and defensiveness on ACTH and cortisol responses to behavioral challenges. *International Journal of Psychophysiology, 37,* 257–265.

Al'Absi, M., Hatsukami, D., & Davis, G. (2005). Attenuated adrenocorticotropic responses to stress predict early relapse. *Psychopharmacology, 181,* 107–117.

Allen, M. T., Stoney, C. M., Owens, J. F., & Matthews, K. A. (1993). Hemodynamic adjustments to laboratory stress: The influence of gender and personality. *Psychosomatic Medicine, 55,* 505–517.

Andersson, K., Eneroth, P., & Agnati, L. F. (1981). Nicotine-induced increases of noradrenaline turnover in discrete noradrenaline nerve terminal systems of the hypothalamus and the median eminence of the rat and their relationship to changes in the secretion of adenohypophyseal hormones. *Acta Physiologica Scandanavica, 113*(2), 227–231.

Atkinson, H. C., & Waddell, B. J. (1997). Circadian variation in basal plasma corticosterone and adrenocorticotropin in the rat: Sexual dimorphism and changes across the estrous cycle. *Endocrinology, 138*(9), 3842–3848.

Back, S. E., Brady, K. T., Jackson, J. L., Salstrom, S., & Zinzow, H. (2005). Gender differences in stress reactivity among cocaine-dependent individuals. *Psychopharmacology (Berl), 180*(1), 169–176.

Back, S. E., Waldrop, A. E., Saladin, M. E., Yeatts, S. D., Simpson, A., McRae, A. L., et al. (2008). Effects of gender and cigarette smoking on reactivity to psychological and pharmacological stress provocation. *Gender and Cigarette Smoking. Psychoneuroendocrinology, 33,* 560–568.

Balfour, D. J. (1989). Influence of nicotine on the release of monoamines in the brain. *Progress in Brain Research, 79,* 165–172.

Becker, J. B. (1999). Gender differences in dopaminergic function in striatum and nucleus accumbens. *Pharmacology, Biochemistry, and Behavior, 64*(4), 803–812.

Becker, J. B., Molenda, H., & Hummer, D. L. (2001). Gender differences in the behavioral responses to cocaine and amphetamine. Implications for mechanisms mediating gender differences in drug abuse. *Annual NY Academy of Sciences, 937,* 172–187.

Bepko, C. (1991). Disorders of power: Women and addiction in the family. In M. McGoldrick, C. M. Anderson, & F. Walsh (Eds.), *Women in families: A framework for family therapy* (pp. 406–426). New York: Norton.

Blanchard, D. C. (1998) Stress-related psychopathology as a vulnerability factor in drug-taking: The role of sex. In C. L. Weatherington & A. B. Roman (Eds.), *Drug addiction research and the health of women* (pp. 151–164). Washington, DC: National Institute on Drug Abuse.

Brady, K. T., & Sinha, R. (2005). Co-occurring mental and substance use disorders: The neurobiological effects of chronic stress. *American Journal of Psychiatry, 162*(8), 1483–1493.

Brady, K. T., Waldrop, A. E., McRae, A. L., Back, S. E., Saladin, M. E., Upadhyaya, H. P., et al. (2006). The impact of alcohol dependence and posttraumatic stress disorder on cold pressor task response. *Journal of Studies on Alcohol, 67*(5), 700–706.

Brebner, J. (2003). Gender and emotions. *Personality and Individual Differences, 34,* 387–394.

Breese, G. R., Chu, K., Dayas, C. V., Funk, D., Knapp, D. J., Koob, G. F., et al. (2005). Stress enhancement of craving during sobriety: A risk for relapse. *Alcoholism: Clinical and Experimental Research*, 29(2), 185–195.

Carroll, K. M., Sinha, R., Nich, C., Babuscio, T., & Rounsaville, B. J. (2002). Contingency management to enhance naltrexone treatment of opioid dependence: A randomized clinical trial of reinforcement magnitude. *Experimental and Clinical Psychopharmacology*, 10, 54–63.

Carroll, M. E., Anderson, M. M., & Morgan, A. D. (2007). Higher locomotor response to cocaine in female (vs. male) rats selectively bred for high (HiS) and low (LoS) saccharin intake. *Pharmacology, Biochemistry, and Behavior*, 88(1), 94–104.

Chaplin, T., Hong, K.-I., Bergquist, K., & Sinha, R. (2007). Sex differences in stress- and alcohol cue-induced craving and emotion in social drinkers. *Alcoholism: Clinical and Experimental Research*, 31(6), 603.

Costa, A., Bono, G., Martignoni, E., Merlo, P., Sances, G., & Nappi, G. (1996). An assessment of hypothalamo–pituitary–adrenal axis functioning in non-depressed, early abstinent alcoholics. *Psychoneuroendocrinology*, 21(3), 263–275.

Dai, X., Thavundayil, J., & Gianoulakis, C. (2002). Response of the hypothalamic–pituitary–adrenal axis to stress in the absence and presence of ethanol in subjects at high and low risk of alcoholism. *Neuropsychopharmacology*, 27(3), 442–452.

Del Rio, G., Velardo, A., Menozzi, R., Zizzo, G., Tavernari, V., Venneri, M. G., et al. (1998). Acute estradiol and progesterone administration reduced cardiovascular and catecholamine responses to mental stress in menopausal women. *Neuroendocrinology*, 67(4), 269–274.

Deroche, V., Marinelli, M., Maccari, S., Le Moal, M., Simon, H., & Piazza, P. V. (1995). Stress-induced sensitization and glucocorticoids. I. Sensitization of dopamine-dependent locomotor effects of amphetamine and morphine depends on stress-induced corticosterone secretion. *Journal of Neuroscience*, 15(11), 7181–7188.

Deutch, A. Y., & Roth, R. H. (1990). The determinants of stress-induced activation of the prefrontal cortical dopamine system. *Progress in Brain Research*, 85, 367–402.

Donny, E. C., Caggiula, A. R., Rowell, P. P., Gharib, M. A., Maldovan, V., & Booth, S., et al. (2000). Nicotine self-administration in rats: Estrous cycle effects, sex differences and nicotinic receptor binding. *Psychopharmacology*, 151, 392–405.

Dorn, L. D., Burgess, E. S., Susman, E. J., von Eye, A., DeBellis, M. D., Gold, P. W., et al. (1996). Response to oCRH in depressed and nondepressed adolescents: Does gender make a difference? *Journal of the American Academy of Child and Adolescent Psychiatry*, 35, 764–773.

Earle, T. L., Linden, W., & Weinberg, J. (1999). Differential effects of harassment on cardiovascular and salivary cortisol stress reactivity and recovery in women and men. *Journal of Psychosomatic Research*, 46, 125–141.

Errico, A. L., Parsons, O. A., King, A. C., & Lovallo, W. R. (1993). Attenuated cortisol response to biobehavioral stressors in sober alcoholics. *Journal of Studies on Alcohol*, 54(4), 393–398.

Evans, S. M. (2007). The role of estradiol and progesterone in modulating the subjective effects of stimulants in humans. *Experimental and Clinical Psychopharmacology*, 15(5), 418–426. (*)

Evans, S. M., & Foltin, R. W. (2006). Exogenous progesterone attenuates the subjective effects of smoked cocaine in women, but not in men. *Neuropsychopharmacology*, 31(3), 659–674.

Evans, S. M., Haney, M., & Foltin, R. W. (2002). The effects of smoked cocaine during the follicular and luteal phases of the menstrual cycle in women. *Psychopharmacology (Berl)*, 159, 397–406.

Faraday, M. M., Blakeman, K. H., & Grunberg, N. E. (2005). Strain and sex alter effects of stress and nicotine on feeding, body weight, and HPA axis hormones. *Pharmacology, Biochemistry, and Behavior*, 80(4), 577–589.

Faraday, M. M., O'Donoghue, V. A., & Grunberg, N. E. (2003). Effects of nicotine and stress on locomotion in Sprague–Dawley and Long–Evans male and female rats. *Pharmacology, Biochemistry, and Behavior*, 74(2), 325–333.

Fillmore, K. M., Golding, J. M., & Leino, E. V. (1997). Patterns and trends in women's and men's drinking. In R. W. Wilsnack & S. C. Wilsnack (Eds.), *Gender and alcohol: Individual and social perspectives* (pp. 21–48). New Brunswick, NJ: Rutgers Center of Alcohol Studies.

Fischer, A. H., Mosquera, P. M. R., van Vianen, A. E. M., & Manstead, A. S. R. (2004). Gender and culture differences in emotion. *Emotion, 4,* 87–94.

Fox, H. C., Berquist, K. L., Hong, K. I., & Sinha, R. (2007). Stress-induced and alcohol cue-induced craving in recently abstinent alcohol dependent individuals. *Alcoholism: Clinical and Experimental Research, 31*(3), 395–403.

Fox, H. C., Garcia, M., Kemp, K., Milivojevic, V., Kreek, M. J., & Sinha, R. (2006). Gender differences in cardiovascular and corticoadrenal response to stress and drug-cue in cocaine dependent individuals. *Psychopharmacology, 185*(3), 348–357. (*)

Fox, H. C., Hong, K. A., Paliwal, P., Morgan, P. T., & Sinha, R. (2008a). Altered levels of sex and stress hormones assessed daily over a 28-day cycle in early abstinent cocaine dependent females. *Psychopharmacology, 195,* 527–536.

Fox, H. C., Hong, K.-I., Siedlarz, K. M., & Sinha, R. (2008b). Enhanced sensitivity to stress and drug/alcohol craving in abstinent cocaine dependent individuals compared to social drinkers. *Neuropsychopharmacology, 33,* 796–805.

Fox, H. C., & Sinha, R. (2007, July). *Gender differences in neurobiological response to stress and alcohol cues: implications for treatment and relapse.* Paper presented at the Annual Meetings of the Research Society of Alcoholism, Chicago, IL.

Fox, H. C., Talih, M., Malison, R., Anderson, G. M., Kreek, M. J., & Sinha, R. (2005). Frequency of recent cocaine and alcohol use affects drug craving and associated responses to stress and to drug-related cues. *Psychoneuroendocrinology, 30,* 880–891.

Frankenhaeuser, M., von Wright, M. R., Collins, A., von Wright, J., Sedvall, G., & Swahn, C. G. (1978). Sex differences in psychoneuroendocrine reactions to examination stress. *Psychosomatic Medicine, 40,* 334–343.

Freed, B. G. (1985). Drug misuse and dependency in women: The meaning and implications of being considered a special population or minority group. *International Journal of the Addictions, 20*(1), 13–62.

Galard, R., Gallart, J. M., Catalan, R., Schwartz, S., Anguello, J. M., & Castellanos, J. M. (1991). Salivary cortisol levels and their correlation with plasma ACTH levels in depressed patients before and after the DST. *American Journal of Psychiatry, 148,* 505–508.

Gianoulakis, C., Dai, X., & Brown, T. (2003). Effect of chronic alcohol consumption on the activity of the hypothalamic–pituitary–adrenal axis and pituitary beta-endorphin as a function of alcohol intake, age, and gender. *Alcoholism: Clinical and Experimental Research, 27*(3), 410–423.

Gianoulakis, C., Krishnan, B., & Thavundayil, J. (1996). Enhanced sensivity of pituitary beta-endorphin to ethanol in subjects at high risk of alcoholism. *Archives of General Psychiatry, 53*(3), 250–257.

Girdler, S. S., & Klatzkin, R. (2007). Neurosteroids in the context of stress: Implications for depressive disorders. *Pharmacology & Therapeutics, 116*(1), 125–139.

Glassman, A. H., Covey, L. S., Dalack, G. W., Stetner, F., Rivelli, S. K., Fleiss, J., et al. (1993). Smoking cessation, clonidine, and vulnerability to nicotine among dependent smokers. *Clinical Pharmacology and Therapeutics, 54*(6), 670–679.

Grant, B. F., Dawson, D. A., Stinson, F. S., Chou, S. P., Dufour, M. C., & Pickering, R. P. (2004). The 12-month prevalence and trends in DSM-IV alcohol abuse and dependence: United States, 1991–1992 and 2001–2002. *Drug and Alcohol Dependence, 74*(3), 223–234.

Green, J. P., Lynn, S. J., & Montgomery, G. H. (2008). Gender-related differences in hypnosis-based treatments for smoking: A follow-up meta-analysis. *American Journal of Clinical Hypnosis, 50*(3), 259–271.

Greenfield, S. F., Trucco, E. M., McHugh, R. K., Lincoln, M., & Gallop, R. J. (2007). The Women's Recovery Group Study: A Stage I trial of women-focused group therapy for substance use disorders versus mixed-gender group drug counseling. *Drug and Alcohol Dependence, 90*(1), 39–47.

Gulinello, M., Gong, Q. H., Li, X., & Smith, S. S. (2001). Short-term exposure to a neuroactive steroid increases alpha4 GABA(A) receptor subunit levels in association with increased anxiety in the female rat. *Brain Research, 910*(1/2), 55–66.

Handa, R. J., Burgess, L. H., Kerr, J. E., & O'Keefe, J. A. (1994). Gonadal steroid hormone receptors and sex differences in the hypothalamo–pituitary–adrenal axis. *Hormones and Behavior*, *28*, 464–476.

Hansen, S., Fahlke, C., Söderpalm, A. H., & Hård, E. (1995). Significance of adrenal corticosteroid secretion for the food restriction-induced enhancement of alcohol drinking in the rat. *Psychopharmacology (Berl)*, *121*(2), 213–221.

Harrod, S. B., Booze, R. M., Welch, M., Browning, C. E., & Mactutus, C. F. (2005). Acute and repeated intravenous cocaine-induced locomotor activity is altered as a function of sex and gonadectomy. *Pharmacology, Biochemistry, and Behavior*, *82*(1), 170–181.

Harrod, S. B., Mactutus, C. F., Bennett, K., Hasselrot, U., Wu, G., Welch, M., et al. (2004). Sex differences and repeated intravenous nicotine: Behavioral sensitization and dopamine receptors. *Pharmacology, Biochemistry, and Behavior*, *78*(3), 581–592.

Heinsbroek, R. P., van Haaren, F., Feenstra, M. G., Boon, P., & van de Poll, N. E. (1991b). Controllable and uncontrollable footshock and monoaminergic activity in the frontal cortex of male and female rats. *Brain Research*, *551*(1/2), 247–255.

Heinsbroek, R. P., van Haaren, F., Feenstra, M. G., van Galen, H., Boer, G., & van de Poll, N. E. (1990). Sex differences in the effects of inescapable footshock on central catecholaminergic and serotonergic activity. *Pharmacology, Biochemistry, and Behavior*, *37*(3), 539–550.

Heinsbroek, R. P., van Haaren, F., van de Poll, N. E., & Steenbergen, H. L. (1991a). Sex differences in the behavioral consequences of inescapable footshocks depend on time since shock. *Physiology & Behavior*, *49*(6), 1257–1263.

Higley, J. D., Hasert, M. F., Suomi, S. J., & Linnoila, M. (1991). Nonhuman primate model of alcohol abuse: Effects of early experience, personality, and stress on alcohol consumption. *Proceedings of the National Academy of Sciences USA*, *88*(16), 7261–7265.

Horrocks, P. M., Jones, A. F., Ratcliffe, W. A., Holder, G., White, A., Holder, R., et al. (1990). Patterns of ACTH and cortisol pulsatility over twenty-four hours in normal males and females. *Clinical Endocrinology (Oxf)*, *32*, 127–134.

Hu, M., Crombag, H. S., Robinson, T. E., & Becker, J. B. (2004). Biological basis of sex differences in the propensity to self-administer cocaine. *Neuropsychopharmacology*, *29*, 81–85.

Inder, W. J., Joyce, P. R., Wells, J. E., Evans, M. J., Ellis, M. J., Mattioli, L., et al. (1995). The acute effects of oral ethanol on the hypothalamic–pituitary–adrenal axis in normal human subjects. *Clinical Endocrinology (Oxf)*, *42*(1), 65–71.

Junghanns, K., Backhaus, J., Tietz, U., Lange, W., Bernzen, J., Wetterling, T., et al. (2003). Impaired serum cortisol stress response is a predictor of early relapse. *Alcohol and Alcoholism*, *38*(2), 189–193.

Junghanns, K., Tietz, U., Dibbelt, L., Kuether, M., Jurth, R., Ehrenthal, D., et al. (2005). Attenuated salivary cortisol secretion under cue exposure is associated with early relapse. *Alcohol and Alcoholism*, *40*(1), 80–85.

Justice, A. J. H., & de Wit, H. (1999). Acute doses of *d*-amphetamine during the early and late follicular phases of the menstrual cycle in women. *Psychopharmacology*, *145*, 67–75.

Justice, A. J. H., & de Wit, H. (2000a). Acute effects of *d*-amphetamine during the early and late follicular phases of the menstrual cycle in women. *Pharmacology, Biochemistry, and Behavior*, *66*(3), 509–515.

Justice, A. J. H., & de Wit, H. (2000b). Acute effects of estradiol pretreatment on the response to d-amphetamine in women. *Neuroendocrinology*, *71*(1), 51–59.

Kajantie, E., & Phillips, D. I. (2006). The effects of sex and hormonal status on the physiological response to acute psychosocial stress. *Psychoneuroendocrinology*, *31*(2), 151–178. (*)

Kauffman, E., Dore, M. M., & Nelson-Zlupko, L. (1995). The role of women's therapy groups in the treatment of chemical dependence. *American Journal of Orthopsychiatry*, *65*(3), 355–363.

Kawakami, S. E., Quadros, I. M., Takahashi, S., & Suchecki, D. (2007). Long maternal separation accelerates behavioural sensitization to ethanol in female, but not in male mice. *Behavioral Brain Research*, *184*(2), 109–116.

Kessler, R. C., Crum, R. M., Warner, L. A., Nelson, C. B., Schulenberg, J., & Anthony, J. C. (1997). Lifetime co-occurrence of DSM-III-R alcohol abuse and dependence with other psychiatric disorders in the National Comorbidity Survey. *Archives of General Psychiatry*, *54*(4), 313–321.

Kirschbaum, C., Kudielka, B. M., Gaab, J., Schommer, N. C., & Hellhammer, D. H. (1999). Impact of gender, menstrual cycle phase, and oral contraceptives on the activity of the hypothalamus–pituitary–adrenal axis. *Psychosomatic Medicine, 61*, 154–162.

Kirschbaum, C., Prüssner, J. C., Stone, A. A., Federenko, I. , Gaab, J., Lintz, D., et al. (1995). Persistent high cortisol responses to repeated psychological stress in a subpopulation of healthy men. *Psychosomatic Medicine, 57*(5), 468–474.

Kirschbaum, C., Wust, S., & Hellhammer, D. (1992). Consistent sex differences in cortisol responses to psychological stress. *Psychosomatic Medicine, 54*, 648–657.

Koob, G. F., & Le Moal, M. (2005). Plasticity of reward neurocircuitry and the 'dark side' of drug addiction. *Nature Neuroscience, 8*(11), 1442–1444.

Kudielka, B. M., Hellhammer, J., Hellhammer, D. H., Wolf, O. T., Pirke, K. M., Varadi, E., et al. (1998). Sex differences in endocrine and psychological responses to psychosocial stress in healthy elderly subjects and the impact of a 2-week dehydroepiandrosterone treatment. *Journal of Clinical Endocrinology and Metabolism, 83*, 1756–1761.

Kudielka, B. M., & Kirschbaum, C. (2005). Sex differences in HPA axis responses to stress: A review. *Biological Psychology, 69*, 113–132. (*)

Kutscher, S., Heise, D. J., Banger, M., Saller, B., Michel, M. C., Gastpar, M., et al. (2002). Concomitant endocrine and immune alterations during alcohol intoxication and acute withdrawal in alcohol-dependent subjects. *Neuropsychobiology, 45*(3), 144–149.

Lamblin, F., & De Witte, P. (1996). Adrenalectomy prevents the development of alcohol preference in male rats. *Alcohol, 13*(3), 233–238.

Lieber, C. S. (1997). Gender differences in alcohol metabolism and susceptibility. In R. W. Wilsnack & S. C. Wilsnack (Eds.), *Gender and alcohol: Individual and social perspectives* (pp. 77–89). New Brunswick, NJ: Rutgers Center of Alcohol Studies.

Lindheim, S. R., Legro, R. S., Morris, R. S., Wong, I. L., Tran, D. Q., Vijod, M. A., et al. (1994). *Journal of the Society for Gynecologic Investigation, 1*(1), 79–83.

Lovallo, W. R., Dickensheets, S. L., Myers, D. A., Thomas, T. L., & Nixon, S. J. (2000). Blunted stress cortisol response in abstinent alcoholic and polysubstance-abusing men. *Alcoholism: Clinical and Experimental Research, 24*(5), 651–658.

Lynch, W. J. (2006). Sex differences in vulnerability to drug self-administration. *Experimental Clinical Psychopharmacology, 14*(1), 34–41.

Lynch, W. J., Arizzi, M. N., & Carroll, M. E. (2002). Effects of sex and the estrous cycle on regulation of intravenously self-administered cocaine in rats. *Psychopharmacology, 152*(2), 132–139.

Lynch, W. J., & Carroll, M. E. (1999). Sex differences in the acquisition of intravenously self-administered cocaine and heroin in rats. *Psychopharmacology (Berl), 144*(1), 77–82.

Matthews, K. A., Gump, B. B., & Owens, J. F. (2001). Chronic stress influences cardiovascular and neuroendocrine responses during acute stress and recovery, especially in men. *Health Psychology, 20*, 403–410.

McCance-Katz, E. F., Hart, C. L., Boyarsky, B., Kosten, T., & Jatlow, P. (2005). Gender effects following repeated administration of cocaine and alcohol in humans. *Substance Use and Misuse, 40*(4), 511–528.

McCormick, C. M., & Mathews, I. Z. (2007). HPA function in adolescence: Role of sex hormones in its regulation and the enduring consequences of exposure to stressors. *Pharmacology, Biochemistry, and Behavior, 86*(2), 220–233.

Mello, N. K. (1988). Effects of alcohol abuse on reproductive function in women. *Recent Developments in Alcoholism, 6*, 253–276.

Moran, M. H., Goldberg, M., & Smith, S. S. (1998). Progesterone withdrawal: II. Insensitivity to the sedative effects of a benzodiazepine. *Brain Research, 807*(1–2), 91–100.

Nich, C., McCance-Katz, E. F., Petrakis, I. L., Cubells, J. F., Rounsaville, B. J., & Carroll, K. M. (2004). Sex differences in cocaine-dependent individuals' response to disulfiram treatment. *Addictive Behaviors, 29*(6), 1123–1128.

Norman, R. L., Smith, C. J., Pappas, J. D., & Hall, J. (1992). Exposure to ovarian steroids elicits a female pattern of cortisol levels in castrated males macaques. *Steroids, 57*, 37–43.

Ogilvie, K. M., & Rivier, C. (1997). Gender difference in hypothalamic–pituitary–adrenal axis response to alcohol in the rat: Activational role of gonadal steroids. *Brain Research*, 766(1–2), 19–28.

O'Malley, S. S., Krishnan-Sarin, S., Farren, C., Sinha, R., & Kreek, M. J. (2002). Naltrexone decreases craving and alcohol self-administration in alcohol-dependent subjects and activates the hypothalamo–pituitary–adrenocortical axis. *Psychopharmacology* (Berl), 160(1), 19–29.

Perkins, K. A. (2001). Smoking cessation in women: Special consideration. *CNS Drugs*, 15(5), 391–411.

Piazza, P. V., Deroche, V., Deminière, J. M., Maccari, S., Le Moal, M., & Simon, H. (1993). Corticosterone in the range of stress-induced levels possesses reinforcing properties: Implications for sensation-seeking behaviors. *Proceedings of the National Academy of Sciences USA*, 90(24), 11738–11742.

Piazza, P. V., & Le Moal, M. (1997). Glucocorticoids as a biological substrate of reward: Physiological and pathophysiological implications. *Brain Research Reviews*, 25(3), 359–372.

Piazza, P. V., Maccari, S., Deminière, J. M., Le Moal, M., Mormède, P., & Simon, H. (1991). Corticosterone levels determine individual vulnerability to amphetamine self-administration. *Proceedings of the National Academy of Sciences USA*, 88(6), 2088–2092.

Piko, B. F., Wills, T. A., & Walker, C. (2007). Motives for smoking and drinking: Country and gender differences in samples of Hungarian and U.S. high school students. *Addictive Behaviors*, 32(10), 2087–2098.

Pomerleau, O. F., & Pomerleau, C. S. (1990). Cortisol response to a psychological stressor and/or nicotine. *Pharmacology, Biochemistry, and Behavior*, 36(1), 211–213.

Prasad, C., & Prasad, A. (1995). A relationship between increased voluntary alcohol preference and basal hypercorticosteronemia associated with an attenuated rise in corticosterone output during stress. *Alcohol*, 12(1), 59–63.

Quinones-Jenab, V. (2006). Why are women from Venus and men from Mars when they abuse cocaine? *Brain Research*, 1126(1), 200–203.

Rivier, C. (1999). Gender, sex steroids, corticotropin-releasing factor, nitric oxide, and the HPA response to stress. *Pharmacology, Biochemistry, and Behavior*, 64(4), 739–751.

Roca, C. A., Schmidt, P. J., & Rubinow, D. R. (1999). Gonadal steroids and affective illness. *The Neuroscientist*, 5(4), 227–237.

Roelfsema, F., Pincus, S. M., & Veldhuis, J. D. (1998). Patients with Cushing's disease secrete adrenocorticotropin and cortisol jointly more asynchronously than healthy subjects. *Journal of Clinical Endocrinology and Metabolism*, 83, 688–692.

Roelfsema, F., van den Berg, G., Frolich, M., Veldhuis, J. D., van Eijk, A., Buurman, M. M., & Etman, B. H. (1993). Sex-dependent alteration in cortisol response to endogenous adrenocorticotropin. *Journal of Clinical Endocrinology Metabolism*, 77, 234–240.

Roth, M. E., & Carroll, M. E. (2004). Sex differences in the acquisition of IV methamphetamine self-administration and subsequent maintenance under a progressive ratio schedule in rats. *Psychopharmacology*, 172, 443–449.

Rounsaville, B. J., Anton, S. F., Carroll, K., Budde, D., Prusoff, B. A., & Gawin, F. (1991). Psychiatric diagnoses of treatment-seeking cocaine abusers. *Archives of General Psychiatry*, 48(1), 43–51.

Russell, M., Light, J. M., & Gruenewald, P. J. (2004). Alcohol consumption and problems: The relevance of drinking patterns. *Alcoholism: Clinical and Experimental Research*, 28(6), 921–930.

Russo, S. J., Jenab, S., Fabian, S. J., Festa, E. D., Kemen, L. M., & Quinones-Jenab, V. (2003). Sex differences in the conditioned rewarding effects of cocaine. *Brain Research*, 970(1–2), 214–220.

Sarnyai, Z., Mello, N. K., Mendelson, J. H., Erös-Sarnyai, M., & Mercer, G. (1996). Effects of cocaine on pulsatile activity of hypothalamic–pituitary–adrenal axis in male rhesus monkeys: Neuroendocrine and behavioral correlates. *Journal of Pharmacology Experimental Therapeutics*, 277(1), 225–234.

Sarnyai, Z., Shaham, Y., & Heinrichs, S. C. (2001). The role of cortocotropin-releasing factor in drug addiction. *Pharmocological Reviews*, 53(2), 209–243.

Schleifer, L. A., Justice, A. J., & de Wit, H. (2002). Lack of effects of acute estradiol on mood in postmenopausal women. *Pharmacology, Biochemistry, and Behavior*, 71, 71–77.

Seeman, T. E., Singer, B., Wilkinson, C. W., & McEwen, B. (2001). Gender differences in age-related changes in HPA axis reactivity. *Psychoneuroendocrinology, 26,* 225–240.

Seyler, L. E., Jr., Fertig, J., Pomerleau, O., Hunt, D., & Parker, K. (1984). The effects of smoking on ACTH and cortisol secretion. *Life Sciences, 34*(1), 57–65.

Shaham, Y., Erb, S., & Stewart, J. (2000). Stress-induced relapse to heroin and cocaine seeking in rats: A review. *Brain Research Review, 33*(1), 13–33.

Shalev, U., Grimm, J. W., & Shaham, Y. (2002). Neurobiology of relapse to heroin and cocaine seeking: A review. *Pharmacological Reviews, 54*(1), 1–42.

Sinha, R. (2001). How does stress increase risk of drug abuse and relapse? *Psychopharmacology (Berl), 158,* 343–59.

Sinha, R., Fox, H. C., Paliwal, P., Hong, K. A., Morgan, P. T., & Bergquist, K. L. (2007). Sex steroid hormones, stress response and drug craving in cocaine dependent women: Implications for relapse susceptibility. *Experimental and Clinical Psychopharmacology, 15*(5), 445–52. (*)

Sinha, R., Fox, H. C., Hong, K. A. Bergquist, K. L., Bhagnagan, Z., & Siedlarz, K. M. (2008). Enhanced negative emotion and alcohol craving, and altered physiological responses following stress and cue exposure in alcohol dependent individuals. *Neuropsychopharmacology,* June 18 (Epubahead of print).

Sinha, R., Fuse, T., Aubin, L. R., & O'Malley, S. S. (2000). Psychological stress, drug-related cues and cocaine craving. *Psychopharmacology (Berl), 152,* 140–148.

Sinha, R., Garcia, M., Paliwal, P., Kreek, M. J., & Rounsaville, B. J. (2006). Stress-induced cocaine craving and hypothalamic–pituitary–adrenal responses are predictive of cocaine relapse outcomes. *Archives of General Psychiatry, 63*(3), 324–331.

Sinha, R., & Rounsaville, B. J. (2002). Sex differences in depressed substance abusers. *Clinical Psychiatry, 63*(7), 616–627.

Sinha, R., Talih, M., Malison, R., Cooney, N., Anderson, G. M., & Kreek, M. J. (2003). Hypothalamic–pituitary–adrenal axis and sympatho–adreno–medullary responses during stress-induced and drug cue-induced cocaine craving states. *Psychopharmacology (Berl), 170,* 62–72.

Smith, C. J., & Norman, R. L. (1987). Influence of the gonads on cortisol secretion in female rhesus macaques. *Endocrinology, 121*(6), 2192–2188.

Smith, S. S., Gong, Q. H., Li, X., Moran, M. H., Bitran, D., Frye, C. A., & et al. (1998). Withdrawal from 3alpha-OH-5alpha-pregnan-20-One using a pseudopregnancy model alters the kinetics of hippocampal GABAA-gated current and increases the GABAA receptor alpha4 subunit in association with increased anxiety. *Journal of Neuroscience, 18*(14), 5275–5284.

Sofuoglu, M., Babb, D. A., & Hatsukami, D. K. (2002). Effects of progesterone treatment on smoked cocaine response in women. *Pharmacology, Biochemistry, and Behavior, 72*(1–2), 431–435.

Sofuoglu, M., Dudish-Poulsen, S., Nelson, D., Pentel, P. R., & Hatsukami, D. K. (1999). Sex and menstrual cycle differences in the subjective effects from smoked cocaine in humans. *Experimental and Clinical Psychopharmacology, 7*(3), 274–283.

Sofuoglu, M., Mitchell, E., & Kosten, T. R. (2004). Effects of progesterone treatment on cocaine responses in male and female cocaine users. *Pharmacology, Biochemistry, and Behavior, 78*(4), 699–705.

Sonne, S. C., Back, S. E., Diaz Zuniga, C., Randall, C. L., & Brady, K. T. (2003). Gender differences in individuals with comorbid alcohol dependence and post-traumatic stress disorder. *American Journal of Addiction, 12*(5), 412–423.

Sorg, B. A., & Steketee, J. D. (2002). Mechanisms of cocaine-induced sensitization. *Progress in Neuropsychopharmacology and Biological Psychiatry, 16*(6), 1003–1012.

Sorocco, K. H., Lovallo, W. R., Vincent, A. S., & Collins, F. L. (2006). Blunted hypothalamic–pituitary–adrenocortical axis responsivity to stress in persons with a family history of alcoholism. *International Journal of Psychophysiology, 59*(3), 210–217.

Stewart, J. (2000). Pathways to relapse: The neurobiology of drug- and stress-induced relapse to drug-taking. *Journal of Psychiatry and Neuroscience, 25*(2), 125–136.

Stroud, L. R., Salovey, P., & Epel, E. S. (2002). Sex differences in stress responses: Social rejection versus achievement stress. *Biological Psychiatry, 52*(4), 318–327.

Teoh, S. K., Lex, B. W., Mendelson, J. H., Mello, N. K., & Cochin, J. (1992). Hyperprolactinemia and macrocytosis in women with alcohol and polysubstance dependence. *Journal of Studies on Alcohol, 53*(2), 176–182.

Terner, J. M., & de Wit, H. (2006). Menstrual cycle phase and responses to drugs of abuse in humans. *Drug and Alcohol Dependence, 84*(1), 1–13.

Tersman, Z., Collins, A., & Eneroth, P. (1991). Cardiovascular responses to psychological and physiological stressors during the menstrual cycle. *Psychosomatic Medicine, 53*(2), 185–197.

Turnbull, J. E., & Gomberg, E. S. (1991). The structure of drinking-related consequences in alcoholic women. *Alcoholism: Clinical and Experimental Research, 15*, 29–38.

van Haaren, F., & Meyer, M. E. (1991). Sex differences in locomotor activity after acute and chronic cocaine administration. *Pharmacology, Biochemistry, and Behavior, 39*(4), 923–927.

Walter, H., Dvorak, A., Gutierrez, K., Zitterl, W., & Lesch, O. M. (2005). Gender differences: Does alcohol affect females more than males? *Neuropsychopharmacology (Hung), 7*(2), 78–82.

Wand, G. S., & Dobs, A. S. (1991). Alterations in the hypothalamic–pituitary–adrenal axis in actively drinking alcoholics. *Journal of Clinical Endocrinology and Metabolism, 72*(6), 1290–1295.

Ward, A. S., Haney, M., Fischman, M. W., & Foltin, R. W. (1997). Binge cocaine self-administration in humans: Intravenous cocaine. *Psychopharmacology (Berl), 132*(4), 375–381.

White, T. L., Justice, A. J., & de Wit, H. (2002). Differential subjective effects of *d*-amphetamine by gender, hormone levels, and menstrual cycle phase. *Pharmacology, Biochemistry, and Behavior, 73*(4), 729–741.

Wisniewski, A. B., Brown, T. T., John, M., Cofranceso, J., Jr., Golub, E. T., Ricketts, E. P., et al. (2006). Cortisol levels and depression in men and women using heroin and cocaine. *Psychoneuroendocrinology, 31*(2), 250–255.

Wileyto, E. P., Patterson, F., Niaura, R., Epstein, L. H., Brown, R. A., Audrain-McGovern, J., et al. (2005). Recurrent event analysis of lapse and recovery in a smoking cessation clinical trial using bupropion. *Nicotine Tobacco Research, 7*(2), 257–268.

Wilsnack, S. (1996). Patterns and trends in women's drinking: Recent findings and some implications for prevention. In J. Howard, S. Martin, P. Mail, M. Hilton, & E. Taylor (Eds.), *Women and alcohol: Issues for prevention research monograph #32* (NIH Pub No. 96-3817, pp. 19–63). Bethesda, MD: U.S. Department of Health and Human Services, Public Health Service, National Institutes of Health, National Institute on Alcohol Abuse and Alcoholism.

Yoshimura, S., Sakamoto, S., Kudo, H., Sassa, S., Kumai, A., & Okamoto, R. (2003). Sex-differences in adrenocortical responsiveness during development in rats. *Steroids, 68*(5), 439–445.

Young, E. A. (1995). The role of gonadal steroids in hypothalamic–pituitary–adrenal axis regulation. *Critical Reviews in Neurobiology, 9*, 371–381.

Zimmer, C., Basler, H. D., Vedder, H., & Lautenbacher, S. (2003). Sex differences in cortisol response to noxious stress. *Clinical Journal of Pain, 19*, 233–239.

CHAPTER 5

Sex Differences in the Transmission of Substance Use Disorders

Amanda Kalaydjian, PhD
Kathleen Ries Merikangas, PhD

Substance use disorders (SUDs), broadly defined, are among the most pervasive psychiatric disorders in society. According to findings from the 2006 National Survey on Drug Use and Health, an annual survey of approximately 67,500 people, approximately 22.6 million persons, or 9.2% of the population ages 12 and older, have had either substance abuse or dependence problems within the past year (Substance Abuse and Mental Health Services [SAMHSA], 2007). Community surveys of the United States have consistently found that substance use disorders are more common in males than in females (Kessler et al., 2005). However, although males are more likely to suffer from substance abuse or dependence (12.3% of males), these problems affect a substantial proportion of women as well (6.3% of women) (SAMHSA, 2007). Of women 12 years and older, past-year abuse of or dependence on illicit drugs was reported by 2.0%, and of alcohol by 5.1%, of respondents (SAMHSA, 2007).

The strikingly high number of women who develop addictions to substances and the high rate at which young girls are being exposed highlight the need to better understand the etiology of SUDs in women. Although the majority of women who engage in recreational and/or experimental substance use will not go on to develop SUDs, it is vital to understand the factors that influence initiation of substance use in women and determine progression to more problematic levels of use. According to a poll conducted by the Harvard School of Public Health/Robert Wood Johnson Foundation and International Communications Research in 2000, Americans view SUDs as one of the most serious public health problems facing our nation. Women face a unique set of issues and consequences with regards to substance use. Accumulating evidence suggests that substance use negatively impacts women's health at higher rates than men (Ashley et al., 1977; Conner et al., 2007). Given the increasing number of women struggling with substance-use-related problems, these issues have a direct and immediate impact on the public health of women across the United States.

The goals of this chapter are (1) to introduce the concepts and challenges of genetic epidemiology of SUDs, (2) to review studies on the genetic epidemiology of SUDs, and (3) to examine whether there are sex differences in the transmission of SUDs in twin and family studies.

BACKGROUND: GENETIC EPIDEMIOLOGY OF SUDs

Genetic Epidemiology

With the increasing success in identifying genetic risk factors for complex disorders, population-based association studies will assume increasing importance in studying the role of genetic risk factors in the etiology and progression of complex human disorders (Khoury & Yang, 1998; Risch, 2000). Results from population-based epidemiological studies will be used to calculate the attributable, relative, and absolute risk of genetic factors identified in family-based linkage and association studies, thereby replacing the concept of heritability—a purely statistical concept—with information about relative risk to an individual and attributable risk in populations. Moreover, population based case–control studies will have an increasing role in the genome-wide search for susceptibility genes underlying complex human disorders.

There is increasing interest in regenerating the field of genetic epidemiology, which is distinguished from its parent disciplines of epidemiology and human genetics in three specific ways: (1) its focus on population-based research; (2) its goal of detecting the joint effects of genes and environment; and (3) the incorporation of the underlying biology of a disease into conceptual models (Merikangas & Risch, 2003).

The four major applications of genetic epidemiology that advance our understanding of SUDs are (1) the establishment of *population-based registries* of SUDs that will be increasingly valuable in validating the numerous genetic tests that will emerge from advances in human genetic research and the Human Genome Project (Lander et al., 2001); (2) identification of *more homogeneous subtypes* of complex disorders through family and high-risk research investigating both biological and contextual factors; (3) investigation of familial patterns among affected and unaffected probands to *estimate strength and mode of genetic transmission*; (4) *quantification of risk* at the levels of the individual and population (i.e., absolute risk, relative risk, attributable risk); and (5) development of a richer conceptualization of *environmental factors* that may be important mediators of expression of genetic risk for SUDs through integration of the tools of genetic epidemiology, behavioral neuroscience, developmental psychology, and neuroscience.

The field of genetic epidemiology focuses on the role of genetic factors that interact with other domains of risk to enhance vulnerability to, or protection against, disease. Genetic epidemiology employs traditional epidemiological study designs to identify explanatory factors for aggregation in groups of relatives ranging from twins to migrant cohorts. Because epidemiology has developed sophisticated designs and analytical methods for identifying disease risk factors, these methods have been extended to include both genes and environmental factors as gene identification proceeds (Kuller, 1979; MacMahon & Trichopoulos, 1996). In general, study designs in genetic epidemiology control for either genetic background while letting the environment vary (e.g., migrant studies, half-siblings, separated twins), or for the environment while allowing variance in the genetic background (e.g., siblings, twins, adopted–nonbiological siblings). Investigations in genetic epidemiology are typically based on a combination of study designs, including family, twin, and adoption studies.

Challenges in the Genetic Epidemiology of Substance Abuse

There are numerous challenges to research and interpretation of studies investigating the genetic epidemiology of substance abuse. These issues are described briefly below.

Phenotypic Definitions

Definitions of the thresholds of the various stages of substance use, including regular use, abuse, and dependence, have been highly controversial. One of the major impediments in elucidating the roles of gene and environment is that the criteria for SUDs in the DSM-IV are often marked by significant overlap, which calls into question whether these diagnoses really account for two fundamentally distinct disorders or whether they may be better explained by gradations of a single disorder on a continuum of severity. Phenotypic definition becomes especially problematic when studies use different measurement tools to reach diagnoses. For example, twin studies of smoking have examined diverse components of smoking, including use, frequency, quantity, age at onset, continued use, current use, current frequency, dependence, severity, and ability to quit (Heath & Madden, 1995); however, the consistency of these measures vary greatly by study. Finally, because the definitions of abuse and dependence are often influenced by cultural, social, and personal factors, aggregation of research across countries can be misleading and lead to biased and incorrect conclusions.

Age/Developmental Stage

Results from twin studies suggest that different factors may exert influence at distinct stages of development, and/or that certain developmental periods are more sensitive than others. For example, McGue et al. (1994) revealed far greater heritability of drug use disorders among males with an early age of onset compared to either females or those with a later age of onset. Since exposure to drugs generally occurs during early adolescence, the above-cited data, which were derived from adult samples, are necessarily susceptible to the biases of all retrospective studies. Further research on the joint influences of genetic, environmental, and developmental factors on persistence and dependence as individuals pass through the risk period for the development of substance dependence is warranted and promises to clarify the influences of age and developmental level in the etiology of SUDs.

Cohort and Generation Effects

One key source of complexity in studying the familial transmission of SUDs is the dramatic changes in availability and patterns of substance use in the general population as well as within specific subgroups. For example, whereas alcohol has been readily available during the past several decades, and cannabis has been somewhat stable as well, crack cocaine and ecstasy have been widely available only during the past decade. These differences contribute to the difficulty in discriminating exposed but unaffected relatives from those who were never exposed to a particular drug—an issue that poses major methodological challenges (Neale, Aggen, Maes, Kubarych, & Schmitt, 2006). Within-generation comparisons are more likely to control for exposure to specific substances. However, siblings are often responsible for the initiation of other siblings into substance use, and this could lead to overestimation of heritability.

Environmental Influences

The development of SUDs is heavily reliant on a myriad of environmental agents. Expression of an SUD is dependent upon environmental factors of exposure to the substance, family dynamics, peer interaction, temperament features, socioeconomic-related factors, and cultural norms, which all interact with the individual's genetic makeup to influence phenotypic expression (Avenevoli, Conway, & Merikangas, 2005; Brook, Brook, Gordon, Whiteman, & Cohen, 1990; Brook, Whiteman, Gordon, Nomura, & Brook, 1986; Brown, 1989; Simcha-Fagan & Schwartz, 1986). Because the development of an SUD is so heavily influenced by the gene–environment interaction and correlation, it is often tricky to disentangle genetic and environmental processes. Interestingly, a recent twin study reported heritability estimates from Norway (low illicit drug use) that were similar to those reported in the United States and Australia (high illicit drug use), thereby suggesting that heritability is unaffected by drug availability (Kendler, Aggen, Tambs, & Reichborn-Kjennerud, 2006).

Spouse Concordance

The tendency for spouses to be concordant for substance use is another issue that must be integrated in the evaluation of genetic evidence (Grant et al., 2007). Merikangas, Rounsaville, and Prusoff (1992) reported that more than 90% of interviewed opioid-dependent proband spouses had a history of opioid dependence. Furthermore, a strong association between rates of drug abuse in adult siblings of opioid abusers and the number of parents with SUDs was demonstrated. It is therefore critical that spouse concordance be incorporated into genetic analyses of SUDs.

Polysubstance Use

Another important factor in examining the role of genetic factors in SUDs is the tendency for substance abusers to misuse multiple substances, both simultaneously and longitudinally (Merikangas, Stolar, et al., 1998; Mirin, Weiss, Griffin, & Michael, 1991). One twin study of substance use revealed moderate heritability for the frequency of use and the tendency to use numerous illicit substances ($h^2 = .32$) (Jang, Livesley, & Vernon, 1995).

Comorbidity with Psychopathology

The comorbidity between substance use and psychiatric disorders is well documented. Some of the largest and most consistent findings have been reported between SUDs and antisocial personality disorder, mood disorders, and anxiety disorders (Compton, Conway, Stinson, Colliver, & Grant, 2005; Conway, Compton, Stinson, & Grant, 2006; Kessler et al., 1996; Regier et al., 1990). Ross, Glaser, and Germanson (1988) found that 78% of their treatment sample of patients with SUDs met DSM-III criteria for a lifetime comorbid psychiatric disorder.

SUMMARY OF GENETIC EPIDEMIOLOGICAL STUDIES OF SUDs

Despite the dramatic advances generated by the sequencing of human genes (Human Genome Project) and progress in the molecular biology of gene expression, the identification of specific genetic vulnerability factors for the development of SUDs will require a complex series of studies of multiple domains influencing susceptibility to SUDs. Unlike Mendelian diseases, wherein a specific gene mutation is directly associated with susceptibility to a particular disease, SUDs are multifactorial disorders that require environmental exposure to a particular substance as well as several different classes of genes involved in the metabolism and central nervous system (CNS) effects of substances. Whereas socioenvironmental factors play a key role in the initial use of a substance, an interaction between individual biological, physiological, psychological, and environmental processes are associated with the progression to more problematic use.

Family Studies

The family study design illustrates the magnitude of aggregation within families as well as the patterns of transmission of SUDs. This method compares the prevalence of a disorder in first-degree relatives of cases to the prevalence of the disorder in first-degree relatives of controls, who are often matched to cases on key characteristics such as age, gender, and psychiatric disorder. By nature, family studies encompass not only genetic effects but environmental and genetic–environmental effects as well. For example, assortative mating, which refers to the tendency of individuals to mate with others of similar traits, is a complex effect that has been shown to occur in families with alcohol dependence (Merikangas, 1990; Schuckit, Smith, Eng, & Kunovac, 2002; Schuckit, Tipp, & Kelner, 1994).

Through decades of research, the family study method has provided critical information regarding the aggregation of SUDs within families. Familial aggregation of alcoholism is well established (for reviews of alcoholism, see McGue, 1994; Merikangas, 1990). One of the most recent studies involved families ascertained through the Collaborative Study on the Genetics of Alcoholism (Collaborative Study) in which 8,296 relatives of probands with alcohol dependence and 1,654 controls reported lifetime risk rates for DSM-IV alcohol dependence of 28.8% and 14.4% in relatives of probands and controls, respectively (Nurnberger et al., 2004). This twofold increase in the risk of alcohol dependence is comparable to estimates reported from a previous family study conducted in the greater New Haven, Connecticut, area (Merikangas, Stolar, et al., 1998). Interestingly, DSM-IV alcohol abuse did not cluster in families (Nurnberger et al., 2004).

Although there has been less systematic research on the familial aggregation of drug use disorders, there is accumulating evidence that these disorders aggregate within families. Family history and uncontrolled family studies (Compton, Cottler, Ridenour, Ben-Abdallah, & Spitznagel, 2002; Croughan, 1985; Gfroerer, 1987; Meller, Rinehart, Cadoret, & Troughton, 1988; Mirin et al., 1991; Mirin, Weiss, Michael, & Griffin, 1988; Rounsaville et al., 1991), as well as controlled studies of first-degree relatives of people who abuse drugs (Bierut et al., 1998; Merikangas, Stolar, et al., 1998), consistently demonstrate that the rates of drug use disorders are elevated among relatives of those who abuse drugs compared to that of controls. The New Haven family study (Merikangas, Stolar, et al., 1998) found an eightfold increased risk of drug use disorders among relatives of probands with drug use disorders, as compared with relatives of psychiatric and unaffected controls (Merikangas, Stolar, et al., 1998). They also found evidence of specificity of familial aggregation of the predominant drug of abuse (Merikangas, Stolar, et al., 1998). However, there is also evidence of cross-transmission of addictive behaviors. Recent results from the Collaborative Study reported a twofold increase in the risk for any DSM-III-R diagnosis of nonalcohol, non-nicotine substance dependence in relatives of probands with alcohol dependence as compared to controls (Nurnberger et al., 2004). Although the influence of gender in the familial transmission of SUDs is unclear, several family studies examining sex differences in transmission are described in a later section.

High-Risk Studies

High-risk studies are a subset of family studies that examine the offspring of parents with SUDs. These studies provide valuable information on the order of onset and patterns of transitions across substance categories, as well as on risk factors for the development of SUDs. Several high-risk studies of children of people with alcohol dependence have demonstrated increased risk of alcoholism in these offspring (Chassin, Rogosch, & Barrera, 1991; Hill & Hruska, 1992; Johnson, Leonard, & Jacob, 1989; Merikangas, Dierker, & Szatmari, 1998b; Reich, Earls, Frankel, & Shayka, 1993; Schuckit & Smith, 1996; Sher, Walitzer, Wood, & Brent, 1991). A longitudinal study conducted by Chassin and colleagues (Chassin, Pitts, DeLucia, & Todd, 1999) also indicated that the effects of parental alcoholism on young-adult SUDs was specific and unique, above and beyond the effects of other parental psychopathology. An intriguing result to arise out of these studies is the association between a low level of response to alcohol in the children of parents with alcohol dependence and the development of alcohol use disorders, which has been especially noted for sons of those with alcohol dependence (Li, 2000; Schuckit & Smith, 1996). A recent study examined this phenomenon in women specifically by comparing daughters with, versus without, parents with alcohol dependence. They found that, similar to sons, daughters of parents with alcohol dependence were also more likely to have a low level of response to alcohol (Eng, Schuckit, & Smith, 2005), which could be one mechanism that increases their risk of developing alcohol dependence in the future.

Unlike the wealth of literature on the children of parents with alcohol dependence, there have been very few controlled studies of the offspring of parents who abuse drugs. Available studies have yielded consistent findings regarding an increased risk of SUDs among offspring of parents with SUDs compared to those of nonsubstance abusers (Martin et al., 1994; Merikangas, Dierker, et al., 1998; Moss, Majumder, & Vanyukov, 1994). In an 8-year follow-up study, offspring of individuals with SUDs had a twofold increased risk for any SUD and a threefold increased risk for alcohol and marijuana abuse or dependence compared to offspring of control parents (Merikangas & Avenevoli, 2000). Hopfer and colleagues (Hopfer, Stallings, Hewitt, & Crowley, 2003) also reported parent–child transmission for marijuana use, abuse, and dependence. Additionally, there is evidence of specificity of transmission, such that adolescents are particularly likely to use the same illicit drug as their parents.

High-risk studies are particularly informative for prevention efforts because they aid in the identification of premorbid vulnerability factors that serve as sources of identification for children at risk for particular disorders. One candidate risk factor is behavioral disinhibition, a trait-like dysfunction in the ability to control behavior that is socially undesirable or has adverse consequences (Gorenstein & Newman, 1980). Recent analyses of family study data similarly support a common neurobehavioral disinhibition factor underlying the risk for drug abuse and dependence, which includes a prominent component of impaired executive decision making in youths at risk for drug abuse. Unfortunately, these studies, and many others like them, were limited to boys; therefore, it remains to be determined if these same results apply to young girls as well.

There are numerous other mechanisms through which parents may convey an increased risk of SUDs to their offspring, including (1) serving as negative role models for the use/abuse of substances and using substances as a coping mechanism (Brook et al., 1986); (2) positive expectancies of the effects of substances (Conway, Swendsen, & Merikangas, 2003); and (3) making available and tolerating substance use in the home (Hawkins, Catalano, & Miller, 1992). Moreover, adolescents with a family history of SUDs are more likely to associate with deviant peers than those without a familial loading (Kandel & Andrews, 1987), indicating interplay between familial and peer influences. However, the manner in which gender may influence the impact of these factors on risk for SUDs is unclear.

Another consideration is that nearly all of the high-risk studies reveal that different risk factors may be involved across the different "stages" of development of SUDs. Whereas individual characteristics and peer influences strongly influence exposure to, and initial patterns of, substance use, family history and psychopathology play a more salient role in the transition to problematic alcohol use and dependence (Avenevoli et al., 2005; Cadoret, Troughton, O'Gorman, & Heywood, 1986). Studies of the differential influence of gender across stages of SUDs are lacking but necessary to gain further insight into unique and common factors in the development of SUDs in high-risk boys and girls.

Twin Studies

Although family and high-risk studies have been helpful in showing that genes may be involved in the development of SUDs, twin studies can provide actual estimates of heritability. Twin studies are informative because identical (monozygotic [MZ]) twins share 100% of their genes, whereas fraternal (dizygotic [DZ]) twins share, on average, 50% of their genes. If genetic factors play an important role in substance use and disorders, then studies of twins should find greater similarity between MZ than DZ twins, assuming that the influence of familial environment on substance use outcomes is equal for MZ and DZ twins. The aggregate twin study data are remarkably consistent in demonstrating that genetic factors play a far greater role in the etiology of more severe patterns of substance use, particularly abuse or dependence, as compared to initial use or early stages of use, which appear to be more strongly determined by environmental influences (Fowler et al., 2007; Kendler & Prescott, 1998b; Rhee et al., 2003; Tsuang et al., 1996). Twin studies have examined general substance use, abuse, and dependence (Grove et al., 1990; Jang et al., 1995; Kendler, Karkowski, Neale, & Prescott, 2000; Pickens et al., 1991), as well as a diverse range of specific substances, including nicotine, caffeine, sedatives, cannabis, cocaine, stimulants, hallucinogens, and opiates (Claridge, Ross, & Hume, 1978; Gurling, Grant, & Dangl, 1985; Heath et al., 1993; Heath & Madden, 1995; Kendler, Karkowski, & Prescott, 1999; Kendler et al., 2000; Kendler & Prescott, 1998a, 1998b; Pedersen, 1981; True et al., 1997; True et al., 1999; Tsuang et al., 1998).

Historically, many twin studies have focused on male twin pairs, which limits the conclusions that can be drawn regarding any differences in heritability of SUDs across the sexes. Table 5.1 gives a summary of recent population-based twin studies of drug dependence that included both men and women. The tetrachoric correlations reflect the correlations in the inferred underlying liability for the development of drug abuse between twins. The results of these studies have been highly consistent in demonstrating the role of genetic factors in the etiology of SUDs. However, the extent of genetic influence differs according to the trait definition employed, as well as the age, sex, and sample source.

Of the studies reviewed in Table 5.1, heritability estimates range from 0 to 87% in males and from 0 to 77% in the females, with a median of 53% and 55%, respectively. The influence of gender across substances is detailed in "Sex Differences in the Genetics of SUDs." The approximately twofold larger correlation between MZ as compared to DZ twins reflects the contributions of genetic factors to the specific substance phenotype. Unique environmental factors play a major role in SUDs in these samples, but, surprisingly, common environmental influences are low. These studies demonstrate the complex interplay (both interactions and correlations) between genetic and environmental factors in the etiology of SUDs.

TABLE 5.1. Population-Based Twin Studies of Abuse/Dependence of Specific Drugs Conducted in the Last 10 Years

| | | | Tetrachoric correlations | | | | Components of variance | | | | | |
| | | | Monozygotic | | Dizygotic | | Addictive genetic | | Common environment | | Unique environment/ error | |
Substance	Author(s) and year	Sample	Male	Female	Male	Female	Male	Female	Male	Female	Male	Female
Alcohol	Heath et al. (1997)[a]	ANH & MRC	0.68	0.58	0.20	0.29	0.64	0.64	0.03	0.01	0.33	0.35
Marijuana	Prescott et al. (1999)[b]	VETR	0.55	0.67	0.32	0.55	0.56	0.66	0.00	0.00	0.44	0.34
Stimulants	Agrawal et al. (2005)	VATSPSUD	—	—	—	—	0.31	0.36	0.00	0.00	0.69	0.64
	Agrawal et al. (2007)[c]	ATR	—	—	—	—	0.68	0.55	0.14	0.16	0.18	0.29
	Kendler et al. (2006)[d]	NIPHTP	0.77	0.77	0.31	0.31	0.77	0.77	0.00	0.00	0.23	0.23
	Lynskey et al. (2002)[e]	ATR	0.70	0.59	0.35	0.51	0.45	—	0.23	0.56	0.32	0.44
	Agrawal et al. (2005)	VATSPSUD	—	—	—	—	0.53	0.00	0.00	0.99	0.47	0.01
Sedatives	Lynskey et al. (2007)[d]	ATR	—	—	—	—	0.65	0.65	0.08	0.08	0.28	0.28
	Agrawal et al. (2005)	VATSPSUD	—	—	—	—	0.08	0.38	0.00	0.00	0.92	0.62
Cocaine	Agrawal et al. (2005)	VATSPSUD	—	—	—	—	0.00	0.35	0.28	0.00	0.72	0.65
	Kendler et al. (2000)	VETR	0.77	—	0.37	—	0.79	—	0.00	—	0.21	—
	Kendler & Prescott (1998)[f]	VETR	—	0.68	—	0.08	—	0.65	—	0.00	—	0.35

Note. ANH&MRC, Australian National Health and Medical Research Council; ATR, Australian Twin Register; NIPHTP, Norwegian Institute of Public Health Twin Panel; VATSPSUD, Virginia Adult Twin Study of Psychoactive and Substance Use Disorders; VETR, Vietnam Era Twin Registry.

[a]Sample also included 754 unlike-sex pairs.

[b]Study used DSM-IV criteria.

[c]Sample diagnosed as having abuse or dependence problems.

[d]Best-fitting model was obtained when components of variance were constrained to equality across the sexes; thus sex-specific estimates reported here are identical.

[e]Sample also included 655 unlike-sex pairs and 753 (377 female and 376 male) single twins.

[f]Study examined dependence without abuse.

Adoption Studies

The classic adoption studies of Cadoret and colleagues (Cadoret, 1992; Cadoret et al., 1986; Cadoret, Yates, Troughton, Woodworth, & Stewart, 1995, 1996) have also been highly informative in elucidating the role of genetic factors in the development of SUDs. Although data on biological parents are often limited with respect to specific patterns of substance use and abuse, their studies provide the strongest evidence, to date, that genetic factors play an important role in the liability to drug abuse. The work identifies two major biological/genetic pathways to the development of drug abuse in adoptees: one that is driven by substance abuse in the biological parent and is limited to drug abuse and dependence in the adoptee; and another that appears to be an expression of underlying aggressiveness and related to antisocial personality disorder (ASPD) in the biological parent (Cadoret et al., 1995, 1996). Although the previous studies by Cadoret and colleagues (Cadoret et al., 1995, 1996) were gender-specific, a follow-up analysis indicated that there were no sex differences in the development of SUDs in adoptees. For both men and women, they found that substance use and problems are elevated in adopted-away offspring of parents who have combined ASPD and SUD as compared to either ASPD or SUD alone (Langbehn et al., 2004).

SEX DIFFERENCES IN THE GENETICS OF SUDs

Expectations for Sex Differences in Transmission of Disease

There are several possible explanations for sex differences in the genetic propensity to express a disorder that can be tested in genetic epidemiological studies. Among diseases with clear-cut Mendelian modes of transmission, including autosomal dominant, autosomal recessive, or X-linked, there are predictable ratios of affected status among male and female probands and relatives. The sex ratio is expected to be equal for most autosomal disorders, whereas sex differences are a characteristic of X-linked diseases, such as color blindness and hemophilia. An X-linked recessive disease only manifests in women, whereas X-linked dominant disorders are manifest in all male offspring and half of the female offspring of an affected parent.

There are also predictable patterns for complex disorders if sex differences are involved in transmission. The sex effect is treated as a differential threshold, with the less commonly affected sex having the higher threshold. Accumulation of more genetic and/or environmental factors is required for the disorder to become manifest at the higher threshold. Because such individuals have increased genetic and/or environmental loading for the disorder, they have more factors to transmit to their relatives. Therefore, the relatives of probands with the higher threshold are more likely to be affected with the disorder. In the case of SUDs, relatives of female probands with SUDs would be expected to exhibit greater rates of SUDs themselves than those of male probands with SUDs, if the sex difference was attributable to genetic factors. Data from both twin and family studies can be used to examine whether genetic factors underlie the sex difference in SUDs. In the next section we review the evidence from twin and family studies on sex differences in the heritability of SUDs.

Sex Differences in Twin Studies of SUDs

Table 5.1 lists 13 population-based twin studies that investigated heritability of SUDs in both male and female twin pairs. In general, there are few sex differences in the heritability of most of the substances evaluated, with a high additive genetic contribution, moderate unique environmental contribution, and nearly no effect of the common environment for alcohol (Heath et al., 1997; Prescott & Kendler, 1999), marijuana (Agrawal et al., 2007; Agrawal, Neale, Jacobson, Prescott, & Kendler, 2005; Kendler et al., 2006; Lynskey et al., 2002), stimulants (Lynskey et al., 2007), and cocaine (Kendler et al., 2000; Kendler & Prescott, 1998b). The twin study that did find significant sex differences in the heritability of particular SUDs reported greater heritability among males for stimulant dependence, and among females for sedative and cocaine dependence (Agrawal et al., 2005). Studies of adolescent substance use generally found a greater contribution of common and unique environmental factors as compared to genetic factors. Similar to the adult studies, there are few sex differences in the role of genetic factors in SUDs (Hopfer et al., 2003). For example, a recent study that used structural equation modeling to investigate the genetic and environmental influences on tobacco initiation, regular tobacco use and nicotine dependence found no sex differences for the sources of variation or causal paths in males and females (Maes et al., 2004). The lack of consistent sex effects in the heritability estimates of SUDs from twin studies suggests that the male preponderance of SUDs is unlikely to be attributable to genetic factors.

FAMILY STUDIES OF SEX DIFFERENCES IN THE TRANSMISSION OF SUDs

Two controlled family studies compared patterns of familial transmission of SUDs among male and female probands (Bierut et al., 1998; Merikangas, Dierker, et al., 1998; Merikangas, Stolar, et al., 1998). In the former study both alcohol abuse and dependence were familial among females, whereas only dependence aggregated among the relatives of males with alcohol dependence (Merikangas, Stolar, et al., 1998). This finding suggests that the relatives of females may have a lower threshold for expression of SUDs than those of males. However, there was no sex of proband effect in the familial aggregation of either alcohol abuse or dependence (Merikangas, Stolar, et al., 1998) or cannabis, cocaine, or opioid abuse or dependence (Merikangas, Dierker, et al., 1998). Likewise, Bierut et al. (1998) did not find that the relatives of female probands had higher rates of marijuana dependence, cocaine dependence, or habitual smoking, despite the significantly lower rates of all of these conditions among female compared to male relatives.

In summary, although there are higher rates of some types of drug abuse and dependence in males, evidence from twin and controlled family studies does not suggest that the sex difference is related to genetic factors underlying these conditions. Therefore, the genes that underlie SUDs do not differ among men and women, suggesting that other nongenetic environmental factors underlie the sex differences in SUDs.

FUTURE DIRECTIONS

One of the most important observations of this work is the lack of controlled family studies of SUDs that specifically investigate sex differences in risk factors and correlates. There is also a lack of sufficient data on sex differences from high-risk studies, adoption studies, and twin studies of specific substances aside from alcohol and cannabis. Prospective studies that examine sex-specific exposure to environmental factors, as well as those that investigate biological factors underlying sex differences at all stages of the substance use trajectory, would be highly informative. SUDs result from a highly complex interaction of multiple environmental, biological, and genetic factors. Therefore, future studies that incorporate a range of potential etiological and risk factors may be more successful in identifying sex-specific factors that inform our understanding of the etiology and treatment of substance use disorders.

KEY POINTS

- Aggregate evidence from family and high-risk studies, twin studies, and adoption studies demonstrates that SUDs are strongly familial and that genetic factors are influential in the progression to dependence on most substances, whereas environmental factors have stronger impact in substance exposure and initiation.
- Although women have lower rates of SUDs than men, evidence from twin and family stud-

ies suggests that genetic factors are not associated with the sex difference in the prevalence of these conditions. This finding suggests that nongenetic environmental factors are likely to explain why women have lower rates of most SUDs.
- Data from the twin studies suggest that both environmental factors common to twin pairs as well as those that influence only one member of a twin pair are both influential in substance use and progression.

REFERENCES

Asterisks denote recommended readings.

Agrawal, A., Lynskey, M. T., Bucholz, K. K., Martin, N. G., Madden, P. A., & Heath, A. C. (2007). Contrasting models of genetic co-morbidity for cannabis and other illicit drugs in adult Australian twins. *Psychological Medicine, 37*(1), 49–60.

Agrawal, A., Neale, M. C., Jacobson, K. C., Prescott, C. A., & Kendler, K. S. (2005). Illicit drug use and abuse/dependence: Modeling of two-stage variables using the CCC approach. *Addictive Behaviors, 30*(5), 1043–1048. (*)

Ashley, M. J., Olin, J. S., le Riche, W. H., Kornaczewski, A., Schmidt, W., & Rankin, J. G. (1977). Morbidity in alcoholics. Evidence for accelerated development of physical disease in women. *Archives of Internal Medicine, 137*(7), 883–887.

Avenevoli, S., Conway, K. P., & Merikangas, K. R. (2005). Familial risk factors for substance use disorders. In J. Hudson & R. Rapee (Eds.), *Current thinking on psychopathology and the family.* New York: Elsevier.

Bierut, L. J., Dinwiddie, S. H., Begleiter, H., Crowe, R. R., Hesselbrock, V., Nurnberger, J. I., Jr., et al. (1998). Familial transmission of substance dependence: Alcohol, marijuana, cocaine, and habitual smoking—A report from the Collaborative Study on the Genetics of Alcoholism. *Archives of General Psychiatry, 55*(11), 982–988.

Brook, J. S., Brook, D. W., Gordon, A. S., Whiteman, M., & Cohen, P. (1990). The psychosocial etiology of adolescent drug use: A family interactional approach. *Genetic Social and General Psychology Monographs, 116*(2), 111–267.

Brook, J. S., Whiteman, M., Gordon, A. S., Nomura, C., & Brook, D. W. (1986). Onset of adolescent drinking: A longitudinal study of intrapersonal and interpersonal antecedents. *Advances in Alcohol and Substance Abuse, 5*(3), 91–110.

Brown, S. A. (1989). Life events of adolescents in relation to personal and parental substance abuse. *American Journal of Psychiatry, 146*(4), 484–489.

Cadoret, R. J. (1992). Genetic and environmental factors in initiation of drug use and the transition to abuse. In M. Blantz & R. Pickens (Eds.), *Vulnerability to drug abuse.* Washington, DC: American Psychological Association.

Cadoret, R. J., Troughton, E., O'Gorman, T. W., & Heywood, E. (1986). An adoption study of genetic and environmental factors in drug abuse. *Archives of General Psychiatry, 43*(12), 1131–1136.

Cadoret, R. J., Yates, W. R., Troughton, E., Woodworth, G., & Stewart, M. A. (1995). Adoption study demonstrating two genetic pathways to drug abuse. *Archives of General Psychiatry, 52*(1), 42–52.

Cadoret, R. J., Yates, W. R., Troughton, E., Woodworth, G., & Stewart, M. A. (1996). An adoption study of drug abuse/dependency in females. *Comprehensive Psychiatry, 37*(2), 88–94.

Chassin, L., Pitts, S. C., DeLucia, C., & Todd, M. (1999). A longitudinal study of children of alcoholics: Predicting young adult substance use disorders, anxiety, and depression. *Journal of Abnormal Psychology, 108*(1), 106–119.

Chassin, L., Rogosch, F., & Barrera, M. (1991). Substance use and symptomatology among adolescent children of alcoholics. *Journal of Abnormal Psychology, 100*(4), 449–463.

Claridge, G., Ross, E., & Hume, W. I. (1978). *Sedative drug tolerance in twins.* Oxford, UK: Pergamon Press.

Compton, W. M., Conway, K. P., Stinson, F. S., Colliver, J. D., & Grant, B. F. (2005). Prevalence, correlates, and comorbidity of DSM-IV antisocial personality syndromes and alcohol and specific drug use disorders in the United States: Results from the National Epidemiologic Survey on Alcohol and Related Conditions. *Journal of Clinical Psychiatry, 66*(6), 677–685.

Compton, W. M., Cottler, L. B., Ridenour, T., Ben-Abdallah, A., & Spitznagel, E. L. (2002). The specificity of family history of alcohol and drug abuse in cocaine abusers. *American Journal of Addiction, 11*(2), 85–94.

Conner, K. R., Hesselbrock, R. M., Meldrum, S. C., Schuckit, M. A., Bucholz, K. K., Gamble, S. A., et al. (2007). Transitions to, and correlates of, suicidal ideatun, plans, and unplanned and planned suicide attempts among 3,729 men and women with alcohol dependence. *Journal of Studies on Alcohol and Drugs, 68*(5), 654–662.

Conway, K. P., Compton, W., Stinson, F. S., & Grant, B. F. (2006). Lifetime comorbidity of DSM-IV mood and anxiety disorders and specific drug use disorders: Results from the National Epidemiologic Survey on Alcohol and Related Conditions. *Journal of Clinical Psychiatry, 67*(2), 247–257.

Conway, K. P., Swendsen, J. D., & Merikangas, K. R. (2003). Alcohol expectancies, alcohol consumption, and problem drinking: The moderating role of family history. *Addictive Behaviors, 28*(5), 823–836.

Croughan, J. L. (1985). The contributions of family studies to understanding drug abuse. In L. Robins (Ed.), *Studying drug abuse*. New Brunswick, NJ: Rutgers University Press.

Eng, M. Y., Schuckit, M. A., & Smith, T. L. (2005). The level of response to alcohol in daughters of alcoholics and controls. *Drug and Alcohol Dependence, 79*(1), 83–93.

Fowler, T., Lifford, K., Shelton, K., Rice, F., Thapar, A., Neale, M. C., et al. (2007). Exploring the relationship between genetic and environmental influences on initiation and progression of substance use. *Addiction, 102*(3), 413–422.

Gfroerer, J. (1987). Correlation between drug use by teenagers and drug use by older family members. *American Journal of Drug and Alcohol Abuse, 13*(1–2), 95–108.

Gorenstein, E. E., & Newman, J. P. (1980). Disinhibitory psychopathology: A new perspective and a model for research. *Psychological Review, 87*(3), 301–315.

Grant, J. D., Heath, A. C., Bucholz, K. K., Madden, P. A., Agrawal, A., Statham, D. J., et al. (2007). Spousal concordance for alcohol dependence: Evidence for assortative mating or spousal interaction effects? *Alcoholism: Clinical and Experimental Research, 31*(5), 717–728. (*)

Grove, W. M., Eckert, E. D., Heston, L., Bouchard, T. J., Jr., Segal, N., & Lykken, D. T. (1990). Heritability of substance abuse and antisocial behavior: A study of monozygotic twins reared apart. *Biological Psychiatry, 27*(12), 1293–1304.

Gurling, H. M., Grant, S., & Dangl, J. (1985). The genetic and cultural transmission of alcohol use, alcoholism, cigarette smoking and coffee drinking: A review and an example using a log linear cultural transmission model. *British Journal of Addiction, 80*(3), 269–279.

Hawkins, J. D., Catalano, R. F., & Miller, J. Y. (1992). Risk and protective factors for alcohol and other drug problems in adolescence and early adulthood: Implications for substance abuse prevention. *Psychological Bulletin, 112*(1), 64–105.

Heath, A. C., Bucholz, K. K., Madden, P. A., Dinwiddie, S. H., Slutske, W. S., Bierut, L. J., et al. (1997). Genetic and environmental contributions to alcohol dependence risk in a national twin sample: Consistency of findings in women and men. *Psychological Medicine, 27*(6), 1381–1396.

Heath, A. C., Cates, R., Martin, N. G., Meyer, J., Hewitt, J. K., Neale, M. C., et al. (1993). Genetic contribution to risk of smoking initiation: Comparisons across birth cohorts and across cultures. *Journal of Substance Abuse, 5*(3), 221–246.

Heath, A. C., & Madden, P. A. F. (1995). Genetic influences on smoking behavior. In J. R. Turner, L. R. Cardon, & J. K. Hewitt (Eds.), *Behavior genetic approaches in behavioral medicine* (pp. 45–67). New York: Plenum Press. (*)

Hill, S. Y., & Hruska, D. R. (1992). Childhood psychopathology in families with multigenerational alcoholism. *Journal of the American Academy of Child and Adolescent Psychiatry, 31*(6), 1024–1030.

Hopfer, C. J., Stallings, M. C., Hewitt, J. K., & Crowley, T. J. (2003). Family transmission of marijuana use, abuse, and dependence. *Journal of the American Academy of Child and Adolescent Psychiatry, 42*(7), 834–841. (*)

Jang, K. L., Livesley, W. J., & Vernon, P. A. (1995). Alcohol and drug problems: A multivariate behavioural genetic analysis of co-morbidity. *Addiction, 90*(9), 1213–1221.

Johnson, S., Leonard, K. E., & Jacob, T. (1989). Drinking, drinking styles and drug use in children of alcoholics, depressives, and controls. *Journal of Studies on Alcohol, 50*(5), 427–431.

Kandel, D. B., & Andrews, K. (1987). Processes of adolescent socialization by parents and peers. *International Journal of the Addictions, 22*(4), 319–342.

Kendler, K. S., Aggen, S. H., Tambs, K., & Reichborn-Kjennerud, T. (2006). Illicit psychoactive substance use, abuse, and dependence in a population-based sample of Norwegian twins. *Psychological Medicine, 36*(7), 955–962.

Kendler, K. S., Karkowski, L., & Prescott, C. A. (1999). Hallucinogen, opiate, sedative, and stimulant use and abuse in a population-based sample of female twins. *Acta Psychiatrica Scandanavica, 99*(5), 368–376.

Kendler, K. S., Karkowski, L. M., Neale, M. C., & Prescott, C. A. (2000). Illicit psychoactive substance use, heavy use, abuse, and dependence in a U.S. population-based sample of male twins. *Archives of General Psychiatry, 57*(3), 261–269.

Kendler, K. S., & Prescott, C. A. (1998a). Cannabis use, abuse, and dependence in a population-based sample of female twins. *American Journal of Psychiatry, 155*(8), 1016–1022.

Kendler, K. S., & Prescott, C. A. (1998b). Cocaine use, abuse, and dependence in a population-based sample of female twins. *British Journal of Psychiatry, 173*, 345–350.

Kessler, R. C., Berglund, P., Demler, O., Jin, R., Merikangas, K. R., & Walters, E. E. (2005). Lifetime prevalence and age-of-onset distributions of DSM-IV disorders in the National Comorbidity Survey Replication. *Archives of General Psychiatry, 62*(6), 593–602.

Khoury, M. J., & Yang, Q. (1998). The future of genetic studies of complex human diseases: An epidemiologic perspective. *Epidemiology, 9*(3), 350–354.

Kuller, L. H. (1979). The role of population genetics in the study of the epidemiology of cardiovascular risk factors. *Progress in Clinical and Biological Research, 32*, 489–495.

Lander, E. S., Linton, L. M., Birren, B., Nusbaum, C., Zody, M. C., Baldwin, J., et al. (2001). Initial sequencing and analysis of the human genome. *Nature, 409*(6822), 860–921.

Langbehn, D. R., Brinkman, R. R., Falush, D., Paulsen, J. S., Hayden, M. R., & International Huntington's Disease Collaborative Group. H. s. D. C. (2004). A new model for prediction of the age of onset and penetrance for Huntington's disease based on CAG length. *Clinical Genetics, 65*(4), 267–277.

Li, T. K. (2000). Pharmacogenetics of responses to alcohol and genes that influence alcohol drinking. *Journal of Studies on Alcohol, 61*(1), 5–12.

Lynskey, M. T., Grant, J. D., Li, L., Nelson, E. C., Bucholz, K. K., Madden, P. A., et al. (2007). Stimulant use and symptoms of abuse/dependence: Epidemiology and associations with cannabis use—A twin study. *Drug and Alcohol Dependence, 86*(2–3), 147–153.

Lynskey, M. T., Heath, A. C., Nelson, E. C., Bucholz, K. K., Madden, P. A., Slutske, W. S., et al. (2002). Genetic and environmental contributions to cannabis dependence in a national young adult twin sample. *Psychological Medicine, 32*(2), 195–207.

MacMahon, B., & Trichopoulos, D. (1996). *Epidemiology: Principles and methods.* Boston: Brown.

Maes, H. H., Sullivan, P. F., Bulik, C. M., Neale, M. C., Prescott, C. A., Eaves, L. J., et al. (2004). A twin study of genetic and environmental influences on tobacco initiation, regular tobacco use, and nicotine dependence. *Psychological Medicine, 34*(7), 1251–1261.

Mann, K., Batra, A., Gunthner, A., & Schroth, G. (1992). Do women develop alcoholic brain damage more readily than men? *Alcoholism: Clinical and Experimental Research, 16*(6), 1052–1056.

Martin, C. S., Earleywine, M., Blackson, T. C., Vanyukov, M. M., Moss, H. B., & Tarter, R. E. (1994). Aggressivity, inattention, hyperactivity, and impulsivity in boys at high and low risk for substance abuse. *Journal of Abnormal Child Psychology, 22*(2), 177–203.

McGue, M. (1994). Genes, environment, and the etiology of alcoholism. In R. Zucker, G. Boyd, & J. Howard (Eds.), *The development of alcohol problems: Exploring the biopsychosocial matrix.* Rockville, MD: U.S. Department of Health and Human Services: Research Monograph No. 26.

Meller, W. H., Rinehart, R., Cadoret, R. J., & Troughton, E. (1988). Specific familial transmission in substance abuse. *International Journal of the Addictions*, 23(10), 1029–1039.

Merikangas, K. R. (1990). The genetic epidemiology of alcoholism. *Psychological Medicine*, 20(1), 11–22.

Merikangas, K. R., & Avenevoli, S. (2000). Implications of genetic epidemiology for the prevention of substance use disorders. *Addictive Behaviors*, 25(6), 807–820. (*)

Merikangas, K. R., Dierker, L. C., & Szatmari, P. (1998). Psychopathology among offspring of parents with substance abuse and/or anxiety disorders: A high-risk study. *Journal of Child Psychology and Psychiatry*, 39(5), 711–720.

Merikangas, K. R., & Risch, N. (2003). Will the genomics revolution revolutionize psychiatry? *American Journal of Psychiatry*, 160(4), 625–635. (*)

Merikangas, K. R., Rounsaville, B. J., & Prusoff, B. A. (1992). Familial factors in vulnerability to substance abuse. In M. D. Glantz & R. W. Picken, (Eds.), *Vulnerability to drug abuse* (pp. 75–98). Washington, DC: American Psychological Association.

Merikangas, K. R., Stolar, M., Stevens, D. E., Goulet, J., Preisig, M. A., Fenton, B., et al. (1998). Familial transmission of substance use disorders. *Archives of General Psychiatry*, 55(11), 973–979.

Mirin, S. M., Weiss, R. D., Griffin, M. L., & Michael, J. L. (1991). Psychopathology in drug abusers and their families. *Comprehensive Psychiatry*, 32(1), 36–51.

Mirin, S. M., Weiss, R. D., Michael, J., & Griffin, M. L. (1988). Psychopathology in substance abusers: Diagnosis and treatment. *American Journal of Drug and Alcohol Abuse*, 14(2), 139–157.

Moss, H. B., Majumder, P. P., & Vanyukov, M. (1994). Familial resemblance for psychoactive substance use disorders: Behavioral profile of high risk boys. *Addictive Behaviors*, 19(2), 199–208.

Neale, M. C., Aggen, S. H., Maes, H. H., Kubarych, T. S., & Schmitt, J. E. (2006). Methodological issues in the assessment of substance use phenotypes. *Addictive Behaviors*, 31(6), 1010–1034.

Nurnberger, J. I., Jr., Wiegand, R., Bucholz, K., O'Connor, S., Meyer, E. T., Reich, T., et al. (2004). A family study of alcohol dependence: Coaggregation of multiple disorders in relatives of alcohol-dependent probands. *Archives of General Psychiatry*, 61(12), 1246–1256.

Pedersen, N. (1981). Twin similarity for usage of common drugs. *Progress in Clinical and Biological Research*, 69(Pt. C), 53–59.

Pickens, R. W., Svikis, D. S., McGue, M., Lykken, D. T., Heston, L. L., & Clayton, P. J. (1991). Heterogeneity in the inheritance of alcoholism: A study of male and female twins. *Archives of General Psychiatry*, 48(1), 19–28.

Prescott, C. A., & Kendler, K. S. (1999). Genetic and environmental contributions to alcohol abuse and dependence in a population-based sample of male twins. *American Journal of Psychiatry*, 156(1), 34–40.

Quitkin, F. M., Rifkin, A., Kaplan, J., & Klein, D. F. (1972). Phobic anxiety syndrome complicated by drug dependence and addiction: A treatable form of drug abuse. *Archives of General Psychiatry*, 27(2), 159–162.

Regier, D. A., Farmer, M. E., Rae, D. S., Locke, B. Z., Keith, S. J., Judd, L. L., et al. (1990). Comorbidity of mental disorders with alcohol and other drug abuse: Results from the Epidemiologic Catchment Area (ECA) Study. *Journal of the American Medical Association*, 264(19), 2511–2518.

Reich, W., Earls, F., Frankel, O., & Shayka, J. J. (1993). Psychopathology in children of alcoholics. *Journal of the American Academy of Child and Adolescent Psychiatry*, 32(5), 995–1002.

Rhee, S. H., Hewitt, J. K., Young, S. E., Corley, R. P., Crowley, T. J., & Stallings, M. C. (2003). Genetic and environmental influences on substance initiation, use, and problem use in adolescents. *Archives of General Psychiatry*, 60(12), 1256–1264.

Risch, N. J. (2000). Searching for genetic determinants in the new millennium. *Nature*, 405(6788), 847–856.

Ross, H. E., Glaser, T. B., & Germanson, T. (1988). The prevalence of psychiatric disorders in patients with alcohol and other drug problems. *Archives of General Psychiatry*, 45(11), 1023–1031.

Rounsaville, B. J., Kosten, T. R., Weissman, M. M., Prusoff, B., Pauls, D., Anton, S. F., et al. (1991). Psychiatric disorders in relatives of probands with opiate addiction. *Archives of General Psychiatry*, 48(1), 33–42.

Schuckit, M. A., & Smith, T. L. (1996). An 8-year follow-up of 450 sons of alcoholic and control subjects. *Archives of General Psychiatry, 53*(3), 202–210.

Schuckit, M. A., Smith, T. L., Eng, M. Y., & Kunovac, J. (2002). Women who marry men with alcohol-use disorders. *Alcoholism: Clinical and Experimental Research, 26*(9), 1336–1343.

Schuckit, M. A., Tipp, J. E., & Kelner, E. (1994). Are daughters of alcoholics more likely to marry alcoholics? *American Journal of Drug and Alcohol Abuse, 20*(2), 237–245.

Sher, K. J., Walitzer, K. S., Wood, P. K., & Brent, E. E. (1991). Characteristics of children of alcoholics: Putative risk factors, substance use and abuse, and psychopathology. *Journal of Abnormal Psychology, 100*(4), 427–448.

Simcha-Fagan O., & Schwartz, J. (1986). Neighborhood and delinquency: An assessment of contextual effects. *Criminology, 24,* 667–703.

Substance Abuse and Mental Health Services Administration. (2007, September). *SAMHSA's latest national survey on drug use and health.* Retrieved November 20, 2007, from *oas.samhsa.gov/ NSDUHLatest.htm.*

True, W. R., Heath, A. C., Scherrer, J. F., Waterman, B., Goldberg, J., Lin, N., et al. (1997). Genetic and environmental contributions to smoking. *Addiction, 92*(10), 1277–1287.

True, W. R., Xian, H., Scherrer, J. F., Madden, P. A., Bucholz, K. K., Heath, A. C., et al. (1999). Common genetic vulnerability for nicotine and alcohol dependence in men. *Archives of General Psychiatry, 56*(7), 655–661.

Tsuang, M. T., Lyons, M. J., Eisen, S. A., Goldberg, J., True, W., Lin, N., et al. (1996). Genetic influences on DSM-III-R drug abuse and dependence: A study of 3,372 twin pairs. *American Journal of Medical Genetics, 67*(5), 473–477.

Tsuang, M. T., Lyons, M. J., Meyer, J. M., Doyle, T., Eisen, S. A., Goldberg, J., et al. (1998). Co-occurrence of abuse of different drugs in men: The role of drug-specific and shared vulnerabilities. *Archives of General Psychiatry, 55*(11), 967–972. (*)

Weiss, R. D., Pope, H. G., Jr., & Mirin, S. M. (1985). Treatment of chronic cocaine abuse and attention deficit disorder, residual type, with magnesium pemoline. *Drug and Alcohol Dependence, 15*(1–2), 69–72.

CHAPTER 6

Sex Differences and Neurotransmitter Systems in Addiction

Teresa A. Pigott, MD
Maryann H. Walker, PhD
Scott A. Teitelbaum, MD
Ching-ju Lu, MPH

Substances of abuse are chemically diverse and associated with different behavioral effects, but they all likely share a common final pathway that involves the brain reward system. Numerous investigators have conceptualized the addictive process as a "hijacking" of the brain's reward pathways with subsequent occurrence of specific, measurable changes in the brain (Lubman, Yucel, & Pantelis, 2004; Volkow et al., 2006).

Whereas gender differences in prevalence rates, clinical characteristics, and clinical course have been identified, much less attention has been focused on potential gender differences in the neurobiological mechanisms that underlie substance use disorders. This is surprising since the brain regions considered to be most important in addiction (e.g., amygdala, hippocampus, prefrontal cortex) are sexually dimorphic in terms of structure and function (Cahill, 2006). Pre-clinical data also suggest that neurotransmitter systems, including those with particular importance to addictive disorders, such as monoamines, gamma-aminobutyric acid (GABA), and opioids, are sexually dimorphic (Craft, 2003).

This chapter focuses on the proposed role of neurotransmitter systems in the neurobiology of addiction, with special attention given to the potential role of gender in these processes. The neurobiology of four of the most prevalent drugs of abuse (i.e., opioids, cocaine, alcohol, and cannabis) are reviewed in this chapter.

OPIOID DEPENDENCE

Epidemiology and Gender

There has been an alarming increase in opioid use in the U.S. since 1995. Data from the 2004 National Survey on Drug Use and Health (NSDUH; Substance Abuse and Mental Health Services Administration [SAMHSA], 2005) revealed that nonmedical use of prescription pain relievers (opioid analgesics) was the drug category with the largest number of new users in the past year. Historically, men have had a higher risk than women for opiate dependence. However, a comparison of females versus males enrolled in methadone maintenance treatment (MTT) programs revealed that females had greater illness severity, elevated rates of medical and psychiatric comorbidity, and a less favorable outcome than their male counterparts (Chatham, Hiller, Rowan-Szal, Joe, & Simpson, 1999). There is much less of a gender difference in prevalence rates for prescription opioid dependence, with the male-to-female ratio estimated at 1.5:1. This difference disparity may be related to the fact that women are more likely to be prescribed opiate medications than males (Simoni-Wastila, 2000).

Neurotransmission and Gender Effects

Enkaphalin, beta-endorphin, and dynorphin are endogenous "opioid-like" peptides identified within the central nervous system (CNS) that interact with the opiate receptor sites. There are mu-opiate, delta-opiate, and kappa-opiate receptors. Classic morphine-like opioid compounds as well as the endogenous opioid, beta-endorphin, bind preferentially to the mu-opiate receptor site. Stimulation of the mu-opiate receptor is associated with supraspinal analgesia, acute euphoria, and physical dependence as well as other effects associated with opioid analgesics, such as respiratory depression and myosis (Stine, 1998). Chronic opioid administration is associated with the development of tolerance, sensitization, and physical dependence. Although the exact neural mechanisms that underlie these processes remain undetermined, considerable data implicate two specific neuroanatomical pathways: (1) the mesolimbic dopamine system, and (2) noradrenergic pathways originating within the locus coeruleus (LC). The mesolimbic dopamine system is widely recognized as integral to the brain's reward system (Wise, 1989) and is also considered the critical neuroanatomical locus in mediating the reinforcing effects of opioids.

Norepinephrine also appears to have a key role in the rewarding effects of opioids (Ventura, Alcaro, & Puglisi-Allegra, 2005). The LC, the primary noradrenergic nucleus within the brain, has a major role in the development of opioid dependence and opioid withdrawal. There is emerging data that glutamate and other excitatory amino acid neurotransmitters are involved in the pharmacological action of opioids and subsequent changes at the N-methyl-D-aspartate (NMDA) receptor site are critical in the development of opioid-induced tolerance, sensitization and physical dependence (Trujillo, 2002).

The stress response is reported to be profoundly altered during chronic opioid administration. Dependence on opioids is linked to a reduced stress response, followed by a relatively overactive stress response in the context of acute opioid withdrawal states. Early exposure to physical and/or psychological trauma has also been posited to induce physiological alterations in the stress response that may further enhance addiction vulnerability once opioids are administered (Stimmel & Kreek, 2000).

Animal models of drug abuse have identified several sex-determined differences in behavioral response to opioids. Whereas opiate intake appears to be similar in male and female rodents in short-term self-administration models, female rodents consume greater levels of heroin and morphine than male rodents when long-term and/or extended access conditions are permitted (Carroll, Campbell, & Heideman, 2001). Thus, sex differences in opiate intake may be significantly influenced by the access conditions and may also become more pronounced over time (Lynch, Roth, & Carroll, 2002). There is also evidence of sex differences in opioid-related relapse; female rats have a greater response than male rats to the reintroduction of fentanyl after a period of abstinence (Klein, Popke, & Grunberg, 1997). Female rats also demonstrate evidence of greater hyperanalgesia effects than male rats when administered subanalgesic doses of the mu-opioid receptor agonist, morphine. Recent studies conducted in rats suggest that the observed sex differences in pain sensitivity and opiate anal-gesia may be directly attributable to testosterone exposure during early development (Craft, Mogil, & Aloisi, 2004). Early testosterone deprivation increased pain sensitivity in neonate male rats, but this effect could be reversed with testosterone treatment during adulthood. Female rats given testosterone as neonates showed reduced sensitivity to pain; however, fur-ther administration of testosterone in adulthood had no effect. Early testosterone exposure also influenced rats' sensitivity to morphine-induced analgesia during adulthood. Male rats deprived of testosterone as neonates were less sensitive to morphine than normal males, and females given testosterone as neonates were more sensitive to morphine than control females (Craft et al., 2004).

There is also some evidence of gender differences in kappa-opiate receptor function in rats. Administration of kappa-opiate receptor agonists has been reported to induce greater antinociceptive responses in female than male rats, and subanalgesic doses of kappa-receptor agonists are also reported to elicit hyperanalgesia to a greater extent in male than female rats. These findings suggest that the sexual dimorphism observed is directly attributable to the type of opioid receptor predominantly activated by the opioid (Holtman & Wala, 2006).

Numerous studies have reported that women have a higher prevalence of chronic pain states and demonstrate lower pain thresholds than males (Graven-Nielsen & Arendt-Nielsen, 2007). Some laboratory studies also suggest that females have greater analgesic response to mu-opioid agonists but not to kappa-agonist-antagonists. In fact, men often require a 30–40% greater dose of mu-opiate receptor agonists than women in order to achieve a similar level of pain relief. This finding of increased sensitivity to opiate analgesia suggests that females may be at greater risk for adverse event occurrence (e.g., respiratory depression) when administered the same dose as males (Pleym, Spigset, Kharasch, & Dale, 2003). How-ever, some studies conducted in clinical samples have reported contrasting results. Female patients administered kappa-opiate agonist antagonists following oral surgery showed more robust analgesia than males (Fillingim & Gear, 2004). Female gonadal hormones have a significant impact on pain perception and as a result, pain threshold and pain tolerance vary with the stage of the menstrual cycle (Graven-Nielsen & Arendt-Nielsen, 2007).

Summary

In summary, while men are more likely to meet criteria for an opiate use disorder than women, this difference may, in part, reflect differences in exposure and opportunity rather than overall vulnerability. There is considerable evidence that opioid abuse results in disrup-tion of the endogenous opioid system and profound molecular and neurochemical alterations. Much of what is known about potential gender differences in opiate response is derived from animal data. Animal models indicate that female rats consume greater levels of heroin and morphine when long-term and/or extended access conditions are permitted. Female rats also demonstrate evidence of greater vulnerability to the reinforcing effects of opiates during the reinstatement phase of addiction. Human studies reveal that women have lower pain thresh-olds and demonstrate enhanced sensitivity and greater analgesic response when administered mu-opioid agonists. Neuroimaging studies conducted in healthy subjects have identified gen-der differences in the mu-opioid system response to pain, but the differences appear to be limited to the low estrogen phase of the menstrual cycle. This finding along with the animal data provide further support for the importance of estrogen and other gonadal hormones in modulating endogenous opioid neurotransmission and stress responses in humans. Addi-tional investigations appear warranted to further explore the sex differences already detected in the endogenous opioid system, pain perception, and opioid analgesia.

COCAINE DEPENDENCE

Epidemiology and Gender

Although the lifetime prevalence rate for cocaine use in the United States remains significantly higher in men, the number of women using cocaine has increased rapidly over the last decade (Leigh & Jimenez, 2002). In fact, results from the 2005 NSDUH indicate that nearly 40% of Americans who use cocaine are women (SAMHSA, 2005). Although most data suggest that males have greater rates of exposure to cocaine, the sexes progress to cocaine use at an equal rate once exposure occurs (Van Etten & Anthony, 1999).

Neurotransmission and Gender Effects

Cocaine has potent effects on the brain's neural reward circuitry, including the mesolimbic and mesocortical dopaminergic pathways involving the nucleus accumbens (NAcc), ventral tegmental area (VTA), ventral palladium, and prefrontal cortex (PFC). Self-administration of cocaine results in increased extracellular dopamine in the NAcc (Pettit & Justice, 1989). Moreover, cocaine intake behavior is sensitive to concentrations of dopamine in the NAcc as well as the amygdala. Injection of a dopaminergic neurotoxin into the mesolimbic–mesocortical dopaminergic pathways attenuates self-administration of cocaine in animals. Data from both cloning and expression studies demonstrate that the dopamine transporter (DAT) is the site where cocaine binds and elicits its primary pharmacological actions within the brain.

Several different dopamine receptor subtypes, including the D_1, D_2, and D_3 receptors, are implicated as modulators of cocaine's actions within the brain. The D_2 receptor appears to mediate cocaine's stimulatory and rewarding properties, and the D_3 receptor is reported to mediate sensitization and facilitation of cocaine-induced stimulation (Koob & Le Moal, 1997). Female rats were reported to have a more robust cocaine-induced motor response than male rats (Festa et al., 2006). Cocaine-induced motor responses in rats are reportedly linked to D_1 receptor activation. Since male but not female rats show reduced D_1 binding levels in the caudate putamen, the finding of increased cocaine-induced behavioral response in female rats suggests that they have greater sensitivity to D_1 receptor blockade relative to the males rats (Festa et al., 2006). Although preliminary, these results suggest that gender differences exist in dopamine-mediated behavioral responses to acute cocaine administration.

There is also evidence that glutamate, an excitatory neurotransmitter, is critical in mediating cocaine's actions within the brain (Kalivas, 2004). Glutamatergic neurons are present in the neural pathways that interconnect the PFC, amygdala, NAcc, and VTA. Glutamatergic mechanisms appear to be particularly instrumental in mediating the persistent neural adaptations that occur during chronic cocaine (and other addictive drug) administration. Cocaine releases glutamate through a dopamine-dependent mechanism in the VTA and stimulates the formation of glutamatergic synapses in the NAcc.

The serotonin (5-hydroxytryptamine [5-HT]) neurotransmitter system is also implicated in cocaine's rewarding and aversive properties. In rat models self-administration of cocaine is enhanced by stimulation of the 5-HT_{1B} receptor. In contrast, activation of the 5-HT_{1A} or the 5-HT_{2C} receptor results in reduced self-administration of cocaine. Data from microdialysis studies also suggest that cocaine has modulatory effects on the opioid neuropeptide system, especially dynorphin activity. Dynorphin and other kappa-opioid receptor agonists reportedly lower dopamine concentrations in the NAcc. The dynorphin–kappa-opioid receptor system appears to have an essential compensatory role in attenuating cocaine-induced dopamine surges (Kreek, Schluger, Borg, Gunduz, & Ho, 1999). Animal data suggest that psychostimulants activate cocaine and amphetamine-regulated transcript (CART) cells in the NAcc, and the CART peptide has been proposed as a novel target for cocaine's actions (Hurd, Svenson, & Ponten, 1999). Gender differences have been reported in the expression of CART messenger ribonucleic acid (mRNA) levels, with male in comparison to female rats having higher levels of CART mRNA in the NAcc shell at baseline. Following acute cocaine administration, male rats demonstrate elevated CART mRNA levels in the central amygdala (Fagergren & Hurd, 1999).

Preclinical studies have identified gender differences in cocaine response, with female rats demonstrating greater sensitivity to the behavioral effects of acute and chronic cocaine administration, as measured by locomotor (ambulation, rearing, and stereotypic) responses (Festa & Quinones-Jena, 2004). Since specific gonadal hormone receptor sites have been identified throughout the CNS, including many of the brain regions considered to be targets for cocaine's rewarding properties, the brain is now widely recognized as one of the specific target tissues for estrogen, progestin, and the androgens. Moreover, binding of gonadal hormones to gonadal hormone receptor sites in the mesolimbic brain region has been associated with important alterations within the neurotransmitter systems located in that region. For example, binding of estrogen to the gonadal hormone receptor site has been linked to a significant increase in density of 5-HT_{2A} binding sites in the anterior frontal, cingulate, and NA regions, as well a significant increase in D_2 receptors in the striatum (Fink, Sumner, Rosie, Grace, & Quinn, 1996). As reviewed by Becker and Hu (2008), exogenous estradiol administration in female rats can act directly on the striatum to induce changes in dopamine release and dopamine receptor activity and can also enhance dopamine release by direct effects at the NAcc. Estradiol's action at the striatal neurons is reported to be dependent upon a G-protein coupled receptor (Mermelstein, Becker, & Surmeier, 1996). Microdialysis studies also indicate that estradiol affects GABAergic neurons and, according to Becker and Hu (2008), estradiol rapidly inhibits GABA release from the intrinsic striatal neurons as a direct effect. In contrast, estradiol's ability to enhance DA release is an indirect action that occurs as a consequence of dopamine's release from GABA-mediated inhibition.

With estrogen's effects on dopamine and other neurotransmitters in mind, there has been considerable interest in the potential impact of gonadal hormones and fluctuations on cocaine-induced responses in both animal and human studies. Preclinical studies have consistently identified gender differences in cocaine response that appear to be directly attributable to the influence of gonadal sex hormones, especially estrogen. For example, female rats exhibit the lowest cocaine-induced behavioral response during the diestrous phase, when estrogen levels are slowly rising and progesterone levels are also low (Walker, Nelson, Smith, & Kuhn, 2002). In contrast, higher levels of cocaine-induced locomotor activity occur during the proestrous (both estrogen and progesterone levels peak and then slowly decline) and estrous (both estrogen and progesterone levels decline) phases in female rats. Estradiol also facilitates the acquisition of cocaine self-administration in female, but not male, rats. Interestingly, concurrent administration of progesterone in female rats is reported to counteract the facilitatory effect of estradiol on cocaine self-administration (Jackson, Robinson, & Becker, 2006). Chronic cocaine administration studies have failed to detect a consistent relationship between estrous cycle phase and behavioral responses. One study found no relationship between estrous cycle phase and cocaine-induced behavioral responses (Booze, Wood, Welsh, Berry, & Mactutus, 1999), and others found that the estrous cycle was interrupted by chronic cocaine administration (King et al., 1990). A more recent study used a shorter duration of cocaine administration and found that only the diestrous phase revealed evidence of sensitization to cocaine-induced behavioral responses (Sell, Thomas, & Cunningham, 2002). Female rats in estrous, relative to nonestrous females or male rats, also have greater responses to reinstatement of cocaine after a period of abstinence (Kippin et al., 2005).

Acute and chronic cocaine administration is associated with reduced behavioral responses in female rats after gonadectomy (Chin et al., 2002; Walker et al., 2001). In contrast, gonadectomy in male rats is not associated with reductions in cocaine-induced locomotor responses (Chin et al., 2002). These findings suggest that estrogen and progesterone are particularly important in modulating cocaine-induced behavioral responses in female rats. Moreover, ovariectomized female rats that receive both estrogen and progesterone are consistently reported to have augmented cocaine-induced locomotor activity, in comparison to ovariectomized female rats without such replacement therapy (Quinones-Jenab et al., 2000). These preclinical findings suggest that female gonadal hormones are important modulators of cocaine-induced behavioral responses, with estrogen increasing and progesterone either decreasing or having a negligible effect on cocaine-induced locomotor activity in rodents (Festa & Quinones-Jena, 2004).

Similar to preclinical findings, human studies indicate significant differences in response to cocaine administration between female and male subjects. For instance, several studies conducted in subjects who abuse cocaine have reported that females, relative to males, report more intense craving, increased depressive symptomatology, and overall greater responsiveness to cocaine-related cues (Elman, Karlsgodt, & Gastfriend, 2001). Females with cocaine abuse are also reported to experience greater levels of anxiety than their male counterparts after intranasal administration of cocaine (Kosten et al., 1996).

Several studies have examined the potential impact of menstrual cycle phase on response to cocaine. In a comparison of female (n = 7) and male (n = 7) subjects with occasional use of cocaine, intranasal administration of cocaine resulted in relatively lower peak plasma levels of cocaine in women. Women took significantly longer to report cocaine-related subjective effects and also endorsed less episodes of intense euphoria or dysphoria than men. Although female subjects had significantly higher peak plasma cocaine levels during the follicular phase, no difference in cocaine-related subjective effects were detected between the follicular and luteal phases of the menstrual cycle in the same report (Lukas et al., 1996). In a study of acute intravenous cocaine administration conducted in men (n = 12) and women (n = 22) who abuse cocaine, no differences in cocaine's pharmacokinetic and pharmacodynamic effects were detected. Moreover, there was no evidence of significant differences in cocaine plasma concentrations or in cocaine-related subjective effects between the follicular and luteal phases of the menstrual cycle in the female subjects (Mendelson et al., 1999). However, females had less desire and an attenuated subjective response to smoked cocaine during the luteal in comparison to follicular phase (Sofuoglu, Duidish-Poulsen, Nelson, Pentel, & Hatsukami, 1999). Additionally, women with cocaine dependence (n = 11) who smoked cocaine had increased heart rate and endorsed more positive feelings during the follicular phase than the luteal phase. Females reporting dysphoric mood during the luteal phase also reported improvement in mood after administration of cocaine (Evans, Haney, & Foltin, 2002). Since the luteal phase is characterized by relatively high levels of progesterone relative to the follicular phase of the menstrual cycle, these findings suggest that progesterone may attenuate the subjective effects of cocaine. These findings also suggest that gender and menstrual cycle influences on cocaine's effects may vary significantly as a function of the route of administration.

There is some preliminary data suggesting that exogenous hormone administration may influence cocaine-induced effects. Women (n = 7) with occasional cocaine use who were on triphasic oral contraceptive pills were challenged with an acute dose of intranasal cocaine and placebo. There were no differences in cocaine-induced subjective, physiological, or plasma cocaine and metabolite levels during the times equivalent to the follicular and luteal phases of the menstrual cycle (Kouri, Lundahl, Borden, McNeil, & Lukas, 2002). However, females who abused cocaine ($n = 5$), when given an acute dose of progesterone (vs. placebo) prior to smoked cocaine administration, experienced an attenuation of cocaine's subjective effects (Sofuoglu, Babb, & Hatsukami, 2002). In a more recent study (Evans & Foltin, 2006) administration of progesterone during the follicular phase in women with cocaine dependence ($n = 11$) attenuated the positive subjective effects of smoked cocaine, whereas only minimal changes in the positive subjective effects of smoked cocaine were observed after progesterone administration in men with cocaine dependence ($n = 10$).

Cocaine dependence has also been associated with enhanced sensitivity to stress and increased hypothalamic–pituitary–adrenal (HPA) axis reactivity. Responses to stress-induced versus neutral imagery and cocaine-related cues were compared in a group of females with cocaine dependence and low ($n = 5$), moderate ($n = 9$), and high ($n = 5$) progesterone levels, respectively. The high-progesterone in comparison to low-progesterone group of females with cocaine dependence demonstrated significantly lower stress-induced and drug-cue-induced cocaine craving, reduced anxiety levels, and lower systolic and diastolic blood pressure levels. These findings are consistent with previous preclinical and clinical studies suggesting that progesterone attenuates the behavioral effects of cocaine (Sinha et al., 2007).

The same researchers also conducted a study using similar methodology in a group of recently abstinent women with cocaine dependence ($n = 25$) and men ($n = 25$). Men showed significantly higher levels of adrenocorticotropin hormone (ACTH) cortisol, and systolic blood pressure at baseline and in response to stress-induced imagery, neutral imagery, and cocaine-related cues. Women had significantly higher basal heart rate and prolactin levels in comparison to men. No gender differences in response to stress-induced imagery or cocaine-related cues were detected during the study (Fox et al., 2006). Another study examined stress, sex steroid hormone levels, mood, and cocaine craving across the menstrual cycle in females with cocaine dependence ($n = 10$) and female control subjects ($n = 10$). The females with cocaine dependence demonstrated significantly higher levels of both cortisol and progesterone across the menstrual cycle and significantly lower estradiol–progesterone (E2/P) ratios, compared to female controls. They also showed significantly increased negative mood ratings compared to controls. There was no evidence that the intensity of cocaine craving varied across the menstrual cycle (Fox, Hong, Paliwal, Morgan, & Sinha, 2008).

Neuroimaging studies have been particularly illuminating in the investigation of potential neural correlates of cocaine abuse and dependence in humans. Cerebral perfusion abnormalities have been identified in human subjects after acute cocaine administration and also in chronic users of cocaine, relative to control subjects. For example, an early single photon emission computerized tomography (SPECT) study reported that males with cocaine dependence ($n = 13$), relative to male controls ($n = 13$), had significant alterations in cerebral perfusion (Levin et al., 1994). Males with cocaine dependence were also much more likely to have cerebral perfusion abnormalities than females with cocaine dependence ($n = 13$). In fact, no significant differences were detected in cerebral perfusion patterns between females with cocaine dependence and female controls (Levin et al., 1994). However, another SPECT study used procaine-induced limbic regional cerebral blood flow (rCBF) responses to compare females with cocaine dependence ($n = 10$) and female controls ($n = 10$); this more recent SPECT study revealed that the females with cocaine dependence had markedly muted and distinctly different procaine-induced limbic responses in comparison to female controls (Adinoff et al., 2003).

Several neuroimaging studies have identified gender differences in regional brain function in subjects with cocaine dependence. In addition to finding reduced rCBF in the bilateral and medial orbitofrontal cortex (OFC) in abstinent (11–28 days) subjects with cocaine dependence ($n = 35$), relative to control subjects ($n = 37$), a recent positron emission tomagraphy (PET) study also reported evidence of gender-related differences in rCBF activity in the subjects with cocaine dependence. Males with cocaine dependence had reduced rCBF in the bilateral OFC, whereas females with cocaine dependence had reduced rCBF in the medial OCF region. Additional gender differences in regional activity levels were also identified (males: reduced rCBF in the bilateral anterolateral temporal cortex and anterior cingulated regions; females: reduced rCBF in the bilateral superior frontal gyri region) in the same study (Adinoff et al., 2006).

Several different types of neuroimaging studies have identified gender differences in regional brain activity in response to drug-related cues. A SPECT study conducted during a period of acute abstinence compared rCBF patterns in a group of males and females with cocaine dependence and control subjects. Males with cocaine dependence demonstrated reduced rCBF in the anterior cingulate and frontal brain regions, relative to male controls, whereas females with cocaine dependence had increased rCBF in the posterior cingulate region, in compared to female controls (Tucker, Browndyke, Gottschalk, Cofrancesco, & Kosten, 2004). Kilts, Gross, Ely, and Dexler (2004) used PET imaging to investigate neural response to cocaine-related versus neutral imagery in a group of females with cocaine dependence ($n = 8$) and males with cocaine dependence ($n = 8$). The females responded to cocaine-related imagery, versus neutral imagery, with increased activation of the superior temporal gyrus, dorsal anterior and posterior cingulate cortex, NAcc area, and the central sulcus regions. However, the cocaine-related activation of the amygdala, insula, OFC, and ventral cingulate cortex regions was significantly less in the females than in the males. Females with cocaine dependence also responded to the cocaine-related imagery with diffuse and widely distributed activation of the frontal cortical regions, as compared to the males with cocaine dependence.

In addition to the gender differences reported in drug-cue-induced regional brain activity, there is also evidence of sex differences in response to stressful stimuli. For example, a functional magnetic resonance imaging (fMRI) study compared responses to stressful images and drug-cue-related stimuli in men ($n = 5$) and women ($n = 6$) with cocaine dependence. The men demonstrated greater activation of the left uncus and right claustrum areas in response to the drug cue; none of the brain areas in the men demonstrated greater response to stress-induced than drug-cue-induced stimuli. In contrast, the women revealed greater stress-induced activation in the right medial and superior frontal gyri and no brain area revealed greater activation in response to drug cues than to stressful stimuli (Li, Kemp, et al., 2005). The same group also used fMRI and stressful versus neutral guided imagery tasks to compare stress responses in male ($n = 17$) and female ($n = 10$) abstinent subjects with cocaine dependence. The females again demonstrated greater responses to stressful stimuli than to drug-induced cues. The females relative, to the males, demonstrated greater stress-induced activation in numerous frontolimbic regions, including the left middle frontal, anterior cingulate, inferior frontal cortices and insula, and right cingulate cortex regions. In addition, the stress-induced change in activity within the left anterior cingulate and right posterior cingulate cortical areas was inversely correlated with changes in craving rating scores (Li, Kosten, et al., 2005). These preliminary results suggest that sex differences may exist in stress- and drug-cue-associated brain activation responses in subjects with cocaine dependence.

Summary

In summary, the number of women using cocaine has increased rapidly over the last decade, and women are reported to progress more rapidly to cocaine dependence than men. There are also data suggesting that women report greater intensity of cocaine craving during periods of abstinence and also may have greater disease severity than men. Data from both pre-clinical and clinical studies reveal gender differences in behavioral and subjective responses to cocaine administration that are, at least partially, due to the influence of gonadal hormones. Estrogen appears to augment cocaine-induced behavioral responses, and progesterone, in turn, exhibits primarily inhibitory effects on cocaine-induced behavioral responses in females. Some preliminary data indicate that testosterone may attenuate cocaine-induced behavioral responses in male rats, but human data are lacking. The estrous cycle has modulatory influences on cocaine-induced locomotor activity in female rats. Although there is also some evidence that the menstrual cycle can influence the subjective effects of cocaine in women, this effect appears to vary as a function of the route of administration. Several neuroimaging studies have identified gender differences in regional brain function in subjects with cocaine dependence at rest and also in response to drug-related cues as well as stressful imagery. Additional investigations are needed to further examine gender differences in cocaine-induced behavioral responses, with particular attention on the potential influence of gonadal hormones on the neurobiological basis of cocaine addiction.

ALCOHOL DEPENDENCE

Epidemiology and Gender

Alcohol dependence is one of the most serious public health problems in the United States and is twice as common in men than in women (SAMHSA, 2007). In the United States, 11.7% of men versus 3.4% of women, ages 18 and older, report heavy alcohol use, as defined as five or more drinks on one occasion on 5 or more days in the past month (SAMHSA, 2006). Although women are less likely than men to abuse or develop dependence to alcohol, research suggests an increased vulnerability of women to the physiological consequences of drinking (Chou, 1994). The course of alcohol dependence becomes telescoped in women, with later onset but more rapid progression of disease and earlier expression of the long-term secondary effects of alcohol on internal organs (Diehl et al., 2007). Women are also at greater risk for adverse physiological effects of alcohol and more likely to develop alcohol-related illnesses (Greenfield, 2002).

Neurotransmission and Gender Effects

Whereas gender differences in disease progression from initiation to potential relapse is fairly well established, research on the neural bases of these differences is significantly lacking (Becker & Hu, 2008). Alcohol changes the structure and function of the hydrophobic pockets of cellular proteins. Alcohol-sensitive proteins include ion channels, neurotransmitter receptors, and signal transduction enzymes (Kenna, McGeary, & Swift, 2004). Neurotransmitter systems with roles in alcohol dependence include GABA (GABA-A, GABA-B receptors), glutamate (NMDA, alpha-amino-3-hydroxyl-5-methyl-4-isoxazole propionic acid [AMPA] kainite receptors), dopamine [D_1, D_2, D_3, D_4, receptors], 5-HT (several receptors, especially 5-HT_3), and endogenous opioids (mu-, sigma-, kappa-opioid receptors) (Wilkens, 2007).

Alcohol withdrawal is characterized by CNS hyperactivity and sympathetic arousal symptoms, including tremors, anxiety, agitation, nausea and vomiting, headache, sweating, and increased blood pressure, heart rate, and seizure susceptibility (Devaud, Risinger, & Selvage, 2006; Wilkens, 2007). Data suggest significant sex differences in seizure susceptibility in the preclinical setting (Devaud, Alele, Chadda, & Ritu, 2003; Devaud & Chadda 2001). Female rats, in comparison to male rats, are reported to have reduced response to convulsant-like stimulants during alcohol withdrawal (Devaud et al., 2006). Women also are less likely to experience alcohol-induced seizures during withdrawal, as shown in a retrospective chart review of 1,179 hospitalized patients (Wojnar, Wasilewski, Matsumoto, & Cedro, 1997). Clinical data also suggests that women report fewer DSM-IV withdrawal symptoms, as compared to men, when the groups were matched for variables of alcohol consumption (Deshmukh et al., 2003).

The HPA axis and endogenous opioid system influence alcohol consumption, and chronic alcohol abuse alters the activity of both systems. Both gender and age differences have been reported in the activity of the HPA axis under basal conditions, in response to stress, and after acute alcohol challenge (Devaud et al., 2003). There is also evidence that chronic alcohol-consumption-induced alteration in HPA and beta-endorphin activity occurs as a function of the severity of alcohol abuse, gender, and age. For example, heavy drinking has been associated with lower plasma ACTH and beta-endorphin levels and higher plasma cortisol levels than in nondrinkers; moreover, the heavy-drinking-induced decreases in plasma ACTH and beta-endorphin levels were reported as more pronounced in females than males in the 30–44 and 45–60 age groups (Gianoulakis, Dai, & Brown, 2003). These findings suggest that stress-induced responses may be gender-specific and associated with differential alterations in GABA-ergic and glutamergic systems in men versus women that are further amplified in the context of alcoholism (Devaud et al., 2006).

Some neuroimaging studies suggest that there are gender differences in the consequences of alcohol dependence. Schweinsburg and colleagues (2003) examined differences in brain metabolism utilizing proton magnetic resonance spectroscopy. They found that although men and women showed comparable amounts of neuronal loss, women with alcohol dependence showed a significantly greater loss than women without alcohol dependence, as compared to the difference seen between males with and without alcohol dependence. On the other hand, in Wang and colleagues' (2003) study of alcohol intoxication of healthy controls, men demonstrated significantly greater decrease in brain glucose metabolism as compared to women. The authors argued that the dampened sensitivity to the effects of acute alcohol administration on brain glucose metabolism in females suggests a gender difference in the influence of alcohol on GABA-ergic neurotransmission.

Summary

In summary, although clinical data on gender differences in the neurobiology of alcohol abuse and dependence are limited, gender differences in the metabolism of alcohol and physical morbidity of long-term alcohol abuse are well established. Women are more susceptible to the immediate effects of alcohol intoxication and are more likely to suffer the health consequences of prolonged abuse, such as cardiac disorders, brain atrophy, and liver disease. Most of the literature available on the gender differences in alcohol use disorders is in animal models; clinical data are significantly lacking, and essential, to a greater understanding of alcohol addiction in women.

CANNABIS DEPENDENCE

Epidemiology and Gender

Cannabis (marijuana) is the most widely produced plant-based illicit drug worldwide and the most commonly used illicit drug in the United States. The National Epidemiologic Survey on Alcohol and Related Conditions (NESARC) indicated that rates of DSM-IV cannabis abuse and dependence have increased significantly over the past decade with the lifetime prevalence rate estimated at 1.5% (2.2% males vs. 0.8% females) (Compton, Grant, Colliver, Glantz, & Stinson, 2004).

Neurotransmission and Gender Effects

The psychoactive properties of cannabis are mediated by the interaction of delta-9-tetrahydrocannibol (Δ9-THC) with the cannabinoid 1 (CB_1) receptors located within the central brain reward circuits, particularly within the neural circuitry of the VTA and the NAcc. There is also evidence that cannabinoid actions at the CB_1 receptor impact the 5-HT system. Since CB_1 receptors are codistributed with 5-HT transporter proteins in the amygdala, some investigators have suggested that cannabinoid-induced activation of the CB_1 receptor may result in reduced 5-HT release, with a subsequent acute dysphoric response (Ashton, Darlington, & Smith, 2006). Chronic cannabinoid administration has also been linked to up-regulation of 5-HT_{2A} receptor activity and concurrent down-regulation of 5-HT_{1A} receptor activity in another report. Since these particular 5-HT abnormalities are also present in depressive states, this finding may help explain the common association between chronic cannabis exposure and increased risk of depression (Hill, Sun, Tse, & Gorzalka, 2006).

It is not yet known whether consistent sex differences exist in cannabinoid-induced behavioral or physiological responses. Most of the data available are preclinical in nature. In rats, cannabinoid receptor density (Rodriguez de Fonseca, Ramos, Bonnin, & Fernandez-Ruiz, 1993) transcription and signal transduction (Mize & Alper, 2000) are influenced by sex hormones, implying a difference in male and female responses to cannabinoids. As reviewed by Craft (2005), preclinical data indicate gender differences in hypothermic, antinociceptive, and motoric effects of cannabinoids. Although D9-THC and other cannabinoid agonists elicit antinociceptive effects in both sexes, these effects are stronger in females (Romero et al., 2002). There is one report of greater D9-THC-induced hypothermia in female than male rats (Borgen, Lott, & Davis, 1973). The effect of cannabinoids on motor response in rats is less consistent and apparently dependent on the specific motor activity investigated. However, female rats are reported to be more sensitive than male rats to cannabinoid-induced locomotor activation, catalepsy, and horizontal locomotion reductions (Wiley, 2003; Tseng, Harding, & Craft, 2004).

Cannabinoids also are reported to elicit opposing actions related to sexual behavior in female versus male rats. For example, cannabinoids, when administered in relatively low acute doses, facilitate sexual receptivity in female rats (Mani, Mitchell, & O'Malley, 2001), whereas they impair sexual behavior in male rats at both low and high doses (Murphy, Gher, Steger, & Bartke, 1994). However, studies have demonstrated that cannabinoid administration in female rats is associated with suppression of sexual and nesting behaviors, as well as delayed ovulation and parturition (Frischknecht, Sieber, & Waser, 1982). Similarly, mice also demonstrate evidence of tolerance to the suppressive effects of cannabinoids on sexual and other social behaviors, presumably by attenuating release of luteinizing hormone (LH) from the pituitary (Frischknecht et al., 1982; Wenger, Ledent, Csernus, & Gerendai, 2001).

Subchronic Δ9-THC exposure produced greater impairment in spatial learning in female rats than their male counterparts (Cha, Jones, Kuhn, Wilson, & Swartzwelder, 2007). In addition, female rats exhibited greater self-administration of a synthetic cannabinoid, as compared to males (Fattore et al., 2007), suggesting differential reward systems between genders. However, a recent report also revealed evidence of some potential strain and gender differences in cannabis self-administration in rats. Both Long–Evans (LE) and Lister–hooded (LH) rats were found to self-administer a synthetic cannabinoid agonist (WIN 55,212-2), whereas Sprague–Dawley rats did not. Moreover, the female LE and LH rat strains self-administered greater amounts of WIN 55,212-2 than the male LE and LH rat strains, and ovariectomy was found to abolish the sex difference. Based on these findings the authors speculated that estrogen may have a permissive role in the reinforcing properties of cannabis administration (McGregor & Arnold, 2007). There is also evidence that Δ9-THC exposure differentially regulates opioid gene expression in female and male rats due to the interaction of estrogens (Corchero, Fuentes, & Manzanares, 2002). The endocannabinoid, anandamide, has been reported to be more potent in reversing mesenteric vasculature contractions induced by norepinephrine in female rats than in male rats in another study (Peroni et al., 2004).

Differences in cannabinoid pharmacokinetics have been reported in rodent studies. The metabolism of Δ9-THC in the liver is significantly different between humans and rats. In rats, females primarily metabolize Δ9-THC in the liver to its active metabolite, 11-hydroxy-Δ9-THC, whereas males metabolize it into multiple metabolites. Adult male rats also have a greater proportion of body fat than female rats, and it is mostly distributed within the peritoneal cavity. Since cannabinoids are highly lipophilic, body fat distribution would be expected to have a substantial influence on the distribution of cannabinoids throughout the body; in fact, female rats are reported to have greater brain tissue concentrations of Δ9-THC and its metabolites, compared to male rats, after the same amount of Δ9-THC exposure (Tseng et al., 2004).

There are very limited data concerning cannabinoids and potential impact of gender in humans. There is some evidence that Δ9-THC pharmacokinetics may differ between men and women, although the route of administration also appears to be a confounding variable. After oral administration of cannabis, women were reported to reach peak plasma concentrations of Δ9-THC more rapidly and to have higher Δ9-THC maximal plasma concentrations than men in one report (Nadulski et al., 2005). However, after smoked cannabis, Δ9-THC plasma concentrations were similar between men and women in several other reports (Mathew, Wilson, & Davis, 2003). No gender differences in subjective effects after smoking cannabis were noted in the same report (Mathew et al., 2003). However, women reported greater dizziness and experienced a greater drop in mean arterial blood pressure than men is one study (Mathew et al., 2003). Women also showed a more reduced tachycardic response than men after smoking THC (Cochetto, Owens, Perez-Reyes, DiGuiseppi, & Miller, 1981). Women with cannabis dependence were reported to have evidence of greater visuospatial memory deficits during a period of abstinence than similarly tested men with cannabis dependence during abstinence (Pope, Jacobs, Mialet, Yurgelun-Todd, & Gruber, 1997). Although sex differences in central cannabinoid receptors have not been examined, CB_1 receptor protein expression in leukocytes was found to be greater in women than in men (Onaivi et al., 1999). The effect of Δ9-THC, the endocannabinoid anandamide, and the synthetic cannabinoid receptor agonist WIN 55,212-2 on platelet 5-HT uptake and membrane microviscosity was examined in subjects with cannabis-dependent ($n = 19$) and in control subjects ($n = 20$). Opposite effect of cannabis on the 5-HT uptake efficiency was observed in men and women, with women having lower 5-HT uptake in response to chronic cannabis administration (Velenovská & Fisar, 2007).

Very little information is available concerning the potential influence of female gonadal hormones on cannabis effects in humans. A group of young women using cannabis ($n = 30$) prospectively completed daily ratings concerning mood, use of cannabis and alcohol, and sexual activity over three consecutive menstrual cycles. Women who had "heavy" cannabis use consistently reported more negative and fewer positive moods than those with "light" cannabis use. Cannabis consumption was a stronger predictor of mood than the menstrual cycle phase (Lex, Griffin, Mello, & Mendelson, 1989). There was no significant association between the amounts of daily cannabis use and the phase of the menstrual cycle (Griffin, Mendelson, Mello, & Lex, 1986). Cannabis dependence has been reported to suppress ovulation and to alter LH, follicle-stimulating hormone, and estrogen levels in women (Lee, Oh, & Chung, 2006). Smoking a single 1-g cannabis cigarette (containing 1.8% Δ9-THC) induced a 30% suppression of plasma LH levels in women during the luteal phase of the menstrual cycle, whereas smoking a placebo cigarette resulted in no change in LH in one report (Mendelson et al., 1986). In contrast, the same researchers also demonstrated that LH levels in post-menopausal women (n = 10), after smoking a single 1-g cannabis cigarette (containing 1.8% Δ9-THC), were not different from the placebo cigarette (Mendelson, Mello, et al., 1985). Chronic cannabis use has been associated with increased prolactin levels and galactorrhea in women and gynecomastia in men (Ashton, 1999). However, there is also evidence that cannabis induces acute suppression of plasma prolactin levels in females.

Summary

In summary, males have a higher prevalence rate of cannabis use disorders than females. Several endogenous cannabinoids have been isolated in the past 15–20 years, as well as two endogenous cannabinoid receptors, CB_1 and CB_2. Preclinical data suggest that female rats are more sensitive to cannabis-induced behavioral (locomotor, hypothermic, antinociceptive) effects than male rats. There are also preliminary data suggesting that female rats self-administer cannabis more than male rats, although some recent data revealed evidence of potential strain differences in cannabis self-administration in rats. Some of the gender effects may also be largely attributable to pharmacokinetic differences in cannabis metabolism, since female rats are reported to have greater brain tissue concentrations of Δ9-THC and its metabolites, compared to male rats after the same amount of Δ9-THC exposure. There are also preliminary data suggesting that cannabinoid receptor density, transcription, and signal transduction may be influenced by gonadal hormones, with perhaps estrogen having a permissive role in the reinforcing properties of cannabis administration. There are very limited data concerning cannabinoids and potential impact of gender in humans. The few studies that have examined potential gender differences in cannabis-induced subjective or physiological responses have generally failed to detect major differences. Little information is also available concerning the potential influence of female gonadal hormones on cannabis response in humans. One prospective study in females with cannabis use failed to detect any significant relationship between mood, menstrual cycle phase, and cannabis consumption. Further investigations are clearly needed.

KEY POINTS

- Gender differences are noted through all phases of drug abuse and dependence, from initiation to relapse.
- The neurobiological bases of these gender differences remain largely unknown. Empirical data are primarily based on animal models of addiction; it is uncertain whether these data can be translated to the humans.
- Gender differences in opioid addiction have been detected in the endogenous opioid system, pain perception, and opioid analgesia; however, much of the research has been conducted in the animal model.
- Gender differences exist in behavioral and subjective responses to cocaine administration, and these differences are at least partially due to the influence of female gonadal hormones.

Estrogen appears to augment cocaine-induced behavioral responses, and progesterone exhibits primarily inhibitory effects on cocaine-induced behavioral responses.

• Gender differences in the metabolism of alcohol and in the physical morbidity of long-term alcohol abuse are well-established, with females being more susceptible to the immediate effects of alcohol intoxication and more likely to suffer the health consequences of prolonged abuse. Differences in withdrawal effects and seizure susceptibility suggest a lower risk to females as compared to males.

• Preclinical data suggest that females are more sensitive to cannabis-induced behavioral effects and are more likely to self-administer cannabis as compared to males. These effects may be due to pharmacokinetic differences, as female rats have greater brain tissue concentrations of $\Delta 9$-THC and its metabolites after the same amount of $\Delta 9$-THC exposure.

REFERENCES

Asterisks denote recommended readings.

Adinoff, B., Devous, M. D., Best, S. E., Harris, T. S., Chandler, P., Frock, S. D., et al. (2003). Regional cerebral blood flow in female cocaine-addicted subjects following limbic activation. *Drug and Alcohol Dependence*, 71(3), 255–268.

Adinoff, B., Williams, M. J., Best, S. E., Harris, T. S., Chandler, P., & Devous, M. D., Sr. (2006). Sex differences in medial and lateral orbitofrontal cortex hypoperfusion in cocaine-dependent men and women. *Gender Medicine*, 3(3), 206–222.

Ashton, C. H. (1999). Adverse effects of cannabis and cannabinoids. *British Journal of Anesthesia*, 83, 637–649.

Ashton, J. C., Darlington, C. L., & Smith, P. F. (2006). Co-distribution of the cannabinoid CB1 receptor and the 5-HT transporter in the rat amygdale. *European Journal of Pharmacology*, 537(1–3), 70–71.

Becker, J. B., & Hu, M. (2008). Sex differences in drug abuse. *Frontiers in Neuroendocrinology*, 29, 36–47. (*)

Booze, R. M., Wood, M. L., Welch, M. A., Berry, S., & Mactutus, C. F. (1999). Estrous cyclicity and behavioral sensitization in female rats following repeated intravenous cocaine administration. *Pharmacology, Biochemistry, and Behavior*, 64, 605–610.

Borgen, L. A., Lott, G. C., & Davis, W. M. (1973). Cannabis-induced hypothermia: A dose–effect comparison of crude marihuana extract and synthetic D9-tetrahydrocannibinol in male and female rats. *Research Communications in Chemical Pathology and Pharmacology*, 5, 621–626.

Cahill, L. (2006). Why sex matters for neuroscience. *Nature Reviews Neuroscience*, 7, 477–484.

Carroll, M. E., Campbell, U. C., & Heideman, P. (2001). Ketaconazole suppresses food restriction-induced increases in heroin self-administration in rats: Sex differences. *Experimental and Clinical Psychopharmacology*, 9, 307–316.

Cha, Y. M., Jones, K. H., Kuhn, C. M., Wilson, W. A., & Swartzwelder, H. S. (2007). Sex differences in the effects of D-tetrahydrocannabinol on spatial learning in adolescent and adult rats. *Behavioural Pharmacology*, 18, 563–569.

Chatham, L. R., Hiller, M. L., Rowan-Szal, G. A., Joe, G. W., & Simpson, D. D. (1999). Gender differences at admission and follow-up in a sample of methadone maintenance clients. *Substance Use and Misuse*, 34(8), 1137–1165.

Chin, J., Sternin, O., Wu, H. B. K., Burrell, S., Lu, D., Jenab, S., et al. (2002). Endogenous gonadal hormones modulate behavioral and neurochemical responses to acute and chronic cocaine administration. *Brain Research*, 945, 123–130.

Chou, S. P. (1994). Sex differences in morbidity among respondents classified as alcohol abusers and/or dependent: Results of a national study. *Addiction*, 89(1), 87–93.

Cochetto, D. M., Owens, S. M., Perez-Reyes, M., DiGuiseppi, S., & Miller, L. L. (1981). Relationship between plasma delta-9-tetrahydrocannibinol concentration and pharmacologic effects in man. *Psychopharmacology, 75,* 158–164.

Compton, W. M., Grant, B. F., Colliver, J. D., Glantz, M. D., & Stinson, F. S. (2004). Prevalence of marijuana use disorders in the United States. *Journal of the American Medical Association, 291*(17), 2114–2121.

Corchero, J., Fuentes, J. A., & Manzanares, J. (2002). Gender differences in proenkephalin gene expression response to delta 9-tetrahydrocannabinol in the hypothalamus of the rat. *Journal of Psychopharmacology, 16*(4), 283–289.

Craft, R. M. (2003). Sex differences in opioid analgesia: "From mouse to man." *Clinical Journal of Pain, 19,* 175–186. (*)

Craft, R. M. (2005). Sex differences in the behavioral effects of cannabinoids. *Life Sciences, 77,* 2471–2478. (*)

Craft, R. M., Mogil, J. S., & Aloisi, A. M. (2004). Sex differences in pain and analgesia: The role of gonadal hormones. *European Journal of Pain, 8,* 397–411.

Deshmukh, A., Rosenbloom, M. J., Sassoon, S., O'Reilly, A., Pfefferbaum, A., & Sullivan, E. V. (2003). Alcoholic men endorse more DSM-IV withdrawal symptoms than alcoholic women matched in drinking history. *Journal of Studies on Alcohol, 64*(3), 375–379.

Devaud, L. L., Alele, P., & Ritu, C. (2003). Sex differences in the central nervous system actions of ethanol. *Critical Reviews in Neurobiology, 15,* 41–59. (*)

Devaud, L. L., & Chadda, R. (2001). Sex differences in rats in the development of and recovery from ethanol dependence assessed by changes in seizure susceptibility. *Alcoholism: Clinical and Experimental Research, 25,* 1689–1696.

Devaud, L. L., Risinger, F. O., & Selvage, D. (2006). Impact of the hormonal milieu on the neurobiology of alcohol dependence and withdrawal. *The Journal of General Psychology, 33*(4), 337–356.

Diehl, A., Croissant, B., Batra, A., Mundle, G., Nakovics, H., & Mann, K. (2007). Alcoholism in women: Is it different in onset and outcome compared to men? *European Archives of Psychiatry and Clinical Neuroscience, 257,* 344–351.

Elman, I., Karlsgodt, K. H., & Gastfriend, D. R. (2001). Gender differences in cocaine craving among non-treatment-seeking individuals with cocaine dependence. *American Journal of Drug and Alcohol Abuse, 27*(2), 193–202.

Evans, S. M., & Foltin, R. W. (2006). Exogenous progesterone attenuates the subjective effects of smoked cocaine in women, but not in men. *Neuropsychopharmacology, 31*(3), 659–674.

Evans, S. M., Haney, M., & Foltin, R. W. (2002). The effects of smoked cocaine during the follicular and luteal phases of the menstrual cycle in women. *Psychopharmacology, 159,* 397–406.

Fagergren, P., & Hurd, Y. L. (1999). Mesolimbic gender differences in peptide CART mRNA expression: Effects of cocaine. *Neuroreport, 10*(16), 3449–3452.

Fattore, L., Spanos, M. S., Altea, S., Angius, F., Fadda, P., & Fratta, W. (2007). Cannabinoid self-administration in rats: Sex differences and influence of ovarian cycle. *British Journal of Pharmacology, 152,* 795–804.

Festa, E. D., Jenab, S., Weiner, J., Nazarian, A., Niyomchai, T., Russo, S. J., et al. (2006). Cocaine-induced sex differences in D_1 receptor activation and binding levels after acute cocaine administration. *Brain Research Bulletin, 68*(4), 277–284.

Festa, E. D., & Quinones-Jenab, V. (2004). Gonadal hormones provide the biological basis for sex differences in behavioral responses to cocaine. *Hormones and Behavior, 46*(5), 509–519. (*)

Fillingim, R. B., & Gear, R. W. (2004). Sex differences in opioid analgesia: Clinical and experimental findings. *European Journal of Pain, 8*(5), 413–425.

Fink, G., Sumner, B. E., Rosie, R., Grace, O., & Quinn, J. P. (1996). Estrogen control of central neurotransmission: Effect on mood, mental state, and memory. *Cellular and Molecular Neurobiology, 16*(3), 325–344.

Fox, H. C., Garcia, M., Jr., Kemp, K., Milivojevic, V., Kreek, M. J., & Sinha, R. (2006). Gender differences in cardiovascular and corticoadrenal response to stress and drug cues in cocaine dependent individuals. *Psychopharmacology (Berl), 185*(3), 348–357.

Fox, H. C., Hong, K. A., Paliwal, P., Morgan, P. T., & Sinha, R. (2008). Altered levels of sex and stress steroid hormones assessed daily over a 28-day cycle in early abstinent cocaine-dependent females. *Psychopharmacology (Berl)*, *195*(4), 527–536.

Frischknecht, H. R., Sieber, B., & Waser, P. G. (1982). Effects of multiple, chronic, and early hashish exposure on mating behavior, nest-building, and gestation in mice. *Comparative Biochemistry and Physiology*, *72C*, 363–368.

Gianoulakis, C., Dai, X., & Brown, T. (2003). Effect of chronic alcohol consumption on the activity of the hypothalamic–pituitary–adrenal axis and pituitary beta-endorphin as a function of alcohol intake, age, and gender. *Alcoholism: Clinical and Experimental Research*, *27*(3), 410–423.

Graven-Nielsen, T., & Arendt-Nielsen, L. (2007). Gender differences in response to pain. *Ugeskrift for Laeger*, *169*(25), 2425–2427.

Greenfield, S. F. (2002). Women and alcohol use disorders. *Harvard Review of Psychiatry*, *10*(2), 76–85.

Griffin, M. L., Mendelson, J. H., Mello, N. K., & Lex, B. W. (1986). Marihuana use across the menstrual cycle. *Drug and Alcohol Dependence*, *18*(2), 213–224.

Hill, M. N., Sun, J. C., Tse, M. T., & Gorzalka, B. B. (2006). Altered responsiveness of serotonin receptor subtypes following long-term cannabinoid treatment. *International Journal of Neuropsychopharmacology*, *9*(3), 277–286.

Holtman, J. R., Jr., & Wala, E. P. (2006). Characterization of the antinociceptive effect of oxycodone in male and female rats. *Pharmacology, Biochemistry, and Behavior*, *83*(1), 100–108.

Hurd, Y. L., Svenson, P., & Ponten, M. (1999). The role of dopamine, dynorphin, and CART systems in the ventral striatum and amygdala in cocaine abuse. *Annals of the New York Academy of Sciences*, *877*, 499–506.

Jackson, L. R., Robinson, T. E., & Becker, J. B. (2006). Sex differences and hormonal influences on acquisition of cocaine self-administration in rats. *Neuropsychopharmacology*, *31*(1), 129–138.

Kalivas, P. W. (2004). Recent understanding in the mechanisms of addiction. *Current Psychiatry Reports*, *6*, 347–351.

Kenna, G. A., McGeary, J. E., & Swift, R. M. (2004). Pharmacotherapy, pharmacogenomics, and the future of alcohol dependence treatment. *American Journal Heath-Systems Pharmacy*, *61*(21), 2272–2279.

Kilts, C. D., Gross, R. E., Ely, T. D., & Drexler, K. P. (2004). The neural correlates of cue-induced craving in cocaine dependent women. *American Journal of Psychiatry*, *161*, 233–241.

King, T. S., Schenken, R. S., Kang, I. S., Javors, M. A., & Riehl, R. M. (1990). Cocaine disrupts estrous cyclicity and alters the reproductive neuroendocrine axis in the rat. *Neuroendocrinology*, *51*, 15–22.

Kippin, T. E., Fuchs, R. A., Mehta, R. H., Case, J. M., Parker, M. P., Bimonte-Nelson, H. A., et al. (2005). Potentiation of cocaine-primed reinstatement of drug seeking in female rats during estrus. *Psychopharmacology (Berl)*, *182*(2), 245–252.

Klein, L. C., Popke, J. E., & Grunberg, N. E. (1997). Sex differences in effects of predictable and unpredictable footshock on fentanyl self-administration in rats. *Experimental and Clinical Psychopharmacology*, *5*, 99–106.

Koob, G. F., & Le Moal, M. (1997). Drug abuse: Hedonic homeostatic dysregulation. *Science*, *278*(5335), 52–58.

Kosten, T. R., Kosten, T. A., McDougle, C. J., Hameedi, F. A., McCance, E. F., Rosen, M. I., et al. (1996). Gender differences in response to intranasal cocaine administration to humans. *Biological Psychiatry*, *39*, 147–148.

Kouri, E. M., Lundahl, L. H., Borden, K. N., McNeil, J. F., & Lukas, S. E., (2002). Effects of oral contraceptives on acute cocaine responses in female volunteers. *Pharmacology, Biochemistry, and Behavior*, *74*, 173–180.

Kreek, M. J., Schluger, J., Borg, L., Gunduz, M., & Ho, A. (1999). Dynorphin A1-13 causes elevation of serum levels of prolactin through an opioid receptor mechanism in humans: Gender differences and implications for modulation of dopaminergic tone in the treatment of addictions. *Journal of Pharmacology and Experimental Therapeutics*, *288*(1), 260–269.

Lee, S. Y., Oh, S. M., & Chung, K. H. (2006). Estrogenic effects of marijuana smoke condensate and cannabinoid compounds. *Toxicology and Applied Pharmacology*, *214*(3), 270–278.

Leigh, W. A., & Jimenez, M. A. (Eds.). (2002). *Women of color health data book* (2nd ed., NIH Publication No. 02-4247). Washington, DC: U.S. Office of Research on Women's Health.

Levin, J. M., Holman, B. L., Mendelson, J. H., Teoh, S. K., Garada, B., Johnson, K. A., et al. (1994). Gender differences in cerebral perfusion in cocaine abuse: Technetium-99m-HMPAO SPECT study of drug-abusing women. *Journal of Nuclear Medicine, 35*(12), 1902–1909.

Lex, B. W., Griffin, M. L., Mello, N. K., & Mendelson, J. H. (1989) Alcohol, marijuana, and mood states in young women. *International Journal of the Addictions, 24*(5), 405–424.

Li, C. S., Kemp, K., Milivojevic, V., & Sinha, R. (2005). Neuroimaging study of sex differences in the neuropathology of cocaine abuse. *Gender Medicine, 2*(3), 174–182.

Li, C. S., Kosten, T. R., & Sinha, R. (2005). Sex differences in brain activation during stress imagery in abstinent cocaine users: A functional magnetic resonance imaging study. *Biolological Psychiatry, 57*(5), 487–494. (*)

Lubman, D. I., Yucel, M., & Pantelis, C. (2004). Addiction, a condition of compulsive behavior? Neuroimaging and neuropsychological evidence of inhibitory dysregulation. *Addiction, 99,* 1491–1502.

Lukas, S. E., Sholar, M. B., Lundahl, L. H., Lamas, X., Kouri, E., Wines, J. D., et al. (1996). Sex differences in plasma cocaine levels and subjective effects after acute cocaine administration in human volunteers. *Psychopharmacology, 125,* 346–356.

Lynch, W. J., Roth, M. E., & Carroll, M. E. (2002). Biological basis of sex differences in drug abuse: Preclinical and clinical studies. *Psychopharmacology, 164,* 121–137. (*)

Mani, S. K., Mitchell, A., & O'Malley, B. W. (2001). Progesterone receptor and dopamine receptors are required in D-tetrahydrocannibinol modulation of sexual receptivity in female rats. *Proceedings of the National Academy of Sciences, 98,* 1249–1254.

Mathew, R. J., Wilson, W. H., & Davis, R. (2003). Postural syncope after marijuana: A transcranial Doppler study of the hemodynamics. *Pharmacology, Biochemistry, and Behavior, 75,* 309–318.

McGregor, I. S., & Arnold, J. C. (2007). Cannabis reward: Biased towards the fairer sex? *British Journal of Pharmacology, 152*(5), 562–564.

Mendelson, J. H., Cristofaro, P., Ellingboe, J., Benedikt, R., & Mello, N. K. (1985). Acute effects of marihuana on luteinizing hormone in menopausal women. *Pharmacology, Biochemistry, and Behavior, 23*(5), 765–768.

Mendelson, J. H., Mello, N. K., & Ellingboe, J. (1985). Acute effects of marihuana smoking on prolactin levels in human females. *Journal of Pharmacology and Experimental Therapeutics, 232*(1), 220–222.

Mendelson, J. H., Mello, N. K., Ellingboe, J., Skupny, A. S., Lex, B. W., & Griffin, M. (1986). Marijuana smoking suppresses luteinizing hormone in women. *Journal of Pharmacology and Experimental Therapeutics, 237*(3), 862–866.

Mendelson, J. H., Mello, N. K., Sholar, M. B., Siegel, A. J., Kaufman, M. J., Levin, J. M., et al. (1999). Cocaine pharmacokinetics in men and in women during the follicular and luteal phases of the menstrual cycle. *Neuropsychopharmacology, 21*(2), 294–303.

Mermelstein, P. G., Becker, J. B., & Surmeier, D. J. (1996). Estradiol reduces calcium currents in rat neostriatal neurons through a membrane receptor. *Journal of Neuroscience, 16,* 595–604.

Mize, A. L., & Alper, R. H. (2000). Acute and long-term effects of 17beta-estradiol on G(i/o) coupled neurotransmitter receptor function in the female rat brain as assessed by agonist-stimulated [35S] GTPgammaS binding. *Brain Research, 859,* 326–333.

Murphy, L. L., Gher, J., Steger, R. W., & Bartke, A. (1994). Effects of D9-tetrahydrocannibinol on copulatory behavior and neuroendocrine responses of male rats to female conspecifics. *Pharmacology, Biochemistry, and Behavior, 48,* 1011–1017.

Nadulski, T., Pragst, F., Weinberg, G., Roser, P., Schnelle, M., Fronk, E. M., et al. (2005). Randomized double-blind, placebo-controlled study about the effects of cannabidiol on the pharmacokinetics of delta9-tetrahydrocannabinol after oral application of THC versus standardized cannabis extract. *Therapeutic Drug Monitoring, 27,* 799–810.

Onaivi, E. S., Chaudhuri, G., Abaci, A. S., Parker, M., Manier, D. H., Martin, P. R., et al. (1999). Expression of cannabinoid receptors and their gene transcripts in human blood cells. *Progress in Neuropsychopharmacology and Biological Psychiatry, 23,* 1063–1077.

Peroni, R. N., Orliac, M. L., Becu-Villalobos, D., Huidobro-Toro, J. P., Adler-Graschinsky, E., & Celuch, S. M. (2004). Sex-linked differences in the vasorelaxant effects of anandamide in vascular mesenteric beds: Role of oestrogens. *European Journal of Pharmacology, 493,* 151–160.

Pettit, H. O., & Justice, J. B., Jr. (1989). Dopamine in the nucleus accumbens during cocaine self-administration as studied by in vivo microdialysis. *Pharmacology, Biochemistry, and Behavior, 34*(4), 899–904.

Pleym, H., Spigset, O., Kharasch, E. D., & Dale, O. (2003). Gender differences in drug effects: Implications for anesthesiologists. *Acta Anaesthesiologica Scandanavica, 47*(3), 241–259.

Pope, H. G., Jacobs, A., Mialet, J.-P., Yurgelun-Todd, D., & Gruber, S. (1997). Evidence for a sex-specific residual effect of cannabis on visuospatial memory. *Psychotherapy and Psychosomatics, 66,* 179–184.

Quinones-Jenab, V., Perrotti, L. I., Ho, A., Jenab, S., Schlussman, S. D., Franck, J., et al. (2000). Cocaine affects progesterone plasma levels in female rats. *Pharmacology, Biochemistry, and Behavior, 66,* 449–453.

Rodriguez de Fonseca, F., Ramos, J. A., Bonnin, A., & Fernandez-Ruiz, J. J. (1993). Presence of cannabinoid binding sites in the brain from early postnatal ages. *NeuroReport, 4,* 135–138.

Romero, E. M., Fernandez, B., Sagredo, O., Gomez, N., Uriguen, L., Guaza, C., et al. (2002). Antinociceptive, behavioural and neuroendocrine effects of CP 55,940 in young rats. *Developmental Brain Research, 136,* 85–92.

Schweinsburg, B. C., Alhassoon, O. M., Taylor, M. J., Gonzalez, R., Videen, J. S., Brown, G. G., et al. (2003). Effects of alcoholism and gender on brain metabolism. *American Journal of Psychiatry, 160,* 1180–1183.

Sell, S. L., Thomas, M. L., & Cunningham, K. A. (2002). Influence of estrous cycle and estradiol on behavioral sensitization to cocaine in female rats. *Drug and Alcohol Dependence, 67,* 281–290.

Simoni-Wastila, L. (2000). The use of abusable prescription drugs: The role of gender. *Journal of Women's Health and Gender-Based Medicine, 9*(3), 289–297.

Sinha, R., Fox, H., Hong, K. I., Sofuoglu, M., Morgan, P. T., & Bergquist, K. T. (2007). Sex steroid hormones, stress response, and drug craving in cocaine-dependent women: Implications for relapse susceptibility. *Experimental and Clinical Psychopharmacology, 15*(5), 445–452. (*)

Sofuoglu, M., Babb, D. A., & Hatsukami, D. K. (2002). Effects of progesterone treatment on smoked cocaine response in women. *Pharmacology, Biochemistry, and Behavior, 72,* 431–435.

Sofuoglu, M., Duidish-Poulsen, S., Nelson, D., Pentel, P. R., & Hatsukami, D. K. (1999). Sex and menstrual cycle differences in the subjective effects from smoked cocaine in humans. *Experimental and Clinical Psychopharmacology, 7,* 274–283.

Stimmel, B., & Kreek, M. J. (2000). Neurobiology of addictive behaviors and its relationship to methadone maintenance. *Mt. Sinai Journal of Medicine, 67*(5–6), 375–380.

Stine, S. M. (1998). Opiate dependence and current treatments. In E. F. McCance-Katz & T. R. Kosten (Eds.), *New treatments for chemical addiction* (pp. 75–111). Washington, DC: American Psychiatric Association.

Substance Abuse and Mental Health Services Administration. (2005). *Results from the (2004) National Survey on Drug Use and Health: National findings* (Office of Applied Studies, National Survey Drug Use Health, Series H-28, DHHS Publication No. SMA 05-4062). Rockville, MD: Author.

Substance Abuse and Mental Health Services Administration. (2006). National Survey on Drug Use and Health. Retrieved March 27, 2008, from *www.oas.samhsa.gov/NSDUH/2k6NSDUH/tabs/Sect2peTabs43to84.htm#Tab2.46B*

Substance Abuse and Mental Health Services Administration. (2007). *The NSDUH report: Gender differences in alcohol use and alcohol dependence or abuse: 2004 and 2005* (Office of Applied Studies). Rockville, MD.

Trujillo, K. A. (2002). The neurobiology of opiate tolerance, dependence, and sensitization: Mechanisms of NMDA receptor-dependent synaptic plasticity. *Neurotoxicity Research, 4*(4), 373–391.

Tseng, A. H., Harding, J. W., & Craft, R. M. (2004). Pharmacokinetic factors in sex differences in D-tetrahydrocannabinol-induced behavior effects in rats. *Behavioural Brain Research, 154,* 77–83.

Tucker, K. A., Browndyke, J. N., Gottschalk, P. C., Cofrancesco, A. T., & Kosten, T. R. (2004). Gender-specific vulnerability for rCBF abnormalities among cocaine abusers. *NeuroReport*, *15*(5), 797–801.

Van Etten, M. L., & Anthony, J. C. (1999). Comparative epidemiology of initial drug opportunities and transitions to first use: Marijuana, cocaine, hallucinogens, and heroin. *Drug and Alcohol Dependence*, *54*, 117–125.

Velenovská, M., & Fisar, Z. (2007). Effect of cannabinoids on platelet serotonin uptake. *Addiction Biology*, *12*(2), 158–166.

Ventura, R., Alcaro, A., & Puglisi-Allegra, S. (2005). Prefrontal cortical norepinephrine release is critical for morphine-induced reward, reinstatement and dopamine release in the nucleus accumbens. *Cerebral Cortex*, *15*(12), 1877–1886.

Volkow, N. D., Wang, G. J., Telang, F., Fowler, J. S., Logan, J., Childress, A. R., et al. (2006). Cocaine cues and dopamine in dorsal striatum: Mechanism of craving in cocaine addiction. *Journal of Neuroscience*, *26*(24), 6583–6588.

Walker, Q. D., Cabassa, J., Kaplan, K. A., Li, S. T., Haroon, J., Spohr, H. A., et al. (2001). Sex differences in cocaine-stimulated motor behavior: Disparate effects of gonadectomy. *Neuropsychopharmacology*, *25*, 118–130.

Walker, Q. D., Nelson, C. J., Smith, D., & Kuhn, C. M. (2002). Vaginal lavage attenuates cocaine stimulated activity and establishes place preference in rats. *Pharmacology, Biochemistry, and Behavior*, *73*, 743–752.

Wang, G. J., Volkow, N. D., Fowler, J. S., Franceschi, D., Wong, C. T., Pappas, N. R., et al. (2003). Alcohol intoxication induces greater reductions in brain metabolism in male than in female subjects. *Alcoholism, Clinical and Experimental Research*, *27*(6), 909–917.

Wenger, T., Ledent, C., Csernus, V., & Gerendai, I. (2001). The central cannabinoid receptor inactivation suppresses endocrine reproductive functions. *Biochemical and Biophysical Research Communications*, *284*, 363–368.

Wiley, J. L. (2003). Sex-dependent effects of D-tetrahydrocannabinol on locomotor activity in mice. *Neuroscience Letters*, *352*, 77–80.

Wilkens, J. N. (2007). *Neurobiology and pharmacotherapy for alcohol dependence: Treatment options. In identifying and treating patients with alcohol dependence in your practice: Pharmacotherapeutic and psychosocial interventions.* Retrieved April 10, 2008, from *www.medscape.com/viewprogram/6694_pnt*.

Wise, R. A. (1989). The brain and reward. In J. M. Lieberman & S. J. Cooper (Eds.), *The neuropharmacological basis of reward* (pp. 377–424). Oxford, UK: Oxford University Press.

Wojnar, M., Wasilewski, D., Matsumoto, H., & Cedro, A. (1997). Differences in the course of alcohol withdrawal in women and men: A Polish sample. *Alcoholism: Clinical and Experimental Research*, *21*(8), 1351–1355.

CHAPTER 7

Sex Differences in Pharmacokinetics and Pharmacodynamics

C. Lindsay DeVane, PharmD

The pharmacotherapy of women with substance use disorders (SUDs), as with any disorder, should necessarily include a consideration of the contribution sex differences play in pharmacokinetics and pharmacodynamics. This is especially important since prescribing guidelines and dispositional parameters for many drugs were developed over decades of studies conducted predominantly in young adult males (Merkatz, Temple, Sobel, et al., 1993). Women generally weigh less than men, so drugs dosed on an average milligram daily basis will tend to result in higher levels in women than the same dose given to an average male. In addition, sex differences have been observed in the activity of many drug-metabolizing enzymes and transporters mediating the clearance of both drugs of abuse as well as the medications used in treating addiction. Such differences can impact the variability in drug response, potentially causing either exaggerated or diminished drug effects in relation to expectations based on normative data obtained from males. This chapter summarizes sex-determined differences that have a potential influence on drug pharmacokinetics. Some fundamental principles of drug disposition are discussed; detailed reviews are available elsewhere (e.g., see Anderson, 2005; Anthony & Berg, 2002; DeVane, 2009; Meibohm, Beierle, & Derendorf, 2002). Research findings are reviewed that differentiate drug disposition and/or response by sex, especially when clinical significance is apparent for women with addictions.

SEX DIFFERENCES IN PHARMACOKINETICS

Basic Description of Drug Disposition

The field of pharmacokinetics divides the study of drug disposition into *absorption, distribution in the body, metabolism* (i.e., elimination), and *excretion* (renal excretion of drug or metabolites). Mathematical parameters are used to describe these processes and allow predictions of the time course of drug concentration in the body following administration of single or multiple doses. Table 7.1 is a list of the most commonly estimated pharmacokinetic parameters and an explanation of their meaning. Pharmacokinetic studies generally estimate population mean values of these parameters under highly controlled conditions, and the

TABLE 7.1. Pharmacokinetic Parameters Useful to Differentiate Sex Differences in Drug Disposition

Parameter	Abbreviation	Range of values	Explanation/application
Bioavailability	F	0 to 1.0	Usually interpreted to be the proportion of an oral dose of drug that reaches the systemic circulation intact (i.e., neither passes out of the gastrointestinal tract unabsorbed nor is metabolized in the gut wall or liver).
Absorption rate constant	Ka	Measured as reciprocal time; for example, 0.5 hr^{-1} means 50% is absorbed in 1 hour	A measure of the speed or rate at which drug is absorbed and appears in the circulation.
Maximum concentration in plasma	Cmax	Any concentration value above zero	Usually observed early during a dosage interval and may correlate with appearance of clinical effects.
Time of maximum concentration	Tmax	Any time after a drug dose	Tmax values generally reflect the rate of drug absorption, with earlier values in a dosage interval implying faster absorption.
Apparent volume of distribution	Vd	Plasma volume as a minimum; any value possible, reported as L or L/kg.	Relates the drug concentration measured in blood or plasma to the volume of the body that would be necessary to hold all of the administered drug at the same concentration; Vd should not be interpreted to reflect the extent of physical distribution.
Plasma protein binding	F_B or ff	Fraction bound (F_B) or free fraction (ff); can be any value between 0 and 1.0	The proportion of drug in the plasma that circulates bound to proteins or that circulates unbound.
Area under the plasma concentration vs. time curve	AUC	Any value greater than zero measured as concentration × time	An overall measure of systemic drug exposure; essential measure for estimating oral clearance.
Clearance	Cl	Measured in volume of blood or plasma completely cleared of drug over some interval of time; may be normalized to body weight (e.g., L/kg/hr)	Best overall measure of the ability of the body to eliminate drug over time; can be used to predict the amount of drug accumulation in the body upon chronic dosing.
Elimination rate constant	Kel	Similar to Ka except relates amount of drug eliminated over a measure of time; for example, 0.5 hr^{-1} means 50% eliminated in 1 hour	Commonly used to calculate elimination half-life as a more easily understood parameter.
Half-life	$t_{1/2}$	Any time value greater than zero	The time required for drug concentration or the amount of drug in the body to be reduced by 50%.
Extraction ratio	E	0 to 1	The proportion of drug passing through the liver or other eliminating organ that is taken up for elimination; along with blood flow to the organ, E is a primary determinant of clearance.

Note. Data from DeVane (2009).

deviation of drug behavior in any individual patient encountered in clinical practice from the population average can be substantial.

The success of any pharmacological therapy depends upon many factors but critically on (1) choosing the correct drug for the indication; (2) the dosage regimen design, including the route of administration; and (3) the specific formulation to be given. Most therapeutic drugs in addiction medicine are taken by mouth because of the convenience offered by the oral route of administration. As a drug dose is released from its pharmaceutical formulation following oral administration, a portion of the absorbed amount may be extracted into the liver and metabolized. Gut wall extraction and metabolism generally occur to a lesser extent. The remainder that escapes metabolism during the first pass through the gut and liver reaches the systemic circulation. The absorbed drug is transported and distributed, often attached to plasma proteins, to organs and tissues containing molecular targets; this is the point at which sex differences may influence pharmacological response. Drug molecules transiting through the body will eventually be extracted by the liver and metabolized and/or be eliminated by renal excretion. The efficiency of this extraction process, along with blood flow to the kidneys and liver, determines the rate of drug clearance by the body.

When the same milligram daily dose is given repeatedly, a steady-state situation ensues whereby the amount of drug that is introduced into the body each day equals the amount that is eliminated each day. However, rarely (with the exception of a constant rate intravenous infusion) is a steady-state reflected by a true plateau of drug concentration in the blood that can be measured during a pharmacokinetic study. For a substantial period of time during a dosage interval, the processes of absorption, distribution, and elimination occur simultaneously. Drug concentration in blood or plasma is almost always changing over time. Thus a sex difference in any of the multiple physiological factors that influence drug disposition could alter the time course of the drug as it passes through the body. For this reason, subtle differences between women and men in pharmacokinetics can be difficult to detect, and many are likely yet undiscovered. Table 7.2 summarizes some sex differences reported in drug transporters, drug-metabolizing enzymes, and plasma drug-binding proteins.

Absorption

The pharmacokinetic models used to study drug absorption focus on the effects of membrane permeability, dosage form release or dissolution rate of drug into the gastrointestinal (GI) tract, gastric emptying time (GI transit), and first-pass elimination. The first two factors are not thought to be influenced by sex. GI transit time is slower in females than males (Chen, Coong, Chang, et al., 1995; Sadik, Abrahamsson, & Stotzer, 2003) and is thought to be due to an inhibitory effect of estrogen on gastric emptying (Coskun, Sevine, Tevetoglu, et al., 1995). Although the results of bioavailability studies are not consistent, conditions that decrease small-intestinal transit time are expected to decrease drug absorption. Opioids delay GI transit, which may alter the rate of absorption of orally administered drugs. Methyl-naltrexone attenuated a morphine-induced delay in GI transit and reversed the lower bioavailability of acetaminophen caused by morphine alone, compared to placebo—an effect apparently independent of sex (Murphy, Sutton, Prescott, et al., 1997). Alterations in GI transit time have been observed in pregnancy but not consistently during the menstrual cycle (Caballero-Plascenia, Valenzuela-Barranco, Martin-Ruiz, et al., 1999; Singer & Brandt, 1991). Nevertheless, hormonal-induced changes may contribute to intrasubject variability in drug absorption. In conclusion, sex does not appear to be a significant influence on total drug absorption, but absorption rate may be slightly slower in women.

Drug molecules encounter a barrier to absorption following release from an oral dosage

TABLE 7.2. Sex Differences in Drug Transporters, Drug-Metabolizing Enzymes, and Plasma Drug-Binding Proteins

	Gender-specific activity	Comments	References
Drug transporters			
P-glycoprotein (P-gp)	F < M or F = M	Potentially greater gastrointestinal absorption of substrates	Lown et al. (1997); Schuetz et al. (1995); Paine et al. (2005)
Breast cancer resistance protein (BCRP)	F < M	Possible sex-specific variability in pharmacokinetics of BCRP substrates	Merino et al. (2005)
Drug-metabolizing enzymes			
CYP1A2	F < M	Lower clearance of CYP1A2 substrates for clozapine and olanzapine shown	Relling et al. (1992); Ou-Yang et al. (2000); Haring et al. (1989); Lane et al. (1999)
CYP2A6	F > M	Influences nicotine metabolism	Xu et al. (2004); Benowitz et al. (2002)
CYP2B6	F > M	Influences bupropion metabolism	Lamba et al. (2003)
CYP2C9	F = M	Sparse data to suggest sex differences	Anderson (2005)
CYP2C19	F = M	Oral contraceptives may decrease activity; ethnic differences	Hagg et al. (2001); Sviri et al. (1999); Tamminga et al. (1999)
CYP2D6	F > M	Inconsistent findings	McCune et al. (2001); Tamminga et al. (1999)
CYP2E1	F < M	Higher ethanol in women due to other factors	Lucas et al. (1995); Baraona et al. (2001)
CYP3A4	F > M or F = M	Conclusions confounded by overlap of substrate specificity with P-gp	Hunt et al. (1992); Cummins et al. (2002)
UDPGT	F < M		Liston et al. (2001); de Leon (2003)
Plasma proteins			
Albumin	F = M; decreases with age in both	Increased free fraction of drugs with age	Bailey & Briggs (2004); Verbeeck et al. (1984)
Alpha-1-acid glycoprotein	F < M	Decreases induced by estrogen treatment	Tuck et al. (1997); Wiegratz et al. (2003)

formulation by the action of efflux transporters, which minimize or prevent passage across the endothelial cells of the GI tract. These cells contain several drug transporters as well as drug-metabolizing enzymes. The most thoroughly studied transporter is the *ABCB1* gene product known as P-glycoprotein (P-gp). The normal function of this protein is to efflux its substrates back into the GI tract, an energy-requiring process that displays both sex and genetic variability. The reports of sex differences in P-gp expression have not been consistent. Schuetz, Furuya, Schuetz, et al. (1995) reported that women had a significantly higher level of P-gp than men from innumochemical analysis of messenger ribonucleic acid (mRNA) in 41 hepatic tissue samples. In contrast, women have been found to have lower expression of P-gp in the gut wall than men (Lown, Mayo, Leichman, et al., 1997). The results of duodenal biopsies from 45 women and 48 men found a 10-fold variability in P-gp expression and no sex difference (Paine, Hart, Ludington, et al., 2005). A sex difference in P-gp content or activity would predict a change in drug efflux into the GI tract of P-gp substrates. The overall effect could be a change in hepatic extraction and presystemic metabolism and an alteration in oral drug bioavailability. Experimental support for a clinically significant effect of a sex difference in P-gp on drug bioavailability is lacking, but the impact of P-gp on drug absorption is likely to be highly substrate dependent. Human data for other drug transporters are sparse.

Apart from sex differences in drug transporters, genetic variability in transporter expression may influence drug dosage requirements in either sex. For example, our group showed that transgenic mice lacking the gene encoding for P-gp had dramatically higher brain concentration of methadone, compared to genetically intact animals (Wang, Ruan, Taylor, et al., 2004). This finding implies that individuals with single nucleotide polymorphisms (SNPs), coding for reduced P-gp activity might require different maintenance doses of methadone. Coller, Barratt, Dahlen, et al. (2006) found that patients with a wild-type, or normal, halotype for several P-gp (SNPs) required higher methadone dose requirements than those with a defective allele. This genetic consequence may be especially important in the pregnant patient with an opioid dependence, as P-gp appears to influence transplacental passage of methadone (Nanovskaya, Nekhayeva, Karunaratne, et al., 2005). Our recognition is increasing of the importance of placental transporter proteins in the psychopharmacological treatment of the pregnant patient (Wang, Newport, Stowe, et al., 2007). While it is well recognized that increases in methadone clearance during pregnancy generally result in a need for cautious increased maintenance dosing (Wolff, Boys, Rostami-Hodjegan, et al., 2005), the genotype of both the mother and the fetus for relevant enzymes and transporters becomes an important pharmacokinetic variable in individualizing pharmacotherapy for the pregnant woman with an addiction.

Distribution

The systemic circulation is not the target site of action for drugs of abuse or their drug therapies. The distribution of drugs to tissues beyond the systemic circulation is dependent upon a variety of factors that include plasma protein and tissue binding, body composition and weight, and organ blood flow. With few exceptions in psychopharmacology, such as lithium and gabapentin, drugs circulate and are distributed to their sites of action bound to plasma proteins. Drug-binding proteins in plasma are principally albumin for acidic drugs and alpha-1-acid glycoprotein (AAG) for basic drugs. Plasma albumin concentration decreases with advanced age in both men and women. AAG concentration has been reported to increase with age, but the increase is less in females. Plasma albumin concentration appears to be unaffected by sex, whereas the concentration of AAG is slightly lower in females, compared with males (Kishino, Nomura, Di, et al., 1995; Routledge, Stargel, Kitchell, et al., 1981).

Sex differences in drug protein binding have been investigated for a variety of prototypic acidic and basic drugs (Routledge, Stargel, Kitchell, et al., 1981). AAG concentration in 245 healthy subjects was significantly lower in women than men (0.67 ± 0.16 mg/ml vs. 0.78 ± 0.18 mg/ml) (Kishino et al., 1995), but no significant difference was found in the unbound fraction when using disopyramide as a test drug. The plasma protein binding of chlorpromazine, propranolol, meperidine, desipramine, salicylic acid, and phenytoin was determined in 35 males and 29 females by Verbeeck, Cardinal, and Wallace (1984). The free fractions of basic and acidic drugs showed a negative correlation with plasma protein levels. Only for salicylic acid was there a statistically significant difference between females and males. Treatment with estrogen, in the form of either oral contraceptives or estrogen replacement therapy, decreased the concentration of AAG by 18–37% (Tuck, Holleran, & Bergland, 1997; Walle, Fagan, Topmiller, et al., 1994; Wiegratz, Kutschera, Lee, et al., 2003). The protein decrease was reflected by an decrease in the bound percentage of propranolol in plasma by approximately 2%. The significance for pharmacotherapy is unclear but is likely to be marginal for small differences in drug protein binding. Most reviews of plasma protein-binding data conclude that the clinical significance of any sex differences in protein binding is minimal or questionable (Bailey & Briggs, 2004; Beierle, Meibohm, & Devendorf, 1999; Harris, Benet, & Schwartz, 1995).

Metabolism

Drug and xenobiotic elimination are fundamental processes essential to life. The vast number of organic and inorganic compounds in the environment would quickly overwhelm humans and other living organisms with an unbearable amount of substances toxic to various organs if sufficient means were unavailable to keep such toxins to a tolerable load. Although nutrients and minerals, such as iron, are essential in maintaining physiological integrity, in sufficient quantity they also become toxic.

The principal pathways of biotransformation that affect drugs are traditionally separated into Phase I and Phase II reactions. Phase I reactions are biotransformations of chemical groups on the drug molecule. Phase II reactions attach or conjugate the drug to an endogenous or exogenous substrate to make a larger molecule more easily eliminated by glomerular filtration. Phase I reactions introduce oxygen into the drug molecule or hydrolyze esters or amides. They frequently, but not always, precede Phase II reactions. Multiple families of enzymes are available to serve this function. The resulting primary metabolite can be further metabolized, if necessary, by Phase II reactions, which generally create more hydrophilic (water-soluble) molecules. Of the principle enzymes for drug metabolism, the cytochrome P450 (CYP) families involved in Phase I oxidations and the uridine glucuronyl-transferase (UGT) families involved in Phase II conjugations have received the most study for sex differences.

The CYP isoenzymes are a heterogeneous group of over 30 heme-containing oxidative enzymes located predominantly in the endoplasmic reticulum of hepatocytes (Shimada, Yamazaki, Mimura, et al., 1994). Some enzyme content is also located in extrahepatic tissues, including the brain and along the GI tract (Paine et al., 2006). This enzyme content is responsible for Phase I metabolism of a wide variety of endogenous and exogenous substrates, including fatty acids, prostaglandins, steroids, carcinogens/procarcinogens, and drugs. The P450 enzymes are involved in metabolism of at least 80% of all available drugs. Eight CYP enzymes are recognized as the most important for human drug metabolism: CYP1A2,

CYP2A6, CYP2B6, CYP2C9, CYP2C19, CYP2D6, CYP2E1, and CYP3A4. Sex-related differences have been investigated for each of these.

Other enzyme systems include the flavin-containing mono-oxygenases (FMOs) of at least five isoenzyme families in humans and the UGTs of which UGT1 and UGT2 are the most important subfamilies for drug metabolism (Liston, Markowitz, & DeVane, 2001). Other non-P450 enzymes are the methyltransferases and sulfotransferases, but sex-determined differences have been less well studied for these than for the CYP isozymes.

The activity of CYP1A2 shows a broad variability across women and men. Its activity has frequently been phenotyped using caffeine metabolism evaluated as various metabolite ratios in urine. Studies in European American, African American, and Chinese populations are consistent in finding CYP1A2 activity to be lower in women than men (Ou-Yang, Huang, Wang, et al., 2000; Relling, Lin, Ayers, et al., 1992). However, no major interethnic differences were found in CYP1A2 activity, using phenacetin as a metabolite probe, between European American and Chinese women (Bartoli, Xiasdong, Gatti, et al., 1996). These studies suggest that a slower clearance and higher plasma concentration of CYP1A2 substrates would occur in females. In samples from 148 patients, plasma concentrations of clozapine, a CYP1A2 substrate, in males were only 69% of the concentrations in female patients when normalized for dose and body weight (Haring, Meise, Humpel, et al., 1989). Data from a larger sample of 2,648 males and 1,127 females predicted a 17% higher plasma clozapine concentration in females (Rostami-Hodjegan, Amin, Spencer, et al., 2004). Like clozapine, olanzapine is a CYP1A2 substrate, and females accumulate higher plasma concentrations due to a 30% lower clearance than males, but there were no demonstrated differences in effectiveness or adverse events (Physicians' Desk Reference, 2005).

CYP1A2 is highly inducible. In response to treatment with St. Johns wort, CYP1A2 appeared to be induced only in females and not males (Wenk, Todesco, & Krahenbuhl, 2004). It is also induced by cigarette smoking but inhibited by oral contraceptives (Rasmussen, Brix, Kyvik, et al., 2002). In clozapine patients, females who smoke had lower clozapine plasma concentrations, compared to females who did not smoke (Haring et al., 1989).

CYP2A6 appears to be the major P450 involved in human nicotine metabolism to cotinine (Messina et al., 1997). Its activity is highly variable both in *in vitro* investigations using human liver microsomes (Messina, Tyndale, & Sellers, 1997) and in humans phenotyped using coumarin as a specific and selective CYP2A6 substrate. Xu, Huang, Zhu, et al. (2004) found the activity to vary 300-fold between Chinese women (*n* = 57) and men (*n* = 63). The CYP2A6 activity of females was higher than those of males, but there was no sex-related difference in the incidence of poor metabolizers. These results are consistent with the findings of Benowitz, Lessov-Schlaggar, Swan, et al. (2002), who reported that clearance of nicotine was significantly higher in women than in men. In addition, clearance was higher among women taking oral contraceptives than in those who were not taking oral contraceptives. Women who were perimenopausal or postmenopausal were not different from men.

Drugs related to substance abuse or treatment are among the 70 or more identified substrates of CYP2B6, including bupropion, nicotine, and 3,4-methylenedioxymethamphetamine (MDMA). In human liver microsomes, the activity of CYP2B6 varied more than 100-fold, with females having higher amounts of CYP2B6 mRNA, protein expression, and activity than males (Lamba, Lamba, Yasuda, et al., 2003). Because CYP2B6 is the major enzyme responsible for conversion of bupropion to its primary metabolite, hydroxybupropion, sex-related differences should emerge in the pharmacokinetics of bupropion. Previously, no significant sex difference was found in bupropion disposition (Hsyu, Singh, Giargiari, et al., 1997). However, Stewart, Berkel, Parish, et al. (2001) found differences between female and male adolescents treated with bupropion in a smoking cessation trial, with females demonstrating a greater AUC, Vd, and elimination half-life than males. These differences are opposite what would be expected based on the finding of greater CYP2B6 activity in microsomes (Lamba et al., 2003); however, clearance, when normalized for body weight, did not differ.

CYP2C9 and CYP2C19 together comprise about 25% of the total immunoquantified P450 content of the liver (Shimada et al., 1994). Both are involved in the metabolism of clinically important drugs and have been investigated for sex differences in their activity. A lack of data exists to document a sex-dependent difference in the activity of CYP2C9 (Anderson, 2005). The data for CYP2C19 are inconsistent due to a confounding effect by oral contraceptives. Sviri, Shpizen, Leitersdorf, et al. (1999) found that female subjects had a significantly lower activity of 2C19, as measured by mephenytoin excretion in 140 Jewish Israeli subjects, as did Tamminga, Wemer, Oosterhuis, et al. (1999) in a larger study of Dutch volunteers. In European Scandinavian volunteers (330 males and 281 females), phenotyping using mephenytoin yielded no significant sex difference (Hagg, Spigset, & Dahlqvist, 2001). There appear to be minor ethnic group differences in CYP2C19 activity between females and males and greater divergence in the frequency of genetically determined poor metabolizers, with an incidence of 15–25% in Asian populations compared with 2–5% in European American and African American populations (Bertilsson, 1995).

CYP2D6 is a well-studied isoform of the CYP P450s and is involved in the metabolism of many widely prescribed drugs. Poor activity of the enzyme, reflected by a poor metabolizer phenotype, has been extensively documented to occur with a frequency of 5–10% in European American populations and 1% of Asian and African American populations, but the frequency does not appear to differ by sex (Bertillson, 1995). Several studies of activity in the extensive (i.e., normal) metabolizer phenotype have reported conflicting results. Three studies using widely accepted phenotyping methods found no difference in 2D6 activity by sex (Kashuba, Natziger, & Kearns, 1998; Llerena, Cobaleda, Martinez, et al., 1996; McCune, Lindley, Decker, et al., 2001), but the results of other studies support a finding of a slight increase in activity in women (Hagg et al., 2001; Labbe, Sirois, Pilote, et al., 2000; Tamminga et al., 1999).

The importance of CYP2E1 for women and addiction lies in recognition that this inducible enzyme is the CYP isoform responsible for the metabolism of ethanol. Other enzymes that are responsible for the oxidative metabolism of ethanol are alcohol dehydrogenase and aldehyde dehydrogenase. Women have a lower activity of CYP2E1 than men but this difference disappears in people with alcohol dependence (Lucas, Menez, Girre, et al., 1995). A sex difference in ethanol pharmacokinetics, leading to high blood alcohol in women, is due to lower first-pass metabolism associated with lower gastric alcohol dehydrogenase rather than hepatic oxidation (Baraona, Abittan, Dohmen, et al., 2001).

CYP3A4, of all the P450s, is thought to be involved in the metabolism of the largest number of drugs and a large number of psychoactive drugs (von Moltke, Greenblatt, Schmider, et al., 1995). A number of studies has found that females, on average, have greater clearance of CYP3A4 substrates, implying a greater enzyme activity. Some *in vitro* data, using microsomal preparations from human male and female liver samples, support a greater activity in women (Hunt, Westerkam, & Stave, 1992). Although a number of studies suggests a trend toward higher clearance of CYP3A4 substrates in women (Fleishaker, Hulst, Ekernas, et al., 1992; Hulst, Fleishaker, Peter, et al., 1994; Schroeder, Cho, Pollack, et al., 1998), a substantial amount of data suggest that no sex difference exists (Gammans, Westrick, Shea, et al., 1989; Kashuba, Bertino, & Rocci, 1998; Kirkwood, Moore, Hayes, et al., 1991). The discrepancies may be partly accounted for by women's lower hepatic P-gp levels (Schuetz et al., 1995). Because P-gp is an efflux transporter that serves to exclude its substrates from intracellular access, a lower activity in women may lead to higher intrahepatocyte access and metabolism of drugs that are both P-gp and 3A4 substrates (Cummins, Wu, & Benet, 2002). This situation would decrease measured AUC and lead to a greater clearance, making it appear as if CYP3A4 activity were higher.

The major Phase II metabolic process, and one of the most common pathways in the formation of hydrophilic drug metabolites, is that of UGTs. The importance of glucuronidation in psychopharmacology is increasingly recognized, but Phase II enzymes are less well studied for sex differences than the CYP families (de Leon, 2003; Liston et al., 2001). The UGT1 and UGT2 subfamilies represent the most important of the UGTs for human drug metabolism. Buprenorphine, morphine, naloxone, and naltrexone may be partially metabolized by UGT1A3 and UGT2B7. Clozapine and olanzapine are substrates for UGT1A4 and as well as CYP1A2. Genetic polymorphism has been demonstrated for several UGTs, although the consequences of mutations for drug clearance are less well understood compared to the P450s. Multiple UGTs appear to be involved in the metabolism of many drugs, implying a lower substrate specificity than with the major CYP isozymes. Sex differences have been found, with clearance lower in women for acetaminophen, oxazepam, temazepam, and propranolol (Abernethy, Divoll, Greenblatt, et al., 1982; Divoll, Greenblatt, Harmatz, et al., 1981; Greenblatt, Divoll, Harmatz, et al., 1980; Walle, Walle, Cowart, et al., 1989). Lower activity of UGTs could also contribute to the higher clozapine and olanzapine concentrations in women due to an additive effect with CYP1A2.

Excretion

Renal excretion of drugs is the summation of the amount that undergoes glomerular filtration, plus that excreted by tubular secretion, minus the amount undergoing tubular reabsorption. Women have approximately 10% lower glomerular filtration rate than men. The majority of drugs used to treat addiction to drugs of abuse, as well as the abused drugs, undergo extensive metabolism (Table 7.3), with only small proportions of their total body clearance contributed by excretion of unmetabolized drug. Acamprosate is an exception; it is not metabolized and undergoes complete renal clearance. Its disposition does not differ between females and males (Saivin, Hulot, Chabac, et al., 1998).

SEX DIFFERENCES IN PHARMACODYNAMICS

Sex differences in pharmacodynamics have not been studied as thoroughly as pharmacokinetic differences, in part because of the greater difficulty in quantifying pharmacodynamic effects (Gandhi, Aweeka, Greenblatt, et al., 2004). Sex-related differences in pharmacodynamic response to drugs of abuse or their treatments could occur in several circumstances (Lynch, Roth, & Carroll, 2002). Pharmacokinetic differences between females and males can lead to different drug concentrations in plasma, and presumably at sites of action in the brain, to produce different degrees of pharmacological response. This outcome would be most likely when the magnitude of pharmacological response is dependent on the drug concentration. Alternatively, the biology of a drug's molecular targets might differ between women and men, leading to sex differences in pharmacodynamics with or without any difference in plasma drug concentration. Few studies involving drugs of abuse have been reported in which sex differences in pharmacokinetics and pharmacodynamics were simultaneously investigated, so only a few examples can be given.

The major elimination pathways for some drugs of abuse and drugs used in the treatment of addictions are listed in Table 7.3. For these drugs, sex-determined differences in

TABLE 7.3. Major Elimination Pathways for Drugs of Abuse and Treatment Drugs

	Elimination pathways
Drugs of abuse	
Alcohol	Alcohol dehydrogenase, aldehyde dehydrogenase, CYP2E1
Codeine	CYP2D6, CYP3A4, UGT2B4, UGT2B7
Cocaine	Pseudocholinesterase, carboxylesterase-1 (hCE-1), carboxylesterase-2 (hCE-2); CYP3A4; FMO
Heroin	hCE-2; hCE-1; pseudocholinesterase
Marijuana	CYP2C9, CYP3A4
MDMA	CYP2D6, CYP1A2, CYP2B6, CYP3A4, sulfotransferases; UGTs
Methamphetamine	CYP2D6
Methadone	CYP2B6, CYP3A4
Morphine	UGT1A3, UGT2B7, CYP3A4, CYP2C8
Nicotine	CYP1A2, Renal clearance = 15%
Oxycodone	CYP2D6
Treatment drugs	
Acamprosate	Renal clearance = 100%
Buprenorphone	CYP3A4, UGT1A3, UGT2B7, UGT 1A1
Bupropion	CYP2B6
Naloxone	UGT1A3, UGT2B7
Naltrexone	UGT1A3, UGT2B7, UGT1A1

Note. CYP, cytochrome P450; UGT, uridine glucuronyltransferase.

the activity of enzymes and transporters (Table 7.2) can be compared with their elimination pathways to predict whether or not a sex difference in disposition might occur, which could influence pharmacodynamic response. An implication of differences in CYP2A6 activity in females (Table 7.2) is that sex-related differences in nicotine clearance could affect smoking behavior. Previously, no significant difference was found in the number of cigarettes smoked per day or carbon dioxide levels between the sexes (Zeman, Hiraki, Sellers, et al., 2002), but females had significantly lower nicotine levels than male smokers. A faster nicotine metabolism in females was confirmed by Johnstone, Benowitz, Cargill, et al. (2006), who also found smoking behavior to be influenced by CYP2A6 genotype.

Sex differences have been found in morphine analgesia, with greater morphine potency but slower speed of onset and offset in women than men (Sarton, Olofsen, Romberg, et al., 2000). However, no sex difference was found in plasma concentrations of morphine and its metabolites following intravenous morphine infusion in healthy female and male volunteers. This finding implies that opioid receptor differences exist according to sex that influence the apparent differences in pharmacodynamic effects.

CYP2B6 is the principle enzyme involved in bupropion metabolism. CYP2B6 can also metabolize nicotine and is highly polymorphic, with over 100 variants described (Zanger, Klein, Saussele, et al., 2007). One mutant form, CYP2B6*6, has been associated with decreased bupropion metabolism in human liver samples (Hesse, He, Krishnaswamy, et al., 2004). Lee, Gepson, Hoffmann, et al. (2007) found that subjects in a bupropion smoking cessation trial who were homozygous or heterozygous for CYP2B6*6 variants had higher abstinence rates than patients with the CYP2B6*1 wild-type genotype at the end of treatment or at the 6-month follow-up period. Plasma drug concentrations were not reported.

In seven women and seven men who were occasional cocaine users, an intranasal dose of cocaine resulted in higher peak cocaine plasma concentrations and more intense subjective effects in men and occurred earlier (Lukas, Sholar, Lundahl, et al., 1996). In spite of these differences, peak heart rate increases did not differ between women and men suggesting women may have been more sensitive to the cardiovascular effects of cocaine.

IMPLICATIONS FOR WOMEN AND ADDICTION

Sex-determined differences related to specific enzymes and/or transporters have been documented that can contribute to alterations in several pharmacokinetic processes. Most often these differences appear as subtle changes in drug clearance or plasma concentrations. The impact on pharmacodynamic effects is often unclear. The genetic polymorphisms resulting in pronounced changes in activity of a drug-metabolizing enzyme, as occurs with CYP2D6, appear to have a greater likelihood of influencing pharmacodynamic response in an individual patient than inherent differences in sex-determined enzyme activity. The normal degree of variability in the activity of enzymes in either sex far exceeds the differences in mean activity between women and men. In addition, the variability in pharmacodynamic response for many drugs appears to exceed pharmacokinetic variability.

A factor that obscures sex-dependent differences in drug clearance is the existence of multiple pathways of elimination for most drugs. Even though a sex difference may exist in one metabolic pathway, a lack of difference in a secondary pathway may minimize an overall difference in clearance between women and men. In a cross-over study, 10 men and 8 women took either triazolam or zolpidem (Greenblatt, Harmatz, von Moltke, et al., 2000). Weight-normalized clearance of triazolam was higher in women than in men, but zopidem clearance was lower in women than men. Triazolam is nearly completely dependent upon CYP3A4 for its elimination and higher enzyme activity in women (Table 7.2) might explain the higher clearance, although the difference in women and men was not significant. Zolpidem is cleared predominantly by CYP3A4 but also to a lesser degree by CYP2C9 and CYP1A2 (von Moltke, Greenblatt, Granda, et al., 1999), which could contribute to a lower overall clearance due to the lower CYP1A2 activity reported in females (Relling et al., 1992).

Despite the expanding database documenting sex differences in pharmacokinetics, sex-specific dosage recommendations are available for only a few drugs. Research in this field needs to combine pharmacokinetic and pharmacodynamic evaluations in the same study along with appropriate genotyping when genetic contributions to drug disposition or response are suspected. Sex differences in drug abuse exist, and further research is needed to elucidate the mechanisms for the observed differences.

KEY POINTS

- Sex differences have been observed in the activity of many drug-metabolizing enzymes and transporters that mediate the disposition of both drugs of abuse and the medications used in treating addictions.
- The normal degree of variability in the activity of enzymes in either sex far exceeds the differences in mean activity between women and men.
- Sex differences in pharmacodynamics have not been as thoroughly investigated as pharmacokinetic differences. Such differences can impact the variability in drug response, potentially causing either exaggerated or diminished drug effects in relation to expectations based on data obtained in young adult males (the population most frequently studied during drug development).
- Future research in pharmacogenetics is likely to uncover more bases for sex differences in drug response and lead to better treatment recommendations.

REFERENCES

Asterisks denote recommended readings.

Abernethy, D. R., Divoll, M., Greenblatt, D. J., et al. (1982). Obesity, sex, and acetaminophen disposition. *Clinical Pharmacology and Therapeutics, 31,* 783–790.

Anderson, G. D. (2005). Sex and racial differences in pharmacological response: Where is the evidence: Pharmacogenetics, pharmacokinetics, and pharmacodynamics. *Journal of Women's Health, 14,* 19–29. (*)

Anthony, M., & Berg, M. J. (2002). Biologic and molecular mechanisms for sex differences in pharmacokinetics, pharmacodynamics, and pharmacogenetics: Part II. *Journal of Women's Health and Gender-Based Medicine, 11,* 617–629. (*)

Bailey, D. N., & Briggs, J. R. (2004). The binding of selected therapeutic drugs to human serum alpha-1 acid glycoprotein and to human serum albumin in vitro. *Therapeutic Drug Monitoring, 26,* 40–43.

Baraona, E., Abittan, C. S., Dohmen, K., et al. (2001). Gender differences in pharmacokinetics of alcohol. *Alcoholism: Clinical and Experimental Research, 225,* 502–507.

Bartoli, A., Xiaodong, S., Gatti, G., et al. (1996). The influence of ethnic factors and gender on CYP1A2-mediated drug disposition: A comparative study in Caucasian and Chinese subjects using phenacetin as a marker substrate. *Therapeutic Drug Monitoring, 18,* 586–591.

Beierle, I., Meibohm, B., & Derendorf, H. (1999). Gender differences in pharmacokinetics and pharmacodynamics. *International Journal of Clinical Pharmacology and Therapeutics, 37,* 529–547.

Benowitz, N. L., Lessov-Schlaggar, C. N., Swan, G. E., et al. (2002). Female sex and oral contraceptive use accelerate nicotine metabolism. *Clinical Pharmacology and Therapeutics, 79,* 480–488. (*)

Bertilsson, L. (1995). Geographical/interracial differences in polymorphic drug oxidations: Current state of knowledge of cytochrome P450 (CYp. 2D6 and 2C19). *Clinical Pharmacokinetics, 29,* 192.

Caballero-Plascencia, A. M., Valenzuela-Barranco, M., Martin-Ruiz, J. L., et al. (1999). Are there changes in gastric emptying during the menstrual cycle? *Scandinavian Journal of Gastroenterology, 34,* 772–776.

Chen, T. S., Doong, M. L., Chang, F. Y., et al. (1995). Effects of sex steroid hormones on gastric emptying and gastrointestinal transit in rats. *American Journal of Physiology: Gastrointestinal and Liver Physiology, 268,* G171–176.

Coller, J. K., Barratt, D. T., Dahlen, K., et al. (2006). ABCB1 genetic variability and methadone dosage requirements in opioid-dependent individuals. *Clinical Pharmacology and Therapeutics, 80,* 682–690.

Coskun, T., Sevine, A., Tevetoglu, I., et al. (1995). Delayed gastric emptying in conscious male rats following chronic estrogen and progesterone treatment. *Research in Experimental Medicine, 195,* 49–54.

Cummins, C. L., Wu, C. Y., & Benet, L. Z. (2002). Sex-related differences in the clearance of cytochrome P450 3A4 substrates may be caused by P-glycoprotein. *Clinical Pharmacology and Therapeutics, 72,* 474–489.

de Leon, J. (2003). Glucuronidation enzymes, genes, and psychiatry. *International Journal of Neuropsychopharmacology, 6,* 57–72.

DeVane, C. L. (2009). Principles of pharmacokinetics and pharmacodynamics. In A. F. Schatzberg & C. B. Nemeroff (Eds.), *American Psychiatric Publishing textbook of psychopharmacology* (4th ed.). Arlington, VA: American Psychiatric Publishing.

Divoll, M., Greenblatt, D. J., Harmatz, J. S., et al. (1981). Effect of age and gender on disposition of temazepam. *Journal of Pharmacological Sciences, 70,* 1104–1107.

Fleishaker, J. C., Hulst, L. K., Ekernas, S.-A., et al. (1992). Pharmacokinetics and pharmacodynamics of adinazolam and N-desmethyladinazolam after oral and intravenous dosing in healthy young and elderly volunteers. *Journal of Clinical Psychopharmacology, 12,* 403–414.

Gandhi, M., Aweeka, F., Greenblatt, R. M., et al. (2004). Sex differences in pharmacokinetics and pharmacodynamics. *Annual Review of Pharmacology and Toxicology, 44,* 499–523.

Greenblatt, D. J., Divoll, M., Harmatz, J. S., et al. (1980). Oxazepam kinetics: Effects of age and sex. *Journal of Pharmacology and Experimental Therapeutics, 215,* 86–91.

Greenblatt, D. J., Harmatz, J. S., von Moltke, L. L., et al. (2000). Comparative kinetics and response to the benzodiazepine agonists triazolm and zolpidem: Evaluation of sex-dependent differences. *Journal of Pharmacology and Experimental Therapeutics, 293,* 435–443.

Hagg, S., Spigset, O., & Dahlqvist, R. (2001). Influence of gender and oral contraceptives on CYP2D6 and CYP2C19 activity in healthy volunteers. *British Journal of Clinical Pharmacology, 51,* 69–173.

Haring, C., Meise, U., Humpel, C., et al. (1989). Dose-related plasma levels of clozapine: Influence of smoking behavior, sex, and age. *Psychopharmacology, 99*(Suppl. 1), S38–S40.

Harris, R. Z., Benet, L. Z., & Schwartz, J. B. (1995). Gender effects in pharmacokinetics and pharmacodynamics. *Drugs, 50,* 222–239.

Hesse, L. M., He, P., Krishnaswamy, S., et al. (2004). Pharmacogenetic determinants of interindividual variability in bupropion hydroxylation by cytochrome P450 2B6 in human liver microsomes. *Pharmacogenetics, 14,* 225–238.

Hulst, L. K., Fleishaker, J. C., Peter, G. R., et al. (1994). Effect of age and gender on triliazad pharmacokinetics in humans. *Clinical Pharmacology and Therapeutics, 55,* 378–384.

Hunt, C. M., Westerkam, W. R., & Stave, G. M. (1992). Effect of age and gender on the activity of human hepatic CYP3A. *Biochemical Pharmacology, 44,* 275–283.

Hsyu, P.-H., Singh, A., Giargiari, T. D., et al. (1997). Pharmacokinetics of bupropion and its metabolites in cigarette smokers versus nonsmokers. *Journal of Clinical Pharmacology, 37,* 737–743.

Johnstone, E., Benowitz, N., Cargill, A., et al. (2006). Determinants of the rate of nicotine metabolism and effects on smoking behavior. *Clinical Pharmacology and Therapeutics, 80,* 319–330.

Kashuba, A. D., Bertino, J. S., Jr., Rocci, M. L., et al. (1998). Quantification of 3-month intraindividual variability and the influence of sex and menstrual cycle phase on CYP3A activity as measured by phenotyping with intravenous midazolam. *Clinical Pharmacology and Therapeutics, 64,* 269–277.

Kashuba, A. D., Nafziger, A. N., Kearns, G. L., et al. (1998). Quantification of intraindividual variability and the influence of menstrual cycle phase on CYP2D6 activity as measured by dextromethorphan phenotyping. *Pharmacogenetics, 8,* 403–410.

Kirkwood, C., Moore, A., Hayes, P., et al. (1991). Influence of menstrual cycle and gender on alprazolam pharmacokinetics. *Clinical Pharmacology and Therapeutics, 50,* 404–409.

Kishino, S., Nomura, A., Di, Z. S., et al. (1995). Alpha-1-acid glycoprotein concentration and the protein binding of disopyramide in healthy subjects. *Journal of Clinical Pharmacology, 35,* 510–514.

Labbe, L., Sirois, C., Pilote, S., et al. (2000). Effect of gender, sex hormones, time variables, and physiological urinary pH on apparent CYP2D6 activity as assessed by metabolic ratios of marker substrates. *Pharmacogenetics, 10,* 425–438.

Lamba, V., Lamba, J., Yasuda, K., et al. (2003). Hepatic CYP2B6 expression: Gender and ethnic differences and relationship to CYP2B6 genotype are CAR (constitutive androstane receptor) expression. *Journal of Pharmacology and Experimental Therapeutics, 307,* 906–922.

Lane, H.-Y., Chang, Y.-C., Chang, W.-H., et al. (1999). Effects of gender and age on plasma levels of clozapine and its metabolites: Analyzed by critical statistics. *Journal of Clinical Psychiatry, 60,* 36–40.

Lee, A. M., Jepson, C., Hoffmann, E., et al. (2007). CYP2B6 genotype alters abstinence rates in a bupropion smoking cessation trial. *Biological Psychiatry, 62,* 635–641.

Liston, H. L., Markowitz, J. S., & DeVane, C. L. (2001). Drug glucuronidation in clinical psychopharmacology. *Journal of Clinical Psychopharmacology, 21,* 500–515.

Llerena, A., Cobaleda, J., Martinez, C., et al. (1996). Interethnic differences in drug metabolism: Influence of genetic and environmental factors on debrisoquine hydroxylation phenotype. *European Journal of Drug Metabolism and Pharmacokinetics, 21,* 129–138.

Lown, K. S., Mayo, R. R., Leichman, A. B., et al. (1997). Role of intestinal–glycorotein (mdr1) in interpatient variation in the oral bioavailability of cyclosporine. *Clinical Pharmacology and Therapeutics, 62,* 248–260.

Lucas, D., Menez, C., Girre, C., et al. (1995). Cytochrome P450 2E1 genotype and chlorzoxazone metabolism in healthy and alcoholic Caucasian subjects. *Pharmacogenetics, 5*, 298.

Lukas, S. E., Sholar, M., Lundahl, L. H., et al. (1996). Sex differences in plasma cocaine levels and subjective effects after acute cocaine administration in human volunteers. *Psychopharmacology, 125*, 346–354.

Lynch, W. J., Roth, M. E., & Carroll, M. E. (2002). Biological basis of sex differences in drug abuse: Preclinical and clinical studies. *Psychopharmacology, 164*, 121–137. (*)

McCune, J. S., Lindley, C., Decker, J. L., et al. (2001). Lack of gender difference and large intrasubject variability in cytochrome P450 activity measured by phenotyping with dextromethorphan. *Journal of Clinical Pharmacology, 41*, 723–731.

Meibohm, B., Beierle, I., & Derendorf, H. (2002). How important are gender differences in pharmacokinetics? *Clinical Pharmacokinetics, 41*, 329–342. (*)

Merino, G., van Herwaarden, A. E., Wagenaar, E., et al. (2005). Sex-dependent expression and activity of the ATP binding cassette transporter breast cancer resistance protein (BCRP/ABCG2) in liver. *Molecular Pharmacology, 67*, 1765–1771.

Merkatz, R. B., Temple, R., Sobel, S., et al. (1993). Women in clinical trials of new drugs: A change in Food and Drug Administration Policy. *New England Journal of Medicine, 329*, 292–296.

Messina, E. S., Tyndale, R. F., & Sellers, E. M. (1997). A major role for CYP2A6 in nicotine C-oxidation by human liver microsomes. *Journal of Pharmacology and Experimental Therapeutics, 282*, 1608–1614.

Murphy, D. B., Sutton, J. A., Prescott, L. F., et al. (1997). Opioid-induced delay in gastric emptying. *Anesthesiology, 87*, 765–770.

Nanovskaya, T., Nekhayeva, I., Karunaratne, N., et al. (2005). Role of P-glycoprotein in transplacental transfer of methadone. *Biochemical Pharmacology, 69*, 1869–1878.

Ou-Yang, D.-S., Huang, S.-L., Wang, W., et al. (2000). Phenotypic polymorphism and gender-related differences of CYP1A2 activity in a Chinese population. *British Journal of Clinical Pharmacology, 49*, 141–151.

Paine, M. F., Hart, H. L., Ludington, S. S., et al. (2006). The human intestinal cytochrome P450 "pie." *Drug Metabolism and Disposition, 34*, 880–886.

Paine, M. F., Ludington, S. S., Chen, M.-L., et al. (2005). Do men and women differ in proximal small intestinal CYP3A or P-glycoprotein expression? *Drug Metabolism and Disposition, 33*, 426–433.

Physicians' Desk Reference. (2005). Zyprexa Monograph, Eli Lilly & Co., 2005.

Rasmussen, B. B., Brix, T. H., Kyvik, K. O., et al. (2002). The interindividual differences in the 3-demethylation of caffeine alias CYP1A2 is determined by both genetic and environmental factors. *Pharmacogenetics, 12*, 473–478.

Relling, M., Lin, J., Ayers, G., et al. (1992). Racial and gender differences in N-acetyltransferase, xanthine oxidase, and CYP1A2 activities. *Clinical Pharmacology and Therapeutics, 52*, 643–658.

Rostami-Hodjegan, A., Amin, A. M., Spencer, E. P., Lennard, M. S., Tucker, G. T., & Flanagan, R. J. (2004). Influence of dose, cigarette smoking, age, sex, and metabolic activity on plasma clozapine concentrations: A predictive model and nomograms to aid clozapine dose adjustment and to assess compliance in individual patients. *Journal of Clinical Psychopharmacology, 24*, 70–78.

Routledge, P. A., Stargel, W. W., Kitchell, B. B., et al. (1981). Sex-related differences in the plasma protein binding of lignocaine and diazepam. *British Journal of Clinical Pharmacology, 11*, 245–250.

Sadik, R., Abrahamsson, H., & Stotzer, P. O. (2003). Gender differences in gut transit shown with a newly developed radiological procedure. *Scandinavian Journal of Gastroenterology, 38*, 36–42.

Saivin, S., Hulot, T., Chabac, S., et al. (1998). Clinical pharmacokinetics of acamprosate. *Clinical Pharmacokinetics, 35*, 331–345.

Sarton, E., Olofsen, E., Romberg, R., et al. (2000). Sex differences in morphine analgesia. *Anesthesiology, 93*, 1245–1254.

Schroeder, T. J., Cho, M. J., Pollack, G. M., et al. (1998). Comparison of two cyclosporine formulations in healthy volunteers: Bioequivalence of the new Sang-35 formulations and Neoral. *Journal of Clinical Pharmacology, 38*, 807–814.

Schuetz, E. G., Furuya, K. N., & Schuetz, J. D. (1995). Interindividual variation in expression of P-glycoprotein in normal human liver and secondary hepatic neoplasms. *Journal of Pharmacology and Experimental Therapeutics, 275,* 1011–1018.

Shimada, T., Yamazaki, H., Mimura, M., et al. (1994). Interindividual variations in human liver cytochrome P-450 enzymes involved in the oxidation of drugs, carcinogens, and toxic chemicals: Studies with liver microsomes of 30 Japanese and 30 Caucasians. *Journal of Pharmacology and Experimental Therapeutics, 270,* 414–423.

Singer, A. J., & Brandt, L. J. (1991). Pathophysiology of the gastrointestinal tract during pregnancy. *American Journal of Gastroenterology, 86,* 1695–1712.

Stewart, J. J., Berkel, H. J., Parish, R. C., et al. (2001). Single-dose pharmacokinetics of bupropion in adolescents: Effects of smoking status and gender. *Journal of Clinical Pharmacology, 41,* 770–778.

Sviri, S., Shpizen, S., Leitersdorf, E., et al. (1999). Phenotypic–genotypic analysis of CYP2C19 in the Jewish Israeli population. *Clinical Pharmacology and Therapeutics, 65,* 275–282.

Tamminga, W. J., Wemer, J., Oosterhuis, B., et al. (1999). CYP2D6 and CYP2C19 activity in a large population of Dutch healthy volunteers: Indications for oral contraceptive-related gender differences. *European Journal of Clinical Pharmacology, 55,* 177–184.

Tuck, C. H., Holleran, S., & Bergland, L. (1997). Hormonal regulation of lipoprotein(a) levels: Effects of estrogen replacement therapy on lipoprotein(a) and acute phase reactants in postmenopausal women. *Arteriosclerosis, Thrombosi, and Vascular Biology, 17,* 1822–1829.

Verbeeck, R. K., Cardinal, J. A., & Wallace, S. M. (1984). Effect of age and sex on the plasma binding of acidic and basic drugs. *European Journal of Clinical Pharmacology, 27,* 91–97.

von Moltke, L. L., Greenblatt, D. J., Granda, B. W., et al. (1999). Zolpidem metabolism in vitro: Responsible cytochromes, chemical inhibitors, and in vivo correlations. *British Journal of Clinical Pharmacology, 48,* 89–97.

von Moltke, L. L., Greenblatt, D. J., Schmider, J., et al. (1995). Metabolism of drugs by cytochrome P450 3A isoforms: Implications for drug interactions in psychopharmacology. *Clinical Pharmacokinetics, 29*(Suppl. 1), 33–43.

Walle, T., Walle, U. K., Cowart, D., et al. (1989). Pathway-selective sex differences in the metabolic clearance of propranolol in human subjects. *Clinical Pharmacology and Therapeutics, 46,* 257–263.

Walle, U. K., Fagan, T. C., Topmiller, M. J., et al. (1994). The influence of gender and sex steroid hormones on the plasma binding of propranolol enantiomers. *British Journal of Clinical Pharmacology, 37,* 21–25.

Wang, J.-S., Newport, D. J., Stowe, Z. N., et al. (2007). The emerging importance of transporter proteins in the psychopharmacological treatment of the pregnant patient. *Drug Metabolism Reviews, 39,* 723–746. (*)

Wang, J.-S., Ruan, Y., Taylor, R. M., et al. (2004). Brain penetration of methadone (r)- and (S)-enantiomers is greatly increased by P-glycoprotein deficiency in the blood–brain barrier of Abcb1 gene knockout mice. *Psychopharmacology, 173,* 132–138.

Wenk, M., Todesco, L., & Krahenbuhl, S. (2004). Effect of St. John's wort on the activities of CYP1A2, CYP3A4, CYP2D6, N-acetyltransferase 2, and xanthine oxidase in healthy males and females. *British Journal of Clinical Pharmacology, 57,* 495–499.

Wiegratz, E., Kutschera, K., Lee, J. H., et al. (2003). Effect of four different oral contraceptives on various sex hormones and serum-binding globulins. *Contraception, 67,* 25–32.

Wolff, K., Boys, A., Rostami-Hodjegan, A., et al. (2005). Changes to methadone clearance during pregnancy. *European Journal of Clinical Pharmacology, 61,* 763–768.

Xu, P., Huang, S.-L., Zhu, R.-H., et al. (2004). Phenotypic polymorphism of CYP2A6 activity in a Chinese population. *European Journal of Clinical Pharmacology, 58,* 333–337.

Zanger, U. M., Klein, K., Saussele, T., Blievernicht, J., Hofmann, M. H., & Schwab, M. (2007). Polymorphic CYP2B6: Molecular mechanisms and emerging clinical significance. *Future Medicine—Pharmacogenomics, 8,* 743–759.

Zeman, M. V., Hiraki, L., & Sellers, E. M. (2002). Gender differences in tobacco smoking: Higher relative exposure to smoke than nicotine in women. *Journal of Women's Health and Gender-Based Medicine, 1*(1), 147–152.

CHAPTER 8

Gender, Cognition, and Addiction

Simona Sava, MD, PhD
Alexandra McCaffrey, BA
Deborah A. Yurgelun-Todd, PhD

Cognition or cognitive functioning is broadly defined as mental processing and includes attention, learning, memory, comprehension, reasoning, language, and decision making. Gender differences in cognitive abilities have been described in a number of domains, including spatial and verbal processing and mathematical reasoning (Jansen-Osmann & Heil, 2007; Kimura, 2000; Spelke, 2005). It has been suggested that these differences in functional capacity are associated with biological influences. At the beginning of life, the Y chromosome and subsequently the testes and the male gonadal hormones are responsible for producing the male phenotype in the developing embryo. Initially the brain is neither male nor female, but the presence of testosterone secreted by the gonads will result in a male phenotype in the central nervous system (Breedlove, 1992). The brain areas that show the most robust gender dimorphism are regions related to reproductive physiology and behaviors, such as the sexually dimorphic nucleus of the preoptic area, anteroventral periventricular nucleus, or the spinal nucleus of the bulbocavernosus (J. A. Morris, Jordan, & Breedlove, 2004). However, the influence of gonadal hormones on the brain is not limited to reproduction-relevant areas or to developmental years but is also evident in adulthood (McCarthy & Konkle, 2005). It is well documented that cognitive function is subserved by a wide range of brain regions and networks, and gonadal steroid hormones have been thought to have a modulatory influence on a number of these brain areas. For example, substantial research has focused on the hormonal modulation of the number of neurons and synaptic connectivity in the hippocampus (Isgor & Sengelaub, 1998; Leranth, Petnehazy, & MacLusky, 2003; Woolley & McEwen, 1992), a medial temporal lobe structure involved in learning and memory processes. For years, the dominant view was that males perform better than females on tests of spatial information processing and mathematical thinking, while females were thought to have a performance advantage on verbal-based tests. This chapter focuses on the evidence that supports or refutes the hypothesis that there are gender differences in cognitive abilities and discusses the interaction of potential gender differences in cognition and substance use disorders (SUDs).

GENDER DIFFERENCES IN COGNITIVE ABILITIES

Gender Differences in Spatial Ability

As noted above, spatial processing is one of the cognitive domains that is frequently described as demonstrating sexual bias. Spatial ability however is not a unitary domain, but rather it is composed of several dimensions, such as learning and memory for location and identity of objects, spatial relationships between different objects, ability to mentally rotate objects, and ability to navigate through an environment. Together, these component functions allow an individual to function within the spatial environment. To determine what processes may contribute to a gender difference we review the findings from studies that have determined these functions.

Object Location and Object Identity Memory

This section discusses a series of human studies investigating memory for object location and object identity. Object location memory is the process of remembering a particular object's position in space, or within a given spatial array (Silverman & Eals, 1992). When testing for object location memory, participants are asked to identify instances of items being moved (or unmoved) based on their memory of the original array. A number of studies investigating the memory for object location report a female advantage on this task (Crook, Youngjohn, & Larrabee, 1990; Sharps, Welton, & Price, 1993; Silverman & Eals, 1992). However, other studies either found no gender difference (Dabbs, Chang, Strong, & Milun, 1998; Epting & Overman, 1998) or reported that males performed better than females (Postma, Jager, Kessels, Koppeschaar, & van Honk, 2004). Several components of the task, including type of object, encoding context, type of memory tested (recognition vs. recall), and scoring method (based on accuracy, speed of completion, and/or distance) varied among these investigations and likely contributed to the magnitude and direction of the gender differences in performance. In a recent meta-analysis of 86 effect sizes from 36 studies, Voyer and colleagues (Voyer, Postma, Brake, & Imperato-McGinley, 2007) found that males perform better than females when the test score is based on distance, and when the objects in question are masculine in nature. Gender differences in favor of females, however, have been illustrated in virtually all other study designs of object location memory, particularly when accuracy is used as the performance score (De Goede & Postma, 2008; Voyer et al., 2007). Previous studies also indicate that females begin to significantly outperform males in these tasks at as early as age 13 years (Voyer et al., 2007), suggesting that the neurodevelopmental and neuroendocrinological effects of puberty may play a role in the gender differences found in object location memory.

A separate but related cognitive skill that contributes to object location memory is the ability to recognize objects that have been seen before. Memory for object identity or object recall refers to the ability to identify an item, independent of its location in space. Similar to object location tasks, participants performing object identity tasks are initially asked to study an array of items set before them. A new array is then presented, and participants need to identify which objects are old, and which are new (Silverman & Eals, 1992). As with object location memory, females have often been shown to outperform males at this task (Eals & Silverman, 1994; Levy, Astur, & Frick, 2005; McGivern et al., 1998). However, other studies have found no significant gender difference in object identity memory (De Goede & Postma, 2008; Postma et al., 2004; Voyer et al., 2007). Object identity memory has been hypothesized to be a component of location memory, given that to remember the location of all particular objects in an array, one has to remember the positions where the objects were placed, the identity of the objects, and the association between objects and positions (Postma et al., 2004). Although no gender difference was found in the ability to link objects to positions (Postma & De Haan, 1996; Postma et al., 2004), males have been reported to be better at identifying positions (Postma et al., 2004). The discussion above raises an important issue, specifically that cognitive tasks are complex and likely composed of a number of processing components. For each cognitive task there could be components that often show the predicted gender differences in performance, others that show a reversal of the expected gender differences, and others that are sex neutral. Depending on the relative contribution of these processing subcomponents to the performance score, gender differences in performance could emerge on tasks that draw more heavily on gender-dimorphic cognitive processes.

Mental Rotation

Mental rotation is defined as the practice of imagining an object to rotate or turn in three-dimensional space. Tests of mental rotation often consist of illustrations of two- or three-dimensional figures that are to be mentally turned, and then matched to their correct counterparts found in an array of comparison figures (Jansen-Osmann & Heil, 2007). Many studies have shown that during adulthood men perform better than women on tests of mental rotation (Astur, Tropp, Sava, Constable, & Markus, 2004; Collins & Kimura, 1997), and it is thought that the gender differences in performance may arise, at least in part, because of the influence of sex steroid hormones. In women, performance on mental rotation tasks varies with their menstrual cycle: testosterone has a positive influence, while estradiol has a negative influence on performance (Hausmann, Slabbekoorn, Van Goozen, Cohen-Kettenis, & Gunturkun, 2000).

However, the largest male advantage in performance is found on paper-pencil timed mental rotation tests, when participants are presented with four or five comparison figures (Voyer, 1997). Interestingly, when the task parameters are changed by replacing the two- or three-dimensional abstract figures with drawings of animals or cards, removing the time constraints of the test, or reducing the number of comparison figures, the gender differences in performance are sometimes smaller or they disappear (Jansen-Osmann & Heil, 2006; Voyer, 1997). This suggests that factors other than the sex hormones, such as response style (Butler et al., 2006), differential experience and socialization (Baenninger & Newcombe, 1989), or strategy choice (Bryden, George, & Inch, 1990), can affect performance on the mental rotation tasks.

Virtual Navigation

The Morris water maze task is commonly used in rodent literature to investigate learning and memory and hippocampal function (Astur, Ortiz, & Sutherland, 1998; Astur et al., 2004; R. Morris, 1984),as well as gender differences in spatial navigation. Virtual versions of the water maze task have been developed for human testing, and a number of studies have shown repeatedly that males navigate more efficiently than females in a virtual water maze (Astur et al., 1998; Astur et al., 2004). In this task, subjects are placed in a round virtual water maze and learn to escape from the water by navigating to a submerged platform. Good performance requires subjects to remember the location of the submerged platform in relation to other cues in the room, therefore forming a spatial representation of the environment (O'Keefe & Conway, 1978). The male advantage for this ability has been shown to be maintained in real-world navigation as well (Saucier, Green, Leason, MacFadden, Bell, & Elias, 2002). However, a close examination of the cognitive demands for navigational tasks in humans shows that the differences in performance between men and women are found in the initial phases of learning the task and they disappear with training (Astur et al., 2004; Baenninger & Newcombe, 1989; Schmitzer-Torbert, 2007), suggesting that gender differences are limited to the acquisition process, and with sufficient training males and females can reach similar levels of performance. It has been proposed that the gender difference in the acquisition rate may be due in part to the fact that men and women are using different navigation strategies to solve the task (Astur et al., 2004). In virtual environments (Sandstrom, Kaufman, & Huettel, 1998) as well as in real-world settings (Saucier, MacFadden, et al., 2002), women often rely on landmark information to navigate, whereas men use landmarks and the geometry of the environment to navigate to the goal location. Landmarks are prominent objects or visually distinct features of the environment that can provide guidance for finding the route to the goal location. When using a landmark strategy, the participant is learning the location of the goal by relating it to a known landmark or visual scene. When the landmarks are stable (i.e., not moved between trials), this strategy can be successfully used to navigate to a known location. Integrating the information about landmarks with information related to the geometry of the environment (i.e., information about the shape, length, and angles of the environment) allows for greater flexibility and better performance in situations when landmarks are removed, or navigation to a novel location is required (Foo, Warren, Duchon, & Tarr, 2005). Moreover, areas of the medial temporal lobe are differentially involved in processing landmark or spatial information (Ekstrom & Bookheimer, 2007). Other navigational strategies can be used, such as the response strategy, which takes into account body movements such as right or left turns. The response strategy does not require learning about the spatial layout of the environment, and both genders seem to be equally likely to use it to solve a navigational task (Schmitzer-Torbert, 2007). Interestingly, the striatum, and not the medial temporal lobe, is involved in response-based navigation (Etchamendy & Bohbot, 2007). As with the mental rotation, the strategy used to solve a virtual navigation task is important when investigating gender differences in spatial performance.

Gender Differences in Mathematical Reasoning

A second broad category of cognitive functions that has been reported to show sex differences is mathematical reasoning. Several functional brain systems contribute to abstract mathematical thinking. Elizabeth Spelke (2005) identifies five such systems. The first system represents small number of objects; the second represents larger, approximate numerical magnitudes; the third consists of quantifiers and number words; the fourth and the fifth systems refer to representation of environmental geometry and landmarks, respectively. No consistent gender differences have been found in the ability to represent small number of objects in infancy or the acquisition of the quantifier language system during early childhood (Spelke, 2005). Similarly, boys and girls younger than age 16 years perform equally well on tests of geometric representation, landmark navigation, or mental rotation, indicating that no clear-cut innate gender difference exists in these abilities (Leplow et al., 2003; Roberts & Bell, 2002). Gender differences are found in more complex quantitative tasks and generally emerge during or after elementary school years, suggesting that societal factors play a role in the development of gender differences in these cognitive domains. When identified, gender differences are small and could be attributed to the application of different cognitive strategies of solving a task. Overall, males and females show equal ability to master new and challenging mathematical concepts (Lubinski, Webb, Morelock, & Benbow, 2001; Webb, Lubinski, & Benbow, 2002).

Gender Differences in Verbal Ability

Research has long pointed to gender differences favoring females in cognitive tests of verbal ability (Denno, Meijs, Nachshon, & Aurand, 1982; Halpern, 1986; Maccoby & Jacklin, 1974). In particular, women have been found to perform better on verbal fluency tasks, speed of articulation, and verbal memory tasks (Kimura, 2000). These results, combined with findings by Flannery et al. (Flannery, Liederman, Daly, & Schultz, 2000), suggest that reading disorders are approximately twice as common in boys as in girls and have led to focused study of the neural underpinnings of this gender difference in verbal processing. One hypothesis is that the female advantage in verbal processing is due to the fact that language functions are being performed bilaterally in the female brain. In other words, males predominantly use the left hemisphere for verbal processing, whereas females use both hemispheres to perform the same tasks (Dorion et al., 2000; Gur et al., 2000; McGlone, 1980). This hypothesis could also explain the reported advantage that males exhibit in visuospatial tasks, given that in this model, the right hemisphere of the female brain would be forced to "compete" between spatial and verbal processing (Dorion et al., 2000; Levy, 1969; McGlone, 1980). Performance indicating left lateralization in males and bilateral response in females has been found in studies involving visual word learning, phonological rhyming tasks, verb generation, picture naming, and semantic decision making (Chen et al., 2007; Gur et al., 2000; Shaywitz et al., 1995; Vikingstad et al., 2000), while auditory phonological or comprehension task have yielded more conflicting results (Coney, 2002; Sommer, Aleman, Bouma, & Kahn, 2004). Similar to findings from studies of visuospatial ability, the cognitive strategies used by males and females during verbal processing could be different (Breitenstein et al., 2005). Alternatively, gender differences in neural pathway activation during verbal processing could be a result of anatomical differences in the brain of males and females. For example, the isthmus segment of the corpus callosum is larger in females, and this could result in a higher interhemispheric connectivity in women compared to men (Steinmetz, Staiger, Schlaug, Huang, & Jancke, 1995).

Summary

To summarize, existing data support the existence of a male advantage in spatial processing, particularly in mental rotation and spatial navigation and a female advantage in performance on verbal ability tasks. Several factors may contribute to these differences. Gonadal hormones affect hippocampal morphology, and the hippocampus is involved in spatial processing. Moreover, gender differences tend to emerge after puberty. Therefore, it is possible that the gender differences in spatial ability are mediated by the sex hormones via the hippocampus. Figure 8.1 shows an example of the differential activation in the medial temporal lobe during spatial navigation in males and females. Although males show bilateral activation in the hippocampus and associated medial temporal lobe structures during learning in a virtual water maze task, females only show activation in the right medial temporal lobe. Males and females were equally proficient at learning the task, therefore the difference in the pattern of brain activation cannot be attributed to differences in performance. The images represent averaged activation data from eight males and eight females collected in our laboratory (Sneider, Sava, Rogowska, Gruber, & Yurgelun-Todd, 2008).

Another important factor that likely contributes to gender differences in cognitive abilities is the different strategies that males and females use to solve a task. Depending on the particular requirements of a task, the different strategies used by males and females could be equally effective and result in no gender differences in performance, or one gender could use a less efficient strategy that results in a lower performance. However, it is important to note

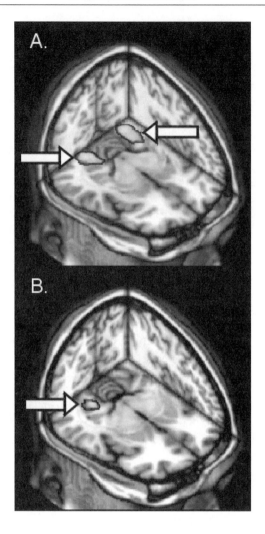

FIGURE 8.1. While learning to navigate in a virtual environment, males (A) and females (B) show different patterns of activation in the parahippocampal gyrus, an area located in the medial temporal lobe. In males, the parahippocampal gyrus is bilaterally activated, while in females only the right parahippocampal cortex shows activation (Sava, Sneider, & Yurgelun-Todd, 2007).

that even when performance at the beginning of training is different, males and females can reach similar levels of performance with sufficient training.

GENDER DIFFERENCES AND ADDICTION

Over the past few decades, research has showed that SUDs may result in cortical and sub-cortical damage, as well as impairments across a number of cognitive domains, including attention, decision making, memory, and problem solving (Cunha, Nicastri, Gomes, Moino, & Peluso, 2004; Gruber, Silveri, & Yurgelun-Todd, 2007; Tucker et al., 2004; Vik, Cellucci, Jarchow, & Hedt, 2004). Although there is substantial research on gender differences in the epidemiology, progression, and treatment of addiction, the study of gender differences in cognitive abilities in patients who are addicted is still in its infancy. To date, very few studies have investigated the role of gender in mediating the effects of drug abuse and addiction on cognitive processing (Gruber & Yurgelun-Todd, 2000). For the most part, research studies have either focused on one gender or have not reported the results by gender. In the remainder of this chapter we review studies that report gender effects on cognition across a variety of cognitive tasks and abused substances, and discusses the challenges in conducting research in this field. One important aspect of cognitive functioning in drug addiction is distinguishing between the acute intoxication and the residual effects of chronic drug abuse. To ensure that the acute effects of the drug do not affect cognitive performance at the time of testing, one has to implement a period of *abstinence* from using the drug. During the abstinence period the drug is eliminated from the body, and any impairments on cognitive tasks would not be due to acute intoxication. However, participant who are addicted who stop taking illicit substances are likely to experience withdrawal symptoms, which may also have a negative impact on cognitive processing. Furthermore, recovery of the drug-induced neurotoxic effects might occur after the participants stop the drug intake, and the recovery might occur at different rates for different drugs. These factors need to be carefully controlled when designing experiments.

Studies of gender differences in cognitive processing in SUDs have produced conflicting results. A number of studies have reported that *women have fewer cognitive impairments* associated with drug use (Bolla, McCann, & Ricaurte, 1998; Ersche, Clark, London, Robbins, & Sahakian, 2006). More than two decades ago, it was shown that chronic alcohol use was associated with deficits in visuospatial learning in men, but not in women (Fabian, Parsons, & Sheldon, 1984). More recently, a study investigating the effects of ecstasy on cognition in recently abstinent users (Bolla et al., 1998) found that ecstasy use was associated with impairment in immediate verbal memory and delayed visual memory, and that men had greater dose-related deficits than women on vocabulary scores, despite having relatively less impairment of serotoninergic function (Reneman et al., 2001).

Ersche and colleagues investigated gender differences in current amphetamine and opiate users, and nonusing healthy comparison participants on a battery of tests that included a cognitive rule-learning set-shifting task, a test of spatial planning, a test of geometric pattern and spatial location learning, and a delayed pattern recognition memory task (Ersche et al., 2006). Similar to findings in the general population as highlighted in the first part of the chapter, the control group showed gender differences in visuospatial test performance, with males having higher accuracy on the delayed pattern recognition memory. Males also performed better than females on the first trial of the geometric pattern and spatial location learning. However, in amphetamine and opiate users the relationship was reversed: female users performed better than male users, and no different than female controls. These results are consistent with the perspective that visuospatial memory impairments associated with drug use are more pronounced in males, possibly due to the neuroprotective effect of estrogen in females (Dluzen & McDermott, 2004; Myers, Anderson, & Dluzen, 2003; Yu & Liao, 2000). The study of Ersche and colleagues (2006) described above also tested former amphetamine and opiate users after an average of 8 years of abstinence. Despite the long abstinence period, former drug users performed similarly to current drug users, and the female advantage was maintained. However, both groups were impaired compared to controls on all tests except for the rule-learning set-shifting task.

Other studies found *impaired performance in females or no gender differences* in cognitive abilities in participants addicted to ecstasy and alcohol (Glenn & Parsons, 1992; Medina, Shear, & Corcoran, 2005). One study investigated nine cognitive dimensions in 31 men and 34 women using ecstasy: premorbid intelligence, selective and sustained attention, working memory, inhibition of overlearned responses, sequencing and psychomotor speed, problem solving and reasoning, visual and verbal fluency, visual memory, and verbal memory (Medina et al., 2005). Participants were tested after an average of 15 days of abstinence from using ecstasy. The authors found that ecstasy exposure was related to poorer verbal learning and memory ability in a dose-dependent manner, while no relationship was observed for measures of attention or executive function. The only gender difference was found on performance on a design fluency task, where increased lifetime ecstasy use was associated with better design fluency scores among men, and poorer performance among the women, possibly due to an increase in the speed of performance among men. Another study investigated speed and accuracy to complete tests of verbal skill, learning and memory, problem solving, and perceptual-motor skills in male and female alcoholics and controls (Glenn & Parsons, 1992). Although the participants who were alcoholic had lower efficiency ratios (defined as accuracy/time to complete a task) than controls in all four of the cognitive domains investigated, no gender difference was reported, suggesting that the male and female alcoholics had similar deficits as a result of chronic alcohol consumption.

For the purpose of this chapter, we are also asking whether gender affects the extent to which the cognitive impairments observed in individuals who are drug dependent are affected by abstinence. Compared to nonusers, former ecstasy users still present psycho-pathology and cognitive impairments after 5 months of abstinence, and both genders are equally affected (Thomasius et al., 2003). A recent study of male and female alcoholic individuals at 3 weeks postdetoxification found that the alcoholic group performed more poorly than the controls on tests of motor speed, visuospatial processing, working memory, spatial planning, and problem solving (Flannery et al., 2007). However, when data was analyzed for gender differences in controls and patients who were alcoholics, it was found that female alcoholic patients had greater response latencies than male alcoholic patients and male and female controls, and lower performance on a hippocampal-dependent visual working memory task. Moreover, the female alcoholics had lower performance on problem-solving tasks when compared to the other three groups (Flannery et al., 2007). Findings from an adolescent cohort of heavy alcohol users provide some insight into how cognitive impairments emerge. During adolescence, female alcohol users show a different pattern of brain activation compared to controls on a hippocampal-dependent working memory task, despite having no impairment in performance (Caldwell et al., 2005). The participants in this study were current alcohol users and were not instructed to abstain from drinking before testing; therefore, there was variability in the length of abstinence period. It has been suggested that in initial stages of heavy alcohol use, reorganization of neuronal networks could compensate for the alcohol-related subtle neuronal dysfunction in adolescent girls; however, if increased alcohol consumption continues, the compensation might no longer be possible and decreases in performance might emerge (Caldwell et al., 2005).

Performance on hippocampal and prefrontal cortex-dependent tasks has also been shown to be impaired in female heroin users who had been abstinent for 3 months. Specifically, female heroin users exhibited impaired egocentric spatial ability in a map-following task, and lower working memory performance on map and picture memory tasks when compared to male and female nonusers, and male heroin users (Wang et al., 2007). The gender differences in performance on spatial tasks have been related to the organizational effects of the gonadal hormones on the brain development during the embryonic and neonatal period (Romeo, Richardson, & Sisk, 2002), as well as their activational effects during adolescence and adulthood (Hajszan, Milner, & Leranth, 2007). Chronic abuse of opiates, such as heroin, may lead to changes in dopaminergic neurotransmission (Alexander, DeLong, & Strick, 1986). The detrimental effect of heroin on hippocampal function in women could be the result of an interaction of the heroin-induced dopaminergic system dysfunction and gonadal hormone activity on the hippocampal neurons (Wang et al., 2007). One study that investigated performance of heavy and light cannabis users after a period of 19 hours of abstinence found that female heavy cannabis users were shown to be more impaired than female light cannabis users on a spatial memory task, while this pattern was not present in males (Pope, Jacobs, Mialet, Yurgelun-Todd, & Gruber, 1997). This suggests that cannabis use might have different effects on cognitive processing of males and females.

Taken together, these results suggest that the cognitive impairments related to drug use might recover at different rates for males and females, and the drug of choice (i.e., ecstasy, amphetamine, opiate, or alcohol) and patterns of use might affect the recovery rate. Therefore, when studying the cognitive consequences of drug use, it is important to test males and females and analyze the data by gender.

SUMMARY

The research reviewed in this chapter suggests that gender differences can be found in some cognitive domains, such as spatial and verbal processing. However, the differences in performance are generally small, and significant overlap exists between the performance range of males and females on any given task. Moreover, manipulating subtle aspects of the tasks employed, like the duration of training, can affect the magnitude of the observed gender difference in performance. Interestingly, the hippocampus and the medial temporal lobe may undergo long-lasting structural changes as a consequence of chronic drug use (Nestler, 2001, 2002) and functions that require intact medial temporal lobe, like visuospatial learning and working memory, are often found to be differentially affected in males and females who are drug addicts (Caldwell et al., 2005; Ersche et al., 2006; Fabian et al., 1984; Flannery et al., 2007; Wang et al., 2007). This suggests that the medial temporal lobe function is not only modulated by gonadal hormones (Driscoll, Hamilton, Yeo, Brooks, & Sutherland, 2005; Saucier et al., 2002) but also might be particularly sensitive to the effects of illicit drug use.

The effects of stress on development of SUDs are well documented (Frone, 2008; Kreek, Nielsen, Butelman, & LaForge, 2005; Sinha, 2007), and gender-specific cognitive response to stressors could differentially contribute to the development of SUDs. Sustained elevated glucocorticoid levels associated with chronic stress have been shown to damage hippocampal neurons (McEwen, 2000; Sapolsky, 2000), and these data are consistent with the observations that individuals who are chronically stressed frequently display memory impairments. Alterations in hippocampal function may lead to decreased hippocampal inhibition over the hypothalamic–pituitary–adrenal axis, which in turn would further increase glucocorticoid levels and neuronal damage. Stress can induce neuroadaptations in stress circuits that could lead to increased salience of drug and drug-related stimuli when the participant is exposed to "stress" contexts (Robinson & Berridge, 2000; Sinha, 2001). It has been shown that elevated cortisol levels can have different effects on the cognitive functioning in males and females (McCormick, Lewis, Somley, & Kahan, 2007; Nakayama, Takahashi, Wakabayashi, Oono, & Radford, 2007), but the interaction of stress, gender, and substance use, and its effects on cognition are not well understood and need to be addressed in future studies.

Although some gender differences may be biologically driven (i.e., caused by the action of sex hormones on the brain), other factors, such as differences in cognitive strategies applied to solve a task, are also likely to contribute to the observed differences in performance. Research done in chronic drug users has yielded mixed results. Animal studies generally report greater neurotoxic effects in males after exposure to drugs, particularly in the case of substances that affect dopaminergic and serotoninergic transmission (Heller, Bubula, Lew, Heller, & Won, 2001; Wagner, Tekirian, & Cheo, 1993), whereas estrogen is hypothesized to have a neuroprotective effect (Dluzen & McDermott, 2004). Human studies also showed that chronic use of dopaminergic and serotoninergic drugs has more detrimental effects on male brains (Kaufman et al., 2001; Kim et al., 2005). However, the neuroprotective effects of estrogen in females cannot be the only factor affecting the gender differences in participants who are addicted, because females have been shown to be more impaired than males on some tasks. It is likely that the performance on any cognitive task is affected by an interaction of the hormonal milieu, drug use patterns (i.e., type of drug, duration of use, age at the onset of use), and the time of testing (ongoing addiction vs. abstinence and withdrawal), as well as the premorbid intellectual ability of the participant. Although more research is needed to understand the interaction of gender and addiction on cognitive processing, existing data underscores the importance of studying individual component processes of complex tasks and including male and female participants in future studies.

KEY POINTS

- Gender differences seem to exist in spatial and verbal processing, but the magnitude of the differences in performance is generally small and varies across tasks.
- The magnitude and direction of gender differences in cognition can be different in participants who are addicted when compared to the general population. Specifically, amphetamine and opiate use seem to produce more cognitive impairments in men than in women, while other drugs (such as alcohol and ecstasy) might have different gender-specific effects related to particular cognitive dimensions.
- The specific effects of drug use on cognition depend on the drug of choice, the time of testing, and gender.
- Although hormonal influences can contribute to the variability observed in cognitive processing in participants who are addicted, more research is necessary to understand what other factors contribute to the observed gender differences.

REFERENCES

Asterisks denote recommended readings.

Alexander, G. E., DeLong, M. R., & Strick, P. L. (1986). Parallel organization of functionally segregated circuits linking basal ganglia and cortex. *Annual Review of Neuroscience, 9,* 357–381.

Astur, R. S., Ortiz, M. L., & Sutherland, R. J. (1998). A characterization of performance by men and women in a virtual Morris water task: A large and reliable sex difference. *Behavioural Brain Research, 93*(1/2), 185–190.

Astur, R. S., Tropp, J., Sava, S., Constable, R. T., & Markus, E. J. (2004). Sex differences and correlations in a virtual Morris water task, a virtual radial arm maze, and mental rotation. *Behavioural Brain Research, 151*(1/2), 103–115.

Baenninger, M., & Newcombe, N. (1989). The role of experience in spatial test performance: A meta-analysis. *Sex Roles, 20,* 327–344.

Bolla, K. I., McCann, U. D., & Ricaurte, G. A. (1998). Memory impairment in abstinent MDMA ("Ecstasy") users. *Neurology, 51*(6), 1532–1537.

Breedlove, S. M. (1992). Sexual dimorphism in the vertebrate nervous system. *Journal of Neuroscience, 12*(11), 4133–4142.

Breitenstein, C., Jansen, A., Deppe, M., Foerster, A. F., Sommer, J., Wolbers, T., et al. (2005). Hippocampus activity differentiates good from poor learners of a novel lexicon. *Neuroimage*, *25*(3), 958–968.

Bryden, M. P., George, J., & Inch, R. (1990). Sex differences and the role of figural complexity in determining the rate of mental rotation. *Perceptual and Motor Skills*, *70*, 467–477.

Butler, T., Imperato-McGinley, J., Pan, H., Voyer, D., Cordero, J., Zhu, Y. S., et al. (2006). Sex differences in mental rotation: Top-down versus bottom-up processing. *Neuroimage*, *32*(1), 445–456.

Caldwell, L. C., Schweinsburg, A. D., Nagel, B. J., Barlett, V. C., Brown, S. A., & Tapert, S. F. (2005). Gender and adolescent alcohol use disorders on BOLD (blood oxygen level dependent) response to spatial working memory. *Alcohol and Alcoholism*, *40*(3), 194–200.

Chen, C., Xue, G., Dong, Q., Jin, Z., Li, T., Xue, F., et al. (2007). Sex determines the neurofunctional predictors of visual word learning. *Neuropsychologia*, *45*(4), 741–747.

Collins, D. W., & Kimura, D. (1997). A large sex difference on a two-dimensional mental rotation task. *Behavioral Neuroscience*, *111*(4), 845–849.

Coney, J. (2002). Lateral asymmetry in phonological processing: Relating behavioral measures to neuroimaged structures. *Brain and Language*, *80*(3), 355–365.

Crook, T. H., 3rd, Youngjohn, J. R., & Larrabee, G. J. (1990). The Misplaced Objects Test: A measure of everyday visual memory. *Journal of Clinical and Experimental Neuropsychology*, *12*(6), 819–833.

Cunha, P. J., Nicastri, S., Gomes, L. P., Moino, R. M., & Peluso, M. A. (2004). [Neuropsychological impairments in crack cocaine-dependent inpatients: preliminary findings]. *Revista Brasileira de Psiquiatria*, *26*(2), 103–106.

Dabbs, J. M., Chang, E.-L., Strong, R. A., & Milun, R. (1998). Spatial ability, navigation strategy, and geographic knowledge among men and women. *Evolution and Human Behavior*, *19*, 89–98.

De Goede, M., & Postma, A. (2008). Gender differences in memory for objects and their locations: A study on automatic versus controlled encoding and retrieval contexts. *Brain and Cognition*, *66*(3), 232–242.

Denno, D., Meijs, B., Nachshon, I., & Aurand, S. (1982). Early cognitive functioning: sex and race differences. *International Journal of Neuroscience*, *16*(3/4), 159–172.

Dluzen, D. E., & McDermott, J. L. (2004). Developmental and genetic influences upon gender differences in methamphetamine-induced nigrostriatal dopaminergic neurotoxicity. *Annals of the New York Academy of Sciences*, *1025*, 205–220.

Dorion, A. A., Chantome, M., Hasboun, D., Zouaoui, A., Marsault, C., Capron, C., et al. (2000). Hemispheric asymmetry and corpus callosum morphometry: A magnetic resonance imaging study. *Neuroscience Research*, *36*(1), 9–13.

Driscoll, I., Hamilton, D. A., Yeo, R. A., Brooks, W. M., & Sutherland, R. J. (2005). Virtual navigation in humans: The impact of age, sex, and hormones on place learning. *Hormones and Behavior*, *47*(3), 326–335.

Eals, M., & Silverman, I. (1994). The hunter-gatherer theory of spatial sex differences: Proximate factors mediating the female advantage in recall of object arrays. *Ethology and Sociobiology*, *15*, 95–105.

Ekstrom, A. D., & Bookheimer, S. Y. (2007). Spatial and temporal episodic memory retrieval recruit dissociable functional networks in the human brain. *Learning and Memory*, *14*(10), 645–654.

Epting, L. K., & Overman, W. H. (1998). Sex-sensitive tasks in men and women: a search for performance fluctuations across the menstrual cycle. *Behavioral Neuroscience*, *112*(6), 1304–1317.

Ersche, K. D., Clark, L., London, M., Robbins, T. W., & Sahakian, B. J. (2006). Profile of executive and memory function associated with amphetamine and opiate dependence. *Neuropsychopharmacology*, *31*(5), 1036–1047.

Etchamendy, N., & Bohbot, V. D. (2007). Spontaneous navigational strategies and performance in the virtual town. *Hippocampus*, *17*(8), 595–599.

Fabian, M. S., Parsons, O. A., & Sheldon, M. D. (1984). Effects of gender and alcoholism on verbal and visual-spatial learning. *Journal of Nervous and Mental Disease*, *172*(1), 16–20.

Flannery, B., Fishbein, D., Krupitsky, E., Langevin, D., Verbitskaya, E., Bland, C., et al. (2007). Gender differences in neurocognitive functioning among alcohol-dependent Russian patients. *Alcoholism, Clinical and Experimental Research*, *31*(5), 745–754.

Flannery, K. A., Liederman, J., Daly, L., & Schultz, J. (2000). Male prevalence for reading disability is found in a large sample of black and white children free from ascertainment bias. *Journal of the International Neuropsychological Society, 6*(4), 433–442.

Foo, P., Warren, W. H., Duchon, A., & Tarr, M. J. (2005). Do humans integrate routes into a cognitive map? Map- versus landmark-based navigation of novel shortcuts. *Journal of Experimental Psychology: Learning, Memory, and Cognition, 31*(2), 195–215.

Frone, M. R. (2008). Are work stressors related to employee substance use? The importance of temporal context assessments of alcohol and illicit drug use. *Journal of Applied Psychology, 93*(1), 199–206.

Glenn, S. W., & Parsons, O. A. (1992). Neuropsychological efficiency measures in male and female alcoholics. *Journal of Studies on Alcohol, 53*(6), 546–552.

Gruber, S., & Yurgelun-Todd, D. (2000). Neuropsychological correlates of substance abuse. In M. J. Kaufman (Ed.), *Brain imaging in substance abuse: Research, clinical, and forensic applications* (pp. 199–230). New York: Elsevier Science. (*)

Gruber, S. A., Silveri, M. M., & Yurgelun-Todd, D. A. (2007). Neuropsychological consequences of opiate use. *Neuropsychology Review, 17*(3), 299–315.

Gur, R. C., Alsop, D., Glahn, D., Petty, R., Swanson, C. L., Maldjian, J. A., et al. (2000). An fMRI study of sex differences in regional activation to a verbal and a spatial task. *Brain and Language, 74*(2), 157–170.

Hajszan, T., Milner, T. A., & Leranth, C. (2007). Sex steroids and the dentate gyrus. *Progress in Brain Research, 163*, 399–816. (*)

Halpern, D. F. (1986). *Sex differences in cognitive abilities*. Hillsdale, NJ: Erlbaum.

Hausmann, M., Slabbekoorn, D., Van Goozen, S. H., Cohen-Kettenis, P. T., & Gunturkun, O. (2000). Sex hormones affect spatial abilities during the menstrual cycle. *Behavioral Neuroscience, 114*(6), 1245–1250.

Heller, A., Bubula, N., Lew, R., Heller, B., & Won, L. (2001). Gender-dependent enhanced adult neurotoxic response to methamphetamine following fetal exposure to the drug. *Journal of Pharmacology and Experimental Therapeutics, 298*(2), 769–779.

Isgor, C., & Sengelaub, D. R. (1998). Prenatal gonadal steroids affect adult spatial behavior, CA1 and CA3 pyramidal cell morphology in rats. *Hormones and Behavior, 34*(2), 183–198.

Jansen-Osmann, P., & Heil, M. (2006). Violation of pure insertion during mental rotation is independent of stimulus type, task, and subjects' age. *Acta Psychologica, 122*(3), 280–287.

Jansen-Osmann, P., & Heil, M. (2007). Suitable stimuli to obtain (no) gender differences in the speed of cognitive processes involved in mental rotation. *Brain and Cognition, 64*(3), 217–227. (*)

Kaufman, M. J., Levin, J. M., Maas, L. C., Kukes, T. J., Villafuerte, R. A., Dostal, K., et al. (2001). Cocaine-induced cerebral vasoconstriction differs as a function of sex and menstrual cycle phase. *Biological Psychiatry, 49*(9), 774–781.

Kim, S. J., Lyoo, I. K., Hwang, J., Sung, Y. H., Lee, H. Y., Lee, D. S., et al. (2005). Frontal glucose hypometabolism in abstinent methamphetamine users. *Neuropsychopharmacology, 30*(7), 1383–1391.

Kimura, D. (2000). *Sex and cognition*. Cambridge, MA: MIT Press.

Kreek, M. J., Nielsen, D. A., Butelman, E. R., & LaForge, K. S. (2005). Genetic influences on impulsivity, risk taking, stress responsivity and vulnerability to drug abuse and addiction. *Nature Neuroscience, 8*(11), 1450–1457.

Leplow, B., Lehnung, M., Pohl, J., Herzog, A., Ferstl, R., & Mehdorn, M. (2003). Navigational place learning in children and young adults as assessed with a standardized locomotor search task. *British Journal of Psychology, 94*(Pt. 3), 299–317.

Leranth, C., Petnehazy, O., & MacLusky, N. J. (2003). Gonadal hormones affect spine synaptic density in the CA1 hippocampal subfield of male rats. *Journal of Neuroscience, 23*(5), 1588–1592.

Levy, J. (1969). Possible basis for the evolution of lateral specialization of the human brain. *Nature, 224*(5219), 614–615.

Levy, L. J., Astur, R. S., & Frick, K. M. (2005). Men and women differ in object memory but not performance of a virtual radial maze. *Behavioral Neuroscience, 119*(4), 853–862.

Lubinski, D., Webb, R. M., Morelock, M. J., & Benbow, C. P. (2001). Top 1 in 10,000: A 10-year follow-up of the profoundly gifted. *Journal of Applied Psychology, 86*(4), 718–729.

Maccoby, E. E., & Jacklin, C. N. (1974). *The psychology of sex differences*. Stanford, CA: Stanford University Press.

McCarthy, M. M., & Konkle, A. T. (2005). When is a sex difference not a sex difference? *Frontiers in Neuroendocrinology, 26*(2), 85–102. (*)

McCormick, C. M., Lewis, E., Somley, B., & Kahan, T. A. (2007). Individual differences in cortisol levels and performance on a test of executive function in men and women. *Physiology and Behavior, 91*(1), 87–94.

McEwen, B. S. (2000). Effects of adverse experiences for brain structure and function. *Biological Psychiatry, 48*(8), 721–731.

McGivern, R. F., Mutter, K. L., Anderson, J., Wideman, G., Bodnar, M., & Huston, P. J. (1998). Gender and differences in incidental learning and visual recognition memory: Support for a sex difference in unconscious environmental awareness. *Personality and Individual Differences, 25*(2), 223–232.

McGlone, J. (1980). Sex differences in human brain asymmetry: A critical survey. *Behavioral and Brain Sciences, 3*, 215–263.

Medina, K. L., Shear, P. K., & Corcoran, K. (2005). Ecstasy (MDMA) exposure and neuropsychological functioning: A polydrug perspective. *Journal of the International Neuropsychological Society, 11*(6), 753–765.

Morris, J. A., Jordan, C. L., & Breedlove, S. M. (2004). Sexual differentiation of the vertebrate nervous system. *Nature Neuroscience, 7*(10), 1034–1039.

Morris, R. (1984). Developments of a water-maze procedure for studying spatial learning in the rat. *Journal of Neuroscience Methods, 11*(1), 47–60.

Myers, R. E., Anderson, L. I., & Dluzen, D. E. (2003). Estrogen, but not testosterone, attenuates methamphetamine-evoked dopamine output from superfused striatal tissue of female and male mice. *Neuropharmacology, 44*(5), 624–632.

Nakayama, Y., Takahashi, T., Wakabayashi, A., Oono, H., & Radford, M. H. (2007). Sex differences in the relationship between cortisol levels and the Empathy and Systemizing Quotients in humans. *Neuroendocrinology Letters, 28*(4), 445–448.

Nestler, E. J. (2001). Neurobiology. Total recall-the memory of addiction. *Science, 292*(5525), 2266–2267.

Nestler, E. J. (2002). Common molecular and cellular substrates of addiction and memory. *Neurobiology of Learning and Memory, 78*(3), 637–647.

O'Keefe, J., & Conway, D. H. (1978). Hippocampal place units in the freely moving rat: Why they fire where they fire. *Experimental Brain Research, 31*(4), 573–590.

Pope, H. G., Jr., Jacobs, A., Mialet, J. P., Yurgelun-Todd, D., & Gruber, S. (1997). Evidence for a sex-specific residual effect of cannabis on visuospatial memory. *Psychotherapy and Psychosomatics, 66*(4), 179–184.

Postma, A., & De Haan, E. H. (1996). What was where? Memory for object locations. *Quarterly Journal of Experimental Psychology. A Human Experimental Psychology, 49*(1), 178–199.

Postma, A., Jager, G., Kessels, R. P., Koppeschaar, H. P., & van Honk, J. (2004). Sex differences for selective forms of spatial memory. *Brain and Cognition, 54*(1), 24–34.

Reneman, L., Booij, J., de Bruin, K., Reitsma, J. B., de Wolff, F. A., Gunning, W. B., et al. (2001). Effects of dose, sex, and long-term abstention from use on toxic effects of MDMA (ecstasy) on brain serotonin neurons. *Lancet, 358*(9296), 1864–1869.

Roberts, J. E., & Bell, M. A. (2002). The effects of age and sex on mental rotation performance, verbal performance, and brain electrical activity. *Developmental Psychobiology, 40*(4), 391–407.

Robinson, T. E., & Berridge, K. C. (2000). The psychology and neurobiology of addiction: an incentive-sensitization view. *Addiction, 95*(Suppl. 2), S91–S117.

Romeo, R. D., Richardson, H. N., & Sisk, C. L. (2002). Puberty and the maturation of the male brain and sexual behavior: Recasting a behavioral potential. *Neuroscience and Biobehavioral Reviews, 26*(3), 381–391.

Sandstrom, N. J., Kaufman, J., & Huettel, S. A. (1998). Males and females use different distal cues in a virtual environment navigation task. *Brain Research. Cognitive Brain Research, 6*(4), 351–360.

Sapolsky, R. M. (2000). The possibility of neurotoxicity in the hippocampus in major depression: a primer on neuron death. *Biological Psychiatry, 48*(8), 755–765.

Saucier, D. M., Green, S. M., Leason, J., MacFadden, A., Bell, S., & Elias, L. J. (2002). Are sex differences in navigation caused by sexually dimorphic strategies or by differences in the ability to use the strategies? *Behavioral Neuroscience, 116*(3), 403–410.

Schmitzer-Torbert, N. (2007). Place and response learning in human virtual navigation: Behavioral measures and gender differences. *Behavioral Neuroscience, 121*(2), 277–290.

Sharps, M. J., Welton, A. L., & Price, J. L. (1993). Gender and task in the determination of spatial cognitive performance. *Psychology of Women Quarterly, 17*, 71–83.

Shaywitz, B. A., Shaywitz, S. E., Pugh, K. R., Constable, R. T., Skudlarski, P., Fulbright, R. K., et al. (1995). Sex differences in the functional organization of the brain for language. *Nature, 373*(6515), 607–609.

Silverman, I., & Eals, M. (1992). Sex differences in spatial abilities: Evolutionary theory and data. In J. Barkow, I. Cosmides, & J. Tooby (Eds.), *The adapted mind: Evolutionary psychology and the generation of culture* (pp. 533–549). New York: Oxford University Press.

Sinha, R. (2001). How does stress increase risk of drug abuse and relapse? *Psychopharmacology, 158*(4), 343–359.

Sinha, R. (2007). The role of stress in addiction relapse. *Current Psychiatry Reports, 9*(5), 388–395.

Sneider, J. T., Sava, S., Rogowska, J., Gruber, S. A., & Yurgelun-Todd, D. A. (2008). *Sex differences in fMRI activation during spatial navigation.* Poster presented at the Society for Neuroscience Meeting, Washington, DC.

Sommer, I. E., Aleman, A., Bouma, A., & Kahn, R. S. (2004). Do women really have more bilateral language representation than men? A meta-analysis of functional imaging studies. *Brain, 127*(Pt. 8), 1845–1852.

Spelke, E. S. (2005). Sex differences in intrinsic aptitude for mathematics and science?: A critical review. *American Psychologist, 60*(9), 950–958. (*)

Steinmetz, H., Staiger, J. F., Schlaug, G., Huang, Y., & Jancke, L. (1995). Corpus callosum and brain volume in women and men. *NeuroReport, 6*(7), 1002–1004.

Thomasius, R., Petersen, K., Buchert, R., Andresen, B., Zapletalova, P., Wartberg, L., et al. (2003). Mood, cognition and serotonin transporter availability in current and former ecstasy (MDMA) users. *Psychopharmacology, 167*(1), 85–96.

Tucker, K. A., Potenza, M. N., Beauvais, J. E., Browndyke, J. N., Gottschalk, P. C., & Kosten, T. R. (2004). Perfusion abnormalities and decision making in cocaine dependence. *Biological Psychiatry, 56*(7), 527–530.

Vik, P. W., Cellucci, T., Jarchow, A., & Hedt, J. (2004). Cognitive impairment in substance abuse. *Psychiatric Clinics of North America, 27*(1), 97–109, ix.

Vikingstad, E. M., Cao, Y., Thomas, A. J., Johnson, A. F., Malik, G. M., & Welch, K. M. (2000). Language hemispheric dominance in patients with congenital lesions of eloquent brain. *Neurosurgery, 47*(3), 562–570.

Voyer, D. (1997). Scoring procedure, performance factors, and magnitude of sex differences in spatial performance. *American Journal of Psychology, 110*(2), 259–276.

Voyer, D., Postma, A., Brake, B., & Imperato-McGinley, J. (2007). Gender differences in object location memory: A meta-analysis. *Psychonomic Bulletin and Review, 14*(1), 23–38.

Wagner, G. C., Tekirian, T. L., & Cheo, C. T. (1993). Sexual differences in sensitivity to methamphetamine toxicity. *Journal of Neural Transmission: General Section, 93*(1), 67–70.

Wang, J. H., Liu, X. F., Chen, Y. M., Sun, H. Y., Fu, Y., Ma, M. X., et al. (2007). Heroin impairs map-picture-following and memory tasks dependent on gender and orientation of the tasks. *Behavioral Neuroscience, 121*(4), 653–664.

Webb, R. M., Lubinski, D., & Benbow, C. P. (2002). Mathematically facile adolescents with math science aspirations: New perspectives on their educational and vocational development. *Journal of Educational Psychology, 94*, 785–794.

Woolley, C. S., & McEwen, B. S. (1992). Estradiol mediates fluctuation in hippocampal synapse density during the estrous cycle in the adult rat. *Journal of Neuroscience, 12*(7), 2549–2554.

Yu, L., & Liao, P. C. (2000). Estrogen and progesterone distinctively modulate methamphetamine-induced dopamine and serotonin depletions in C57BL/6J mice. *Journal of Neural Transmission, 107*(10), 1139–1147.

The Roles of Sex Differences in the Drug Addiction Process

Amanda Elton, BS
Clinton D. Kilts, PhD

Attempts to compare the neurobiological, developmental, behavioral, social, emotional, psychological, cognitive, and life experiences between men and women have been ongoing for centuries. The focus and outcome of such studies are typically defined as being related to "gender" differences—a misattribution of such differences to the distinction between the continuous variable of masculinity and femininity that defines gender. In fact, the great majority of such studies instead focused on the categorical distinction between the sexes represented by males and females. This discussion, therefore, begins with the recognition that research exploring sex differences is generally conducted under the misnomer of gender differences and thus weakened from the outset by "political correctness" related to the use of the term *sex* as both a biological distinction between males and females and an action. Here we refer to differences between samples of men and women as being related to sex differences and leave the characterization of gender differences to studies that possess sufficient, valid instruments to allow such distinctions.

The following discussion of differences between the sexes in the addiction process is qualified by the fact that such differences are highly multidetermined, and thus such comparisons usually represent broad generalizations. This chapter presents a critical, though not comprehensive, review of the current state of the emerging understanding of sex differences in the neurobiology of the addiction process, as elucidated by neuroimaging technology, and a synthesis of this knowledge into present and future directives for managing drug abuse and addiction in men and women.

In this chapter we adopt a complex view in which sex differences in addiction are seen as more proximally related to sex-dependent interactions between social, developmental, and environmental variables and biological differences rather than to innate biological differences alone. Recent generations of women in the United States have witnessed major changes in developmental pressures, attitudes toward drug use, and their occupational status that unquestionably impact the nature and degree of sex differences in drug abuse and addiction. The neurobiology of sex differences in drug abuse and addiction is viewed here as a consequence of these psychosocial and environmental factors interacting with genetic differences between the sexes.

DRUG ADDICTION

Drug addiction is characterized by pathological motivation for drug-seeking and -use behaviors associated with the inability to inhibit such behaviors in spite of clear adverse consequences (Kalivas & Volkow, 2005). This discussion of the neurobiology of sex differences in drug abuse and addiction is based on a now common view of addiction as a multistage process. This theoretical model of the addiction process extends from initial drug use to the long-term consequences of end-stage addiction and focuses on three stages: *acquisition* of the addicted state, *maintenance* as a chronically relapsing state, and the long-term personal and social *consequences* of end-stage drug addiction. In this model the acquisition of drug abuse and subsequent addiction are mediated by a transition of drug incentives from reinforcing to habit-based. This transition is associated with altered reward sensitivity, a process that is positively and negatively modulated by multiple genetic, psychosocial, and developmental factors (Kandel, Hu, Griesler, & Schaffran, 2007). The acquisition process is mediated by maladaptive alterations in patterns of neural activity in striatal and frontal cortical areas and their modes of functional connectivity. In the second stage of this model, the chronically relapsing nature of the addicted state is maintained by the combination of pathological motivations for drug-related behaviors and diminished behavioral control, with drug use precipitated by conditioned drug cues, stress, and exposure to the drug itself, as well as motivation related to a desire to relieve aversive drug-withdrawal states. Although less studied as a component of the addiction process, the neurobiology of the long-term social and personal expressions of drug addiction is considered here as a third stage, as these factors underlie the immense socioeconomic costs of addiction and are a source of significant sex differences in the addiction process.

The neurobiology of the multistage drug addiction process represents stage-selective alterations in neurotransmitter and receptor levels, as well as alterations in distributed neural processes that influence cognitive, affective, and social functioning. The neurobiology of the transition from initial drug use to compulsive abuse and addiction has been most informatively characterized by the use of animal models based on drug self-administration (Koob & Kreek, 2007). The initial reinforcing or "liking" effects of drugs of abuse are mediated by their actions on dopamine neurotransmission in the ventral striatum, whereas subsequent compulsive drug abuse or "wanting" is attributed to allostatic alterations in reward processes (Ahmed & Koob, 2005) and the engagement of dorsal striatal mechanisms related to habit learning (Everitt & Robbins, 2005). The complex neurobiology of the chronic relapses that characterize addiction is attributed to the associative learning and memory processes related to chronic, intermittent drug abuse, which imbue conditioned drug cues, stressors, and the drug itself with their intense properties as precipitants of relapse. Neurobiological mechanisms that transduce the experience of these relapse factors to drug-seeking and -use behaviors have been informed by animal models (Shalev, Grimm, & Shaham, 2002) and human neuroimaging approaches (Childress et al., 1999; Grant et al., 1996; Risinger et al., 2005; Sinha et al., 2005). Such mechanisms of relapse include limbic and striatal alterations that code the intense drug motivational state often referred to as craving (Kilts et al., 2001) and a disabling of prefrontal cortical functions that represent opponent processes to relapse (R. Z. Goldstein, Volkow, Wang, Fowler, & Rajaram, 2001; Kaufman, Ross, Stein, & Garavan, 2003). The neural mechanisms that mediate the social and personal disabilities associated with end-stage addiction are only now being revealed by the emerging field of social cognition and its neuroscience.

This chapter begins with a brief discussion of sex differences in brain anatomy and physiology. Next, the core topic of sex differences in the neurobiology of the addiction process is discussed, focusing on the three-stage model (acquisition, maintenance by chronic relapse, end-stage expression) of drug addiction. Finally, the topic is summarized by a discussion of the implications of sex differences for the prevention, prognosis, and treatment of drug addiction.

DIFFERENCES BETWEEN THE SEXES IN BRAIN BIOLOGY AND ANATOMY

Behavioral dimorphisms between the sexes are attributed to global and regional brain structural and functional dimorphisms. The following discussion highlights the fact that many of the brain regions exhibiting sexual dimorphisms are the same as those limbic, paralimbic, striatal, and cerebral cortical areas most often implicated in the drug addiction process.

The Role of Sex Hormones

Sex is increasingly recognized as a determinant of variation in the brain and behavior. (Interested readers are directed to Cahill [2006] for a more extensive treatment of this topic.) Historically, the authoritative position on the effects of sex (the biological denotation) on the brain and behavior focused on the role of sex hormones or sex behavior (Levine, 1966). Sex hormones are steroid hormones that can be categorized into two main groups: androgens (predominantly testosterone in humans) and estrogens (primarily17beta-estradiol). They are produced and released by the gonads and, to a lesser extent, the adrenal cortex. Although circulating androgen levels are higher in males and estrogen levels higher in females, it is important to note that these hormones are present in both sexes. Furthermore, sex hormone levels fluctuate through a monthly menstrual cycle in women (or estrus cycle in many other mammals) and vary by season of the year and time of day in men.

In conjunction with certain genes, sex hormones are involved in sexual differentiation of the brain during development and continue to influence complex sex differences throughout life. For fetuses with a Y chromosome, masculinization of the brain begins prenatally with the expression of sex-specific genes (notably the gene *SRY*) that are harbored on the Y chromosome. This genotype results in the development of the testes and the subsequent production of androgens that promote development of masculine structures in the body, including masculinization of the brain. Sex hormone receptors in the brain continue to mediate effects of testosterone on brain and body functions throughout adulthood (reviewed by Alexander & Peterson, 2001). When two X chromosomes are present (with no Y chromosome), testosterone levels remain low, and the resulting phenotype is female. Following sexual differentiation, estrogens continue to affect the brain through long-term changes in gene expression that involve activation of estrogen receptors or immediate modulation of intracellular signaling (Belcher & Zsarnovsky, 2001). Later developmental and functional roles of estrogen in the brain include feminization and masculinization, neuroprotection, mood regulation, reproductive behavior, working memory, and hippocampal-dependent memory (McEwan & Alves, 1999). (For a more thorough treatment of this topic, the interested reader is directed to Alexander & Peterson [2001].)

Despite the critical influence of sex hormones on cell signaling pathways and gene expression throughout life, the long-held belief that sex differences in the brain and behavior are solely due to the actions of sex hormones is increasingly untenable. Nonetheless, the extensive research on the roles of sex hormones in sex differences cannot be entirely ignored, and as such, we refer to pertinent findings in this area throughout the rest of this chapter.

Sexual Dimorphisms of Brain Structure

Sex differences of a structural or functional nature exist at all levels of the neural axis (Shah et al., 2004). Although male and female brains are more anatomically alike than different, numerous brain structures are sexually dimorphic. Such sex differences emerge in a background of immense interindividual variation in human brain morphology and morphometrics and unquestionably contribute to such variation. Structural dimorphisms related to sex have been long recognized in small mammals. In rats, for example, the volume of the CA1, a functionally and anatomically distinct subregion of the hippocampus, is significantly larger in males than in females (reviewed by Cahill, 2006). Similarly, the medial and other nuclei of the amygdala exhibit long-recognized sex differences in morphology and synaptic organization (Cooke & Wooley, 2005). The recent development of high-resolution structural magnetic resonance imaging (MRI) has afforded unique opportunities to extend the analysis of sex differences to human brain morphology and morphometry. Such MRI studies support the existence of significant differences between the sexes in global and regional brain total volume and gray and white matter volume, as well as differences in measures of anatomical connectivity between brain regions. Men have larger total brain volumes than women (Kruggel, 2006; Luders, Steinmetz, & Joncke, 2002), although more robust sex-related dimorphisms are observed for regional gray and white matter brain volumes, when controlling for critical variables of age, education, handedness, and total intracranial volume (Chen, Sachdev, Wen, & Anstey, 2007).

In the limbic system the hippocampus is larger in women than in men (Maller, Reglade-Meslin, Anstey, & Sachdev, 2006). The amygdala, however, is larger in men compared to women (J. M. Goldstein et al., 2001) and is a unique exception to the remarkable degree of structural covariance in the brain of men and women (Mechelli, Friston, Frackowiak, & Price, 2005). Gur, Gunning-Dixon, Bilker, and Gur (2002), however, noted no differences between men and women in amygdalar and hippocampal volumes, highlighting the fact that sex affects brain volumes through complex interactions with other factors.

Human brain structural dimorphisms between the sexes are not limited to subcortical limbic structures. For example, the anterior cingulate cortex (ACC), a brain area prominent in the executive control of attention, memory, motor behavior, motivation, and emotion, exhibits morphometric (quantifiable) and morphological (descriptively characterized) sexual dimorphisms. Women exhibit greater gray matter volumes in the dorsal anterior, posterior, and ventral cingulate cortices (Chen et al., 2007). However, a characterization of sex differences in ACC morphology indicated that men exhibit more profound patterns of hemispheric asymmetry characterized by increased fissurization of the left ACC (Yücel et al., 2001). Women exhibit greater gyrification in the frontal and parietal lobes, compared to men, implying more cortical surface area for these regions (Luders et al., 2004). There are thus prominent sex differences in the morphology and morphometry of cortical and subcortical brain regions implicated in the neurobiology of drug abuse and addiction.

Women exhibit greater volumes than men for the precentral gyrus, orbital frontal cortex, superior frontal gyrus, and lingual gyrus (J. M. Goldstein et al., 2001). These investigators further noted that those brain regions exhibiting higher densities of sex hormone receptors during development or involved in reproductive behavior were significantly more sexually dimorphic than other regions, suggesting that sex hormones play an important developmental role in the expression of sexual dimorphisms of brain structures.

The white matter of the brain exhibits a highly ordered organization in supporting neurotransmission over spatial distances that is estimable using the MRI approach of diffusion tensor imaging (DTI). Sex differences in brain regional white matter organization—a measure of anatomical connectivity—have also been observed (Hsu et al., 2008). Such MRI measures of interregional anatomical and functional connectivity represent a finer-grained characterization of brain organization at the neural circuit and network level and thus offer a useful complement to morphometric and morphological approaches to defining sexual dimorphisms in the human brain.

The cerebral hemispheres are structurally and functionally distinct, and sex differences in hemispheric laterality have been described. In some strains of mice, the males exhibit greater right, compared to left, volumes of the granule layer of the hippocampal dentate gyrus, whereas no such laterality is observed for females (Tabibnia, Cooke, & Breedlove, 1999). In one particular mouse strain that was not sexually dimorphic in this brain region, but where the right granule cell layer is larger than the left in both sexes, it was further shown that a genetic defect that renders the androgen receptors insensitive prevents hippocampal laterality, suggesting a role of androgens in the development of hemispheric differences in mice (Tabibnia et al., 1999). In humans anatomical hemispheric asymmetry tends to be more apparent in men than in women (Good et al., 2001; Gur et al., 1999). In one example, a leftward asymmetry of the inferior parietal lobule was observed in men, whereas in women, the pattern of asymmetry was opposite, though small (Frederiske, Aylward, Barta, & Pearlson, 1999). The extent to which any sex differences in brain structure reflect functional dimorphisms is an important question when considering the potential implications of sex-related dimorphisms for complex behavioral phenotypes such as drug addiction.

Sexual Dimorphisms of Brain Function

Although the physiological significance of sex differences in global and regional brain anatomy and hemispheric lateralization remains unclear, behavioral and *in vivo* functional neuroimaging results suggest that there are functional corollaries of the observed structural dimorphisms that underlie sex-related behavioral dimorphisms. For example, men are generally thought to have superior ability on spatial reasoning tasks, compared to women, a difference mirrored by the observation that performance of a spatial mental rotation task was associated with significant sex differences in the activation and functional connectivity of the ventral ACC (Butler et al., 2007). A seminal positron emission tomography (PET) study (Protopescu et al., 2005) demonstrated a critical role for sex hormones in regulating the resting state activity of the dorsolateral prefrontal cortex. However, sex differences in the neural representation of addiction-related brain functions, associated with reward or incentive processing and inhibitory behavioral control, are selectively discussed here (the interested reader is again referred to Cahill [2006] for a broader treatment of this topic). A relevant recent study used functional MRI (fMRI) to demonstrate that sex steroids significantly modulate the function of the brain reward system, as the neural activity related to reward processing was regulated by menstrual cycle stage and correlated with gonadal steroid hormone levels (Dreher et al., 2007). During the midfollicular phase (days 4–8 after onset of menses) women exhibited a greater magnitude of activation of the amygdala and orbitofrontal cortex during reward anticipation than during the luteal phase (6–10 days after luteinizing hormone surge) (Figure 9.1). Significant sex differences in the response of the putamen and medial prefrontal cortex were also observed for reward anticipation and receipt, respectively (Figure 9.1). These findings suggest a neurobiological basis for the greater subjective response to psychostimulants observed in women in the follicular versus luteal phase of the menstrual cycle (Evans, Haney, & Foltin, 2002; Justice & de Wit, 1999).

Drug addiction is increasingly viewed as a disorder of the neurobiology of self-control processes (Baler & Volkow, 2006). The process of inhibitory control of behavior is frequently modeled in experiments using the stop-signal or go/no-go tasks (Aron & Poldrack,

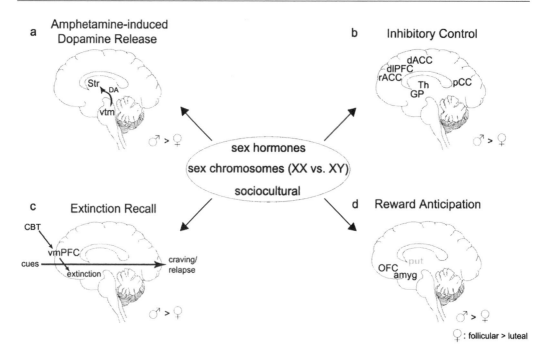

FIGURE 9.1. Sex differences in the behavioral and neural representation of cognitive and dopaminergic substrates of the drug addiction process and its treatment. Results of sex-difference studies using molecular and functional brain imaging approaches are superimposed on a saggital representation of the human brain. (a) PET results illustrating a greater increase in striatal dopamine receptor occupancy (greater dopamine release) following D-amphetamine administration in a sample of healthy men versus women (Munro et al., 2006). The inference from this study is that men exhibit a greater reinforcing response to psychostimulants, which would increase the likelihood of their transitioning from initial drug use to chronic abuse. vtm, midbrain ventral tegmentum; DA, dopamine; Str, striatum. (b) fMRI results illustrating that men exhibit greater activation of cortical, striatal, and thalamic representatives of an inhibitory motor control network in response to a stop-signal task, compared to women. The inference of this study is that there are sex differences in the neural correlates of inhibitory behavioral processes representing opponent mechanisms for pathological drug motivational states associated with addiction. rACC, rostral anterior cingulate cortex; dlPFC, dorsolateral prefrontal cortex; dACC, dorsal anterior cingulate cortex; pCC, posterior cingulate cortex; Th, thalamus; GP, globus pallidus. (c) fMRI results illustrating that men exhibit greater recall of extinction memory than do women (in the late follicular menstrual phase) (Milad et al., 2006, 2007). The inference from this finding is that the ability of extinction-based addiction therapies such as cognitive-behavioral therapy (CBT) to extinguish the association of conditioned drug cues with drug craving and relapse differs for men and women. vmPFC, ventromedial prefrontal cortex. (d) fMRI results illustrating sex and menstrual cycle phase differences in neural activity that encode reward anticipation or processing (Dreher et al., 2007). OFC, orbitofrontal cortex; put, putamen; amyg, amygdala.

2006). Testing a hypothesis that men are more impulsive than women, Li, Huang, Constable, and Sinha (2006) observed that men exhibit significantly greater distributed neural responses to response inhibition demands in a stop-signal task than do women, in spite of comparable task performance. Compared to a sample of healthy women, men exhibited a greater magnitude of neural activation for the striatal, cingulate, and frontal cortical representatives of the inhibitory control network (Li et al., 2006) (Figure 9.1). One inference of this study is that men are more impulsive than women as a result of less efficient neural processing of inhibitory control demands.

There also appear to be relatively consistent differences between the sexes in the hemispheric laterality of amygdalar responses to emotion-processing tasks. Both memory for emotional events (Cahill, 2003; Cahill, Uncapher, Kilpatrick, Alkire, & Turner, 2004) and the perception of facial expressions of emotion (Kilgore & Yurgelun-Todd, 2001; Proverbio, Brignone, Matarazzo, Del Zotto, & Zani, 2006; Williams et al., 2005) are associated with a preferential engagement of the left amygdala in women and the right amygdala in men. Sex-related hemispheric differences in amygdalar function are also exhibited in the resting state and extend to marked differences between the sexes in the hemispheric lateralization of amygdalar functional connectivity (Kilpatrick, Zaid, Pardo, & Cahill, 2006). These sex differences in amygdalar responsivity and connectivity may contribute to the observation that males and females with cocaine addictions exhibit striking differences in the amygdalar response to conditioned drug cues that provoke relapse.

In summary, there appear to be sex differences in the neural processing of rewards as behavioral reinforcers, a difference that is relevant to the role of a disrupted valuation of drug and nondrug rewards in the acquisition of drug abuse and addiction (Robinson & Berridge, 2000), and perhaps relevant to sex differences in the efficacy of reinforcer-based addiction therapies such as contingency management (K. M. Carroll & Onken, 2005). Men and women also differ in the activation of a network of brain regions engaged by demands for inhibitory behavioral control—a difference of clear relevance to sex differences in the ability of behavioral therapies to enhance drug-refusal skills. Finally, it is probable that observed human brain functional dimorphisms reflect sex-related neurochemical dimorphisms. For example, PET studies indicate that women exhibit lower *in vivo* alpha-[^{11}C]methyl--tryptophan uptake, an index of serotonin synthesis, throughout much of the predominantly left cerebral cortex, but not subcortex, compared to men (Sakai et al., 2006).

Although sex hormones are unlikely to account for all observed sexual dimorphisms of brain functional organization, research findings such as that discussed earlier for reward-related neural processing indicate that sex hormones regulate the extent of sex-related functional dimorphisms. For example, although studies show that men tend to perform better on spatial tasks, there are variations within the sexes that depend on sex hormone levels (reviewed by Kimura, 2002). Men with lower levels of testosterone tend to perform better than those with higher levels, whereas women with high testosterone levels have enhanced spatial abilities, compared to women with low testosterone levels. Furthermore, higher estrogen levels decrease the spatial abilities of women while enhancing their performance in areas that are typically female-oriented, such as those requiring fine motor skills and verbal fluency. In fact, enhanced fine motor skills have been reported in women in the midluteal phase, when estrogen levels are highest. The menstrual cycle has also been shown to influence hemispheric functional asymmetry, with higher levels of estrogen resulting in the suppression of right-hemispheric functioning (reviewed by Kimura, 2002). These findings illustrate the need to separately consider the sexes when exploring the functional neuroanatomy of the human brain and how variations in sex hormone levels within the sexes may influence outcomes in studies of sex differences.

Sex Differences in Neurodevelopment and Stress Reactivity

Males and females exhibit a different time course of brain maturation. In a cross-sectional imaging study by De Bellis et al. (2001), significant neurodevelopmental sex differences were observed, wherein age-related decreases in gray matter and increases in white matter were greater in males. The pioneering human neurodevelopment MRI studies of Giedd and colleagues (Giedd, Castellanos, Rajapakse, Vaituzis, & Rapoport, 1997; Giedd et al., 1999) suggest that limbic and frontal cortex gray matter volumes exhibit distinct rates of maturation in adolescent boys and girls. Functionally, electroencephalography (EEG) patterns in boys and girls between 2 months and 16 years of age demonstrate that certain brain regions, including those involved in motor skills, language, and social cognition, develop at different times and in a different sequence for each sex (Hanlon, Thatcher, & Cline, 1999). These sex-related patterns of neurodevelopmental timing suggest that the nature and timing of neurotrophic as well as adverse events (e.g., maltreatment) may differentially affect males and females.

Drug addiction is clearly a stress-sensitive disorder and has even been described as a stress-related disorder (Becker et al., 2007). Therefore, the characterization of sex differences in the neurobiology of the drug addiction process is linked to an understanding of sex differences in the neurobiology of stress reactivity. In this regard, women are generally recognized as having an increased sensitivity to stress and a heightened stress response, compared to men, a sex difference that renders femaleness as a predisposing factor for postpubertal stress-related disorders (Becker et al., 2007). Women exhibit a qualitatively differing emotional response to psychological stress, compared to men (Kelly et al., 2008). Men and women also exhibit a strikingly distinct pattern of neural responses to psychological stress, with men displaying a right prefrontal cortex activation and orbitofrontal cortex deactivation and women displaying a prominent activation of the striatum and paralimbic cortex (Wang et al., 2007). These findings of sex-dependent stress responses predict that men and women with drug addictions would differ in the affective and neural correlates of drug craving precipitated by stressors—a prediction confirmed by recent fMRI studies in men and women with cocaine addictions (see below).

Sex differences in neurodevelopment and stress reactivity converge in modulating the association of early life stress with heightened risk for the development of drug abuse and addiction. Exposure to the stress of famine during the first trimester of gestation was associated with heightened risk for drug addiction later in life, but only for male offspring (Franzek et al., 2008). The severity of traumatic experiences in childhood was associated with increased risk for relapse in women, but not men, following treatment for cocaine addiction (Hyman et al., 2008). It is known that stressful events in childhood can result in an altered stress response system in adulthood (Heim et al., 2000), although sex differences in the relationship between altered stress reactivity as a result of childhood maltreatment and the development of drug addictions and/or risk of relapse in drug addicted populations have not been systematically studied.

SEX DIFFERENCES IN THE CLINICAL ASPECTS OF DRUG ADDICTION

Drug addiction represents one of the most common psychiatric disorders worldwide. Like most psychiatric disorders, drug addiction exhibits marked sex differences in prevalence and symptomatology (Holden, 2005). Men and women with drug use disorders differ in prevalence, course, and outcome. In general, the prevalence rates for drug abuse and addiction are higher in men than women; however, women often exhibit similar rates for select drug addictions or represent a large minority of drug-addicted individuals across samples. For instance, the prevalence of lifetime and current nicotine dependence in the United States is similar for men and women (26 and 14% vs. 23 and 12%, respectively) (Hughes, Helzer, & Lindberg,

2006). In contrast, the prevalence of current crack cocaine abuse in women is one-fourth to one-third that of men (Hope, Hickman, & Tilling, 2005). It is, however, noteworthy that birth year effect studies indicate that sex differences in the prevalence and clinical features of drug abuse and dependence have decreased in recent generations (Holdcraft & Iacono, 2004).

Drug addiction is associated with deficits in cognitive, affective, and social functioning, as well as occupational, relational, and family disabilities. The nature and magnitude of cognitive deficits associated with drug abuse and addiction vary widely among studies and drugs (Jager et al., 2008). In one study of individuals with cocaine addiction the presence of cognitive deficits was dependent on recent drug abstinence, perhaps due to the precognitive effects of acute cocaine use (Woicik et al., 2008). Abstinent men and women who abuse cocaine and who did not fulfill criteria for drug dependence also demonstrated subtle sex differences in cognitive functioning (Rahman & Clarke, 2005). Heroin addiction is associated with sex differences in cognitive disability, with women demonstrating greater impairment and lesser drug-abstinence-related recovery than men (Liu, Li, Wilson, Ma, & Hu, 2005). Sex differences in the nature and magnitude of cognitive deficits associated with drug addiction, however, have not been studied systematically.

Are there are neural correlates of observed sex differences in presentation, course of illness, and treatment outcomes? A recent study of sex differences in fear extinction recall supports possible sex differences in response to extinction-based behavioral therapies for addiction. Using an aversive fear conditioning paradigm and skin conductance response as a measure of the conditioned fear response, a sexual dimorphism was noted in which men exhibited greater subsequent recall of the extinction memory than did women in the late follicular, but not early follicular, phase of the menstrual cycle (Milad et al., 2006). As the ventromedial prefrontal cortex (vmPFC) is involved in the recall of extinction memory (Quirk & Mueller, 2008), these findings suggest that sex hormones regulate vmPFC activity related to extinction recall (Figure 9.1). The inference is that sex differences, perhaps mediated by sex hormones, may exist in the ability to recall therapeutic memory related to extinction-based addiction therapies, and thus these sex differences predict differences in response to such therapies.

Child Maltreatment in Drug-Abusing Populations

Drug-abuse problems are commonly seen in subjects of both sexes with a history of abuse or trauma in childhood. The co-association of childhood physical and sexual abuse and later drug abuse and addiction is undeniable; more than half of all individuals who abuse drugs and enter treatment for drug addiction report a history of childhood abuse or neglect (Min, Farkas, Minnes, & Singer, 2007; Pirard, Sharon, Kang, Angarita, & Gastfriend, 2005). Emotional abuse, emotional neglect, and physical neglect incidence rates have also been reported in drug-abusing populations at levels that are higher than the general population (Medrano, Zule, Hatch, & Desmond, 1999). When considering only female drug abusers, a history of physical or sexual trauma was reported in 55–99% of cases (reviewed by Swan, 1998). A similar female sample reported that 40% had experienced at least one form of childhood abuse, of which 27% had been sexually abused (Brady, Kileen, Saladin, Dansky, & Becker, 1994). Additional samples of treatment-seeking women who were drug abusers reported rates of childhood physical abuse of 28 and 32% and rates of childhood sexual abuse of 31 and 42% (Brems, Johnson, Neal, & Freemon, 2005; Fullilove, Fullilove, Smith, & Winkler, 1993).

It has been estimated that 80% of men who have been sexually abused have problems with alcohol abuse, compared to about 11% of men without a sexual abuse history (Whea-lin, n.d.). In drug abuse treatment programs for men, 13–25% reported having experienced physical abuse, 25% emotional abuse, 6–7% sexual abuse, and 18% multiple types of abuse (Brems et al., 2005; Dunn, Ryan, & Dunn, 1994). Within a group of adolescents who abused drugs, 17% reported that they had been sexually abused, 11% reported physical abuse, and 11% reported both physical and sexual abuse (Stewart, 1994). These studies, and many oth-ers, suggest that a history of childhood maltreatment predisposes victims to drug abuse and addiction later in life.

Childhood maltreatment also predisposes women to adult prostitution (Medrano, Hatch, Zule, & Desmond, 2003; Widom, Weiler, & Cottler, 1999), which is strongly linked to drug abuse and addiction (Nuttbrock, Rosenblum, Magura, Villano, & Wallace, 2004). Sex differ-ences in the prevalence of prostitution associated with drug abuse and addiction also represent a vehicle by which violence, abuse, and disability are perpetuated in women. Thirty-two per-cent of a sample of women with heroin addiction reported trading sex for drugs or money in the past year (El-Bassel, Simoni, Cooper, Gilbert, & Schilling, 2001). The lifetime and 1-year prevalence rates for prostitution in a sample of 1,606 women entering substance abuse treat-ment programs in the United States were 51 and 41%, respectively (Burnette et al., 2008). Women involved in prostitution report high rates of rape, assault, and physical and mental illnesses (Burnette et al., 2008; El-Bassel et al., 2001; El-Bassel & Witte, 2001; Roxburgh, Degenhardt, & Copeland, 2006). A pattern emerges in which early life trauma predisposes women toward drug abuse and addiction as well as recurring trauma in adulthood.

SEX DIFFERENCES IN THE BRAIN BIOLOGY OF THE ADDICTION PROCESS

Males and females exhibit significant behavioral differences in all of the stages of the drug addiction process, from initiation to end-stage addiction (Becker & Hu, 2008). These behav-ioral dimorphisms are associated with sex differences in the emerging neurobiology related to the stages of the addiction process. Sex-linked genes, sex hormones, and psychosocial factors directly and indirectly regulate sex differences in the susceptibility to drug abuse and addiction and in rates of relapse. Understanding the biological mechanisms behind these sex-dependent processes would furnish a better understanding of the drug addiction process in men and women and offer novel sex-specific treatment targets. The following discussion of sex differences in the neurobiology of the drug addiction process is organized by the stage of the addiction process and, within the maintenance stage, the type of relapse precipitant.

Acquisition of Addiction

Although men are more likely than women to suffer from drug addiction, women prog-ress more quickly from initial use to addiction. The decreased relative time for women to become alcohol dependent has been especially well documented (reviewed by Lynch, Roth, & Carroll, 2002). This sex difference in propensity to escalate drug self-administration has been demonstrated in rat and monkey models (Becker & Hu, 2008; Fattore, Spano, Altea, Angius, & Fadda, 2007; Mello, Knudson, & Mendelson, 2007). Animal model and human neuroimaging studies have identified possible brain mechanisms underlying sex differences in the acquisition of drug abuse and addiction. The facilitating effects of drugs of abuse on brain dopamine neurotransmission are consistently offered as the mechanism of action related to the properties of drugs as reinforcers, implicating dopamine as a key mediator of the progression from initial drug use to chronic abuse. Human PET studies using the D_2 dopamine receptor ligand [^{11}C]raclopride support sex differences in amphetamine-induced striatal dopamine release (Munro et al., 2006). Compared to healthy women, men exhibited greater dopamine release in response to amphetamine administration in the ventral striatum, dorsal putamen, and caudate nucleus (Figure 9.1). The observation that men also exhibited greater positive subjective reactions to amphetamine administration supports the relevance of this neurochemical sex difference to a mechanism by which men would exhibit increased vulnerability to the acquisition of psychostimulant abuse and addiction. Also, for the female subjects, amphetamine-induced striatal dopamine release did not differ as a function of menstrual cycle phase (Munro et al., 2006).

These human *in vivo* molecular brain imaging findings are inconsistent with the results of animal model studies of the addiction process that show that female rats acquire drug self-administration more readily than males (Becker & Hu, 2008; Carroll, Lynch, Roth, Morgan, & Cosgrove, 2004; Hu, Crombag, Robinson, & Becker, 2004; Fattore et al., 2007; Lynch & Carroll, 1999). The replication of this sex difference using ovariectomized female rats suggests that there are intrinsic sex differences in the acquisition of cocaine self-administration that are regulated independently of sex hormones (Hu et al., 2004). In addition, estrogen administration enhanced this acquisition process in females, indicating that there are both sex hormone-dependent and -independent mechanisms for increased cocaine sensitivity in female rats (Hu et al., 2004). The sex hormone-dependent mechanism has been attributed to the facilitating influence of estrogen on dopamine neurotransmission. However, the PET study (Munro et al., 2006), mentioned above, suggests that in humans, the facilitating effects of estrogen involve a site of action other than the modulation of psychostimulant-induced increases in extracellular dopamine concentrations. The sex hormone-independent mechanism may involve genes residing on the sex chromosomes that directly influence the sexually dimorphic vulnerability to drug abuse (Davies & Wilkinson, 2006) by influencing behaviors such as habit learning (Quinn, Hitchcott, Umeda, Arnold, & Taylor, 2007).

Relapse and the Maintenance of the Addicted State

Drug addiction is a chronically relapsing disorder. Data concerning sex differences in relapse in humans are inconsistent, plausibly related to possible sex differences in reactivity to different factors (discussed below) known to be associated with relapse (Becker & Hu, 2008; Hser, Evans, & Huang, 2005; Marsh, Cao, & D'Aunno, 2004).

Conditioned Drug Cue–Induced Relapse

Conditioned drug use reminders or cues represent powerful precipitants of drug craving and relapse to drug-seeking and -use behaviors in addicted individuals. In laboratory settings the study of drug cue-induced craving has used diverse forms of drug-cue exposure, including drug-related paraphernalia, videotape/audiotape simulations of drug use, and script-guided mental imagery of drug use behavior, contexts, and reactions. Similar levels of self-rated craving in response to drug cues for men and women have been reported in smokers (Niaura et al., 1998) and alcoholics (Rubonis et al., 1994). However, significant and complex sex differences in reactivity to drug cues have been reported in male and female individuals with cocaine and opiate addictions. In one mixed-sex sample of individuals with cocaine addiction, females exhibited significantly higher self-reported craving responses to cocaine cues, relative to males; however, craving responses of females were not different from other male-only samples (Robbins, Ehrman, Childress, & O'Brien, 1999). Females with heroin addiction exhibited greater drug craving and psychophysiological responses to conditioned drug cues than did a sample of matched males, though differences were dependent on the method of drug cue exposure (Yu et al., 2007). Males with cocaine addiction exhibited comparable craving and greater adrenocorticotropin hormone (ACTH), cortisol, and blood pressure responses to conditioned drug cues compared to a sample of women with cocaine addiction (Fox et al., 2006). These observed sex differences in motivational, neuroendocrine, and cardiovascular reactivity to conditioned drug cues suggest a sexual dimorphism in the neurobiology of cue-induced relapse that would indicate a need for sex-specific therapies for relapse prevention in men and women with drug addictions.

Drug use reminders, which lead to drug craving in drug-dependent individuals, have been associated with local changes in human cerebral blood flow estimates of localized neural activity. Although the majority of such functional neuroimaging studies have focused on drug cue responses in exclusively male or mixed-samples of individuals with drug addiction, several recent studies have focused on female subject. Relative to female, nondependent social drinkers, young (18–24 years) women with alcohol dependence exhibited a greater activation of the subcallosal, anterior cingulate and lateral prefrontal cortex, and insula in response to alcohol cues; the cue-induced subcallosal cortex response was positively correlated with the self-reported craving response (Tapert, Brown, Baratta, & Brown, 2004). The cue responses of a sample of young men with alcohol dependence were not similarly defined and compared. In a study of the neural correlates of cue-induced cocaine craving, Kilts, Gross, Ely, and Drexler (2004) used PET imaging to compare the brain responses to script-guided mental imagery of personal cocaine use in male and female individuals seeking treatment for cocaine addiction. Both sexes demonstrated drug cue-related activation of the ventral striatum, a finding consistent with their comparable drug motivational response to the imagery cue (Figure 9.2). However, compared to men, women exhibited significantly less cue-induced activation of the amygdala, insula, lateral orbitofrontal cortex, postcentral gyrus, and anterior striatum (Figure 9.3). Conversely, women exhibited greater cue-induced activation of the precentral gyrus, inferior frontal cortex, dorsolateral prefrontal cortex, and the dorsal anterior and posterior cingulate cortex (Figure 9.3). The sexes demonstrated opposite drug cue responses in the right amygdala. These sex differences suggest that whereas both sexes exhibited similar neural responses to the incentive motivational properties of drug cues, women in this sample distinctly engaged cortical areas involved in cognitive control that would suppress habit-based cue responses and dampen the drug-cue valuation functions of the amygdala. The resulting inference is that this sex-specific distributed neural response to this precipitant of relapse would render females with cocaine addiction more able to forego a drug-seeking and -use response to drug cues, compared to males. The differences in neural responses of women and men to drug cues may influence their susceptibility to, or may offer sex-specific strategies to prevent, drug cue-induced relapse.

Stress-Induced Relapse

Anecdotal reports and empirical evidence from animal models and human studies support the experience of acute stress as a major risk factor for relapse in individuals with drug addictions. The consistent observation that men and women exhibit qualitatively and quantitatively differing affective and neural responses to stressors (Kelly et al., 2008; Khurana & Devaud, 2007; Wang et al., 2007) supports the presence of sex differences in the susceptibility of individuals with drug addictions to stress-induced relapse. A study of sex differences in the subjective and physiological reactions to psychological and physical stressors in subjects with cocaine addiction found that women responded with higher subjective reports of stress than

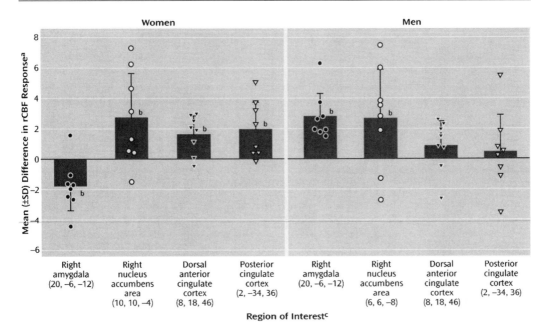

FIGURE 9.2. Sex differences in the neural response of women and men with cocaine dependence to conditioned drug use reminders (Kilts et al., 2004). The ordinate represents the difference if rCBF response for cocaine use versus neutral script imagery for female (*left*) and male (*right*) individuals seeking treatment for cocaine addiction. Brain regions of interest (ROI) on the abscissa represent rCBF for the amygdala (•), nucleus accumbens (○), and dorsal anterior (▼) and posterior (Δ) cingulate cortex (numbers in parentheses represent the stereotaxic location [Talairach] of voxel maxima for each ROI). Asterisks represent significant differences between imagery conditions ($p < .005$). Adapted from Kilts, Gross, Ely, and Drexler (2004). Copyright 2004 by the American Psychiatric Association. Adapted by permission.

men (Back, Brady, Jackson, Salstrom, & Zinzow, 2005). Conversely, men had higher salivary cortisol and heart rate, both at baseline and following stressors, despite reporting levels of stress and anxiety comparable to women. Compared to men, women with drug dependence exhibited enhanced motivation for drug use and relapse in response to negative affect and interpersonal problems (i.e., stressors) (McKay, Rutherford, Cacciola, Kabasakalian-McKay, & Alterman, 1996; Rubonis et al., 1994). These findings suggest that greater stress reactivity in women with drug addictions may make them more likely to use drugs when faced with unpleasant, stressful circumstances.

A recent series of functional neuroimaging studies of brain responses to script-guided stress imagery suggests that cocaine addiction is associated with altered stress responses in distributed brain areas and that prominent sex differences exist. Relative to healthy comparison subjects, individuals with cocaine addiction demonstrated increased stressor-induced activation of the dorsal striatum and lesser stress responses in the anterior cingulate cortex (Sinha et al., 2005). A functional inference from these results is that individuals who are cocaine-dependent respond to stress by engaging brain areas that encode habit-based behaviors and underengage areas involved in the cognitive control of such behaviors. In comparison to males, female subjects with cocaine addiction demonstrated greater activation of the middle/inferior frontal gyri, posterior and middle cingulate cortex, and insula (Li et al., 2005; Figure 9.3). These studies support the idea that females with cocaine addiction differ

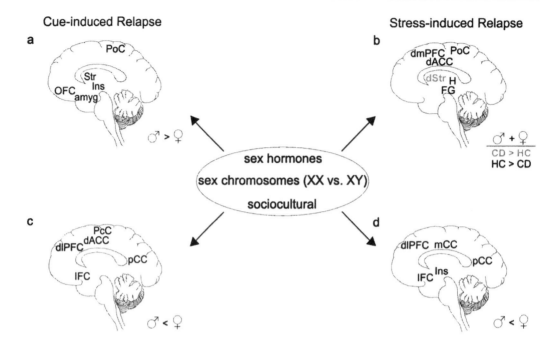

FIGURE 9.3. Sex differences in the neural representation of drug craving induced by relapse factors. Results of sex differences studies using functional brain imaging approaches are superimposed on a saggittal representation of the human brain. PET results from a comparison of rCBF responses for male and female individuals seeking treatment for crack cocaine addiction (Kilts et al., 2004) and illustrating (a) greater drug cue responses in men versus women, and (c) greater drug cue responses for women versus men. OFC, lateral orbitofrontal cortex; amyg, amygdala; Ins, insula; Str, striatum; PoC, postcentral gyrus; dlPFC, dorsolateral prefrontal cortex; IFC, inferior frontal cortex; dACC, dorsal anterior cingulate cortex; PrC, precentral gyrus; pCC, posterior cingulate cortex. fMRI results from (b), a comparison of blood oxygen level-dependent (BOLD) responses between mixed-sex samples of subjects with cocaine dependence (CD) and healthy comparisons (HC) for the contrast of stress mental imagery and baseline conditions (Sinha et al., 2005); and (d), BOLD responses for the contrast of stress mental imagery and baseline conditions in which female individuals seeking treatment for crack cocaine addiction exhibit greater stress responses than male individuals with the same addiction. dmPFC, dorsomedial prefrontal cortex; PoC, postcentral gyrus; daCC, dorsal anterior cingulate cortex; dStr, dorsal striatum; Hi, hippocampus; FG, fusiform gyrus; dlPFC, dorsolateral prefrontal cortex; IFC, inferior frontal cortex; mCC, middle cingulate cortex, pCC, posterior cingulate cortex; Ins, insula.

from their male counterparts in their greater engagement of inhibitory behavioral control processes in response to stress—a neural response in seeming conflict with their presumably greater susceptibility to relapse triggered by stressors. Clearly, more focused and definitive functional neuroimaging studies are needed to define the neurobiology of sex differences in stress-induced relapse in individuals with addictions.

Drug-Induced Relapse

The drug state itself represents another recognized risk factor for relapse to drug-seeking behavior. Several functional neuroimaging studies have localized the neural response to psychostimulants in human drug abusers (Breiter et al., 1997; Risinger et al., 2005). One such study demonstrated that the craving response to passive cocaine administration in a mixed-sex sample of individuals with cocaine addiction was associated with increasing activation of the ventral striatum and parahippocampal gyrus and decreasing activity in the amygdala (Breiter et al., 1997). The craving response to cocaine self-administration in male individuals with cocaine addiction was associated with increasing activation of the ventral anterior cingulate cortex, ventral striatum, cerebellum, and inferior frontal cortex, and with decreasing activity in the superior temporal gyrus, thalamus, and parietal and middle cingulate cortex (Risinger et al., 2005). To date, no such studies have directly compared the neural response related to drug motivational states of men and women addicted to drugs of abuse. Animal models have, however, have provided evidence of sex differences in drug-seeking behavior following noncontingent drug administration. Using the reinstatement animal model of drug relapse, Lynch and Carroll (2000) noted that female rats exhibited a higher rate of drug-seeking behavior following a priming dose of cocaine and that drug self-administration was reinstated at a lower cocaine-priming dose in female compared to male rats.

End-Stage Addiction

The end stage of the addiction process encompasses long-term personal and social costs. The previously mentioned sex differences in functional disabilities, treatment outcomes, and the neurobiology of addiction and relapse support the possibility of sex differences in the long-term consequences of drug addiction with regard to the neurobiological questions. Converging results from multimodal brain imaging approaches comparing male and female individuals with cocaine addiction in the acutely drug-abstinent resting state support significant sex differences in frontal cortical neuropathology. Compared to a within-sex sample of healthy controls, men with cocaine addiction exhibited significantly decreased regional cerebral blood flow (rCBF) in the dorsomedial prefrontal cortex and precentral gyrus, whereas women with cocaine addiction exhibited decreased rCBF in the retrosplenial cortex and no such frontal cortical perfusion deficits (Tucker, Browndyke, Gottschalk, Cofrancesco, & Kosten, 2004). A similar [^{99m}Tc]HMPAO single photon emission computerized tomography (SPECT) imaging study also demonstrated frontal cortical perfusion deficits in male, but not female, subjects with cocaine addiction (Levin et al., 1994). Relative to men, women with cocaine addiction exhibited less evidence of neuronal damage in frontal cortical gray and white matter by *in vivo* magnetic resonance spectroscopy (MRS) (Chang, Ernst, Strickland, & Mehringer, 1999). Whether these sex-specific frontal cortical abnormalities represent trait risk factors or are a consequence of long-term cocaine use is unknown. However, these findings represent a plausible neurobiological mechanism for sexual dimorphism in the global functional impairments related to drug addiction.

GENETIC VARIATION REGULATES THE NEUROBIOLOGY OF THE DRUG ADDICTION PROCESS

This discussion has emphasized the fact that sex differences in the neurobiology of drug abuse and addiction represent the complex contribution of many interactive and individually varying processes. Genetic contributions certainly exist beyond the sex chromosome-linked genes. Genetic variation influences the expression of behavioral characteristics related to stimulus valuation, impulsivity, decision making under risk, stress reactivity, cognitive control, emotionality, and attention, as well as personality traits, drug response, and brain morphology, and thus directly and indirectly influence the drug addiction process (Kreek, Nielson, Butelman, & LaForge, 2005). In recent "imaging genomics" studies, polymorphic variation within autosomal genes has been shown to regulate the neural processing and circuitry representations of complex traits, cognitive processes, and behaviors related to the addiction process (cf. Blasi et al., 2005; Boettiger et al., 2007; Buckholtz, Mattay, Egan, & Weinberger, 2007; Mattay et al., 2003; Passamonti et al., 2006; Yacubian et al., 2007). These complex, multilevel influences of genetic variation on the neurobiology of the addiction process represent an emerging mechanism for the heritability of drug abuse and addiction. It is of note that a polymorphism (*Val158Met*) of the gene encoding catechol-O-methyltransferase (COMT), a variant known to regulate prefrontal cortex function in an allele-dependent manner (Meyer-Lindenberg et al., 2006), is associated with the addiction-relevant personality trait of sensation seeking in women but not men (Lang, Bajbouj, Sander, & Gallinat, 2007). Such sex × COMT genotype interactions support a role for sex-specific genetic determinants of the neurobiology of the drug abuse and addiction process.

IMPLICATIONS FOR PREVENTION AND TREATMENT OF DRUG ADDICTION: FUTURE DIRECTIONS

As alluded to throughout this chapter, the existence of sex differences in familial/social, psychiatric, environmental, and biological factors that underlie the addiction process suggests a need for sex-specific treatment strategies. Here we propose factors to be addressed in the treatment of men and women in either at-risk or addicted populations. Of course, further research would be required to determine the efficacy of such strategies, if implemented.

Early Intervention for At-Risk Populations

The proposed interventions target the intergenerational transmission of drug abuse and addiction. Millions of children in the United States are currently the product of prenatal and postnatal environments characterized by maternal drug abuse and addiction. Children affected by maternal drug addiction confront a high level of developmental risk factors that result in an increased vulnerability to physical, academic, and social/emotional problems (Conners et al., 2004). Early intervention strategies in this at-risk population, in the context of treating mothers with drug addictions, should focus particularly on parenting issues, using methods that have been successful in child maltreatment prevention programs (Peterson, Gable, & Saldana, 1996).

The high rates of childhood abuse and neglect histories in drug-abusing and addicted populations clearly implicate early life trauma as an important risk factor for vulnerability to drug abuse and addiction in adulthood (Dube et al., 2003). Boys and girls differ in the types of childhood maltreatment they experience and in their associated age of onset and severity of drug abuse in adulthood (Hyman et al., 2006). The use of available valid instruments to assess childhood abuse or neglect histories should be a standard component of intake assessments in addiction treatment settings, perhaps particularly for women. As early as possible, females who have been identified as having experienced abuse, neglect, or another form of trauma should receive treatment for their experience with a focus on teaching strategies with which to cope with future stressors.

Addiction Treatment

Current knowledge of sex differences in brain functions related to drug abuse and addiction may be useful in remodeling current substance treatment programs based on the sex of the individual. Men and women with drug addictions differ in the neural representation of drug motivational states provoked by either conditioned drug cues or acute stressors that are associated with relapse. Because women are also more likely to use a drug of abuse in response to stressful situations, stress management and coping techniques may aid relapse prevention in female individuals with drug addictions. The nature of the observed sex differences in the neural response to drug cues suggests that females with addictions may be more responsive to cognitive-behavioral therapy (CBT) approaches that target the extinction of conditioned drug cues by engaging prefrontal cortical processes. Additionally, sex differences in the neural basis of reward processing suggest sex differences in the efficacy of treatment strategies based on incentives such as contingency management or motivational interviewing. Sex differences in brain activity related to inhibitory behavioral control suggest that addiction treatments that target an enabling of the ability to resist the urge to use drugs may differ for each sex. Future substance abuse treatment programs may improve recovery and relapse prevention by incorporating neuroscience findings from sex differences research to develop male-only and female-only treatment groups that utilize sex-specific treatment strategies.

KEY POINTS

- Sex differences in drug addiction are likely due to complex interactions of genes, hormones, and social, developmental, and environmental variables.
- Men and women exhibit structural and functional differences in key brain regions involved in drug addiction.
- A theoretical model of the drug addiction process includes three stages: *acquisition* of the addicted state, *maintenance* as a chronically relapsing state, and the long-term personal and social *consequences* of end-stage drug addiction; sex differences have been observed in all stages of this model.
- Animal model and human neuroimaging studies have identified possible brain mechanisms underlying sex differences in the acquisition of drug abuse and addiction, including dopamine and sex hormone-dependent mechanisms.
- Observations of the neural correlates of drug cue-induced craving suggest that although both sexes exhibit similar neural responses to the incentive motivational properties of drug cues, women engage cortical areas involved in cognitive control that would suppress habit-based cue responses and dampen the drug cue valuation functions of the amygdala.
- The consistent observation that men and women exhibit qualitatively and quantitatively differing affective and neural responses to stressors supports the presence of sex differences in the susceptibility of individuals with drug addictions to stress-induced relapse. Human neuroimaging studies support the idea that female individuals with cocaine addictions differ from their male counterparts in their greater engagement of inhibitory behavioral control processes in response to stress—a neural response in seeming conflict with their presumably greater relapse susceptibility to stressors.
- Animal models of relapse show that females are more susceptible to reinstatement of drug self-administration following a priming dose of the drug.
- Sex differences in functional disabilities, treatment outcomes, and in the neurobiology of addiction and relapse support the possibility of sex differences in the long-term consequences of drug addiction.

REFERENCES

Asterisks denote recommended readings.

Ahmed, S. H., & Koob, G. F. (2005). Transition to drug addiction: A negative reinforcement model based on an allostatic decrease in reward function. *Psychopharmacology, 180*(3), 473–490.

Alexander, G. M., & Peterson, B. S. (2001). Sex steroids and human behavior: Implications for developmental psychopathology. *CNS Spectrums, 6*(1), 75–88. (*)

Aron, A. R., & Poldrack, R. A. (2006). Cortical and subcortical contributions to stop signal response inhibition: Role of the subthalamic nucleus. *Journal of Neuroscience, 26*(9), 2424–2433.

Back, S. E., Brady, K. T., Jackson, J. L., Salstrom, S., & Zinzow, H. (2005). Gender differences in stress reactivity among cocaine-dependent individuals. *Psychopharmacology, 180*, 169–176.

Baler, R. B., & Volkow, N. D. (2006). Drug addiction: The neurobiology of disrupted self-control. *Trends in Molecular Medicine, 12*(12), 559–566.

Becker, J. B., & Hu, M. (2008). Sex differences in drug abuse. *Frontiers in Neuroendocrinology, 29*(1), 36–47.

Becker, J. B., Monteggia, L. M., Perrot-Sinal, T. S., Romeo, R. D., Taylor, J. R., Yehuda, R., et al. (2007). Stress and disease: Is being female a predisposing factor? *Journal of Neuroscience, 27*(44), 11851–11855.

Belcher, S. M., & Zsarnovszky, A. (2001). Estrogenic actions in the brain: Estrogen, phytoestrogens, and rapid intracellular signaling mechanisms. *Journal of Pharmacology and Experimental Therapeutics, 299*, 408–414.

Blasi, G., Mattay, V. S., Bertolino, A., Elvevag, B., Callicott, J. H., Das, S., et al. (2005). Effect of catechol-O-methyltransferase val158met genotype on attentional control. *Journal of Neuroscience, 25*(20), 5038–45.

Boettiger, C. A., Mitchell, J. M., Tavares, V. C., Robertson, M., Joslyn, G., D'Esposito, M., et al. (2007). Immediate reward bias in humans: Fronto-parietal networks and a role for the catechol-O-methyltransferase 158(Val/Val) genotype. *Journal of Neuroscience, 27*, 14383–14391.

Brady, T. K., Kileen, T., Saladin, M. E., Dansky, B. S., & Becker, S. (1994). Comorbid substance abuse and posttraumatic stress disorder: Characteristics of women in treatment. *American Journal on Addictions, 3*, 160–164.

Breiter, H. C., Gollub, R. L., Weisskoff, R. M., Kennedy, D. N., Makris, N., Berke, J. D., et al. (1997). Acute effects of cocaine on human brain activity and emotion. *Neuron, 19*, 591–611.

Brems, C., Johnson, M. E., Neal, D., & Freemon, M. (2004). Child abuse history and substance use among men and women receiving detoxification services. *American Journal of Drug and Alcohol Abuse, 30*(4), 799–821.

Buckholtz, J. W., Meyer-Lindenberg, A., Honea, R. A., Straub, R. E., Pezawas, L., Egan, M. F., et al. (2007). Allelic variation in RGSH impacts functional and structural connectivity in the human brain. *Journal of Neuroscience, 27*(7), 1584–1593.

Burnette, M. L., Lucas, E., Ilgen, M., Frayne, S. M., Mayo, J., & Weitlauf, J. C. (2008). Prevalence and health correlates of prostitution among patients entering treatment for substance use disorders. *Archives of General Psychiatry, 65*(3), 337–344.

Butler, T., Imperato-McGinley, J., Pan, H., Voyer, D., Cunningham-Bussel, A. C., Chang, L., et al. (2007). Sex specificity of ventral anterior cingulate cortex suppression during a cognitive task. *Human Brain Mapping, 28*, 1206–1212.

Cahill, L. (2003). Sex-related influences on the neurobiology of emotionally influenced memory. *Annals of the New York Academy of Sciences, 985*, 163–173.

Cahill, L. (2006). Why sex matters for neuroscience. *Nature Reviews Neuroscience, 7*, 477–484. (*)

Cahill, L., Uncapher, M., Kilpatrick, L., Alkire, M. T., & Turner, J. (2004). Sex-related hemispheric lateralization of amygdala function in emotionally influenced memory: An fMRI investigation. *Learning & Memory, 11*, 261–265.

Carroll, K. M., & Onken, L. S. (2005). Behavioral therapies for drug abuse. *American Journal of Psychiatry, 162*(8), 1452–1460.

Carroll, M. E., Lynch, W. J., Roth, M. E., Morgan, A. D., & Cosgrove, K. P. (2004). Sex and estrogen influence drug abuse. *Trends in Pharmacological Sciences, 25*(5), 273–279.

Chang, L., Ernst, T., Strickland, T., & Mehringer, C. M. (1999). Gender effects on persistent cerebral metabolite changes in the frontal lobes of abstinent cocaine users, *American Journal of Psychiatry, 156*, 716–722.

Chen, X., Sachdev, P. S., Wen, W., & Anstey, K. J. (2007). Sex differences in regional gray matter in healthy individuals aged 44–48 years: A voxel-based morphometric study. *NeuroImage, 36*, 691–699.

Childress, A. R., Mozley, P. D., McElgin, W., Fitzgerald, J., Reivich, M., & O'Brien, C. P. (1999). Limbic activation during cue-induced cocaine craving. *American Journal of Psychiatry, 156*(1), 11–18.

Conners, N. A., Bradley, R. H., Mansell, L. W., Liu, J. Y., Roberts, T. J., Burgdorf, K., et al. (2004). Children of mothers with serious substance abuse problems: An accumulation of risks. *American Journal of Drug and Alcohol Abuse, 30*(1), 85–100.

Cooke, B. M., & Woolley, C. S. (2005). Gonadal hormone dependent structural plasticity of dendrites in the mammalian CNS. *Journal of Neurobiology, 64*, 34–46.

Davies, W., & Wilkinson, L. S. (2006). It is not all hormones: Alternative explanations for sexual differentiation of the brain. *Brain Research, 1126*, 36–45. (*)

De Bellis, M. D., Keshavan, M. S., Beers, S. R., Hall, J., Frustaci, K., Masalehdan, A., et al. (2001). Sex differences in brain maturation during childhood and adolescence. *Cerebral Cortex, 11*(6), 552–557.

Dreher, J.-C., Schmidt, P. J., Kohn, P., Furman, D., Rubinow, D., & Berman, K. F. (2007). Menstrual cycle phase modulates reward-related neural function in women. *Proceedings of the National Academy of Sciences USA, 104*(7), 2465–2470.

Dube, S. R., Felitti, V. J., Dong, M., Chapman, D. P., Giles, W. H., & Anda, R. F. (2003). Childhood abuse, neglect, and household dysfunction and the risk of illicit drug use: The Adverse Childhood Experiences Study. *Pediatrics, 111*(3), 564–572.

Dunn, G. E., Ryan, J. J., & Dunn, C. E. (1994). Trauma symptoms in substance abusers with and without histories of childhood abuse. *Journal of Psychoactive Drugs, 26*, 357–360.

El-Bassel, N., Simoni, J. M., Cooper, D. K., Gilbert, L., & Schilling, R. F. (2001). Sex trading and psychological distress among women on methadone. *Psychology of Addictive Behaviors, 15*(3), 177–184.

El-Bassel, N., & Witte, S. (2001). Drug use and physical and sexual abuse of street sex workers in New York City. *Research for Sex Work, 4*, 31–32.

Evans, S. M., Haney, M., & Foltin, R. (2002). The effects of smoked cocaine during the follicular and luteal phases of the menstrual cycle in women. *Psychopharmacology (Berl), 159*, 397–406.

Everitt, B. J., & Robbins, T. W. (2005). Neural systems of reinforcement for drug addiction: From actions to habits to compulsion. *Nature Neuroscience, 8*, 1481–1489.

Fattore, L., Spano, M. S., Altea, S., Angius, F., & Fadda, P. (2007). Cannabinoid self-administration in rats: Sex differences and the influence of ovarian function. *British Journal of Pharmacology, 152*(5), 795–804.

Fox, H. C., Garcia, M., Jr., Kemp, K., Millivojevic, V., Kreek, M. J., & Sinha, R. (2006). Gender differences in cardiovascular and corticoadrenal response to stress and drug cues in cocaine dependent individuals. *Psychopharmacology, 185*, 348–357.

Franzek, E. J., Spranger, N., Janssens, A. C. J. W., Van Duijn, C. M., & Van De Wetering, B. J. M. (2008). Prenatal exposure to the 1944–45 Dutch "hunger winter" and addiction later in life. *Addiction, 103*, 433–438.

Frederiske, M. E., Lu, A., Aylward, E., Barta, P., & Pearlson, G. (1999). Sex differences in the inferior parietal lobule. *Cerebral Cortex, 9*, 896–901.

Fullilove, M. T., Fullilove, R. E., Smith, M., & Winkler, K. (1993). Violence, trauma, and post-traumatic stress disorder among women drug users. *Journal of Traumatic Stress, 6*, 533–543.

Giedd, J. N., Blumenthal, J., Jeffries, N. O., Castellanos, F. X., Liu, H., Zijdenbos, A., et al. (1999). Brain development during childhood and adolescence: A longitudinal MRI study. *Nature Neuroscience, 2*, 861–863.

Giedd, J. N., Castellanos, F. X., Rajapakse, J. C., Vaituzis, A. C., & Rapoport, J. L. (1997). Sexual dimorphism of the developing human brain. *Progress in Neuro-Psychopharmacology & Biological Psychiatry, 21*, 1185–1201.

Goldstein, J. M., Seidman, L. J., Horton, N. J., Makris, N., Kennedy, D. N., Caviness, V. S., Jr., et al. (2001). Normal sexual dimorphism of the adult human brain assessed by in vivo magnetic resonance imaging. *Cerebral Cortex, 11*, 490–497.

Goldstein, R. Z., Volkow, N. D., Wang, G. J., Fowler, J. S., & Rajaram, S. (2001). Addiction changes orbitofrontal gyrus function: Involvement in response inhibition. *NeuroReport, 12*, 2595–2599.

Good, C. D., Johnsrude, I., Ashburner, J., Henson, R. N., Friston, K. J., & Frackowiak, R. S. (2001). Cerebral asymmetry and the effects of sex and handedness on brain structure: A voxel-based morphometric analysis of 465 normal adult human brains. *Neuroimage, 14*(3), 685–700.

Grant, S., London, E. D., Newlin, D. B., Villemagne, V. L., Liu, X., Contoreggi, C., et al. (1996). Activation of memory circuits during cue-elicited cocaine craving. *Proceedings of the National Academy of Sciences USA, 93*(21), 12040–12045.

Gur, R. C., Gunning-Dixon, F., Bilker, W. B., & Gur, R. E. (2002). Sex differences in temporo-limbic and frontal brain volumes of healthy adults. *Cerebral Cortex, 12*, 998–1003.

Gur, R. C., Turetsky, B. I., Matsui, M., Yan, M., Bilker, W., Hughett, P., et al. (1999). Sex differences in brain gray and white matter in healthy young adults: Correlations with cognitive performance. *Journal of Neuroscience, 19*(10), 4065–4072.

Hanlon, H., Thatcher, R., & Cline, M. (1999). Gender differences in the development of EEG coherence in normal children. *Developmental Neuropsychology, 16*(3), 479–506.

Heim, C., Newport, D. J., Heit, S., Graham, Y. P., Wilcox, M., Bonsall, R., et al. (2000). *Journal of the American Medical Association, 284*(5), 635–636.

Holdcraft, L. C., & Iacono, W. G. (2004). Cross-generational effects on gender differences in psychoactive drug abuse and dependence. *Drug and Alcohol Dependence, 74*, 147–158.

Holden, C. (2005). Sex and the suffering brain. *Science, 308*(5728), 1574.

Hope, V. D., Hickman, M., & Tilling, K. (2005). Capturing crack cocaine use: Estimating the prevalence of crack cocaine use in London using capture-recapture with covariates. *Addiction, 100*(11), 1701–1708.

Hser, Y. I., Evans, E., & Huang, Y. C. (2005). Treatment outcomes among women and men methamphetamine abusers in California. *Journal of Substance Abuse Treatment, 28*(1), 77–85.

Hsu, J.-L., Leemans, A., Bai C.-H., Lee, C.-H., Tsai, Y.-F., Chiu, H.-C., et al. (2008). Gender differences and age-related white matter changes of the human brain: A diffusion tensor imaging study. *Neuroimage, 39*, 566–577.

Hu, M., Crombag, H. S., Robinson, T. E., & Becker, J. B. (2004). Biological basis of sex differences in the propensity to self-administer cocaine, *Neuropsychopharmacology, 29*, 81–85.

Hughes, J., Helzer, J., & Lindberg, S. (2006). Prevalence of DSM/ICD-defined nicotine dependence. *Drug and Alcohol Dependence, 85*(2), 91–102.

Hyman, S. M., Garcia, M., & Sinha, R. (2006). Gender specific associations between types of childhood maltreatment and the onset, escalation and severity of substance use in cocaine dependent adults. *American Journal of Drug and Alcohol Abuse, 32*, 655–664.

Hyman, S. M., Paliwal, P., Chaplin, T. M., Mazure, C. M., Rounsaville, B. J., & Sinha, R. (2008). Severity of childhood trauma is predictive of cocaine relapse outcomes in women but not men. *Drug and Alcohol Dependence, 92*(1–3), 208–216.

Jager, G., de Win, M. M., van der Tweel, I., Schilt, T., Kahn, R. S., van den Brink, W., et al. (2008). Assessment of cognitive brain function in ecstasy users and contributions of other drugs of abuse: Results from an fMRI study. *Neuropsychopharmacology, 33*(2), 247–58.

Justice, J., & de Wit, H. (1999). Acute effects of d-amphetamine during the follicular and luteal phases of the menstrual cycle in women. *Psychopharmacology, 145*, 67–75.

Kalivas, P. W., & Volkow, N. D. (2005). The neural basis of addiction: A pathology of motivation and choice. *American Journal of Psychiatry, 162*(8), 1403–1413.

Kandel, D., Hu, M., Griesler, P., & Schaffran, C. (2007). On the development of nicotine dependence in adolescence. *Drug and Alcohol Dependence, 91*(1), 26–39.

Kaufman, J. N., Ross, T. J., Stein, E. A., & Garavan, H. (2003). Cingulate hypoactivity in cocaine users during a GO-NOGO task as revealed by event-related fMRI. *Journal of Neuroscience, 23,* 7839–7843.

Kelly, M. M., Tyrka, A. R., Anderson, G. M., Price, L. H., & Carpenter, L. L. (2008). Sex differences in emotional and physiological responses to the Trier social stress test. *Journal of Behavior Therapy and Experimental Psychiatry, 39,* 87–98.

Khurana, R. C., & Devaud, L. L. (2007). Sex differences in neurotransmission parameters in response to repeated mild restraint stress exposures in intact male, female and ovariectomised female rats. *Journal of Neuroendocrinology, 19*(7), 511–520.

Kilgore, W., & Yurgelun-Todd, D. (2001). Sex differences in amygdala activation during the perception of facial affect. *NeuroReport, 12,* 2543–2547.

Kilpatrick, L. A., Zaid, D. H., Pardo, J. V., & Cahill, L. F. (2006). Sex-related differences in amygdala functional connectivity during resting conditions. *Neuroimage, 30,* 452–461.

Kilts, C. D., Gross, R. E., Ely, T. D., & Drexler, K. P. G. (2004). The neural correlates of cue-induced craving in cocaine-dependent women. *American Journal of Psychiatry, 161*(2), 233–241.

Kilts, C. D., Schweitzer, J. B., Quinn, C. K., Gross, R. E., Faber, T. L., Muhammad, F., et al. (2001). Neural activity related to drug carving in cocaine addiction. *Archives of General Psychiatry, 58,* 334–341.

Kimura, D. (2002). Sex hormones influence human cognitive pattern. *Neuroendocrinology Letters, 23,* 67–77. (*)

Koob, G., & Kreek, M. J. (2007). Stress, dysregulation of drug reward pathways, and the transition to drug dependence. *American Journal of Psychiatry, 164,* 1149–1159.

Kreek, M. J., Nielson, D. A., Butelman, E. R., & LaForge, K. S. (2005). Genetic influences on impulsivity, risk taking, stress responsivity and vulnerability to drug abuse and addiction. *Nature Neuroscience, 8*(11), 1450–1457.

Kruggel, F. (2006). MRI-based volumetry of head compartments: Normative values of healthy adults. *Neuroimage, 30,* 1–11.

Lang, U. E., Bajbouj, M., Sander, T., & Gallinat, J. (2007). Gender-dependent association of the functional catechol-o-methyltransferase Val158Met genotype with sensation seeking personality trait. *Neuropsychopharmacology, 32,* 1950–1955.

Levin, J. M., Holman, B. L., Mendelson, T. H., Teoh, S. K., Garada, B., Johnson, K. A., et al. (1994). Gender differences in cerebral perfusion in cocaine abuse: Technetium-99m-HMPAO SPECT study of drug using women. *Journal of Nuclear Medicine, 35,* 1902–1909.

Levine, S. N. (1966). Sex differences in the brain. *Scientific American, 214*(4), 84–90.

Li, C.-S. R., Huang, C., Constable, R. T., & Sinha, R. (2006). Gender differences in the neural correlates of response inhibition during a stop signal task. *Neuroimage, 32,* 1918–1929.

Li, C.-S. R., Kosten, T. R., & Sinha, R. (2005). Sex differences in brain activation during stress imagery in abstinent cocaine users: A functional magnetic resonance imaging study. *Biological Psychiatry, 57,* 487–494. (*)

Liu, N., Li, B., Wilson, F. A., Ma, Y., & Hu, X. (2005). Gender effect on the right-left discrimination task in a sample of heroin-dependent patients. *Psychopharmacology, 181,* 735–740.

Luders, E., Narr, K. L., Thompson, P. M., Rex, D. E., Jancke, L., Steinmetz, H., et al. (2004). Gender differences in cortical complexity. *Nature Neuroscience, 7*(8), 799–800.

Luders, E., Steinmetz, H., & Jancke, L. (2002). Brain size and grey matter volume in the healthy human brain. *Neuroreport, 13,* 2371–2374.

Lynch, W. J., & Carroll, M. E. (1999). Sex differences in the acquisition of intravenously self-administered cocaine and heroin in rats. *Psychopharmacology, 144,* 77–82.

Lynch, W. J., & Carroll, M. E. (2000). Reinstatement of cocaine self-administration in rats: Sex differences. *Psychopharmacology, 148,* 196–200.

Lynch, W. J., Roth, M. E., & Carroll, M. E. (2002). Biological basis of sex differences in drug abuse: Preclinical and clinical studies. *Psychopharmacology, 164,* 121–137. (*)

Maller, J. J., Reglade-Meslin, C., Anstey, A. J., & Sachdev, P. (2006). Sex and symmetry differences hippocampal volumetrics: Before and beyond the opening of the crus of the fornix. *Hippocampus, 16,* 80–90.

Marsh, J., Cao, D., & D'Aunno, T. (2004). Gender differences in the impact of comprehensive services in substance abuse treatment. *Journal of Substance Abuse Treatment*, 27(4), 289–300.

Martin-Fardon, R., Ciccocioppo, R., Aujla, H., & Weiss, F. (2008). The dorsal subiculum mediates the acquisition of conditioned reinstatement of cocaine-seeking. *Neuropsychopharmacology*, 33(8), 1827–1834.

Mattay, V. S., Goldberg, T. E., Fera, F., Hariri, A. R., Tessitore, A., Egan, M. F., et al. (2003). Catechol O-methyltransferase val158-met genotype and individual variation in the brain response to amphetamine. *Proceedings of the National Academy of Sciences USA*, 100(10), 6186–6191.

McEwen, B. S., & Alves, S. E. (1999). Estrogen actions in the central nervous system. *Endocrine Reviews*, 20, 279–307.

McKay, J. R., Rutherford, M. J., Cacciola, J. S., Kabasakalian-McKay, R., & Alterman, A. I. (1996). Gender differences in the relapse experience of cocaine patients. *Journal of Nervous and Mental Disease*, 184, 616–622.

Mechelli, A., Friston, K. J., Frackowiak, R. S., & Price, C. J. (2005). Structural covariance in the human cortex. *Journal of Neuroscience*, 25(36), 8303–8310.

Medrano, M. A., Hatch, J. P., Zule, W. A., & Desmond, D. P. (2003). Childhood trauma and adult prostitution behavior in a multiethnic heterosexual drug-using population. *American Journal of Drug & Alcohol Abuse*, 29, 463–486.

Medrano, M. A., Zule, W. A., Hatch, J., & Desmond, D.P . (1999). Prevalence of childhood trauma in a community sample of substance-abusing women. *American Journal of Drug and Alcohol Abuse*, 25(3), 449–462.

Mello, N. K., Knudson, I. M., & Mendelson, J. H. (2007). Sex and menstrual cycle effects on progressive ratio measures of cocaine self-administration in cynomolgus monkeys. *Neuropsychopharmacology*, 32, 1956–1966.

Meyer-Lindenberg, A., Nichols, T., Callicott, J. H., Ding, J., Kolachana, B., Buckholtz, J., et al. (2006). Impact of complex genetic variation in COMT on human brain function. *Molecular Psychiatry*, 11, 867–877.

Milad, M. R., Goldstein, J. M., Orr, S. P., Wedig, M. M., Klibanski, A., Pitman, R. K., et al. (2006). Fear conditioning and extinction: Influence of sex and menstrual cycle in healthy humans. *Behavioral Neuroscience*, 120(6), 1196–1203.

Milad, M. R., Wright, C. I., Orr, S. P., Pitman, R. K., Quirk, G. J., & Rauch, S. L. (2007). Recall of fear extinction in humans activates the ventromedial prefrontal cortex and hippocampus in concert. *Biological Psychiatry*, 62, 446–454.

Munro, C. A., McCaul, M. E., Wong, D. F., Oswald, L. M., Zhou, Y., Brasic, J., et al. (2006). Sex differences in striatal dopamine release in healthy adults. *Biological Psychiatry*, 59, 966–974.

Niaura, R., Shadel, W. G., Abrams, D. B., Monti, P. M., Rohsenow, D. J., & Sirota, A. (1998). Individual differences in cue reactivity among smokers trying to quit: Effect of gender and cue type. *Addictive Behaviors*, 23, 209–224.

Nuttbrock, L. A., Rosenblum, A., Magura, S., Villano, C., & Wallace, J. (2004). Linking female sex workers with substance abuse treatment. *Journal of Substance Abuse Treatment*, 27, 233–239.

Passamonti, L., Fera, F., Magariello, A., Cerasa, A., Gioia, M. C., Muglia, M., et al. (2006). Monoamine oxidase—A genetic variations influence brain activity associated with inhibitory control: New insight into the neural correlates of impulsivity. *Biological Psychiatry*, 59, 334–340.

Peterson, L., Gable, S., & Saldana, L. (1996). Treatment of Maternal addiction to prevent child abuse and neglect. *Addictive Behaviors*, 21(6), 789–801.

Pirard, S., Sharon, E., Kang, S. K., Angarita, G. A., & Gastfriend, D. R. (2005). Prevalence of physical and sexual abuse among substance abuse patients and impact on treatment outcomes. *Drug and Alcohol Dependence*, 78(1), 57–64.

Protopopescu, X., Pan, H., Altemus, M., Tuescher, O., Polanecsky, M., McEwen, B., et al. (2005). Orbitofrontal cortex activity related to emotional processing changes across the menstrual cycle. *Proceedings of the National Academy of Sciences USA*, 102(44), 16060–16065.

Proverbio, A. M., Brignone, V., Matarazzo, S., Del Zotto, M., & Zani, A. (2006). Gender differences in hemispheric asymmetry for face processing. *BMC Neuroscience*, 7, 44.

Quinn, J. J., Hitchcott, P. K., Umeda, E. A., Arnold, A. P., & Taylor, J. R. (2007). Sex chromosome complement regulates habit formation. *Nature Neuroscience, 10*(11), 1398–1400.

Quirk, G. J., & Mueller, D. (2008). Neural mechanisms of extinction learning and retrieval. *Neuropsychopharmacology Reviews, 33,* 56–72.

Rahman, Q., & Clarke, C. D. (2005). Sex differences in neurocognitive functioning among abstinent recreational cocaine users. *Psychopharmacology, 181,* 374–380.

Risinger, R. C., Salmeron, B. J., Ross, T. J., Amen, S. L., Sanfilipo, M., Hoffmann, R. G., et al. (2005). Neural correlates of high and craving during cocaine self-administration using BOLD fMRI. *Neuroimage, 26,* 1097–1108.

Robbins, S. J., Ehrman, R. N., Childress, A. R., & O'Brien, C. P. (1999). Comparing levels of cocaine cue reactivity in male and female outpatients. *Drug and Alcohol Dependence, 53*(3), 223–230.

Robinson, T. E., & Berridge, K. C. (2000). The psychology and neurobiology of addiction: An incentive-sensitization view. *Addiction, 95*(8 Suppl. 2), 91–117.

Roxburgh, A., Degenhardt, L., & Copeland, J. (2006). Posttraumatic stress disorder among female street-based sex workers in the Greater Sydney Area, Australia. *BMC Psychiatry, 6,* 24.

Rubonis, A. V., Colby, S. M., Monti, P. M., Rohsenow, D. J., Gulliver, S. B., & Sirota, A. D. (1994). Alcohol cue reactivity and mood induction in male and female alcoholics. *Journal of Studies on Alcohol, 55,* 487–494.

Sakai, Y., Nishikawa, M., Leyton, M., Benkelfat, C., Young, S. N., & Diksic, M. (2006). Cortical trapping of a-[^{11}C]methyl-L-tryptophan, an index of serotonin synthesis, is lower in females than males. *Neuroimage, 33,* 815–824.

Shah, N. M., Pisapia, J., Maniatis, S., Mendelsohn, M. M., Nemes, A., & Axel, R. (2004). Visualizing sexual dimorphism in the brain. *Neuron, 43,* 313–319.

Shalev, U., Grimm, J. W., & Shaham, Y. (2002). Neurobiology of relapse to heroin and cocaine seeking: A review. *Pharmacological Reviews, 54,* 1–42.

Sinha, R., Lacadie, C., Skudlarski, P., Fulbright, R. K., Rounsaville, B. J., Kosten, T. R., et al. (2005). Neural activity associated with stress-induced cocaine craving: A functional magnetic resonance imaging study. *Psychopharmacology, 183,* 171–180.

Stewart, M. E. (1994). Adolescents in a therapeutic community: Treatment implications for teen survivors of traumatic experiences. *Journal of Psychoactive Drugs, 26,* 409–419.

Sun, W., & Rebec, G. V. (2003). Lidocaine inactivation of ventral subiculum attenuates cocaine-seeking behavior in rats. *Journal of Neuroscience, 23,* 10258–10264.

Swan, N. (1998). Exploring the role of child abuse on later drug abuse: Researchers face broad gaps in information. *NIDA Notes, 13*(2).

Tabibnia, G., Cooke, B. M., & Breedlove, S. M. (1999). Sex difference and laterality in the volume of mouse dentate gyrus granule cell layer. *Brain Research, 827,* 41–45.

Tapert, S. F., Brown, G. G., Baratta, M. V., & Brown, S. A. (2004). fMRI BOLD response to alcohol stimuli in alcohol dependent young women. *Addictive Behaviors, 29*(1), 33–50.

Tucker, K. A., Browndyke, J. N., Gottschalk, P. C., Cofrancesco, A. T., & Kosten, T. R. (2004). Gender-specific vulnerability for rCBF abnormalities among cocaine abusers. *Neuroreport, 15*(5), 797–801. (*)

Wang, J. J., Korczykowski, M., Roa, H. Y., Fan, Y., Pluta, J., Gur, R. C., et al. (2007). Gender difference in neural response to psychological stress. *Social Cognitive and Affective Neuroscience, 2*(3), 227–239.

Whealin, J. (n.d.). *Men and sexual trauma: A National Center for PTSD fact sheet.* Retrieved July 30, 2008, from *www.ncptsd.va.gov/ncmain/ncdocs/fact_shts/fs_male_sexual_assault.html.*

Widom, C. S., Weiler, B. L., & Cottler, L. B. (1999). Childhood victimization and drug abuse: A comparison of prospective and retrospective findings. *Journal of Consulting and Clinical Psychology, 67*(6), 867–880.

Williams, L. M., Barton, M. J., Kemp, A. H., Liddell, B. J., Peduto, A., Gordon, E., et al. (2005). Distinct amygdala-autonomic arousal profiles in response to fear signals in healthy males and females. *Neuroimage, 28,* 618–626.

Witelson, D. F. (1976). Sex and the single hemisphere: Specialization of the right hemisphere for spatial processing. *Science, 193*(4251), 425–427.

Woicik, P. A., Moeller, S. J., Alia-Klein, N., Maloney, T., Lukasik, T. M., Yeliosof, O., et al. (2008). The neuropsychology of cocaine addiction: Recent cocaine use masks impairment. *Neuropsychopharmacology*. Advance online publication 21 May 2008; doi:10.1038/npp.2008 60.

Yacubian, J., Sommer, T., Schroeder, K., Glascher, J., Kalisch, R., Leuenberger, B., et al. (2007). Gene-gene interaction associated with neural reward sensitivity. *Proceedings of the National Academy of Sciences USA, 104*, 8125–8130.

Yu, J., Zhang, S., Epstein, D. H., Fang, Y., Shi, J., Qin, H., et al. (2007). Gender and stimulus difference in cue-induced responses in abstinent heroin users. *Pharmacology, Biochemistry and Behavior, 86*, 485–492.

Yücel, M., Stuart, G. W., Maruff, P., Velakoulis, D., Crowe, S. F., Savage, G., et al. (2001). Hemispheric and gender-related differences in the gross morphology of the anterior cingulated/paracingulate cortex in normal volunteers: An MRI morphometric study. *Cerebral Cortex, 11*, 17–25.

PART III

CO-OCCURRING PSYCHIATRIC DISORDERS

Comorbidity of Substance Use Disorders with Independent Mood and Anxiety Disorders in Women

Results from the National Epidemiologic Survey on Alcohol and Related Conditions

Risë B. Goldstein, PhD, MPH

Substance use, mood, and anxiety disorders are common in adults and associated with considerable economic and psychosocial burdens on affected individuals, their families, and society (Grant et al., 2004; Kessler et al., 1994; Robins, Locke, & Regier, 1991). Moreover, high comorbidity of substance use disorders (SUDs) with mood and anxiety disorders has been well documented in both clinical (Abbott, Weller, & Walker, 1994; Compton et al., 2000; De Wilde, Broekaert, Rosseel, Delespaul, & Soyez, 2007; Magura, Kang, Rosenblum, Handelsman, & Foote, 1998; McCance-Katz, Carroll, & Rounsaville, 1999; Ross, Glaser, & Germanson, 1988; Rounsaville, Weissman, Kleber, & Wilber, 1982; Tómasson & Vaglum, 1998) and epidemiologic (Anthony & Helzer, 1991; Compton, Thomas, Stinson, & Grant, 2007; Conway, Compton, Stinson, & Grant, 2006; Hasin, Stinson, Ogburn, & Grant, 2007; Helzer, Burnam, & McEvoy, 1991; Kessler et al., 1997; Merikangas et al., 1996) samples.

In SUD treatment settings, with men and women considered together, studies conducted over the past 25 years reported lifetime prevalences of mood disorders ranging from 17.7 to 53.9% for major depression, 0.4 to 30.0% for bipolar disorders, and 1.0 to 15.3% for dysthymia. Rates of anxiety disorders ranged from 0.1 to 32.1% for generalized anxiety disorder, 2.7 to 20.4% for social phobia, 1.3 to 19.4% for panic disorder, and 3.5 to 7.0% for simple or specific phobia (Abbott et al., 1994; Brooner, King, Kidorf, Schmidt, & Bigelow, 1997; De Wilde et al., 2007; Magura et al., 1998; Ross et al., 1988; Rounsaville et al., 1982; Rounsaville et al., 1991).

Studies that examined sex-specific lifetime comorbidity with SUDs in addiction treatment settings have found patterns compatible with the sex differences in prevalences of non-SUDs observed in the general population (Brooner et al., 1997; Compton et al., 2000; De Wilde et al., 2007; Griffin, Weiss, Mirin, & Lange, 1989; Hesselbrock, Meyer, & Keener, 1985; Magura et al., 1998; Mann, Hintz, & Jung, 2004; McCance-Katz et al., 1999; Ross,

Glaser, & Stiasny, 1988; Rounsaville et al., 1982, 1991; Tómasson & Vaglum, 1998), though the actual rates were higher. Whether the observed differences were statistically significant or not, women were more likely than men to meet criteria for major depression (19.1 to 69.2% vs. 8.7 to 48.9%), phobias (2.9 to 42.2% vs. 1.9 to 33.7%), dysthymia (4.4 to 21.8% vs. 2.4 to 13.7%), and panic disorder (1.8 to 21.7% vs. 0.5 to 18.4%). With regard to bipolar and generalized anxiety disorders, some of these studies showed no sex differences and others found female excesses.

Studies of lifetime comorbidity of SUDs with mood and anxiety disorders in the general population, based on the Epidemiologic Catchment Area (ECA), the National Comorbidity Survey (NCS), and the National Epidemiologic Survey on Alcohol and Related Conditions (NESARC), show patterns broadly similar to those observed in clinical samples. When men and women with any drug use disorder were considered together, rates ranged from 19.6 to 33.2% for major depression, 5.5 to 12.0% for bipolar disorders, and 10.0 to 11.4% for dysthymia. Rates of anxiety disorders ranged from 10.7 to 22.9% for phobias and 4.2 to 9.0% for panic disorder (Agosti, Nunes, & Levin, 2002; Anthony & Helzer, 1991; Conway et al., 2006). Only Conway et al. (2006) reported a prevalence rate (9.2%) for generalized anxiety disorder. Most studies have reported odds ratios (ORs) measuring associations between SUDs and other psychiatric disorders, or ratios of prevalences in respondents with versus without SUDs, rather than, or in addition to, prevalences. ORs for associations with any lifetime drug use disorder ranged from 3.0 to 5.8 for bipolar disorders, 2.2 to 5.6 for major depression, 2.8 to 4.6 for panic disorder, and 2.2 to 2.7 for phobias (Conway et al., 2006; Merikangas et al., 1996); only Conway et al. (2006) reported ORs for dysthymia (3.6) and generalized anxiety disorder (2.7). ORs (either unadjusted, or adjusted for sociodemographic characteristics) measuring associations with any alcohol use disorder ranged from 2.6 to 6.8 for bipolar disorders, 1.9 to 4.7 for dysthymia, 1.0 to 3.8 for panic disorder, 2.1 to 3.4 for social phobia, 1.1 to 3.4 for major depressive disorder, 1.6 to 2.3 for simple or specific phobia, and 2.1 to 2.2 for generalized anxiety disorder (Hasin et al., 2007; Kessler et al., 1996; Merikangas et al., 1996; Swendsen et al., 1998). Prevalence ratios reported by Helzer et al. (1991) for alcohol abuse and dependence considered together, and Anthony and Helzer (1991) for drug abuse and dependence considered together, from the ECA followed similar patterns. When ORs were examined separately for dependence versus abuse, they were generally larger in association with dependence than with abuse.

In studies based on the NCS and the NESARC reporting sex-specific comorbidity as prevalence rates (Conway et al., 2006; Kessler et al., 1997), consistent with what has been observed in treatment settings and in the general population without SUDs, lifetime rates of mood disorders among individuals with SUDs were higher among women: 30.1 to 48.5% versus 9.0 to 30.1% for major depression; 10.1 to 20.9% versus 3.6 to 11.2% for dysthymia, and 3.8 to 6.8% versus 0.3 to 3.8% for bipolar disorders. Rates of anxiety disorders were also higher among women: 28.2 to 30.7% versus 5.9 to 13.9% for simple or specific phobia, 24.1 to 30.3% versus 10.8 to 19.3% for social phobia; 8.4 to 15.7% versus 2.6 to 8.6% for generalized anxiety disorder; and 7.3 to 12.0% versus 1.6 to 3.6% for panic disorder. ORs from the NCS and the NESARC for mood disorders ranged from 2.3 to 6.7 among women versus 0.3 to 6.2 among men; for bipolar disorders; 1.3 to 4.2 versus 0.7 to 4.1 for dysthymia; and 1.7 to 4.1 versus 0.7 to 3.4 for major depression. For anxiety disorders, the ORs from the NCS and the NESARC ranged from 1.0 to 4.9 versus 0.8 to 6.8 for panic disorder; 1.3 to 3.1 versus 2.6 to 8.6 for generalized anxiety disorder; 1.8 to 2.9 versus 1.0 to 2.9 for social phobia; and 2.2 to 2.6 versus 0.9 to 3.1 for simple or specific phobia. Within studies, ORs did not generally differ significantly by sex, except that Kessler et al. (1997) reported significantly larger ORs among women than men for most mood and anxiety disorders with alcohol abuse. Prevalence ratios reported by Helzer et al. (1991) and Anthony and Helzer (1991) for alcohol and drug use disorders, respectively, based on the ECA survey, followed similar patterns.

The meaning and implications of lifetime comorbidity of SUDs with mood and anxiety disorders have not yet been fully resolved, in part because of differences among diagnostic systems and among studies in the definition and assessment of "primary" or "independent" versus "substance-induced" disorders (Grant et al., 2004; Hasin & Grant, 2002; Kadden, Kranzler, & Rounsaville, 1995; Nunes & Rounsaville, 2006; Raimo & Schuckit, 1998; Schuckit, Tipp, Bergman, et al., 1997; Schuckit, Tipp, Bucholz, et al., 1997). Recent general population studies (Grant et al., 2004; Hasin & Grant, 2002) showed that intoxication and withdrawal effects do not fully explain the comorbidity. Further, when rigorously defined according to the criteria set forth in the fourth edition of the *Diagnostic and Statistical Manual of Mental Disorders* (DSM-IV; American Psychiatric Association, 2000), substance-induced mood and anxiety disorders account for only a small proportion of total prevalence in the general population (Grant et al., 2004). Nevertheless, current comorbidity carries much clearer clinical and public health implications. In addition, assessment of the independence of comorbid disorders from substance use and SUDs is more straightforward because there is no need to rely on retrospective reports of chronological sequences of substance use, abuse, or dependence, versus mood or anxiety symptomatology, that may have occurred long in the past (Grant et al., 2004).

It has only recently been demonstrated (Compton et al., 2007; Hasin et al., 2007) that the considerable comorbidity of specific SUDs with other specific disorders is largely driven by high rates of co-occurrence among other disorders. That is, after adjustment for comorbidity among other disorders, the unique associations of specific SUDs with specific comorbid conditions are more modest than those observed in bivariate analyses or when only sociodemographic characteristics are controlled. Overall prevalences of comorbid conditions provide important evidence to inform clinical practice and public health approaches to case finding. However, unique associations between specific pairs of disorders are also important because they may yield essential clues to the etiology of the index disorder (e.g., drug dependence), the comorbid disorder (e.g., bipolar I disorder), or the co-occurrence of the two. Although both etiological factors and implications of comorbidity may differ between women and men, sex-specific data on unique comorbid associations of SUDs with other specific disorders are not yet available.

Previous general population studies have documented that most individuals with current substance use, mood, or anxiety disorders do not seek treatment or help within a given year (Compton et al., 2007; Grant et al., 2004; Hasin et al., 2007; Kessler, Olfson, & Berglund, 1998; Robins, Locke, & Regier, 1991). Consistent with patterns observed in general medical settings (Weisman, 1994), women seek mental health treatment for mood and anxiety disorders more often than men (Robins et al., 1991; Wang et al., 2005). However, evidence concerning treatment and help seeking for SUDs includes higher utilization by men (Cohen, Feinn, Arias, & Kranzler, 2007; Weisner, Greenfield, & Room, 1995), higher utilization by women (Teesson, Baillie, Lynskey, Manor, & Degenhardt, 2006), and no sex differences (Kessler et al., 2001). In mixed-sex samples individuals with comorbid disorders were more likely to utilize treatment than those with pure disorders (Cohen et al., 2007; Grant et al., 2004; Jacobi et al., 2004; Kessler et al., 1996). However, sex-specific patterns of treatment and help seeking for pure versus comorbid current substance use, mood, and anxiety disorders have not been investigated.

Because of the greater prevalence of SUDs in men, and the larger numbers of men in addiction treatment, the unique features of these disorders and their comorbidity in women have received limited attention in mixed-sex samples. To date, no study has focused specifi-cally on current substance use, mood, and anxiety disorders, their co-occurrences and unique comorbid associations, and associated treatment and help seeking in a large, nationally rep-resentative general population sample of women.

Accordingly, the present report describes 12-month prevalences, comorbidity, and treat-ment utilization for substance use, mood, or anxiety disorders among women in the Wave 1 NESARC (n = 24,575; Grant et al., 2004; Grant, Kaplan, Shepard, & Moore, 2003). With the largest sample of women ascertained to date in a nationally representative epidemiologic sample, and rigorous assessment of substance-induced versus independent mood and anxiety disorders, the NESARC allows precise estimates of the prevalences of comorbid disorders and treatment utilization, as well as important sociodemographic characteristics. In addition, the large sample size facilitates analyses of comorbidity that control for both sociodemo-graphic characteristics and other co-occurring conditions and therefore allow determination of unique associations of specific SUDs with specific mood and anxiety disorders.

METHODS

Sample

The research protocol, including informed consent procedures, was approved by the institu-tional review board of the U.S. Bureau of the Census and the U.S. Office of Management and Budget. As described in detail elsewhere (Grant, Dawson, et al., 2003; Grant et al., 2004), the Wave 1 NESARC was conducted in 2001–2002 by the National Institute on Alcohol Abuse and Alcoholism (NIAAA) and based on a representative sample of the general U.S. population. The target population of the NESARC was adults 18 years and older, residing in households and noninstitutional group quarters. All potential respondents who consented to participate, after receiving written information about the nature of the NESARC, the sta-tistical uses of the data, the voluntary nature of their participation, and the federal laws that rigorously safeguard the confidentiality of identifiable survey information, were interviewed. Face-to-face interviews were conducted with 43,093 respondents, yielding a response rate of 81%. The NESARC oversampled Blacks, Hispanics, and persons 18–24 years old; data were adjusted for oversampling and household- and person-level nonresponse. The weighted data were then further adjusted to represent the civilian U.S. population based on the 2000 Census.

Interviewers and Training

Interviews were conducted by 1,800 professional lay interviewers from the U.S. Bureau of the Census with, on average, 5 years of experience administering health-related surveys. All interviewers completed a 5-day self-study program followed by a 5-day in-person training session at one of the bureau's 12 regional offices. The survey instrument was fully computer-ized with software that included built-in skip, logic, and consistency checks.

Quality of interviewing was assured by regional supervisors who recontacted a random sample of 10% of all respondents by telephone and repeated questions from different parts of the interview to verify answers. In addition, 2,657 respondents were selected randomly for reinterview after their NESARC interviews. Each respondent was readministered one to three complete sections of the NESARC interview. This step served as an additional check on data quality and formed the basis of a further test–retest reliability study (Grant, Kaplan, et al., 2003).

Assessments

The diagnostic interview utilized in the NESARC was the NIAAA Alcohol Use Disorder and Associated Disabilities Interview Schedule—DSM-IV Version (AUDADIS-IV; Grant, Dawson, & Hasin, 2001). Developed to advance measurement of substance use and mental disorders in large-scale surveys, the AUDADIS-IV is a fully structured instrument designed for nonclinician interviewers.

Drug and Alcohol Use Disorder Diagnoses

AUDADIS-IV questions operationalize DSM-IV criteria for drug-specific abuse and dependence for 10 drug classes that are aggregated in this report, as well as alcohol use disorders and nicotine dependence. Consistent with DSM-IV, past-year AUDADIS-IV diagnoses of drug abuse required at least one of the four abuse criteria in the 12 months preceding the interview. AUDADIS-IV drug dependence diagnoses required at least three of the seven DSM-IV dependence criteria to be met for the same specific drug class during the past year. Alcohol abuse and dependence and nicotine dependence diagnoses followed the same algorithms.

Mood and Anxiety Disorders

As described in detail elsewhere (Grant et al., 2004), past-year anxiety (panic disorder with and without agoraphobia, social and specific phobias, and generalized anxiety disorder) and mood (major depressive, dysthymic, bipolar I, and bipolar II) disorder diagnoses in this report are DSM-IV primary, or independent, diagnoses. Consistent with DSM-IV (p. 192), disorders were classified as independent if (1) the respondent had abstained from substance use during the past 12 months; (2) the episodes did not occur in the context of drug or alcohol intoxication or withdrawal; (3) the episodes preceded drug or alcohol intoxication or withdrawal; or (4) the episodes began after intoxication or withdrawal but persisted for more than 1 month after cessation of intoxication or withdrawal (Grant et al., 2004). As reported previously (Grant et al., 2004), however, exclusion of substance-induced disorders among NESARC respondents had virtually no impact on prevalence estimates for mood and anxiety disorders. All mood and anxiety disorders met the DSM-IV clinical significance criterion; major depressive disorder diagnoses also ruled out bereavement. Due to considerations of administration time and respondent burden, posttraumatic stress disorder was assessed in Wave 2.

Treatment and Help Seeking

Respondents were queried separately about their use of treatment or help for alcohol problems, drug problems, and each specific mood or anxiety disorder. Alcohol treatment and help seeking assessed for the 12 months before the NESARC interview covered the following sources: 12-step programs; family service and other social service agencies; emergency departments or crisis centers; alcohol specialty services, including alcohol or drug detoxification wards or clinics, outpatient clinics, outreach programs, and day or partial patient programs; inpatient wards of psychiatric or general hospitals or community mental health facilities; alcohol or drug rehabilitation programs; halfway houses; employee assistance programs; clergy; physicians, psychiatrists, psychologists, social workers, or other health professionals; or other sources of help (Hasin et al., 2007). Drug treatment utilization was defined in parallel fashion, except for the inclusion of methadone maintenance programs as drug specialty services (Compton et al., 2007). Respondents were classified as receiving treatment in the past 12 months for each specific mood and anxiety disorder if they had done any of the following: (1) visited a counselor, therapist, physician, psychologist, or similar person; (2) were hospitalized for at least one night; (3) visited a hospital emergency department; or (4) were prescribed medication for the disorder (Grant et al., 2004).

Reliability and Validity of AUDADIS-IV Diagnoses

As reported in detail elsewhere (Grant et al., 2004), reliability and validity were good to excellent for all SUDs (Canino et al., 1999; Compton, Conway, Stinson, Colliver, & Grant, 2005; Compton, Grant, Colliver, Glantz, & Stinson, 2004; Grant, Dawson, et al., 2003; Grant, Harford, et al., 1995; Hasin, Carpenter, McCloud, Smith, & Grant, 1997; Hasin, Muthén, & Grant, 1997; Hasin & Paykin, 1999; Hasin et al., 2003; Vrasti et al., 1998), and fair to good for mood and anxiety disorders (Canino et al., 1999; Compton et al., 2004, 2005; Conway et al., 2006; Grant, Dawson, et al., 2003; Grant et al., 2004; Grant, Hasin, et al., 2005; Grant, Stinson, et al., 2005).

Statistical Analyses

The analysis sample for this report consists of all female respondents in the Wave 1 NESARC; their sociodemographic characteristics are shown in Table 10.1. Standard contingency table approaches were used to examine prevalences of, and treatment for, past-year substance use, mood, and anxiety disorders. Comorbid associations of each SUD with each mood and anxiety disorder were examined using adjusted ORs with 95% confidence intervals (CIs) derived from multivariable logistic regression models (Hosmer & Lemeshow, 2000). For each comorbid association (e.g., between drug dependence and panic disorder with agoraphobia), the logistic model controlled for age, race/ethnicity, marital status, education, past-year personal income, region and urbanicity of residence, and all additional Axis I (12-month) and II (lifetime) psychiatric diagnoses. Controlling for all other disorders addresses their substantial comorbidity with one another and tests the hypothesis that each index disorder is associated with the pure (noncomorbid) form of the other disorder being examined (Compton et al., 2007; Hasin et al., 2007). All analyses were conducted using SUDAAN (Research Triangle Institute, 2002), a software program that uses Taylor series linearization to adjust for the NESARC's complex sampling design.

RESULTS

Prevalences of SUDs

As shown in Table 10.2, past-year prevalences of any DSM-IV SUD, any alcohol use disorder, and any drug use disorder among women were 5.6%, 4.9%, and 1.2%, respectively. Prevalences of specific drug use disorders ranged from 0.0% for solvent or inhalant use disorders and heroin dependence to 0.6% for cannabis abuse; rates of abuse were greater than those of dependence for alcohol, opioids other than heroin, and cannabis.

Prevalences of Independent Mood and Anxiety Disorders

As shown in Table 10.2, 12-month prevalences of any mood disorder and any anxiety disorder were 11.1% and 14.3%, respectively. Prevalences of specific mood disorders ranged from 0.9% for bipolar II to 6.9% for major depressive disorder, whereas rates of anxiety disorders ranged from 0.8% for panic disorder with agoraphobia to 9.5% for specific phobia.

TABLE 10.1. Sociodemographic Characteristics of Female NESARC Respondents (N = 24,575)

Characteristic	% (SE)[a]	Total n[b]
Age, years		
18–29	21.0% (0.44)	4,849
30–44	30.2% (0.40)	7,525
45–64	30.8% (0.37)	7,100
≥ 65	18.1% (0.37)	5,101
Race or ethnicity		
White	70.7% (1.59)	13,662
Black	12.0% (0.70)	5,204
Native American	2.1% (0.18)	387
Asian or Pacific Islander	4.3% (0.52)	736
Hispanic	10.9% (1.21)	4,586
Marital status		
Married or living with someone as if married	59.1% (0.54)	11,683
Separated, divorced, or widowed	22.7% (0.33)	7,754
Never married	18.3% (0.48)	5,138
Education		
Less than high school	15.4% (0.55)	4,480
High school graduation	29.9% (0.53)	7,283
Some college or more	54.8% (0.61)	12,812
Personal income, U.S.$		
≤ 19,999	60.0% (0.64)	14,592
20,000–34,999	20.7% (0.38)	5,284
35,000–69,999	15.7% (0.44)	3,890
≥ 70,000	3.6% (0.23)	809
Region of residence		
Northeast	19.8% (3.47)	4,734
Midwest	23.0% (3.25)	5,084
South	35.4% (3.30)	9,380
West	21.8% (3.50)	5,377
Urban residence	80.4% (1.63)	20,143

[a]Data are given as percentages of respondents (standard error).
[b]Based on unweighted data.

Co-Occurrence of SUDs with Mood and Anxiety Disorders

Adjusted associations between SUDs and comorbid mood and anxiety disorders are depicted in Table 10.3. Significant comorbid associations included drug dependence with bipolar I disorder (OR = 2.4) and panic disorder with agoraphobia (OR = 2.6).

Prevalences of Mood and Anxiety Disorders among Women with SUDs

As shown in the upper-left corner of Table 10.4, 29.7% of women with any 12-month SUD also had at least one independent 12-month mood disorder, and 26.2% had at least one independent 12-month anxiety disorder. Prevalences of specific mood disorders ranged from 1.0% (bipolar II disorder among women with alcohol abuse) to 29.9% (major depressive

TABLE 10.2. Twelve-Month Prevalence of DSM-IV Substance Use Disorders and Independent Mood and Anxiety Disorders among Women (n = 24,575)

Disorder	Prevalence[a]
Any substance use disorder	5.6% (0.24)
Any substance abuse	3.0% (0.18)
Any substance dependence	2.5% (0.14)
Any alcohol use disorder	4.9% (0.22)
Alcohol abuse	2.6% (0.16)
Alcohol dependence	2.3% (0.13)
Any drug use disorder	1.2% (0.10)
Any drug abuse	0.8% (0.09)
Any drug dependence	0.4% (0.04)
Any mood disorder	11.1% (0.33)
Major depressive disorder	6.9% (0.24)
Dysthymia	1.8% (0.12)
Bipolar I disorder	2.2% (0.13)
Bipolar II disorder	0.9% (0.08)
Any anxiety disorder	14.3% (0.45)
Panic disorder	
With agoraphobia	0.8% (0.07)
Without agoraphobia	2.1% (0.13)
Social phobia	3.3% (0.17)
Specific phobia	9.5% (0.37)
Generalized anxiety disorder	2.8% (0.15)

Note. Consistent with DSM-IV, independent mood and anxiety disorder diagnoses exclude disorders that are substance induced or due to a general medical condition; major depressive disorder diagnoses also rule out bereavement.

[a]Data are given as percentages of respondents (standard error).

disorder among women with drug dependence), whereas rates of specific anxiety disorders ranged from 1.2% (panic disorder with agoraphobia among women with alcohol abuse) to 30.9% (specific phobia among women with drug dependence). Among women with alcohol and drug use disorders, the most common mood disorder was major depressive disorder and the most common anxiety disorder was specific phobia.

Prevalences of SUDs among Women with Mood or Anxiety Disorders

As detailed in Table 10.5, 14.9% of women with any past-year mood disorder had at least one SUD, as did 10.2% of those with any past-year anxiety disorder. Among women with specific mood disorders, the prevalences of comorbid SUDs ranged from 1.5% (drug abuse among those with major depressive disorder) to 13.0% (alcohol dependence among those with bipolar II disorder). Among women with specific anxiety disorders, the prevalences of comorbid SUDs ranged from 1.3% (drug dependence among those with specific phobia) to 8.5% (alcohol dependence among those with panic disorder with agoraphobia). Prevalences of abuse were lower than those of dependence, except for drug abuse versus drug dependence among women with bipolar II disorder (4.6 vs. 2.2%) and specific phobia (1.4 vs. 1.3%). Women who had bipolar I disorder were more likely than those with other mood disorders, and those who had panic disorder with agoraphobia were more likely than those with other anxiety disorders, to have a SUD.

TABLE 10.3. Adjusted Odds Ratios (95% CI) for 12-Month DSM-IV Independent Mood and Anxiety Disorders among Women with a 12-Month DSM-IV Substance Use Disorder

Comorbid disorder	Index disorder: Substance use disorder								
	Any substance use disorder	Any substance abuse	Any substance dependence	Any alcohol use disorder	Alcohol abuse	Alcohol dependence	Any drug use disorder	Any drug abuse	Any drug dependence
Any mood disorder	**1.8 (1.49–2.27)**	1.2 (0.94–1.63)	**2.4 (1.79–3.26)**	**1.7 (1.29–2.10)**	1.2 (0.87–1.61)	**2.0 (1.45–2.86)**	**1.8 (1.23–2.59)**	1.3 (0.81–1.95)	**3.3 (1.58–6.72)**
Major depressive disorder	**1.3 (1.04–1.70)**	1.3 (0.92–1.74)	1.3 (0.92–1.88)	**1.4 (1.06–1.80)**	1.4 (0.98–1.91)	1.3 (0.89–1.96)	0.9 (0.57–1.37)	0.7 (0.41–1.23)	1.2 (0.60–2.32)
Dysthymia	1.1 (0.71–1.79)	1.0 (0.52–2.00)	1.2 (0.64–2.13)	1.2 (0.71–1.88)	1.0 (0.47–2.14)	1.2 (0.64–2.31)	1.4 (0.74–2.71)	1.1 (0.41–2.92)	1.7 (0.72–3.83)
Bipolar I disorder	**1.9 (1.33–2.58)**	1.2 (0.75–2.06)	**2.1 (1.40–3.18)**	1.4 (0.97–2.14)	1.3 (0.70–2.26)	1.5 (0.89–2.43)	**2.1 (1.28–3.51)**	1.6 (0.80–3.34)	**2.4 (1.28–4.69)**
Bipolar II disorder	1.3 (0.85–2.13)	0.9 (0.44–1.70)	1.7 (0.96–2.82)	1.2 (0.72–1.94)	0.6 (0.25–1.20)	1.6 (0.91–2.96)	1.1 (0.48–2.55)	1.4 (0.56–3.32)	0.8 (0.22–2.61)
Any anxiety disorder	1.1 (0.89–1.36)	1.1 (0.81–1.38)	1.1 (0.85–1.47)	1.1 (0.88–1.39)	1.1 (0.83–1.48)	1.1 (0.81–1.46)	1.0 (0.67–1.39)	0.7 (0.45–1.20)	1.5 (0.90–2.41)
Panic disorder									
With agoraphobia	1.2 (0.70–2.01)	1.3 (0.60–2.82)	1.1 (0.59–1.97)	0.9 (0.50–1.66)	1.1 (0.44–2.94)	0.8 (0.42–1.64)	1.8 (0.88–3.47)	0.9 (0.28–2.79)	**2.6 (1.12–5.91)**
Without agoraphobia	1.0 (0.67–1.45)	1.0 (0.55–1.69)	1.0 (0.62–1.62)	1.2 (0.79–1.79)	1.0 (0.56–1.85)	1.3 (0.77–2.14)	0.7 (0.34–1.28)	0.5 (0.19–1.38)	0.9 (0.39–1.93)
Social phobia	1.1 (0.76–1.59)	1.3 (0.84–2.04)	1.0 (0.59–1.51)	0.9 (0.61–1.39)	1.3 (0.78–2.06)	0.7 (0.43–1.26)	1.4 (0.87–2.27)	1.0 (0.51–1.91)	1.9 (1.00–3.70)
Specific phobia	1.0 (0.75–1.21)	1.0 (0.70–1.35)	0.9 (0.69–1.27)	1.0 (0.79–1.35)	1.1 (0.76–1.56)	1.0 (0.71–1.37)	0.9 (0.57–1.33)	0.8 (0.47–1.38)	1.0 (0.53–1.86)
Generalized anxiety disorder	1.0 (0.72–1.44)	0.8 (0.42–1.34)	1.2 (0.81–1.81)	0.9 (0.58–1.33)	0.6 (0.32–1.23)	1.1 (0.66–1.78)	1.2 (0.70–1.97)	1.0 (0.52–2.09)	1.3 (0.65–2.50)

Note. Consistent with DSM-IV, independent mood and anxiety disorder diagnoses exclude disorders that are substance induced or due to a general medical condition; major depressive disorder diagnoses also rule out bereavement. Odds ratios are adjusted for age, marital status, race/ethnicity, past-year income, educational attainment, region and urbanicity of residence, and all additional 12-month Axis I and Axis II diagnoses. Odds ratios that are significantly different from the null value of 1.0 ($p < .05$) are presented in **boldface** type.

TABLE 10.4. Twelve-Month Prevalence of DSM-IV Independent Mood and Anxiety Disorders among Women with a 12-Month DSM-IV Substance Use Disorder

Comorbid disorder	Index disorder: Substance use disorder								
	Any substance use disorder	Any substance abuse	Any substance dependence	Any alcohol use disorder	Alcohol abuse	Alcohol dependence	Any drug use disorder	Any drug abuse	Any drug dependence
Any mood disorder	29.7% (1.60)	19.5% (1.73)	41.8% (2.64)	28.4% (1.71)	18.4% (1.79)	39.4% (2.72)	43.6% (3.37)	31.9% (3.93)	68.0% (5.48)
Major depressive disorder	15.4% (1.29)	11.9% (1.47)	19.7% (2.20)	15.3% (1.36)	12.1% (1.56)	18.9% (2.27)	18.1% (2.68)	12.4% (2.77)	29.9% (5.59)
Dysthymia	4.1% (0.80)	2.4% (0.74)	6.1% (1.50)	4.0% (0.86)	2.2% (0.78)	6.0% (1.60)	8.0% (2.14)	4.6% (2.12)	15.2% (4.54)
Bipolar I disorder	8.7% (0.94)	4.9% (0.94)	13.3% (1.78)	7.7% (0.96)	4.4% (0.93)	11.4% (1.75)	17.2% (2.64)	11.9% (3.01)	28.2% (4.96)
Bipolar II disorder	3.4% (0.58)	1.7% (0.47)	5.4% (1.15)	3.0% (0.61)	1.0% (0.35)	5.3% (1.21)	5.2% (1.41)	5.2% (1.73)	5.3% (2.39)
Any anxiety disorder	26.2% (1.65)	20.1% (1.82)	33.7% (2.53)	25.4% (1.74)	19.6% (1.90)	31.7% (2.57)	34.6% (3.54)	25.0% (3.90)	54.8% (5.66)
Panic disorder									
With agoraphobia	2.5% (0.53)	1.6% (0.54)	3.7% (0.93)	2.0% (0.50)	1.2% (0.51)	3.0% (0.89)	5.8% (1.70)	2.5% (1.31)	12.9% (4.09)
Without agoraphobia	5.0% (0.74)	3.2% (0.76)	7.2% (1.33)	5.1% (0.81)	3.0% (0.79)	7.4% (1.43)	6.3% (1.60)	3.7% (1.54)	11.8% (3.65)
Social phobia	7.7% (1.05)	5.9% (1.11)	9.9% (1.76)	6.7% (1.03)	5.3% (1.06)	8.3% (1.66)	13.8% (2.54)	8.3% (2.23)	25.2% (5.41)
Specific phobia	15.6% (1.32)	12.2% (1.52)	19.6% (2.04)	15.5% (1.47)	12.3% (1.69)	19.0% (2.18)	20.6% (2.98)	15.7% (3.34)	30.9% (5.54)
Generalized anxiety disorder	7.1% (0.86)	3.7% (0.87)	11.3% (1.60)	6.2% (0.88)	2.9% (0.86)	9.8% (1.59)	12.7% (2.34)	8.1% (2.44)	22.3% (4.42)

Note. Consistent with DSM-IV, independent mood and anxiety disorder diagnoses exclude disorders that are substance induced or due to a general medical condition; major depressive disorder diagnoses also rule out bereavement. Data are given as percentages of respondents (standard error).

TABLE 10.5. Twelve-Month Prevalence of DSM-IV Substance Use Disorders among Women with a 12-Month DSM-IV Independent Mood or Anxiety Disorder

Comorbid disorder	Index disorder: Mood or anxiety disorder										
	Any mood disorder	Major depressive disorder	Dysthymia	Bipolar I disorder	Bipolar II disorder	Any anxiety disorder	Panic disorder with agoraphobia	Panic disorder without agoraphobia	Social phobia	Specific phobia	Generalized anxiety disorder
Any substance use disorder	14.9% (0.88)	12.5% (1.01)	12.9% (2.32)	21.9% (2.26)	19.9% (3.27)	10.2% (0.70)	17.4% (3.37)	13.3% (1.88)	12.8% (1.67)	9.1% (0.81)	14.2% (1.64)
Any substance abuse	5.4% (0.54)	5.3% (0.69)	4.1% (1.26)	6.8% (1.33)	5.5% (1.56)	4.3% (0.43)	6.0% (2.06)	4.6% (1.12)	5.4% (1.02)	3.9% (0.50)	4.0% (0.95)
Any substance dependence	9.5% (0.70)	7.3% (0.83)	8.8% (2.02)	15.2% (1.90)	14.4% (3.00)	5.9% (0.56)	11.5% (2.70)	8.7% (1.60)	7.5% (1.32)	5.2% (0.64)	10.3% (1.47)
Any alcohol use disorder	12.5% (0.84)	10.9% (0.98)	11.1% (2.23)	17.1% (2.02)	15.7% (2.97)	8.6% (0.65)	12.3% (2.87)	11.9% (1.81)	9.8% (1.47)	8.0% (0.80)	10.8% (1.50)
Alcohol abuse	4.2% (0.48)	4.5% (0.63)	3.2% (1.13)	5.1% (1.10)	2.7% (0.98)	3.5% (0.38)	3.8% (1.65)	3.7% (0.98)	4.0% (0.83)	3.3% (0.47)	2.7% (0.79)
Alcohol dependence	8.3% (0.68)	6.4% (0.81)	7.9% (1.99)	12.0% (1.78)	13.0% (2.88)	5.2% (0.52)	8.5% (2.44)	8.3% (1.59)	5.8% (1.17)	4.7% (0.63)	8.2% (1.35)
Any drug use disorder	4.9% (0.47)	3.3% (0.50)	5.6% (1.48)	9.6% (1.61)	6.9% (1.88)	3.0% (0.35)	8.9% (2.46)	3.7% (0.95)	5.1% (0.90)	2.7% (0.44)	5.6% (1.02)
Any drug abuse	2.4% (0.37)	1.5% (0.35)	2.2% (1.01)	4.5% (1.27)	4.6% (1.58)	1.5% (0.25)	2.5% (1.32)	1.5% (0.62)	2.1% (0.55)	1.4% (0.31)	2.4% (0.73)
Any drug dependence	2.5% (0.33)	1.7% (0.38)	3.5% (1.10)	5.1% (1.02)	2.2% (1.04)	1.5% (0.25)	6.4% (2.10)	2.3% (0.72)	3.0% (0.75)	1.3% (0.28)	3.2% (0.72)

Note. Consistent with DSM-IV, independent mood and anxiety disorder diagnoses exclude disorders that are substance induced or due to a general medical condition; major depressive disorder diagnoses also rule out bereavement. Data are given as percentages of respondents (standard error).

Treatment Utilization for 12-Month Substance Use, Mood, and Anxiety Disorders

Treatment utilization for total, pure, and comorbid past-year substance use, mood, and anxiety disorders is shown in Table 10.6. Among women with any SUD, 8.5% sought treatment; comparable figures are 29.1% for women with any mood disorder, and 12.4% for women with any anxiety disorder. Drug use disorders were associated with higher rates of treatment utilization than alcohol use disorders. Similarly, dysthymia and major depressive disorder were associated with higher rates of treatment than other mood disorders, and panic disorder, both with and without agoraphobia, was associated with higher rates of treatment than other anxiety disorders. The comorbid forms of alcohol use disorders, major depressive disorder, dysthymia, social and specific phobias, and generalized anxiety disorder were associated with significantly higher rates of treatment than the respective pure disorders. By contrast, women with drug use disorders, bipolar disorders, and panic disorder with and without agoraphobia utilized treatment at similar rates whether their disorders were pure or comorbid.

DISCUSSION

Comorbidity of SUDs with Mood and Anxiety Disorders

Consistent with findings from clinical and epidemiologic studies reviewed in the introduction to this chapter, the present results document high prevalences of specific mood and anxiety disorders among women with SUDs. The observed rates were higher than those in analyses of the NESARC data that included both men and women (Grant et al., 2004), yielding further evidence that comorbid mood and anxiety disorders are more prevalent in women than in men with SUDs. Conversely, and also in line with findings from clinical and general population samples (e.g., Brady & Verduin, 2005; Davis et al., 2006; Gonzalez et al., 2007; Kushner, Abrams, & Borchardt, 2000; Merikangas et al., 1996; Regier et al., 1990), prevalences of comorbid SUDs, particularly dependence disorders, among women with mood or anxiety disorders were higher than among women unselected for mood or anxiety disorders. Nevertheless, they were lower than those observed in analyses of the NESARC sample that included both women and men with mood or anxiety disorders (Grant et al., 2004).

Despite the high *prevalences* of co-occurring specific SUDs and specific mood or anxiety disorders, only the associations of drug dependence with bipolar I and panic disorder with agoraphobia remained significant after adjustment for other comorbid disorders. As was previously reported from the NESARC based on both men and women (Compton et al., 2007; Hasin et al., 2007), these results indicate that much of the comorbidity between specific disorders reflects factors common to these other disorders. Also of note, the 95% CIs around the ORs among women overlapped broadly with, and the point estimates of the ORs were very similar to, those in the mixed-sex NESARC sample. Thus, despite sex differences in the prevalences of comorbid disorders, our findings do not suggest large differences in patterns of comorbid associations between women and men.

Past-Year Treatment Utilization for Pure versus Comorbid Disorders

Regardless of the disorder under consideration, less than half of all affected women sought treatment or help. The overall rates of past-year treatment and help seeking for alcohol (6.5%) and drug (17.7%) use disorders were slightly higher than those observed in the NESARC when women and men were considered together (5.8% and 13.1%, respectively).

TABLE 10.6. Prevalence of Treatment or Help Seeking for Pure versus Comorbid 12-Month Substance Use, Mood, and Anxiety Disorders among Women

Disorder (total number of cases)	Total[a]	Pure[a]	Comorbid[a]	p-value (pure vs. comorbid)
Any substance use disorder (1,264)	8.5% (0.93)	3.1% (1.21)	11.6% (1.23)	< 0.0001
Any alcohol use disorder (1,113)	6.5% (0.83)	2.0% (0.78)	9.2% (1.22)	< 0.0001
Any drug use disorder (280)	17.7% (2.77)	9.7% (8.91)	19.4% (2.85)	0.2873
Any mood disorder (2,710)	29.1% (1.17)	22.0% (1.84)	32.0% (1.48)	0.0001
Major depressive disorder (1,656)	29.7% (1.46)	20.6% (2.24)	33.4% (1.79)	< 0.0001
Dysthymia (430)	31.9% (3.20)	17.8% (5.75)	34.8% (3.56)	0.0204
Bipolar I disorder (552)	21.6% (2.43)	25.4% (6.99)	21.0% (2.35)	0.5465
Bipolar II disorder (227)	2.7% (0.97)	1.4% (0.94)	3.0% (1.18)	0.3028
Any anxiety disorder (3,352)	12.4% (0.70)	5.1% (0.74)	17.1% (1.03)	< 0.0001
Panic disorder				
With agoraphobia (194)	40.9% (4.24)	26.7% (13.1)	42.2% (4.48)	0.2648
Without agoraphobia (466)	29.7% (2.60)	28.6% (5.42)	29.9% (2.97)	0.8332
Social phobia (747)	12.3% (1.47)	0.3% (0.26)	14.7% (1.75)	< 0.0001
Specific phobia (2,230)	3.9% (0.49)	1.2% (0.44)	5.6% (0.74)	< 0.0001
Generalized anxiety disorder (662)	27.0% (2.06)	10.2% (4.69)	28.9% (2.21)	0.0017

[a]Data are given as percentages of respondents (standard error).

However, overall rates of utilization among women with mood or anxiety disorders were similar to those in the mixed-sex sample. Consistent with prior findings from mixed-sex samples (Cohen et al., 2007; Compton et al., 2007; Kessler et al., 1996; Robins et al., 1991), women with comorbid disorders were significantly more likely to have sought help than women with pure disorders, except in the cases of drug use, bipolar, and panic disorders. The small numbers of women with drug use disorders and panic disorder with agoraphobia and the relatively large numerical differences in treatment seeking suggest that statistical power limitations may have constrained the detection of significant differences by pure versus comorbid status. Utilization rates were similar in pure versus comorbid bipolar I and panic disorder without agoraphobia, however, raising the possibility that the relationship of comorbidity, including specific comorbid disorders as well as total burden of illness, to treatment or help seeking may vary over different index disorders. One mechanism possibly underlying such variation may involve the extent to which specific patterns of comorbidity influence affected individuals' perceptions of need for services (Mojtabai, Olfson, & Mechanic, 2002).

Limitations

Limitations of the study include the cross-sectional nature of the data. Longitudinal studies are required to address the causality of the comorbid associations and to identify underlying mechanisms. The recently completed Wave 2 NESARC, which involved a 3-year follow-up of respondents assessed in Wave 1, will yield data bearing importantly on these questions. In addition, considerations of respondent burden forced deferral of the assessment of some DSM-IV disorders and putative risk factors, including posttraumatic stress disorder and adverse childhood experiences, which have been identified in very large proportions of women in addiction treatment (e.g., Charney, Palacios-Boix, & Gill, 2007; Najavits et al.,

2003; Pirard, Sharon, Kang, Angarita, & Gastfriend, 2005; Read, Brown, & Kahler, 2004; Reynolds et al., 2005), until Wave 2.

The NESARC was designed to examine the epidemiology of SUDs and other mental disorders in the general, noninstitutionalized adult population. Although the prevalences of mood and anxiety disorders observed among women with SUDs in the NESARC did not differ greatly from those reported for women in addiction treatment samples, the nature, magnitude, and mechanisms of the unique comorbid associations between specific SUDs and other specific mental disorders may differ in clinically ascertained samples from those observed in the general population because comorbidity itself is associated with treatment entry (Berkson, 1946). Finally, drug use disorders were aggregated across 10 drug categories, in part because of low prevalences of several specific drug use disorders, particularly among women. There may be drug-specific comorbid associations with specific mood or anxiety disorders that were obscured by this aggregation. However, given the rarity of most specific drug use disorders in the general population of women, the sample sizes required to study such drug-specific associations in an epidemiologic survey would be prohibitive.

Clinical Implications

Despite the few unique comorbid associations observed in this study, the high prevalences of co-occurring mood and anxiety disorders among women with SUDs, and of SUDs among women with mood and anxiety disorders, indicate the need for comprehensive assessment of psychiatric disorders in women, regardless of their presenting complaints and the settings (e.g., primary care, mental health, or addiction treatment) in which they are seen. Comprehensive assessment in primary care and mental health settings may be particularly critical because women with SUDs present more frequently than men to settings other than addiction treatment (Chander & McCaul, 2003; Mojtabai, 2005; Weisner & Schmidt, 1992).

In the NESARC sample women appear no less likely than men to seek treatment either for SUDs or for mood or anxiety disorders. Nevertheless, treatment rates among women, particularly for SUDs, are low (8.5%). Previous SUD treatment outcome studies have shown that women respond at least as well as men (Flynn, Joe, Broome, Simpson, & Brown, 2003; Greenfield et al., 2007; Hser, Evans, & Huang, 2005; Weisner, Ray, Mertens, Satre, & Moore, 2003). Nevertheless, traditional SUD treatment programs have been criticized as insufficiently responsive to the unique barriers women face in utilizing services. In addition to high levels of psychiatric comorbidity, these include inadequate funding; needs for obstetrical and gynecological services, child care, and transportation; differential stigmatization of SUDs; discomfort with confrontational treatment approaches; and histories of victimization (Brady & Randall, 1999; Chander & McCall, 2003; Greenfield et al., 2007; Grella, 2003). Although evidence for the superiority of women-only over mixed-sex treatment programs is inconclusive at this point (Brady & Randall, 1999; Chander & McCall, 2003; Green, 2006; Niv & Hser, 2007), it is clear that programs need to implement approaches that effectively address the health disparities manifested in the barriers to care faced by women.

Evidence for effects of specific comorbid mood and anxiety disorders on outcomes of addiction treatment is inconsistent. In mixed-sex samples, major depression and anxiety disorders have been identified as adverse prognostic factors for remission and risk factors for relapse to both substance use and substance dependence (Burns, Teesson, & O'Neill, 2005; Greenfield et al., 1998; Hasin et al., 2002; Kushner et al., 2005). In sex-specific analyses, men with comorbid major depression were dependent on more illicit drugs than men without major depression, whereas women with phobias used fewer illicit drugs than women without phobias, at 1-year posttreatment follow-up (Compton, Cottler, Jacobs, Ben-Abdallah, &

Spitznagel, 2003). Similarly, both men and women with anxiety disorders or with recurrent major depression experienced significantly more lifetime admissions to detoxification than those without (Tómasson & Vaglum, 1998). Conversely, Kranzler, Del Boca, and Rounsaville (1996) found no impact of major depression on most 3-year outcomes of inpatient alcoholism treatment except for lower intensity of drinking in both sexes.

Future research is needed to clarify the prognostic impact of specific mood and anxiety disorders in women and men with SUDs. Further, it is critical to examine whether treatment modalities differ in effectiveness by client sex, patterns of comorbidity, or other characteristics, including sociodemographic and family history variables. Nevertheless, because SUDs and comorbid conditions are severely impairing and disabling in their own rights, treatment providers need to offer evidence-based interventions that address the SUD and comorbid disorders.

In addition to the implications of our findings for treatment research, the identification of unique comorbid associations of drug dependence with bipolar I disorder and panic disorder with agoraphobia indicates the need for etiological research to characterize the nature of these associations, the factors underlying them, and the possible sex specificity of those factors. The longitudinal data obtained in Wave 2 of the NESARC will contribute importantly to this work by allowing identification of factors underlying both onset and course of each disorder. Future research is also indicated to characterize the common factors underlying the co-occurrences among other comorbid disorders in women and men. Further, analyses of the NESARC data are currently in progress to examine associations of childhood adversities and posttraumatic stress disorder with SUDs and other mental disorders, including sex differences. These findings will inform prevention research, including the possible need to tailor specific approaches by sex as well as by targeted comorbid conditions, and thereby more effectively reduce the burdens of SUD, mood disorder, and anxiety disorder morbidity on both women and men.

KEY POINTS

- SUDs, mood disorders, and anxiety disorders are common and frequently comorbid among adult women.
- Among women with any SUD, 12-month prevalence rates of mood disorders and anxiety disorders were 29.7% and 26.2%, respectively
- The most common mood disorder among women with an SUD was major depressive disorder (15.4%).
- The most common anxiety disorder among women with an SUD was specific phobia (15.6%)
- The high prevalences of mood and anxiety disorders among women with SUDs indicate the need for comprehensive assessment of psychiatric disorders by care providers, regardless of whether women are seen in primary care, mental health, or addiction treatment settings.
- Evidence-based treatments for co-occurring SUDs, mood disorders, and anxiety disorders need to be provided to women presenting for care.
- The large majority of women with SUDs do not seek treatment; women with an alcohol use disorder appear to be less likely than women with a drug use disorder to seek treatment.
- Future research is needed to characterize the factors underlying both unique comorbid associations and comorbid associations reflecting common factors related to the co-occurrences among other disorders, as well as to identify optimal treatment and prevention approaches targeting pure and comorbid disorders among both women and men.

ACKNOWLEDGMENTS

The National Epidemiologic Survey on Alcohol and Related Conditions (NESARC) is funded by the National Institute on Alcohol Abuse and Alcoholism (NIAAA) with supplemental support from the National Institute on Drug Abuse (NIDA). This research was supported in part by the Intramural Program of the National Institutes of Health, National Institute on Alcohol Abuse and Alcoholism. I express my appreciation to Bridget F. Grant, PhD, PhD, for her invaluable comments on earlier drafts of this chapter.

DISCLAIMER

The views and opinions expressed in this report are those of the authors and should not be construed to represent the views of sponsoring organizations, agencies, or the U.S. government.

REFERENCES

Asterisks denote recommended readings.

Abbott, P. J., Weller, S. B., & Walker, S. R. (1994). Psychiatric disorders of opioid addicts entering treatment: Preliminary data. *Journal of Addictive Diseases, 13*, 1–11.

Agosti, V., Nunes, E., & Levin, F. (2002). Rates of psychiatric comorbidity among U. S. residents with lifetime cannabis dependence. *American Journal of Drug and Alcohol Abuse, 28*, 643–652.

American Psychiatric Association. (2000). *Diagnostic and statistical manual of mental disorders* (4th ed., text rev.). Washington, DC: Author.

Anthony, J. C., & Helzer, J. E. (1991). Syndromes of drug abuse and dependence. In L. N. Robins & D. A. Regier (Eds.), *Psychiatric disorders in America: The Epidemiologic Catchment Area Study* (pp. 116–154). New York: Free Press.

Berkson, J. (1946). Limitations of the application of fourfold table analysis to hospital data. *Biometrics Bulletin, 2*, 47–53.

Brady, K. T., & Randall, C. L. (1999). Gender differences in substance use disorders. *Psychiatric Clinics of North America, 22*, 241–252. (*)

Brady, K. T., & Verduin, M. L. (2005). Pharmacotherapy of comorbid mood, anxiety, and substance use disorders. *Substance Use and Misuse, 40*, 2021–2041.

Brooner, R. K., King, V. L., Kidorf, M., Schmidt, C. W., & Bigelow, G. E. (1997). Psychiatric and substance use comorbidity among treatment-seeking opioid abusers. *Archives of General Psychiatry, 54*, 71–80.

Burns, L., Teesson, M., & O'Neill, K. (2005). The impact of comorbid anxiety and depression on alcohol treatment outcome. *Addiction, 100*, 787–796.

Canino, G., Bravo, M., Ramírez, R., Febo, V. E., Rubio-Stipec, M., Fernandez, R. L., et al. (1999). The Spanish Alcohol Use Disorder and Associated Disabilities Interview Schedule (AUDADIS): Reliability and concordance with clinical diagnoses in a Hispanic population. *Journal of Studies on Alcohol, 60*, 790–799.

Chander, G., & McCaul, M. E. (2003). Co-occurring psychiatric disorders in women with addictions. *Obstetrics and Gynecology Clinics of North America, 30*, 469–481.

Charney, D. A., Palacios-Boix, J., & Gill, K. J. (2007). Sexual abuse and the outcome of addiction treatment. *American Journal on Addictions, 16*, 93–100.

Cohen, E., Feinn, R., Arias, A., & Kranzler, H. R. (2007). Alcohol treatment utilization: Findings from the National Epidemiologic Survey on Alcohol and Related Conditions. *Drug and Alcohol Dependence, 86*, 214–221.

Compton, W. M., Conway, K. P., Stinson, F. S., Colliver, J. D., & Grant, B. F. (2005). Prevalence and comorbidity of DSM-IV antisocial personality syndromes and specific drug use disorders in the United States: Results from the National Epidemiologic Survey on Alcohol and Related Conditions. *Journal of Clinical Psychiatry, 66*, 677–685.

Compton, W. M., Cottler, L. B., Ben Abdallah, A., Phelps, D. L., Spitznagel, E. L., & Horton, J. C. (2000). Substance dependence and other psychiatric disorders among drug dependent subjects: Race and gender correlates. *American Journal on Addictions*, 9, 113–125.

Compton, W. M., Cottler, L. B., Jacobs, J. L., Ben-Abdallah, A., & Spitznagel, E. L. (2003). The role of psychiatric disorders in predicting drug dependence treatment outcomes. *American Journal of Psychiatry*, 160, 890–895.

Compton, W. M., Grant, B. F., Colliver, J. D., Glantz, M. D., & Stinson, F. S. (2004). Prevalence of marijuana use disorder in the United States: 1991–1992 and 2001–2002. *Journal of the American Medical Association*, 291, 2114–2121.

Compton, W. M., Thomas, Y. F., Stinson, F. S., & Grant, B. F. (2007). Prevalence, correlates, disability, and comorbidity of DSM-IV drug abuse and dependence in the United States: Results from the National Epidemiologic Survey on Alcohol and Related Conditions. *Archives of General Psychiatry*, 64, 566–576. (*)

Conway, K. P., Compton, W., Stinson, F. S., & Grant, B. F. (2006). Lifetime comorbidity of DSM-IV mood and anxiety disorders and specific drug use disorders: Results from the National Epidemiologic Survey on Alcohol and Related Conditions. *Journal of Clinical Psychiatry*, 67, 247–257. (*)

Davis, L. L., Frazier, E., Husain, M. M., Warden, D., Trivedi, M., Fava, M., et al. (2006). Substance use disorder comorbidity in major depressive disorder: A confirmatory analysis of the STAR*D cohort. *American Journal on Addictions*, 15, 278–285.

De Wilde, J., Broekaert, E., Rosseel, Y., Delespaul, P., & Soyez, V. (2007). The role of gender differences and other client characteristics in the prevalence of DSM-IV affective disorders among a European therapeutic community. *Psychiatric Quarterly*, 78, 39–51.

Flynn, P. M., Joe, G. W., Broome, K. M., Simpson, D. D., & Brown, B. S. (2003). Recovery from opioid addiction in DATOS. *Journal of Substance Abuse Treatment*, 25, 177–186.

Gonzalez, J. M., Thompson, P., Escamilla, M., Araga, M., Singh, V., Ferally, N., et al. (2007). Treatment characteristics and illness burden among European Americans, African Americans, and Latinos in the First 2,000 Patients of the Systematic Treatment Enhancement Program for Bipolar Disorder. *Psychopharmacology Bulletin*, 40, 31–46.

Grant, B. F., Dawson, D. A., & Hasin, D. S. (2001). *The Alcohol Use Disorder and Associated Disabilities Interview Schedule—DSM-IV Version*. Bethesda, MD: National Institute on Alcohol Abuse and Alcoholism. Retrieved February 26, 2008, from *www.niaaa.nih.gov*.

Grant, B. F., Dawson, D. A., Stinson, F. S., Chou, P. S., Kay, W., & Pickering, R. (2003). The Alcohol Use Disorder and Associated Disabilities Interview Schedule-IV (AUDADIS-IV): Reliability of alcohol consumption, tobacco use, family history of depression, and psychiatric diagnostic modules in a general population sample. *Drug and Alcohol Dependence*, 71, 7–16.

Grant, B. F., Harford, T. C., Dawson, D. A., Chou, P. S., & Pickering, R. (1995). The Alcohol Use Disorder and Associated Disabilities Interview Schedule (AUDADIS): Reliability of alcohol and drug modules in a general population sample. *Drug and Alcohol Dependence*, 39, 37–44.

Grant, B. F., Hasin, D. S., Stinson, F. S., Dawson, D. A., Chou, S. P., & Ruan, W. J. (2005). Co-occurrence of 12-month mood and anxiety disorders and personality disorders in the U.S.: Results from the National Epidemiologic Survey on Alcohol and Related Conditions. *Journal of Psychiatric Research*, 39, 1–9.

Grant, B. F., Kaplan, K., Shepard, J., & Moore, T. C. (2003). *Source and accuracy statement for Wave 1 of the 2001–2002 National Epidemiologic Survey on Alcohol and Related Conditions*. Bethesda, MD: National Institute on Alcohol Abuse and Alcoholism. Retrieved February 26, 2008, from *www.niaaa.nih.gov*.

Grant, B. F., Stinson, F. S., Dawson, D. A., Chou, S. P., Dufour, M. C., Compton, W., et al. (2004). Prevalence and co-occurrence of substance use disorders and independent mood and anxiety disorders: Results from the National Epidemiologic Survey on Alcohol and Related Conditions. *Archives of General Psychiatry*, 61, 807–816. (*)

Grant, B. F., Stinson, F. S., Hasin, D. S., Dawson, D. A., Chou, S. P., Ruan, W. J., et al. (2005). Prevalence, correlates, and comorbidity of bipolar I disorder and Axis I and II disorders: Results from the National Epidemiologic Survey on Alcohol and Related Conditions. *Journal of Clinical Psychiatry*, 66, 1205–1215.

Green, C. A. (2006). Gender and use of substance abuse treatment services. *Alcohol Research and Health, 29,* 55–62.

Greenfield, S. F., Brooks, A. J., Gordon, S. M., Green, C. A., Kropp, F., McHugh, R. K., et al. (2007). Substance abuse treatment entry, retention, and outcome in women: A review of the literature. *Drug and Alcohol Dependence, 86,* 1–21.

Greenfield, S. F., Weiss, R. D., Muenz, L. R., Vagge, L. M., Kelly, J. F., Bello, L. R., et al. (1998). The effect of depression on return to drinking: A prospective study. *Archives of General Psychiatry, 55,* 259–265.

Grella, C. E. (2003). Effects of gender and diagnosis on addiction history, treatment utilization, and psychosocial functioning among a dually-diagnosed sample in drug treatment. *Journal of Psychoactive Drugs, 35*(Suppl. 1), 169–179.

Griffin, M. L., Weiss, R. D., Mirin, S. M., & Lange, U. (1989). A comparison of male and female cocaine abusers. *Archives of General Psychiatry, 46,* 122–126.

Hasin, D., Carpenter, K. M., McCloud, S., Smith, M., & Grant, B. F. (1997). The Alcohol Use Disorder and Associated Disabilities Interview Schedule (AUDADIS): Reliability of alcohol and drug modules in a clinical sample. *Drug and Alcohol Dependence, 44,* 133–141.

Hasin, D., Liu, X., Nunes, E., McCloud, S., Samet, S., & Endicott, J. (2002). Effects of major depression on remission and relapse of substance dependence. *Archives of General Psychiatry, 59,* 375–380.

Hasin, D., & Paykin, A. (1999). Alcohol dependence and abuse diagnoses: Concurrent validity in a nationally representative sample. *Alcoholism: Clinical and Experimental Research, 23,* 144–150.

Hasin, D. S., & Grant, B. F. (2002). Major depression in 6,050 former drinkers: Association with past alcohol dependence. *Archives of General Psychiatry, 59,* 794–800.

Hasin, D. S., Muthén, B., & Grant, B. F. (1997). The dimensionality of DSM-IV alcohol abuse and dependence: Factor analysis in a clinical sample. In R. Vrasti (Ed.), *Alcoholism: New research perspectives* (pp. 27–39). Munich, Germany: Hogrefe & Hubner.

Hasin, D. S., Schuckit, M. A., Martin, C. S., Grant, B. F., Bucholz, K. K., & Helzer, J. E. (2003). The validity of DSM-IV alcohol dependence: What do we know and what do we need to know? *Alcoholism: Clinical and Experimental Research, 27,* 244–252.

Hasin, D. S., Stinson, F. S., Ogburn, E., & Grant, B. F. (2007). Prevalence, correlates, disability, and comorbidity of DSM-IV alcohol abuse and dependence in the United States: Results from the National Epidemiologic Survey on Alcohol and Related Conditions. *Archives of General Psychiatry, 64,* 830–842. (*)

Helzer, J. E., Burnam, M. A., & McEvoy, L. T. (1991). Alcohol abuse and dependence. In L. N. Robins & D. A. Regier (Eds.), *Psychiatric disorders in America: The Epidemiologic Catchment Area Study* (pp. 81–115). New York: Free Press.

Hesselbrock, M. N., Meyer, R. E., & Keener, J. J. (1985). Psychopathology in hospitalized alcoholics. *Archives of General Psychiatry, 42,* 1050–1055.

Hosmer, D. W., & Lemeshow, S. (2000). *Applied logistic regression* (2nd ed.). New York: Wiley.

Hser, Y.-I., Evans, E., & Huang, Y.-C. (2005). Treatment outcomes among women and men methamphetamine users in California. *Journal of Substance Abuse Treatment, 28,* 77–85.

Jacobi, F., Wittchen, H. U., Holting, C., Höfler, M., Pfister, H., Müller, N., et al. (2004). Prevalence, comorbidity, and correlates of mental disorders in the general population: Results from the German Health Interview and Examination Survey (GHS). *Psychological Medicine, 34,* 597–611.

Kadden, R. M., Kranzler, H. R., & Rounsaville, B. J. (1995). Validity of the distinction between substance-induced and independent depression and anxiety disorders. *American Journal on Addiction, 4,* 107–117.

Kessler, R. C., Aguilar-Gaxiola, S., Berglund, P. A., Caraveo-Anduaga, J. J., DeWit, D. J., Greenfield, S. F., et al. (2001). Patterns and predictors of treatment seeking after onset of a substance use disorder. *Archives of General Psychiatry, 58,* 1065–1071.

Kessler, R. C., Crum, R. M., Warner, L. A., Nelson, C. B., Schulenberg, J., & Anthony, J. C. (1997). Lifetime co-occurrence of DSM-III-R alcohol abuse and dependence with other psychiatric disorders in the National Comorbidity Survey. *Archives of General Psychiatry, 54,* 313–321.

Kessler, R. C., McGonagle, K. A., Zhao, S., Nelson, C. B., Hughes, M., Eshleman, S., et al. (1994).

Lifetime and 12-month prevalence of DSM-III-R psychiatric disorders in the United States: Results from the National Comorbidity Survey. *Archives of General Psychiatry, 51,* 8–19.

Kessler, R. C., Nelson, C. B., McGonagle, K. A., Edlund, M. J., Frank, R. G., & Leaf, P. J. (1996). The epidemiology of co-occurring addictive and mental disorders: Implications for prevention and service utilization. *American Journal of Orthopsychiatry, 66,* 17–31.

Kessler, R. C., Olfson, M., & Berglund, P. A. (1998). Patterns and predictors of treatment contact after first onset of psychiatric disorders. *American Journal of Psychiatry, 155,* 62–69.

Kranzler, H. R., Del Boca, F. K., & Rounsaville, B. J. (1996). Comorbid psychiatric diagnosis predicts three-year outcomes in alcoholics: A posttreatment natural history study. *Journal of Studies on Alcohol, 57,* 619–626.

Kushner, M. G., Abrams, K., & Borchardt, C. (2000). The relationship between anxiety disorders and alcohol use disorders: A review of major perspectives and findings. *Clinical Psychology Review, 20,* 149–171.

Kushner, M. G., Abrams, K., Thuras, P., Hanson, K. L., Brekke, M., & Sletten, S. (2005). Follow-up study of anxiety disorder and alcohol dependence in comorbid alcoholism treatment patients. *Alcoholism: Clinical and Experimental Research, 29,* 1432–1443.

Magura, S., Kang, S.-Y., Rosenblum, A., Handelsman, L., & Foote, J. (1998). Gender differences in psychiatric comorbidity among cocaine-using opiate addicts. *Journal of Addictive Diseases, 17,* 49–61.

Mann, K., Hintz, J., & Jung, M. (2004). Does psychiatric comorbidity in alcohol-dependent patients affect treatment outcome? *European Archives of Psychiatry and Clinical Neuroscience, 254,* 172–181.

McCance-Katz, E. F., Carroll, K. M., & Rounsaville, B. J. (1999). Gender differences in treatment-seeking cocaine abusers: Implications for treatment and prognosis. *American Journal on Addictions, 8,* 300–311.

Merikangas, K. R., Angst, J., Eaton, W., Canino, G., Rubio-Stipec, M., Wacker, H., et al. (1996). Comorbidity and boundaries of affective disorders with anxiety disorders and substance misuse: Results of an international task force. *British Journal of Psychiatry, 168,* 58–67.

Mojtabai, R. (2005). Use of specialty substance abuse and mental health services in adults with substance use disorders in the community. *Drug and Alcohol Dependence, 78,* 345–354.

Mojtabai, R., Olfson, M., & Mechanic, D. (2002). Perceived need and help-seeking in adults with mood, anxiety, or substance use disorders. *Archives of General Psychiatry, 59,* 77–84.

Najavits, L. M., Runkel, R., Neuner, C., Frank, A. F., Thase, M. E., Crits-Cristoph, P., et al. (2003). Rates and symptoms of PTSD among cocaine-dependent patients. *Journal of Studies on Alcohol, 64,* 601–606.

Niv, N., & Hser, Y.-I. (2007). Women-only and mixed-gender drug abuse treatment programs: Service needs, utilization and outcomes. *Drug and Alcohol Dependence, 87,* 194–201.

Nunes, E. V., & Rounsaville, B. J. (2006). Comorbidity of substance use with depression and other mental disorders: From *Diagnostic and Statistical Manual of Mental Disorders,* fourth edition (DSM-IV) to DSM-V. *Addiction, 101*(Suppl. 1), 89–96.

Pirard, S., Sharon, E., Kang, S. K., Angarita, G. A., & Gastfriend, D. R. (2005). Prevalence of physical and sexual abuse among substance abuse patients and impact on treatment outcomes. *Drug and Alcohol Dependence, 78,* 57–64.

Raimo, E. B., & Schuckit, M. A. (1998). Alcohol dependence and mood disorders. *Addictive Behaviors, 23,* 933–946.

Read, J. P., Brown, P. J., & Kahler, C. W. (2004). Substance use and posttraumatic stress disorders: Symptom interplay and effects on outcome. *Addictive Behaviors, 29,* 1665–1672.

Regier, D. A., Farmer, M. E., Rae, D. S., Locke, B. Z., Keith, S. J., Judd, L. L., et al. (1990). Comorbidity of mental disorders with alcohol and other drug abuse: Results from the Epidemiologic Catchment Area (ECA) Study. *Journal of the American Medical Association, 264,* 2511–2518.

Research Triangle Institute. (2002). *Software for Survey Data Analysis, SUDAAN, Version 9.0.* Research Triangle Park, NC: Author.

Reynolds, M., Mezey, G., Chapman, M., Wheeler, B., Drummond, C., & Baldacchino, A. (2005).

Co-morbid post-traumatic stress disorder in a substance misusing clinical population. *Drug and Alcohol Dependence, 77*, 251–258.

Robins, L. N., Locke, B. Z., & Regier, D. A. (1991). An overview of psychiatric disorders in America. In L. N. Robins & D. A. Regier (Eds.), *Psychiatric disorders in America: The Epidemiologic Catchment Area Study* (pp. 328–366). New York: Free Press.

Ross, H. E., Glaser, F. B., & Germanson, T. (1988). The prevalence of psychiatric disorders in patients with alcohol and other drug problems. *Archives of General Psychiatry, 45*, 1023–1031.

Ross, H. E., Glaser, F. B., & Stiasny, S. (1988). Sex differences in the prevalence of psychiatric disorders in patients with alcohol and drug problems. *British Journal of Addictions, 83*, 1179–1192.

Rounsaville, B. J., Anton, S. F., Carroll, K., Budde, D., Prusoff, B. A., & Gawin, F. (1991). Psychiatric diagnoses of treatment-seeking cocaine abusers. *Archives of General Psychiatry, 48*, 43–51.

Rounsaville, B. J., Weissman, M. M., Kleber, H., & Wilber, C. (1982). Heterogeneity of psychiatric diagnosis in treated opiate addicts. *Archives of General Psychiatry, 39*, 161–166.

Schuckit, M. A., Tipp, J. E., Bergman, M., Reich, W., Hesselbrock, V. M., & Smith, T. L. (1997). Comparison of induced and independent major depressive disorder in 2,945 alcoholics. *American Journal of Psychiatry, 154*, 948–957.

Schuckit, M. A., Tipp, J. E., Bucholz, K. K., Nurnberger, J. I., Jr., Hesselbrock, V. M., Crowe, R. R., et al. (1997). The life-time rates of three major mood disorders and four major anxiety disorders in alcoholics and controls. *Addiction, 92*, 1289–1304.

Spitzer, R. L., Endicott, J., & Robins, E. (1978). Research diagnostic criteria: Rationale and reliability. *Archives of General Psychiatry, 35*, 773–782.

Swendsen, J. D., Merikangas, K. R., Canino, G. J., Kessler, R. C., Rubio-Stipec, M., & Angst, J. (1998). The comorbidity of alcoholism with anxiety and depressive disorders in four geographic communities. *Comprehensive Psychiatry, 39*, 176–184.

Teesson, M., Baillie, A., Lynskey, M., Manor, B., & Degenhardt, L. (2006). Substance use, dependence, and treatment seeking in the United States and Australia: A cross-national comparison. *Drug and Alcohol Dependence, 81*, 149–155.

Tómasson, K., & Vaglum, P. (1998). The role of psychiatric comorbidity in the prediction of readmission for detoxification. *Comprehensive Psychiatry, 39*, 129–136.

Vrasti, R., Grant, B. F., Chatterji, S., Üstün, B. T., Mager, D., Olteanu, I., et al. (1998). The reliability of the Romanian version of the alcohol module of the WHO Alcohol Use Disorder and Associated Disabilities Interview Schedule—Alcohol/Drug—Revised (AUDADIS-ADR). *European Addiction Research, 4*, 144–149.

Wang, P. S., Berglund, P., Olfson, M., Pincus, H. A., Wells, K. B., & Kessler, R. C. (2005). Failure and delay in initial treatment contact after first onset of mental disorders in the National Comorbidity Survey Replication. *Archives of General Psychiatry, 62*, 603–613.

Weisman, C. (1994). Women's use of health care. In M. Falik & K. S. Collins (Eds.), *Women's health: The Commonwealth Fund Survey* (pp. 19–48). Baltimore, MD: Johns Hopkins University Press.

Weisner, C., Greenfield, T., & Room, R. (1995). Trends in the treatment of alcohol problems in the U.S. general population, 1979 through 1990. *American Journal of Public Health, 85*, 55–60.

Weisner, C., Ray, G. T., Mertens, J. R., Satre, D. D., & Moore, C. (2003). Short-term alcohol and drug treatment outcomes predict long-term outcome. *Drug and Alcohol Dependence, 71*, 281–294.

Weisner, C., & Schmidt, L. (1992). Gender disparities in treatment for alcohol problems. *Journal of the American Medical Association, 268*, 1872–1876.

CHAPTER 11

Depression and Substance Use Disorders in Women

Helen M. Pettinati, PhD
Jennifer G. Plebani, PhD

Individuals with co-occurring depression and substance use disorders (SUDs) are complicated to treat. The focus of this chapter is on co-occurring mood disorders and SUDs in women. However, we contrast what we know about differences between women and men throughout the chapter in order to accurately portray women with both mood and substance use disorders. We first discuss the scope of the problem of co-occurring depression and substance use, including the historical and contemporary distinction between primary and secondary depression. We then target substance use comorbidity in relation to varying drugs of abuse and co-occurring problems. Next we address treatment options for patients with co-occurring disorders and the implications for recovery. This chapter closes with a discussion of relapse, followed by some suggestions for future research into the co-occurrence of depression and substance use among women.

SCOPE OF THE PROBLEM

Mood disorders, including major depression, bipolar disorder, and dysthymia, occur in approximately 10% of the general population in the United States (National Institute of Mental Health [NIMH], 2007). In addition, up to 50% of adults with a mood disorder have a co-occurring SUD (Wetherington, 2004). With respect to alcohol and drug disorders, recent data find that close to 10% of the general population with an alcohol or drug use disorder will also have a mood disorder. Further, among those who seek treatment for alcohol or drug use, approximately 35–55% will also have a mood disorder (Wetherington, 2004).

Twin studies reveal strong correlations between major depression and alcohol use disorders ($r = .33$) and between major depression and substance use disorders among women ($r = .29$). These correlations are similar to those for men (r's = .35 and .25, respectively) (Kendler, Prescott, Myers, & Neale, 2003). The prevalence rate for major depression among men and women with a 12-month substance use disorder is 14.5%, compared to 6.3% for those respondents without a 12-month substance use disorder (Grant et al., 2004). For both groups with and without a 12-month history, the major depression prevalence rates exclude substance-induced depression. In addition, the odds of having major depression are increased for individuals with an SUD as compared to those without.

Using the data from the Wave 1 of the National Epidemiologic Survey on Alcohol and Related Conditions (NESARC), Grant and colleagues (2004) showed that the odds ratios (ORs) for independent (as opposed to substance-induced) major depression in the general population among those with any substance dependence were 4.1, 3.7, and 9.0, respectively. That the likelihood of having major depression is at least fourfold higher for individuals dependent on any drug or alcohol than for those without suggests that a large number of those with an SUD also have co-occurring major depression. This is borne out in the NESARC data, which show that among past-12-month treatment seekers with an alcohol use disorder, 32.8% had major depression, as did 44.3% of past-12-month treatment seekers with any substance use disorder (Grant et al., 2004).

PRIMARY VERSUS SECONDARY DEPRESSION

The relationship between depression and SUDs is not straightforward for either men or women, with some individuals manifesting depression prior to the development of an SUD (typically called primary depression), and others developing depression as a consequence of chronic drug and/or alcohol use (secondary depression). A third group of individuals develop depression and an SUD concurrently. Substance-induced mood disorders (secondary depression) are the most common psychiatric diagnoses among treatment-seeking individuals with SUDs (Rounsaville, Dolinsky, Babor, & Meyer, 1987).

Generally it has been thought that identifying the etiology of depression in substance-dependent patients is important for determining the best treatment approach (Schuckit, 1985). For example, if the depression is primary, treatment with antidepressant medication has been a common practice (Galanter & Kleber, 1999; Kranzler, Mason, & Modesto-Lowe, 1998; Meyer, 1989). If the depression is secondary, that is, a direct result of substance use, then depressive symptoms are expected to dissipate spontaneously with abstinence, and antidepressant pharmacotherapy may be unnecessary, costly, and burdensome to the patient (Galanter & Kleber, 1999). Clinicians can pursue one or more of several strategies to determine whether a patient's depression is primary or secondary. For example, a family history of, or the presence of risk factors for, depression can be a signal that the patient's major depression is of a primary nature. In addition, clinicians may create a timeline while discussing personal history with the patient, mapping evidence of depression during periods of abstinence, or of a temporal, sequential occurrence of depression preceding substance use—all for the purpose of identifying whether the patient has primary or secondary depression.

The rates of secondary depression among people with alcohol dependence, as reported in the extant literature, vary widely from 10 to 53%, whereas the rates of primary depression appear much less variable, ranging from 2 to 16% (Bronisch, 1990). The variation found in rates of primary and secondary depression is likely the result of differences in patient samples, including sex, in diagnostic criteria, and in the choice of psychiatric assessments used to classify the disorders. Nonetheless, it is difficult to make the differential diagnosis. Table 11.1 lists the symptoms of major depression versus those associated with substance-induced depression, as identified by the text revision of the fourth edition of the *Diagnostic and Statistical Manual of Mental Disorders* (DSM-IV; American Psychiatric Association, 2000). The similarity in symptoms across the two categorical diagnoses illustrates that by applying these criteria alone, there is low confidence in determining whether a patient has a primary or a secondary diagnosis of depression.

TABLE 11.1. Comparison of DSM-IV-TR Symptoms for Major Depressive Disorder versus Substance-Induced Mood Disorder

Major depressive disorder	Substance-induced mood disorder
• Depressed mood	• Depressed mood
• Significantly reduced interest or pleasure in most or all activities	• Significantly reduced interest or pleasure in most or all activities
• Symptoms cause great distress or difficulty in functioning at home, work, or other important areas	• Symptoms cause great distress of difficulty in functioning at home, work, or other important areas
• Fatigue or lack of energy	• Symptoms occur during (or within 4 weeks of) intoxication or withdrawal
• Sleeping too much or too little	
• Change in appetite or weight	
• Trouble concentrating	
• Restlessness	
• Feeling of worthlessness or inappropriate guilt	
• Trouble making decisions	

Note. Data from American Psychiatric Association (2000).

While these differential patterns of determining the etiology of depression are of continued interest in fully characterizing a patient's profile, in recent times using the determination of primary or secondary depression to propose treatment has been questioned. For example, the persistence of depressive symptoms during abstinence is still possible with secondary depression, especially in cases where more permanent drinking-related consequences cannot be reversed (e.g., harm to others that resulted in permanent disability or a death). Also, at least one empirical study has demonstrated an advantage of desipramine over placebo in reducing depressive symptoms in treating secondary depression in patients with alcohol dependence (Mason, Kocsis, Ritvo, & Cutler, 1996; see also Mason & Kocsis, 1991). Finally, Greenfield and colleagues (1998) reported that not treating depression, whether it is primary or secondary, predicted worse treatment outcomes.

DIFFERENTIAL PATTERNS AND PREVALENCE OF CO-OCCURRENCE OF DEPRESSION AND SUDs AMONG MEN VERSUS WOMEN

Prior research has shown that the patterns of co-occurring SUDs and mood disorders differ between men and women. Epidemiological data indicate that women have almost twice the prevalence rate of major depression as do men (20.9 vs. 11.8%, respectively), and that women have a slightly higher odds ratio of having a mood disorder with an SUD than do men (Conway, Compton, Stinson, & Grant, 2006). In addition, data from large-scale studies, such as the Collaborative Study on the Genetics of Alcoholism (Schuckit et al., 1997), have found almost twice as many patients in the secondary as in the primary depression categories (26.4 vs. 15.2%). Interestingly, when examining the data by sex, approximately equal numbers of women have primary and secondary depression (24.7 vs. 24.2%), whereas men have over twice the rate of secondary as they do primary depression (27.4 vs. 10.8%). These data suggest that women may be more likely to "self-medicate" primary depression, whereas men may be more likely to develop depression subsequent to alcohol dependence.

Grant, Hasin, and Dawson (1996) found that primary and secondary depression rates were almost equivalent in a population-based sample (41.0 and 42.5%, respectively).

Although these rates are considerably higher than those found for women by Schuckit et al. (1997), they are similar in that primary and secondary depression rates are comparable; that is, secondary depression rates are not notably higher than primary rates. Epidemiological data on primary versus secondary depression among those with alcohol use disorders reveals that women have higher rates of primary depression and men have higher rates of secondary and concurrent depression, but these differences are not significant (Hanna & Grant, 1997). In contrast, the same data show that women have significantly higher rates of major depression alone (73 vs. 27% for men), whereas men have significantly higher rates of alcohol use disorders alone (65 vs. 35% for women).

Adding to difficulties in identifying correct diagnoses and accurate symptoms, it has also been widely reported that men and women with alcohol dependence exhibit significantly higher Beck Depression Inventory (Beck, Ward, Mendelson, Mock, & Erbaugh, 1961) scores than population norms (18.0, 25.3, and > 9, respectively) (Foster, Peters, & Marshall, 2000). In addition, women seem to develop depressive symptoms prior to developing heavy or problematic drinking (Helzer & Pryzbeck, 1988; Hesselbrock, Meyer, & Keener, 1985; Wilsnack, Klassen, & Wilsnack, 1986). Epidemiological examination of the relationship between depressive history and development of heavy drinking reveals that in women, but not in men, depression predicts subsequent alcohol problems (Moscato et al., 1997). In a study by Moscato and colleagues (1997), data were collected at three time points (1986, 1989, 1993). The OR for developing alcohol problems among women with preexisting depressive symptoms was greatest for Times 1 to 2 (OR = 7.38, 95% confidence interval [CI] = 2.63–20.72), and was significant as well from Times 2 to 3 (OR = 3.17, 95% CI = 1.38–7.31), and from Times 1 to 3 (OR = 4.24, 95% CI = 1.73–10.37). In contrast, alcohol problems were not predictive of subsequent depressive symptoms in women. For men, alcohol problems did not predict subsequent depression, and depression did not predict subsequent alcohol problems.

Data from the Epidemiologic Catchment Area community survey revealed that the odds of developing major depression associated with low, medium, and high levels of alcohol-dependent symptoms were 1.66, 3.98, and 4.32 for women ($p < .001$), and 1.1.9, 2.49, and 2.12 for males ($p = .026$) (Gilman & Abraham, 2001). In contrast, within low, medium, and high baseline depression levels, the 1-year ORs for risk of developing alcohol dependence were 2.75, 3.52, and 7.88 for women and 1.50, 1.41, and 1.05 for men. Data from only the Baltimore cohort of that study revealed a heavy drinking risk 2.6 times greater for women with a history of depressive disorder than for those with no depressive history, and a higher frequency of depressive symptoms elevated the risk for heavy alcohol use (Dixit & Crum, 2000).

Within the primary, secondary, and concurrent depression groups, women were significantly more likely to endorse weight/appetite changes, fatigue, and suicidal ideation/plans/attempts than were men. Within the major depression groups only, women were more likely to endorse weight/appetite changes and fatigue than were men, but there were no differences in the endorsement of suicide-related behaviors. This finding suggests that co-occurring alcohol dependence among depressed women may place them at higher risk for suicidality, solely due to concomitant increases in substance use disorders (Compton, Conway, Stinson, & Grant, 2006).

It has also been reported that women and men with substance dependence exhibit different patterns of co-occurring psychiatric disorders. For example, women with an SUD are more likely to report multiple psychiatric symptoms (e.g., depression and anxiety) than are men (Castel, Rush, Urbanoski, & Toneatto, 2006). In addition, the majority of men (78.3%) and women (86.0%) with a history of alcohol dependence also meet criteria for a psychiatric disorder other than depression (Kessler et al., 1997). One disorder that is commonly seen to co-occur with substance use disorders is posttraumatic stress disorder (PTSD), which often develops along with depressive symptoms in victims of abuse and trauma. A DSM-IV diagnosis of PTSD has a prevalence rate of approximately 8% in the general population, whereas among adolescents with drug dependence, rates climb to 45% for females and 24% for males (Kessler, Sonnega, Bromet, Hughes, & Nelson, 1995). Regardless of sex, higher rates of psychiatric symptoms were correlated with multiple problem substances (cocaine, alcohol, and cannabis) in that study.

One of the problems with reports of prevalence rates and development patterns for co-occurring depression and substance dependence is that data tend to be gathered retrospectively via patient self-report, which adds a potential confound in attempts to elucidate the relationship between the two disorders. Prospective studies reveal that the risk for heavy drinking in women with depressive histories is 2.6 times greater than in women with no history of depressive disorder (Dixit & Crum, 2000). In addition, that study found that a higher frequency of depressive disorders slightly elevated the risk for heavy alcohol use (relative risk = 1.09).

In summary, rates of major depression appear to be rising, suggesting that there will be an increased need for services in the near future for those with depression alone and for those with comorbid depression and SUDs. In a comparative study of the National Longitudinal Alcohol Epidemiologic Survey (NLAES), gathered in 1991–1992, and the National Epidemiologic Survey on Alcohol and Related Conditions (NESARC), gathered in 2001–2002, Compton and colleagues (2006) found that major depression rates for men and women appear to be rising, and that these increases cannot be explained solely by concomitant increases in SUDs.

THE ROLE OF "TELESCOPING" IN TREATMENT-SEEKING WOMEN

Progression from initiation of substance use to an SUD occurs more rapidly in individuals with depression (Rao et al., 1999) and has been specifically discussed in the context of women and alcohol dependence. Referred to as "telescoping" (Hernandez-Avila, Rounsaville, & Kranzler, 2004; Piazza, Vrbka, & Yeager, 1989), the term was defined initially to describe the more rapid progression of women with alcohol dependence to the more serious medical and social consequences, in spite of lower levels of use for shorter durations than men (Piazza et al., 1989). This phenomenon has been also documented among women who abuse substances other than alcohol (Hernandez-Avila et al., 2004). In particular, women were more likely than men to show significantly fewer years between regular use and treatment entry for opioids, cannabis, and alcohol drinking.

SPECIFIC DRUGS OF ABUSE AND DEPRESSION

Below we discuss sex differences in the interaction between specific drugs of abuse—alcohol, nicotine, cocaine, opiates, marijuana, and inhalants—and depressive symptoms.

Alcohol

More women than men have co-occurring mood and alcohol use disorders. Women with co-occurring mood and alcohol use disorders also report higher lifetime rates of physical, sexual, and emotional abuse (Pettinati, Rukstalis, Luck, Volpicelli, & O'Brien, 2000). Those same women were found to drink more frequently prior to treatment entry, as compared to men, although they drank fewer drinks per drinking day than did men. Mann, Hintz, and Jung (2004) found that 65% of female but only 28% of male patients with alcohol dependence had a lifetime history of psychiatric disorders other than alcohol dependence, with women having higher rates of mood and anxiety disorders.

Hanna and Grant (1997) examined the NLAES data to determine if there were any sex differences among individuals with major depressive disorder, alcohol use disorder, or both. Looking at data from 42,862 adult respondents, they derived five categories for respondents of interest: major depressive disorder alone, alcohol use disorder alone, and primary, secondary, and concurrent depression. When examining patterns in primary and secondary depression in men and women with alcohol use disorders, Hanna and Grant found that women had a higher rate of primary depression, whereas men had a higher rate of secondary depression, and the two groups had approximately equal rates of concurrent (no primary or secondary) depression (Hanna & Grant, 1997). In addition, they found that men had higher rates of alcohol use disorders alone, whereas women had higher rates of major depressive disorders (without a substance use disorder).

In characterizing men and women with primary and secondary depression, those with secondary depression were more likely to be older, married, and to have higher socioeconomic status than those with primary depression. In contrast, those with primary depression were more likely to have achieved at least a high school education than those with secondary depression. Those men whose depression appeared to have initiated concurrently with their SUD reported demographic profiles with variable values that fell between primary and secondary depressives on age, proportion married, and percent with a high school education. Among men with alcohol dependence, those with concurrently initiated depression had the lowest socio-economic status in all three types of depression, versus those having never had depression, whereas among women with alcohol dependence, those with concurrently initiated depression reported demographic values (e.g., age, proportion married, and percent with a high school education) that fell between those individuals with primary and secondary depression (Hanna & Grant, 1997).

Among women with alcohol dependence, those with concurrently initiated depression reported the highest levels of daily drinking, followed by those with secondary and then primary depression. Among men with alcohol dependence, those with secondary depression had the highest rates of daily alcohol intake, followed by concurrently initiated and then primary depression. Among both men and women with alcohol dependence, primary, concurrent, and secondary depression onsets were reported at approximate ages of 17, 22, and 26, whereas onsets of alcohol use disorders were reported at approximate ages of 24, 22, and 20 years. In individuals with alcohol dependence and primary or secondary depression, it appears that there is about 6 years between development of one disorder and development of the other. Individuals with major depressive disorder and an alcohol use disorder have nearly twice the rate of lifetime SUDs as do those without concurrent depressive illness, and women with a major depressive disorder and an alcohol use disorder have over five times the rate of lifetime SUDs as do those with only a major depressive disorder. For men with an alcohol use disorder and a major depressive disorder, the rate of lifetime SUDs is almost four times that of men with only an alcohol use disorder. This rate is slightly lower than the rate of lifetime SUDs for women with co-occurring alcohol and mood disorders, and it suggests that depression was more likely to precipitate other drug use among women with alcohol dependence than among men with alcohol dependence (Hanna & Grant, 1997).

Nicotine

People who smoke are more likely to have co-occurring depression than people who do not smoke (Glassman et al., 1990). In addition, depression among individuals with nicotine dependence is a major risk factor for nicotine cessation treatment failure (Anda et al., 1990; Glassman et al., 1988), as well as for posttreatment relapse (Shiffman, 1982). It is possible that there is a biological link between depression and nicotine dependence, as nicotine exerts both direct and indirect effects on the neurotransmitter systems implicated in depression (Hall, Muñoz, Reus, & Sees, 1993). Those who smoke and have a history of major depression are smoke more heavily (Breslau, Kilbey, & Andreski, 1991) and experience more nicotine withdrawal symptoms during cessation attempts (Breslau, Kilbey, & Andreski, 1992; Covey, Glassman, Stetner, & Becker, 1993). Other large-scale studies of the relationship between smoking and depression reveal that individuals with depression are more likely to continue smoking and to smoke with greater intensity than are nondepressed individuals (Friedman, 1996). Individuals with nicotine dependence are also significantly more likely to have alcohol-induced depression than are individuals without current or prior nicotine dependence (Daeppen et al., 2000).

Epidemiological data demonstrate that African American women who smoke have the highest number of depression symptoms (Center for Epidemiologic Studies Depression Scale [CES-D] scores), meaning that they report more depressive symptoms than do European American women or men of either race, regardless of smoking status (Son, Markovitz, Winders, & Smith, 1997). However, further research is needed to evaluate the interrelationship among sex, depression, and nicotine dependence.

Other Drugs of Abuse

Cocaine

Women who present for cocaine treatment typically have significantly higher Beck Depression Inventory (BDI) scores than do with cocaine dependence men, although their depression scores at 6-, 9-, and 12-month posttreatment follow-up are slightly lower than those of men (Wong, Badger, Sigmon, & Higgins, 2002). In another study, among non-treatment-seeking individuals with cocaine abuse, women reported significantly higher total craving scores, more depressive symptoms, and higher family and social problem severity than did men (Elman, Karlsgodt, & Gastfriend, 2001). Although differential sex data are limited, these findings suggest that treatment-seeking women with cocaine dependence have higher severity and greater depression symptom severity than a comparable group of men.

It is unclear whether depression increases cocaine craving, particularly in women. Studies conducted with individuals who have cocaine dependence without comorbid depression found either no difference in outcomes for men and women (Wong et al., 2002) or better outcomes for women than for men (McKay et al., 1996). However, such studies are not focused on outcomes for patients with comorbid depression and cocaine dependence. As such, additional research is required to examine the role of sex differences in treatment outcomes for patients with depression and cocaine dependence.

Opiates

Similar to the findings for cocaine dependence, women with opiate dependence have higher rates of depression. Indeed, depression prevalence among women with opiate dependence was found to be over three times that of men with opiate dependence (28.1 vs. 8.9%). In the same women, suicide attempts were 10 times greater than in their male counterparts (46.9 vs. 4.1 lifetime suicide attempts) (Chiang et al., 2007).

In another study of depression among patients with opiate dependence on methadone maintenance, females had more severe depression scores on the Hamilton Depression Rating Scale than did males (17.6 ± 7 vs. 14.1 ± 7.9, $p = .03$). A subset of women in that study, who were admitted to treatment during pregnancy, had especially high depression scores (20.2 ± 4.1) as compared to nonpregnant women (16.5 ± 7) (Peles et al., 2007). Additional research is required to more fully examine the role of sex differences in treatment outcomes for patients with depression and opiate dependence.

Marijuana

Past-year marijuana use appears to increase the risk for developing depression by about 10% (Harder, Morral, & Arkes, 2006). Other research finds that past-year and lifetime users of marijuana have significantly higher Beck Depression Inventory scores than do individuals with other drug use histories, suggesting a relationship between marijuana and depression (Medina & Shear, 2007). In addition, marijuana use has been associated with suicide attempts (Lynskey et al., 2004) and suicidal behaviors (Fergusson, Horwood, & Swain-Campbell, 2002), which suggests that thorough assessment for mood disorders and suicidal ideation would be appropriate among patients presenting for marijuana treatment. To date, there appears to be no literature specifically addressing sex differences in co-occurring depression and marijuana dependence.

Inhalants

Among users of inhalants, women have higher rates of mood, anxiety, and personality disorders (Wu & Howard, 2007). In addition, users of inhalants have a mood disorder prevalence rate that is almost five times the national average (48 vs. 9.5%, respectively). Within that group, females have a higher prevalence of dysthymia and multiple mood disorders as compared to males (Wu & Howard, 2007). Additional research is required to more fully examine the role of sex differences in treatment outcomes for patients with depression who use inhalants.

TREATMENT OF WOMEN WITH COMORBID DEPRESSION AND SUDs

Where Do Women Present for Treatment?

Women with SUDs often ascribe their drinking or substance use to depression or other problems and are therefore more likely to seek treatment in mental health or general medical settings than in an alcohol or drug treatment facility (Weisner & Schmidt, 1992). A recent review of substance use treatment outcomes in women showed that sex itself was not a significant predictor of treatment retention or outcome (Greenfield et al., 2007). However, that review did demonstrate that there are sex-specific predictors of poorer outcomes, and those predictors include comorbid mood disorders among women.

Treatment Types

Pharmacotherapy

It is typical in clinical practice for patients with depression and an alcohol disorder to be treated either with an antidepressant or counseling or sometimes both. There are relatively few single-site studies of antidepressant pharmacotherapy for the treatment of co-occurring substance dependence and depression (see reviews by Nunes & Levin, 2004; Pettinati, 2004), and only one multisite study of the use of sertraline for comorbid alcohol dependence and major depression (Kranzler et al., 2006). In the multisite study, depressive symptoms and alcohol consumption decreased from pretreatment levels in both the sertraline and placebo groups, with no statistical advantage found for sertraline over placebo. In a review of the smaller single-site antidepressant treatment studies for co-occurring depression and alcohol dependence, antidepressant treatment produced mixed results in its ability to improve mood and/or alcohol dependence (Pettinati, 2004). In the eight studies reviewed, all conducted between 1994 and 2004, only two reported positive outcomes for both drinking and depression. In results taken from a larger placebo-controlled trial, Mason and colleagues (1996) found that 200 mg of desipramine over 24 weeks decreased drinking and improved mood in a subgroup of 28 patients with current depressive disorder. Cornelius and colleagues (1997) found similar positive outcomes for 51 patients enrolled in a trial in which 20–40 mg of fluoxetine over 12 weeks was compared to placebo. By way of contrast, in the three studies that treated patients with 200 mg/day sertraline, Roy (1998) and Moak and colleagues (2003) found a reduction in depression among women only, but no reduction of alcohol use in either males or females, whereas Pettinati and colleagues (2001) found no effect for 200 mg/day sertraline of either reducing depression or alcohol use. In the two studies of nefazodone treatment, one reported a reduction in depression but not alcohol use (Roy-Byrne et al., 2000), whereas the other found a reduction in alcohol use but not depression (Hernandez-Avila et al., 2004). The eighth study, of imipramine, reported a reduction in depressive symptoms but not alcohol use (McGrath et al., 1996). All studies used medication dosages higher than those typically used to treat depression alone.

A meta-analysis of the effect of antidepressants on depression and SUDs, which included a total of 29 double-blind, placebo-controlled studies of patients with both depression and substance use, found that antidepressants other than selective serotonin reuptake inhibitors (SSRIs) had better effects on reducing alcohol or drug use and depressive symptoms for patients with both (Torrens, Fonecsa, Mateu, & Farré, 2005). The same analysis found similar results for patients dependent on alcohol, cocaine, or opioids, and for patients with nicotine dependence with and without depressive histories.

A second meta-analysis of depression treatment among patients with alcohol and drug dependence found that studies with a higher proportion of women ($\geq 40\%$) had significantly smaller effect sizes ($d = 0.20$) than did those with smaller proportions of women ($< 40\%$) ($d = 0.58$, $p = .02$) (Nunes & Levin, 2004). In that meta-analysis, 3 of the 14 trials were comprised of all men and may have skewed the results of the analysis, as those three studies had large effects.

Focusing further on potential sex differences, one of the single-site studies of sertraline for alcohol dependence found that sertraline was more effective than placebo for reducing drinking, but this result was found only among nondepressed patients with no history of (lifetime) depression (Pettinati et al., 2001), and positive outcomes were more likely to occur in women than in men (Pettinati, Dundon, & Lipkin, 2004). It is important to note that patients in that study who were either currently depressed or had lifetime depression did not respond better to sertraline than placebo with regard to reducing depressive symptoms or amount of drinking. A subsequent single-site, double-blind study of sertraline for patients with depression and alcohol dependence found an association between sertraline and reduction of depressive symptoms in women with depression but not in men with alcohol dependence (Moak et al., 2003).

Another study found that antidepressant use was associated with a reduction in drinking by men with depression and alcohol dependence, but was actually related to increased drinking in women with depression and alcohol dependence (Graham & Massak, 2007). Thus this study's results suggest that women with alcohol dependence may increase their drinking in response to certain types of antidepressant therapy.

Of note, little work has been done, to date, to ascertain the effect of other types of pharmacotherapies (i.e., other than antidepressants) on mood and drinking in the comorbid patient population. However, more recently, systematic work (with mixed results) has investigated the treatment of patients with depression and alcohol dependence with a two-pronged medication approach: one for alcohol dependence (e.g., naltrexone) and an antidepressant (for the depression see Oslin, 2005; Pettinati et al., 2007; Salloum, 2007).

Behavioral Treatments

Cognitive-behavioral therapy (CBT) has also shown some efficacy for treating co-occurring substance use and depression when used in conjunction with antidepressant medications (Hesse, 2004). A study of the impact of behavioral counseling and CBT on smoking cessation among individuals with a history of alcohol dependence revealed that those with depressive symptoms had better posttreatment abstinence rates if they had received CBT, whereas those without depressive symptoms fared better with behavioral counseling (Patten, Drews, Myers, Martin, & Wolter, 2002). Sex differences had no significant effect on outcome for either treatment group.

Mixed- versus Women-Only Treatment

Women with comorbid depression and drug or alcohol disorders often have an option to attend either single- or mixed-sex treatment. In two independent studies those in both types of treatment had approximately equivalent Beck Depression Inventory scores and Coopersmith Self-Esteem Inventory scores (Mikesell, Calhoun, & Lottman, 1970), although women who choose to attend women-only treatment had slightly higher depression scores (23 vs. 21, with a score of 19 being the lower cutoff for severe depression), slightly lower self-esteem scores (27 vs. 33, with a score of 70 being a normative score for women), and higher rates of suicide attempts (53 vs. 43%) (Copeland & Hall, 1992). Women-only programs often provide prenatal care and child care and focus on issues more relevant to women (Ashley, Marsden, & Brady, 2003). This focus on parenting and sex-related issues seems to improve treatment outcomes. Women who were able to attend inpatient treatment in a therapeutic community with their children showed improvements in their depression (Schinka et al., 1999).

RELAPSE IN DEPRESSED WOMEN

There are data to suggest that co-occurring depression with alcohol dependence may result in higher relapse rates to drinking or depression, or in some cases lower relapse rates to drinking. However, although depression has often been linked to poorer outcomes among women with substance dependence, the evidence from studies has pointed only to the fact that men with major depression also have poorer drug-treatment outcomes as compared to men without major depression (Compton, Cottler, Jacobs, Ben-Abdallah, & Spitznagel, 2003). In contrast, women with substance dependence and comorbid mood disorders often have comparable treatment outcomes to women without them (cf. Hien, Cohen, Miele, Litt, & Capstick, 2004).

Loosen, Dew, and Prange (1990) found that patients with alcohol dependence and co-occurring depression who had been abstinent for over 2 years, relapsed to drinking after an average of 3.3 years, whereas it was almost 6.8 years abstinent until relapse to drinking in nondepressed patients. In contrast, comorbidity may have a protective effect. In another study, women without comorbid depression had almost twice the alcohol relapse rate of women with comorbid depression (55 vs. 28%, respectively), whereas men showed no difference (40.9 vs. 35.3%, comorbid and noncomorbid relapse rates, respectively) (Mann et al, 2004). In that study, the co-occurrence of major depression was associated with lower drinking intensity in both sexes, which may account in part for the lower relapse rates in women with comorbid depression in that study.

Changes in mood states such as depression are known to precipitate relapse to substance use (Litman, Stapleton, Oppenheim, Peleg, & Jackson, 1983; McKay et al., 2002). In women, such changes are due more often to interpersonal conflicts and social pressure, whereas in men, intrapersonal and interpersonal determinants appear to be equally responsible for relapse (Hodgins, el-Guebaly, & Armstrong, 1995). Needless to say, more research on differences in outcomes between men and women with substance use disorders and depression is needed.

FUTURE DIRECTIONS FOR RESEARCH

Too few studies have evaluated whether differences in pretreatment profiles for men and women affect treatment outcomes, especially with respect to sex-specific treatment responses to the varying types of treatment available to patients with co-occurring depression and substance dependence. Only a few retrospective analyses have attempted to evaluate sex differences in response to treatment. As such, studies comparing demographics, clinical characteristics, and treatment response between male and female patients with co-occurring depression and SUDs are sorely needed. To this end, new studies should be designed so that sex is part of the primary, rather than the secondary, analysis plan. Such studies would need to enroll sufficient women to constitute adequate sample sizes and power to provide the strongest data sets for analysis.

Importantly, preliminary findings from a few studies of a differential treatment response for mood, drinking, or both between men and women treated with certain pharmacological treatments require replication and extension in order to sort out predictable outcome differences due to sex (cf. Pettinati, Dundon, & Lipkin, 2004). Also, further work is needed to determine whether specific psychosocial treatments (e.g., integrated counseling or women-only programs) generate better outcomes for women with co-occurring disorders.

KEY POINTS

- Patients with co-occurring mood and SUDs are more complicated to treat, and there is little research available on sex differences in demographics, clinical presentation, and treatment outcomes.
- Women with an SUD are more likely to present with major depression and/or other Axis I psychiatric disorders than are their male counterparts.
- Women with an SUD are more likely to have primary than secondary depression, score

higher than men on the Beck Depression Inventory, and present with weight and lifetime abuse issues than are their male counterparts.
- Women with comorbid depression and SUDs appear to have a shorter trajectory between years of regular use, problem use, and seeking treatment—a phenomenon known as "telescoping."
- Preliminary findings derived from pharmacotherapy research trials and requiring replication suggest that women with depression and alcohol dependence may respond differentially to some medications than their male counterparts, either in improvement in mood, or reducing drinking, or both.
- CBT and other therapies that can be tailored to address both mood and substance use show better outcomes than nonspecific treatments. Similarly, women-only treatment programs often demonstrate better outcomes than mixed-sex treatment programs.
- In the future, comorbidity studies could better address the interaction of sex, substance dependence, and mood disorders by enrolling enough women for a primary sex-based analysis.

ACKNOWLEDGMENTS

Support for this work was provided in part by the National Institute on Alcohol Abuse and Alcoholism (Grant No. R01-AA09544) and the National Institute on Drug Abuse (Grant No. T32-DA-07241).

REFERENCES

Asterisks denote recommended readings.

American Psychiatric Association. (2000). *Diagnostic and statistical manual of mental disorders* (4th ed., text rev.). Washington, DC: Author.

Anda, R. F., Williamson, D. F., Escobedo, L. G., Mast, E. E., Giovino, G. A., & Remington, P. L. (1990). Depression and the dynamics of smoking: A national perspective. *Journal of the American Medical Association, 264*(12), 1541–1545.

Ashley, O. S., Marsden, M. E., & Brady, T. M. (2003). Effectiveness of substance abuse treatment programming for women: A review. *American Journal of Drug and Alcohol Abuse, 29*, 19–53.

Beck, A. T., Ward, C. H., Mendelson, M., Mock, J., & Erbaugh, J. (1961). An inventory for measuring depression. *Archives of General Psychiatry, 4*, 561–571.

Breslau, N., Kilbey, M., & Andreski, P. (1991). Nicotine dependence, major depression, and anxiety in young adults. *Archives of General Psychiatry, 48*(12), 1069–1074.

Breslau, N., Kilbey, M., & Andreski, P. (1992). Nicotine withdrawal symptoms and psychiatric disorders: Findings from an epidemiologic study of young adults. *American Journal of Psychiatry, 149*(4), 464–469.

Bronisch, T. (1990). Alcoholism and depression. *Progress in Alcohol Research, 2*, 69–99.

Castel, S., Rush, B., Urbanoski, K., & Toneatto, T. (2006). Overlap of clusters of psychiatric symptoms among clients of a comprehensive addiction treatment service. *Psychology of Addictive Behaviors, 20*(1), 28–35.

Chiang, S. C., Chan, H. Y., Chang, Y. Y., Sun, H. J., Chen, W. J., & Chen, C. K. (2007). Psychiatric comorbidity and gender difference among treatment-seeking heroin abusers in Taiwan. *Psychiatry and Clinical Neurosciences, 61*(1), 105–111.

Compton, W., Cottler, L. B., Jacobs, J. L., Ben-Abdallah, A., & Spitznagel, E. L. (2003). The role of psychiatric disorders in predicting drug dependence treatment outcomes. *American Journal of Psychiatry, 60*, 890–895.

Compton, W. M., Conway, K. P., Stinson, F. S., & Grant, B. F. (2006). Changes in the prevalence of major depression and comorbid substance use disorders in the United States between 1991–1992 and 2001–2002. *American Journal of Psychiatry*, *163*(12), 2141–2147.

Conway, K. P., Compton, W., Stinson, F. S., & Grant, B. F. (2006). Lifetime comorbidity of DSM-IV mood and anxiety disorders and specific drug use disorders: Results from the National Epidemiologic Survey on Alcohol and Related Conditions. *Journal of Clinical Psychiatry*, *67*(2), 247–257.

Copeland, J., & Hall, W. (1992). A comparison of women seeking drug and alcohol treatment in a specialist women's and two traditional mixed-sex treatment services. *British Journal of Addiction*, *87*, 1293–1302.

Cornelius, J. R., Salloum, I. M., Ehler, J. G., Jarrett, P. J., Cornelius, M. D., Perel, J. M., et al. (1997). Fluoxetine in depressed alcoholics: A double-blind, placebo controlled trial. *Archives of General Psychiatry*, *54*, 700–705.

Covey, L. S., Glassman, A. H., Stetner, F., & Becker, J. (1993). Effect of history of alcoholism or major depression on smoking cessation. *American Journal of Psychiatry*, *150*, 1546–1547.

Daeppen, J. B., Smith, T. L., Danko, G. P., Gordon, L., Landi, N. A., Nurnberger, J. I., Jr., et al. (2000). Clinical correlates of cigarette smoking and nicotine dependence in alcohol-dependent men and women: The Collaborative Study Group on the Genetics of Alcoholism. *Alcohol and Alcoholism*, *35*(2), 171–175.

Dixit, A. R., & Crum, R. M. (2000). Prospective study of depression and the risk of heavy alcohol use in women. *American Journal of Psychiatry*, *157*(5), 751–758.

Elman, I., Karlsgodt, K. H., & Gastfriend, D. R. (2001). Gender differences in cocaine craving among non-treatment-seeking individuals with cocaine dependence. *American Journal of Drug and Alcohol Abuse*, *27*(2), 193–202.

Fergusson, D. M., Horwood, L. J., & Swain-Campbell, N. (2002). Cannabis use and psychosocial adjustment in adolescence and young adulthood. *Addiction*, *97*(9), 1123–1135.

Foster, J. H., Peters, T. J., & Marshall, E. J. (2000). Quality of life measures and outcome in alcohol-dependent men and women. *Alcohol*, *22*(1), 45–52.

Friedman, G. D. (1996). Depression, smoking, and lung cancer. *American Journal of Epidemiology*, *144*(12), 1104–1106.

Galanter, M., & Kleber, H. D. (1999). *Textbook of substance abuse treatment* (2nd ed., pp. 157–158). Washington, DC: American Psychiatric Association.

Gilman, S. E., & Abraham, H. D. (2001). A longitudinal study of the order of onset of alcohol dependence and major depression. *Drug and Alcohol Dependence*, *63*(3), 277–286.

Glassman, A. H., Helzer, J. E., Covey, L. S., Cottler, L. B., Stetner, F., Tipp, J. E., et al. (1990). Smoking, smoking cessation, and major depression. *Journal of the American Medical Association*, *264*, 1546–1549.

Graham, K., & Massak, A. (2007). Alcohol consumption and the use of antidepressants. *Canadian Medical Association Journal*, *176*(5), 633–637.

Grant, B. F., Hasin, D. S., & Dawson, D. A. (1996). The relationship between DSM-IV alcohol use disorders and DSM-IV major depression: Examination of the primary–secondary distinction in a general population sample. *Journal of Affective Disorders*, *38*, 113–128.

Grant, B. F., Stinson, F. S., Dawson, D. A., Chou, S. P., Dufour, M. C., Compton, W., et al. (2004). Prevalence and co-occurrence of substance use disorders and independent mood and anxiety disorders: Results from the National Epidemiologic Survey on Alcohol and Related Conditions. *Archives of General Psychiatry*, *61*(8), 807–816.

Greenfield, S. F., Brooks, A. J., Gordon, S. M., Green, C. A., Kropp, F., McHugh, R. K., et al. (2007). Substance abuse treatment entry, retention, and outcome in women: A review of the literature. *Drug and Alcohol Dependence*, *86*, 1–21. (*)

Greenfield, S. F., Weiss, R. D., Muenz, L. R., Vagge, L. M., Kelly, J. F., Bello, L. R., et al. (1998). The effect of depression on return to drinking: A prospective study. *Archives of General Psychiatry*, *55*, 259–265.

Hall, S. M., Muñoz, R. F., Reus, V. I., & Sees, K. L. (1993). Nicotine, negative affect, and depression. *Journal of Consulting and Clinical Psychology*, *61*(5), 761–767.

Hanna, E. Z., & Grant, B. F. (1997). Gender differences in DSM-IV alcohol use disorders and major depression as distributed in the general population: Clinical implications. *Comprehensive Psychiatry, 38*(4), 202–212.

Harder, V. S., Morral, A. R., & Arkes, J. (2006). Marijuana use and depression among adults: Testing for causal associations. *Addiction, 101*(10), 1463–1472.

Helzer, J. E., & Pryzbeck, T. R. (1988). The co-occurrence of alcoholism and other psychiatric disorders in the general population and its impact on treatment. *Journal of Studies on Alcohol, 49,* 219–224.

Hernandez-Avila, C. A., Rounsaville, B. J., & Kranzler, H. R. (2004). Opioid-, cannabis-, and alcohol-dependent women show more rapid progression to substance abuse treatment. *Drug and Alcohol Dependence, 74,* 265–272.

Hesse, M. (2004). Achieving abstinence by treating depression in the presence of substance-use disorders. *Addictive Behaviors, 29*(6), 1137–1141.

Hesselbrock, M. H., Meyer, R. E., & Keener, J. J. (1985). Psychopathology in hospitalized alcoholics. *Archives of General Psychiatry, 42,* 1050–1055.

Hien, D. A., Cohen, L. R., Miele, G. M., Litt, L. C., & Capstick, C. (2004). Promising treatments for women with comorbid PTSD and substance use disorders. *American Journal of Psychiatry, 161,* 1426–1432.

Hodgins, D. C., el-Guebaly, N., & Armstrong, S. (1995). Prospective and retrospective reports of mood states before relapse to substance use. *Journal of Consulting and Clinical Psychology, 63*(3), 400–407.

Kendler, K. S., Prescott, C. A., Myers, J., & Neale, M. C. (2003). The structure of genetic and environmental risk factors for common psychiatric and substance use disorders in men and women. *Archives of General Psychiatry, 60*(9), 929–937.

Kessler, R. C., Crum, R. M., Warner, L. A., Nelson, C. B., Schulenberg, J., & Anthony, J. C. (1997). Lifetime co-occurrence of DSM-III-R alcohol abuse and dependence with other psychiatric disorders in the National Comorbidity Survey. *Archives of General Psychiatry, 54*(4), 313–321.

Kessler, R. C., Sonnega, A., Bromet, E., Hughes, M., & Nelson, C. B. (1995). Posttraumatic stress disorder in the National Comorbidity Survey. *Archives of General Psychiatry, 52*(12), 1048–1060.

Kranzler, H. R., Mason, B., & Modesto-Lowe, V. (1998). Prevalence, diagnosis, and treatment of comorbid mood disorders and alcoholism. In H. R. Kranzler & B. Rounsaville (Eds.), *Dual diagnosis and treatment* (pp. 107–136). New York: Marcel Dekker.

Kranzler, H. R., Mueller, T., Cornelius, J., Pettinati, H. M., Moak, D., Martin, P. R., et al. (2006). Sertraline treatment of co-occurring alcohol dependence and major depression. *Journal of Clinical Psychopharmacology, 26*(1), 13–20.

Litman, G. K., Stapleton, J., Oppenheim, A. N., Peleg, M., & Jackson, P. (1983). Situations related to alcoholism relapse. *British Journal of Addiction, 78*(4), 381–389.

Loosen, P. T., Dew, B. W., & Prange, A. J. (1990). Long-term predictors of outcome in abstinent alcoholic men. *American Journal of Psychiatry, 147*(12), 1662–1666.

Lynskey, M. T., Glowinski, A. L., Todorov, A. A., Bucholz, K. K., Madden, P. A., Nelson, E. C., et al. (2004). Major depressive disorder, suicidal ideation, and suicide attempt in twins discordant for cannabis dependence and early-onset cannabis use. *Archives of General Psychiatry, 61*(10), 1026–1032.

Mann, K., Hintz, T., & Jung, M. (2004). Does psychiatric comorbidity in alcohol dependent patients affect treatment outcome? *European Archives of Psychiatry and Clinical Neuroscience, 254*(3), 172–181.

Mason, B. J. (1996). Dosing issues in the pharmacotherapy of alcoholism. *Alcoholism: Clinical and Experimental Research, 20*(Suppl. 7), 10A–16A.

Mason, B. J., & Kocsis, J. H. (1991). Desipramine treatment of alcoholism. *Psychopharmacology Bulletin, 27,* 155–161.

Mason, B. J., Kocsis, J. H., Ritvo, E. C., & Cutler, R. B. (1996). A double-blind, placebo controlled trial of desipramine for primary alcohol dependence stratified on the presence or absence of major depression. *Journal of the American Medical Association, 275,* 761–767.

McGrath, P. J., Nunes, E. V., Stewart, J. W., Goldman, D., Agosti, V., Ocepek-Welikson, K., et al.

(1996). Imipramine treatment of alcoholics with primary depression: A placebo-controlled clinical trial. *Archives of General Psychiatry, 53*, 232–240.

McKay, J. R., Pettinati, H. M., Morrison, R., Feeley, M., Mulvaney, F. D., & Gallop, R. (2002). Relation of depression diagnoses to 2-year outcomes in cocaine-dependent patients in a randomized continuing care study. *Psychology of Addictive Behaviors, 16*(3), 225–235.

McKay, J. R., Rutherford, M. J., Cacciola, J. S., Kabasakalian-McKay, R., & Alterman, A. I. (1996). Gender differences in the relapse experiences of cocaine patients. *Journal of Nervous and Mental Disease, 184*(10), 616–622.

Medina, K. L., & Shear, P. K. (2007). Anxiety, depression, and behavioral symptoms of executive dysfunction in ecstasy users: Contributions of polydrug use. *Drug and Alcohol Dependence, 87*(2–3), 303–311.

Meyer, R. E. (1989). Prospects for a rational pharmacotherapy of alcoholism. *Journal of Clinical Psychiatry, 50*, 403–412.

Mikesell, R. H., Calhoun, L. G., & Lottman, T. J. (1970). Instructional set and the Coopersmith Self-Esteem Inventory. *Psychological Reports, 26*(1), 317–318.

Moak, D. H., Anton, R. F., Latham, P. K., Voronin, K. E., Waid, R. L., & Durazo-Arvizu, R. (2003). Sertraline and cognitive behavioral therapy for depressed alcoholics: Results of a placebo-controlled trial. *Journal of Clinical Psychopharmacology, 23*(6), 553–562.

Moscato, B. S., Russell, M., Zielezny, M., Bromet, E., Egri, G., Mudar, P., et al. (1997). Gender differences in the relation between depressive symptoms and alcohol problems: A longitudinal perspective. *American Journal of Epidemiology, 146*(11), 966–974.

National Institute of Mental Health. (2007). *The numbers count: Mental disorders in America.* Retrieved October 31, 2007, from *www.nimh.nih.gov/health/publications/the-numbers-count-mental-disorders-in-america.shtml#Eating.*

Nunes, E. V., & Levin, F. R. (2004). Treatment of depression in patients with alcohol or other drug dependence: A meta-analysis. *Journal of the American Medical Association, 291*(15), 1887–1896.

Oslin, D. W. (2005). Treatment of late-life depression complicated by alcohol dependence. *American Journal of Geriatric Psychiatry, 13*(6), 491–500.

Patten, C. A., Drews, A. A., Myers, M. G., Martin, J. E., & Wolter, T. D. (2002). Effect of depressive symptoms on smoking abstinence and treatment adherence among smokers with a history of alcohol dependence. *Psychology of Addictive Behaviors, 16*(2), 135–142.

Peles, E., Schreiber, S., Naumovsky, Y., & Adelson, M. (2007). Depression in methadone maintenance treatment patients: Rate and risk factors. *Journal of Affective Disorders, 99*(1–3), 213–220.

Pettinati, H. M. (2004). Antidepressant treatment of co-occurring depression and alcohol dependence. *Biological Psychiatry, 56*(10), 785–792.

Pettinati, H. M., Dundon, W. D., & Lipkin, C. (2004). Gender differences in response to sertraline pharmacotherapy in type A alcohol dependence. *American Journal on Addictions, 13*, 236–247.

Pettinati, H. M., Oslin, D. W., Lynch, K. G., Kampman, K. M., Dundon, W. D., & Gallis, T. (2007). Sertraline and naltrexone for alcohol dependence and depression. *Alcoholism: Clinical and Experimental Research, 31*, 271A, 90.

Pettinati, H. M., Rukstalis, M. R., Luck, G. J., Volpicelli, J. R., & O'Brien, C. P. (2000). Gender and psychiatric comorbidity: Impact on clinical presentation of alcohol dependence. *American Journal of the Addictions, 9*, 242–252.

Pettinati, H. M., Volpicelli, J. R., Luck, G., Kranzler, H., Rukstalis, M., & Cnaan, A. (2001). Double-blind clinical trial of sertraline treatment for alcohol dependence. *Journal of Clinical Psychopharmacology, 21*(2), 143–153.

Piazza, N. J., Vrbka, J. L., & Yeager, R. D. (1989). Telescoping of alcoholism in women alcoholics. *International Journal of the Addictions, 24*(1), 19–28.

Rao, U., Ryan, N. D., Dahl, R. E., Birmaher, B., Rao, R., Williamson, D. E., et al. (1999). Factors associated with the development of substance use disorder in depressed adolescents. *Journal of the American Academy of Child and Adolescent Psychiatry, 38*(9), 1109–1117.

Rounsaville, B. J., Dolinsky, Z. S., Babor, T. F., & Meyer, R. E. (1987). Psychopathology as a predictor of treatment outcome in alcoholics. *Archives of General Psychiatry, 44*, 505–513.

Roy, A. (1998). Placebo-controlled study of sertraline in depressed recently abstinent alcoholics. *Biological Psychiatry, 44,* 633–637.

Roy-Byrne, P. P., Pages, K. P., Russo, J. E., Jaffe, C., Blume, A. W., Kingsley, E., et al. (2000). Nefazodone treatment of major depression in alcohol-dependent patients: A double-blind, placebo-controlled trial. *Journal of Clinical Psychopharmacology, 20,* 129–136.

Salloum, I. M., Douaihy, A., Cornelius, J. R., Kirisci, L., Kelly, T. M., & Hayes, J. (2007). Divalproex utility in bipolar disorder with co-occurring cocaine dependence: A pilot study. *Addictive Behaviors, 32*(2), 410–415.

Schinka, J. A., Hughes, P. H., Coletti, S. D., Hamilton, N. L., Renard, C. G., Urmann, C. F., et al. (1999). Changes in personality characteristics in women treated in a therapeutic community. *Journal of Substance Abuse and Treatment, 16*(2), 137–142.

Schuckit, M. A. (1985). The clinical implications of primary diagnostic groups among alcoholics. *Archives of General Psychiatry, 42,* 1043–1049.

Schuckit, M. A., Tipp, J. E., Bergman, M., Reich, W., Hesselbrock, V. M., Smith, T. L., et al. (1997). Comparison of induced and independent major depressive disorders in 2,945 alcoholics. *American Journal of Psychiatry, 154*(7), 948–957.

Shiffman, S. (1982). Relapse following smoking cessation: A situational analysis. *Journal of Consulting and Clinical Psychology, 50*(1), 71–86.

Son, B. K., Markovitz, J. H., Winders, S., & Smith, D. (1997). Smoking, nicotine dependence, and depressive symptoms in the CARDIA Study: Effects of educational status. *American Journal of Epidemiology, 145*(2), 110–116.

Torrens, M., Fonseca, F., Mateu, G., & Farré, M. (2005). Efficacy of antidepressants in substance use disorders with and without comorbid depression: A systematic review and meta-analysis. *Drug and Alcohol Dependence, 78*(1), 1–22.

Weisner, C., & Schmidt, L. (1992). Gender disparities in treatment for alcohol problems. *Journal of the American Medical Association, 268*(14), 1872–1876.

Wetherington, C. L. (Chair). (2004, May 5). *Drug abuse treatment issues in women: Integrating the science of addiction into psychiatric practice.* Symposium conducted at the 157th annual meeting of the American Psychiatric Association, New York. (*)

Wilsnack, R. W., Klassen, A. D., & Wilsnack, S. C. (1986). Retrospective analysis of lifetime changes in women's drinking behavior. *Advances in Alcohol and Substance Abuse, 5*(3), 9–28.

Wong, C. J., Badger, G. J., Sigmon, S. C., & Higgins, S. T. (2002). Examining possible gender differences among cocaine-dependent outpatients. *Experimental and Clinical Psychopharmacology, 10*(3), 316–323.

Wu, L. T., & Howard, M. O. (2007). Psychiatric disorders in inhalant users: Results from The National Epidemiologic Survey on Alcohol and Related Conditions. *Drug and Alcohol Dependence, 88*(2–3), 146–155.

CHAPTER 12

Gender, Anxiety, and Substance Use Disorders

Kathleen T. Brady, MD, PhD
Karen Hartwell, MD

A number of studies suggests that anxiety disorders, symptoms of anxiety, and substance use disorders (SUDs) commonly co-occur. The interaction between these disorders and symptoms is not unidirectional but, rather, multifaceted and variable. Anxiety disorders may be a risk factor for the development of substance abuse and dependence. In addition, anxiety disorders are likely to modify the presentation and outcome of treatment for SUDs, just as substance use and SUDs are likely to modify the presentation and outcome of treatment for anxiety disorders. Anxiety symptoms also emerge during the course of chronic intoxication and withdrawal. Women appear to have a greater risk of co-occurring anxiety and SUDs, and the etiological relationship between anxiety and substance use may differ somewhat in men and women. In this chapter gender differences in the area of co-occurring SUDs and anxiety disorders are reviewed, including prevalence, diagnostic concerns, and treatment issues. This chapter focuses on panic disorder (PD), generalized anxiety disorder (GAD), social anxiety disorder (SAD), and obsessive–compulsive disorder (OCD). Posttraumatic stress disorder (PTSD) is covered in detail by Hien (Chapter 14, this volume).

EPIDEMIOLOGY

In order to put the prevalence estimates of gender differences in co-occurring SUDs and anxiety disorders in context, an understanding of gender differences in the general prevalence estimates for each independent category of disorders is important. A number of epidemiological studies conducted in the United States over the past 20 years has consistently demonstrated that anxiety disorders are approximately twice as common in women, as compared to men, with some variation in the gender differential for specific anxiety disorders. In the National Comorbidity Study (NCS; Kessler et al., 1994), women were more likely to meet lifetime criteria for PD (5.0 vs. 2.0%), GAD (6.6 vs. 3.6%), simple phobia (15.5 vs. 6.7%), and SAD (15.5 vs. 11.1%). The National Epidemiologic Survey on Alcohol and Related Conditions (NESARC) is the most recent and largest survey study focused on psychiatric disorders and SUDs, with a Wave 1 sample of more than 43,000 adults (Grant, Stinson, et al., 2004). In NESARC, approximately 20% of women and 11.7% of men had a lifetime anxiety disorder with a similar prevalence rate for specific disorders by gender as that found in the NCS (Conway, Compton, Stinson, & Grant, 2006).

In general, epidemiological studies consistently demonstrate that drug and alcohol use disorders are more commonly found in men, as compared to women (Conway et al., 2006; Kessler et al., 1994; Reiger et al., 1990). In NESARC, 12-month prevalence rates of alcohol abuse were almost three times higher in men, compared with women (6.9% men vs. 2.6% women; Grant, Stinson, et al., 2004), and men were twice as likely to meet lifetime DSM-IV criteria for any drug use disorder (13.8% men vs. 7.1% women; Conway et al., 2006). These findings are consistent with past epidemiological surveys in identifying a gender difference for alcohol use disorders as higher than that for drug use disorders (Grant et al., 1994; Kessler et al., 1994). In contrast, the rates of prescription drug abuse in women closely approach that of men. The National Survey on Drug Use and Health reported 12-month prevalence rates of nonmedical use of pain relievers to be 1.4% for males and 1.1% for females ages 18–25, and 0.5% for males and 0.4% for females ages 26 and older (Substance Abuse and Mental Health Services Administration [SAMHSA], 2006). Gender differences in tobacco use and dependence are also substantially less than for other substances of abuse, with only slightly more men than women reporting use of tobacco (13.5% men and 10.2% women) and meeting criteria for past 12-month nicotine dependence (14.1% men vs. 11.5% women; Grant, Hasin, Chou, Stinson, & Dawson, 2004; Steinberg, Akincigil, Delnevo, Crystal, & Carson, 2006). Of interest, a recent study that compared gender differences in alcohol use disorders in birth cohorts reaching adulthood since the 1970s found evidence that the gender gap is closing (Hasin, Stinson, Ogburn, & Grant, 2007). The gender gap in SUDs narrows in adolescents, and there are equal gender rates of illicit drug and alcohol use and greater use of cigarettes and nonmedical use of prescription drugs in girls (SAMSHA, 2006).

These studies also demonstrate that anxiety disorders and SUDs co-occur more commonly than would be expected by chance alone and that this relationship is stronger for women, as compared to men. NESARC was specifically designed to distinguish between independent (i.e., not attributed to withdrawal or intoxication) and substance-induced mood and anxiety disorders. Of respondents with an SUD in the past 12 months, 17.7% also met criteria for an independent anxiety disorder. Approximately 15% of those with any anxiety disorder in the past 12 months had at least one co-occurring SUD (Grant, Stinson, et al., 2004). The relationship between anxiety disorders and drug use disorders (odds ratio [OR] = 2.8) was stronger than the relationship between anxiety and alcohol use disorders (OR = 1.7). Hasin explored both 12-month and lifetime diagnoses using the NESARC data. For an alcohol use disorder, 12-month prevalence was 8.5% and lifetime prevalence was 30.3%. The OR of alcohol use disorders co-occurring with any anxiety disorder was 1.9 for 12-month diagnoses and 10.4 for lifetime diagnoses (Hasin et al., 2007). Associations between drug use disorders and specific anxiety disorders were virtually all significantly positive ($p < .05$). In general, the ORs were more positive for abuse, as compared to dependence, and more positive for women, compared with men, but few significant gender differences were seen. The association between any anxiety disorder and SAD and tranquilizer or opiate use disorders was more significant for women, whereas the relationship between PD and either tranquilizer or cocaine use disorder was more significant for men. Marijuana use disorders were the most common drug use disorder in individuals with anxiety disorders (15.1%), followed by cocaine (5.4%), amphetamine (4.8%), hallucinogen (3.7%), and sedative (2.6%) use disorders (Conway et al., 2006).

DRUG CLASS AND ANXIETY SYMPTOMS

The relationship between anxiety symptoms, anxiety disorders, and SUDs differs between drugs of different classes. The highly comorbid relationship between alcohol and anxiety has received more attention than any other SUD. This focus is probably attributable to the fact that alcohol is legal, readily available, and many individuals with anxiety report using it to relieve anxiety symptoms. However, the relationship between alcohol use and anxiety is complex and probably varies across anxiety disorders. The short-term relief of anxiety via alcohol use, in combination with long-term anxiety induction from chronic drinking and withdrawal, can initiate a feed-forward cycle of increasing anxiety symptoms and alcohol consumption (Kushner, Abrams, & Borchardt, 2000).

There is relatively little research on co-occurring anxiety disorders and cocaine, methamphetamine, and amphetamine use. These agents stimulate noradrenergic systems, and acute intoxication is often associated with anxiety. Because of these anxiogenic effects, it has been postulated that individuals who are vulnerable to anxiety may be less likely to abuse or become dependent on this class of drugs (de Wit, Uhlenhuth, & Johanson, 1986). When anxiety symptoms are reported in individuals with stimulant use disorders, careful attention to the time course of anxiety symptoms relative to stimulant use is critical.

In one large sample (n = 1,016) of individuals with methamphetamine dependence, women reported higher levels of anxiety than did men. Frequency of methamphetamine use was positively associated with severity of both general and phobic anxiety (Zweben et al., 2004). A study of incarcerated women found that methamphetamine was the most common form of drug dependence; about one-fourth of the sample had GAD, PD, or PTSD (Vik, 2007). In a sample of current amphetamine users, one-third of respondents reported that anxiety symptoms had preceded their initiation of amphetamine use. About two-thirds of the sample reported experiencing anxiety since initiation of amphetamines and at least one-half reported panic attacks (Vincent, Schoobridge, Ask, Allsop, & Ali, 1998).

The relationship between anxiety and nicotine use has received much recent attention. In NESARC, 28% of the participants used tobacco products and 25% currently smoked cigarettes. The 12-month prevalence rate of nicotine dependence was 13% in the general population and 25% among individuals with anxiety disorders. The risk of anxiety disorder among individuals with nicotine dependence was more than twice that of any other psychiatric disorder. Conversely, the prevalence rates of nicotine dependence were also increased in individuals with anxiety disorders (p. 40%, SAD 27%, and GAD 33%). No gender differential in these rates was reported (Grant, Hasin, et al., 2004). Despite the strong associations between smoking, nicotine dependence, and anxiety disorders, there has been relatively little investigation of causal connections or treatment. The Development and Assessment of Nicotine Dependence in Youth (DANDY) study followed a cohort of seventh graders for 3.5 years and found a strong association between trait anxiety and all measures of tobacco use and nicotine dependence. A relaxing effect from initial exposure to nicotine, distinct from relief of withdrawal symptoms, was predictive of a sixfold increase in risk for nicotine dependence. Again, no gender differential in this relationship was reported (DiFranza et al., 2004).

The relationship between marijuana and anxiety remains unclear. Some studies suggest that marijuana use increases the long-term risk of anxiety; others find that marijuana use results in acute anxiety symptoms during intoxication only, and that anxiety symptoms can develop as part of marijuana withdrawal (Raphael, Wooding, Stevens, & Connor, 2005). A recent review attempted to determine order of onset and potential causal relationships between marijuana use and anxiety through the examination of seven longitudinal, population-based studies (Moore et al., 2007). After controlling for confounding factors, there was little evidence to suggest that marijuana use predicted long-term anxiety or anxiety disorders, but it was associated with transient anxiety reactions. There were no gender differences reported. Studies suggest that the use of marijuana as a coping strategy may serve to enhance anxiety through an avoidance–anxiety cycle, and users who report coping motives for their use also use marijuana more often (Bonn-Miller, Zvolensky, Bernstein, & Stickle, 2007).

SEX AND THE NEUROBIOLOGY OF SUDs AND ANXIETY DISORDERS

Anxiety disorders have been conceptualized as chronic distress states associated with neurobiological *alterations* in brain stress circuits (McEwen, 2000; Nemeroff, 1996; Sapolsky, Alberts, & Altmann, 1997). On the other hand, chronic drug use is associated with *neuroadaptations* in brain reward pathways that produce secondary psychiatric symptoms, including anxiety, during acute and protracted withdrawal states (Markou, Kosten, & Koob, 1998). With increasing severity of addiction, neuroadaptations in stress and reward circuits may underlie the increasing emotional distress often associated with SUDs (Koob & Le Moal, 1997; Stewart, 2000). A growing body of evidence from basic science and clinical studies implicates common neurobiological pathways and abnormalities as involved in addiction and anxiety disorders. Animal studies have demonstrated that uncontrollable stress increases drug self-administration, and neurobiological correlates of stress appear to mediate this response (Stewart, 2000). Corticotropin-releasing factor (CRF), one of the key hormones involved in the stress response, has been implicated in the pathophysiology of anxiety and addictive disorders (Nemeroff, 1996; Sinha, 2001). In animal models, early life stress and chronic stress result in long-term changes in stress responses that can alter the sensitivity of the dopamine system to stress and increase susceptibility to self-administration of substances of abuse (Meaney et al., 1993; Shalev, Grimm, & Shaham, 2002).

The locus coeruleus–norepinephrine system, the serotonin system, and the GABA–benzodiazepine receptor complex are all implicated in anxiety. Female gonadal hormones, especially estrogen and progesterone, have a regulatory role in the function of these systems. The stress response in the locus coeruleus appears to be attenuated in the presence of estrogen (Kirschbaum, Klauer, Filipp, & Hellhammer, 1995; Lindheim et al., 1992). Animal studies also indicate that estrogen elicits a significant increase in striatal D_2 receptors (Fink, Sumner, Rosie, Grace, & Quinn, 1996). Furthermore, estrogen enhances serotonin function through several actions, including increasing transporter sites and decreasing metabolism (Pigott, 1999), which may explain the decrease in response to selective serotonin reuptake inhibitor (SSRI) treatment in postmenopausal women. Progesterone has anxiolytic effects that have been attributed to its effects on the GABA–benzodiazepine receptor complex (Kroboth & McAuley, 1997; Majewska, 1992). Progesterone acts as an allosteric modulator, enhancing benzodiazepine receptor binding sensitivity and amplifying the pharmacological effects of benzodiazepines. A number of studies has demonstrated an attenuation of the acute effects and self-administration of cocaine by progesterone. In addition, progesterone has a complex metabolic pathway with multiple active metabolites, such as pregnenolone and allopregnenolone. Many of the neuromodulatory effects of progesterone result in antagonism or neutralization of estrogenic actions (Janowsky, Halbreich, & Rausch, 1996; Sherwin, 1991), so the ratio of estrogen to progesterone may be important in determining the cumulative effects. The premenstrual, postpartum, and perimenopausal periods are all characterized by rapid fluctuation in the levels of progesterone and estrogen. Changes in the clinical severity of anxiety symptoms during these periods, particularly PD (Altshuler, Hendrick, & Cohen,

1998; Halbreich, 1997) and OCD have also been reported (Williams & Koran, 1997). In summary, there is much overlap in the neurobiological systems involved in addictions and anxiety disorders. There are also gender differences in these systems that may be due, in part, to the modulatory influence of gonadal hormones. Future work in this area will help us to better understand gender differences in co-occurring anxiety and SUDs and to gender-specific therapies.

SCREENING AND DIFFERENTIAL DIAGNOSIS

Differential diagnosis is one of the most difficult challenges in the area of co-occurring anxiety and SUDs. Substance use and withdrawal can mimic nearly every psychiatric disorder. Substances of abuse have profound effects on neurotransmitter systems involved in the pathophysiology of anxiety disorders and, with chronic use, may unmask a vulnerability or lead to organic changes that manifest as an anxiety disorder. The best way to differentiate substance-induced, transient symptoms of anxiety from anxiety disorders that warrant treatment is through observation of symptoms during a period of abstinence. Transient substance-related states will improve with time. The duration of abstinence necessary for accurate diagnosis remains controversial and is likely to be based on both the diagnosis being assessed and the substance used. For example, long half-life drugs (e.g., some benzodiazepines, methadone) may require several weeks of abstinence for withdrawal symptoms to subside, but shorter-acting substances (e.g., alcohol, cocaine, short half-life benzodiazepines) require shorter periods of abstinence to make valid diagnoses. A family history of anxiety disorder, the onset of anxiety symptoms before the onset of SUD, and sustained anxiety symptoms during lengthy periods of abstinence all suggest an independent anxiety disorder.

Because of the high rate of co-occurrence of anxiety and SUDs, screening patients for both, whether presenting at primary care, substance use, or psychiatric treatment settings, is critical. This is especially important considering that early diagnosis and treatment can improve treatment outcomes. Studies have demonstrated that individuals with co-occurring anxiety and SUDs have a worse outcome than those with either disorder alone. In one 12-year prospective study of 473 individuals with GAD, SAD, or PD, the overall clinical course and probability of recurrence was worsened by comorbid SUDs (Bruce et al., 2005). Another study demonstrated that individuals with a baseline anxiety disorder in treatment for alcohol use disorders were significantly more likely to relapse during follow-up (Kushner et al., 2005). No gender differences were reported in either of these studies. In a large study ($n = 401$) of individuals with drug dependence, GAD predicted more drug dependence diagnoses at 12-month follow-up. Interestingly, outcomes for men were more closely associated with psychiatric status, as compared to outcomes among women. For women, the presence of phobic disorders predicted better treatment outcomes (Compton, Cottler, Jacobs, Ben-Abdallah, & Spitznagel, 2003).

GENERAL TREATMENT CONSIDERATIONS

In general, treatment efforts addressing psychiatric conditions and SUDs have developed in parallel. The integration of services and effective treatments from both fields will be critical to the optimal treatment of individuals with co-occurring disorders. It is important to maximize the use of nonpharmacological treatments. Learning strategies to self-regulate anxiety symptoms can help patients interrupt the cycle of using external agents to combat intolerable subjective states and make it possible for them to acquire alternative coping strategies. Among psychosocial treatments, cognitive-behavioral therapies (CBTs) are among the most effective for both anxiety disorders and SUDs. Some promising pilot work investigating the integration of treatments to develop therapies specifically targeting co-occurring disorders is discussed in the sections that follow, but much work is left to be done.

Progress has been made in developing pharmacotherapeutic treatments for both SUDs and anxiety disorders. The pharmacotherapeutic treatment of specific anxiety disorders is discussed in detail below; here we provide an overview of some general principles. Individuals in recovery can have complex and conflicting feelings and attitudes about the use of medications and may see the need for medications as a sign of defectiveness or failure. It is important to address feelings about taking medications and emphasize the need for medication adherence in a proactive manner.

In cases where the relationship of psychiatric symptoms and substance use is unclear, the risk–benefit ratio of using medications must be carefully considered. Should the decision to use medication be made, treatment should follow routine clinical practice for the treatment of the anxiety disorder, with some exceptions. It is important to pay attention to potential toxic interactions that might occur between the prescription medications and illicit drugs and alcohol in case of relapse. It is also important to use the agent with the least abuse potential. Despite their effectiveness in immediate relief of panic and other anxiety symptoms, benzodiazepines are generally avoided in substance-using populations because of the abuse potential. Benzodiazepines may be considered as adjunctive medication during the early treatment phase when antidepressant activation or latency of onset is an issue. If a benzodiazepine is prescribed to a patient with a co-occurring SUD, limited amounts of medication should be given, and the patient should be closely monitored for relapse. As a rule, benzodiazepines should be considered for chronic treatment only when other pharmacological and nonpharmacological treatment options have been exhausted. If necessary, a benzodiazepine with a low abuse potential such as oxazepam and chlordiazepoxide may be considered.

Because co-occurring anxiety disorders are more commonly seen in women with SUDs, medication treatment of comorbid conditions is likely to be particularly important in this population. In this regard, one study comparing an SSRI (sertraline) to a tricyclic antidepressant (imipramine) in the treatment of depression found that premenopausal women had a preferential response to sertraline (Kornstein et al., 2000). However, in a study of sertraline treatment of nondepressed individuals with alcohol dependence, sertraline treatment reduced drinking in early-onset males, but not in the female groups (Pettinati, Dundon, & Lipkin, 2004). Cornelius and colleagues explored the use of fluoxetine in individuals with depression and alcohol dependence and found significant improvement in both mood and alcohol outcomes (Cornelius et al., 1997). These same agents have demonstrated efficacy in the treatment of many anxiety disorders, so the same principles are likely to apply in the treatment of co-occurring anxiety disorders and SUDs. As such, although evidence does not support the use of antidepressant medications in the absence of psychiatric comorbidity in individuals with SUDs, careful evaluation of psychiatric disorders and appropriate treatment will likely improve outcomes.

Finally, the use of agents targeting substance use specifically, such as naltrexone or disulfiram, as add-on treatment for individuals with comorbid anxiety disorders and SUDs, is underexplored. In one study of 254 outpatients with alcohol dependence and a variety of comorbid psychiatric disorders, Petrakis, Poling, Levinson, Nich, Carroll, Ralevski, and Rounsaville (2005) investigated the efficacy of disulfiram, naltrexone, or their combination in a 12-week randomized trial. Participants treated with either naltrexone or disulfiram had significantly more consecutive weeks of abstinence and fewer drinking days per week. In comparison to naltrexone-treated participants, disulfiram-treated participants reported less craving from pre- to posttreatment. The effects of the medications by specific comorbid psychiatric disorder were not discussed, but active medication was associated with greater symptom improvement (e.g., less anxiety). No clear advantage of combining medications was observed, and there were no gender differences reported.

In the sections that follow, the prevalence rates, differential diagnosis, and treatment of GAD, SAD, OCD, and PD are reviewed. PTSD is covered in Chapter 14 (this volume); simple phobia is not covered because most evidence suggests that this disorder has no specific relationship with SUDs.

GENERALIZED ANXIETY DISORDER

Overview

GAD is a chronic and disabling disorder associated with substantial personal, societal, and economic costs (Ballenger et al., 2001; Grant et al., 2005). Epidemiological studies have consistently demonstrated a 4–6% lifetime prevalence, with women being twice as likely as men to develop GAD. The disorder is highly associated with a number of other psychiatric disorders, including SUDs. In NESARC, individuals with GAD were at significantly increased risk for SUDs, with a lifetime OR of 2.2 for any alcohol use disorder, 2.7 for any drug use disorder, and 2.5 for nicotine dependence (Grant et al., 2005). There were no gender differences in these ORs. As such, consistent with the general population estimates, GAD should be twice as common in women with an SUD, as compared to men. Women with GAD are more likely to develop coexisting diagnoses, particularly dysthymia and depression, and these co-occurring conditions worsen prognosis and reduce the likelihood of remission (Pigott, 2003).

Differential Diagnosis

GAD symptoms have considerable overlap with those of acute intoxication from stimulants and withdrawal from alcohol, opiates, sedative, and hypnotic drugs. Because of this overlap, distinguishing substance-induced anxiety symptoms from GAD can be challenging. The DSM-IV diagnostic criteria of GAD require a 6-month duration of symptoms that is not directly related to the physiological effects of a substance; however individuals with SUDs will have difficulty maintaining abstinence for 6 months, and an earlier diagnosis could be important to successful recovery. Taking a careful history can establish the timing of the GAD relative to the SUD is important. Because both SUDs and GAD can result in significant occupational, social, and health problems, it can be challenging to discern if the impairments are related to the SUD, an independent anxiety disorder, or both. As patients engage in recovery and their functioning improves, ongoing assessment of their anxiety symptoms will provide valuable information regarding diagnosis and need for continued treatment.

Treatment

There is little evidence-based research to guide treatment decisions for individuals with co-occurring GAD and SUDs, and none of the existing evidence leads to gender-specific recommendations. Recent guidelines for the pharmacotherapeutic treatment of GAD from the Canadian Psychiatric Association (2006) suggest that first-line medications include the SSRIs and venlafaxine XR. Paroxetine, escitalopram, and venlafaxine have demonstrated long-term efficacy with increasing response rates over 6 months. Because approximately 20–40% of patients with GAD relapse within 6–12 months after the discontinuation of pharmacotherapy, long-term treatment may be needed. Buspirone has been examined, with mixed results, in the treatment of highly anxious individuals with alcohol dependence (McKeehan & Martin, 2002). It has the advantage of interactings minimally with alcohol (Mattila, Aranko, & Seppala, 1982) and having low abuse potential (Cole, Orzack, Beake, Bird, & Bar-Tal, 1982). Although the SSRIs have not been studied specifically in individuals with co-occurring GAD and SUDs, because they are effective in the treatment of uncomplicated GAD and relatively safe to use in individuals with SUDs, these agents would be a reasonable choice in individuals with co-occurring disorders. Psychosocial treatments are clearly efficacious in the treatment of GAD. CBT has been used most often in combination with SUD treatment, with goals of managing anxious states without medications (McKeehan & Martin, 2002).

SOCIAL ANXIETY DISORDER

Overview

The lifetime prevalence estimates of SAD vary widely, ranging from 3–13%, based on epidemiological and community-based studies (Grant et al., 2005). Most studies report that women have approximately 1.5 times greater prevalence of SAD, as compared to men. In NESARC, the lifetime prevalence of an alcohol use disorder (48%), any drug use disorder (22.3%), and nicotine dependence (33%) in individuals were all approximately double that of individuals without lifetime SAD, but no gender differences were reported (Grant et al., 2005).

Data are relatively limited concerning gender differences in SAD. There are two main subtypes of SAD: a generalized type in which individuals are more disabled and have a broad range of social fears, and a nongeneralized type that involves anxiety limited to specific situations, such as public speaking (Kessler, Stein, & Berglund, 1998). Several studies have suggested that women are more likely to have the generalized subtype of SAD, and that genetic factors play an important role in the development of this subtype (Kendler et al., 1995; Stein et al., 1998).

Differential Diagnosis

Because the age of onset of SAD is usually during childhood or adolescence (Grant et al., 2005), its symptoms typically precede the onset of comorbid SUDs (Carrigan & Randall, 2003). The key symptom, fear of performance or fear of social situations generally, is specific to SAD and not associated with alcohol use or withdrawal.

Treatment

Current treatment recommendations for SAD with comorbid SUDs include the use of SSRIs or beta-blockers in combination with psychosocial treatment. No studies specifically address gender differences in the treatment of SAD, and only a few studies examine treatment options in comorbid populations. Schade and colleagues randomized 96 patients with alcohol dependence and comorbid agoraphobia, PD with agoraphobia, or SAD ($n = 87$) to CBT plus optional fluvoxamine (150 mg/day) versus treatment as usual. Both groups improved in anxiety and alcohol measures, with greater improvement in anxiety outcomes reported by the combined treatment group. Fluvoxamine was not associated with better outcomes (Schade et al., 2005). Two small placebo-controlled studies investigated the use of paroxetine treatment in individuals with co-occurring AUD and SAD; the paroxetine group demonstrated significant improvement in social anxiety. In the other study, although no significant group differences were noted in alcohol use, the paroxetine group reported less use of alcohol to self-medicate anxiety (Book, Thomas, Randall, & Randall, 2008; Randall, Johnson, et al., 2001). There were no gender differences reported in any of the studies cited.

In a study of individual CBT for AUD versus concurrent AUD/SUD therapy, drinking measures improved in both groups; however, those who received concurrent treatment had worse alcohol outcomes. The authors hypothesized that exposure to anxiety-provoking social situations in concurrent treatment may have increased drinking to cope (Randall, Thomas, & Thevos, 2001). Terra and colleagues followed 300 detoxified patients with alcohol dependence, with and without SAD, after they have received standard treatment. No significant differences were found between the two groups in treatment adherence and outcomes. Individuals with SAD who attended Alcoholics Anonymous (AA) chaired meetings less often, were more ashamed of attendance, felt less integrated into the group, and were less likely to feel better after a meeting (Terra et al., 2006). No gender differences were reported in either of these studies. These results suggest that individuals with SAD may need treatment targeting their social anxiety before being able to benefit from group interventions. Individual therapy may be better tolerated than group therapy, and a period of sobriety and skills training may be important before increasing their exposure to social situations.

PANIC DISORDER

Overview

In NESARC, lifetime prevalence of PD (with or without agoraphobia) was 5.1% (Grant et al., 2006). NESARC and other epidemiological studies consistently show that both PD and panic attacks occur twice as frequently in women as men. The 12-month OR of any co-occurring SUD and PD with agoraphobia (OR = 3.1) or without agoraphobia (OR = 2.1) was elevated. For any alcohol use disorder, the 12-month OR of PD with agoraphobia was 2.5 and for PD without agoraphobia was 2.0. For any drug use disorder, the 12-month OR for PD with agoraphobia was 6.0 and for PD without agoraphobia was 3.4. Women with PD are more prone to develop alcohol dependence than men (Andrade, Eaton, & Chilcoat, 1996; Marshall, 1996), and the risk of alcohol dependence is elevated in the relatives of women with PD, suggesting a shared genetic diathesis between panic and alcohol use disorders in women (Fyer et al., 1996; Kendler et al., 1995). In NESARC, the risk of sedative and tranquilizer dependence was elevated in men with PD, as compared to women (Conway et al., 2006).

Women with PD have an elevated risk of developing agoraphobia and other avoidance behaviors (Dick, Bland, & Newman, 1994), as well as other comorbid psychiatric disorders such as GAD and simple phobia (Andrade et al., 1996; Fyer et al., 1996). Women with PD are also particularly vulnerable to somatization disorder and somatic presentations of anxiety (Yonkers et al., 1998). Taken together, these findings suggest that women with PD are likely to have a more complicated clinical course with greater functional impairment, as compared to men.

Differential Diagnosis

Many individuals with alcohol dependence report symptoms caused by alcohol withdrawal that mimic panic attacks and are likely to markedly improve during the first several weeks of abstinence (Schuckit et al., 1997). Alternatively, the self-medication hypothesis suggests that alcohol use may decrease panic symptoms, resulting in persistent use in individuals with PD. The literature concerning the relative order of onset of PD and SUDs is mixed (Cosci, Schruers, Abrams, & Griez, 2007). If a few panic attacks occur early in recovery and decrease in frequency, they may respond to support and reassurance. However, if the panic attacks continue or increase over several weeks of abstinence, the diagnosis of PD should be made. Without treatment, the risk of relapse to alcohol use is increased. In one prospective study of people with alcohol dependence recruited from acute treatment, PD was the most common diagnosis and was predictive of relapse. After 4 months, approximately 50% no longer met diagnostic criteria for any anxiety disorder (Kushner et al., 2005). This finding emphasizes the need to carefully track anxiety symptoms early in recovery and to provide normalizing information to patients about common withdrawal symptoms and the typical course of recovery.

Treatment

According to current guidelines, four classes of medications—SSRIs, tricyclic antidepressants (TCAs), benzodiazepines, and monoamine oxidase inhibitors (MAOIs)—have approximately comparable efficacy in the treatment of PDs (American Psychiatric Association, 1998). As previously discussed, benzodiazepines are generally avoided in individuals with SUDs. Fluoxetine, sertraline, paroxetine, and fluvoxamine—all SSRIs—have demonstrated effectiveness in clinical trials and are likely to be the best choice for individuals with co-occurring PD and SUD.

An extensive body of literature supports the efficacy of CBT in the treatment of PD. Bowen and colleagues conducted a controlled trial of standard alcohol treatment versus combined treatment with CBT for PD plus SUD (Bowen, D'Arcy, Keegan, & Senthilselvan, 2000). At follow-up, improvement of panic symptoms and relapse rates did not differ between the two groups. The authors hypothesized that typical strategies for managing anxiety, such as stress management, relaxation training, and relapse prevention, presented in standard alcohol treatment programs may have interfered with the detection of differences between the two groups.

OBSESSIVE–COMPULSIVE DISORDER

Overview

Data from the Epidemiologic Catchment Area study (Karno, Golding, Sorenson, & Burnam, 1988) indicated that the lifetime prevalence of OCD was 2–3%. Most studies suggest that the lifetime prevalence of OCD is 1.5 times higher in men than women, and men have an earlier onset of illness than women; in addition, the course of illness is more episodic and less severe in women, compared with men (Pigott, 2003). OCD symptoms appear to be substantially influenced by the female reproductive cycle. There is a marked increase in the prevalence of OCD after menarche, and a significant percentage of women with OCD report premenstrual and postpartum worsening of symptoms, suggesting an influence of gonadal hormone level and fluctuation (Williams & Koran, 1997).

The association between OCD and SUDs is less robust than for other anxiety disorders. In the National Comorbidity Survey replication study, OCD was negatively correlated with SUDs (Kessler, Chiu, Demler, Merikangas, & Walters, 2005). In the Collaborative Study on the Genetics of Alcoholism, data from 2,713 alcoholics and 919 controls demonstrated no significant difference in rates of OCD (Schuckit et al., 1997). A number of studies of treatment-seeking samples also suggest a nonsignificant relationship. There do not appear to be gender differences in the relationship between OCD and SUDs.

Differential Diagnosis

Craving in SUDs has been compared to the intrusive recurrent thoughts that drive behavior in OCD (Modell, Glaser, Cyr, & Mountz, 1992). Although these similarities may implicate common neurobiological processes, the thoughts and compulsions in a pure SUD are restricted to alcohol and drug use and/or avoidance of withdrawal symptoms, so differential diagnosis with substance-induced symptoms should not be difficult.

Treatment

There are no controlled studies of pharmacological treatment of co-occurring OCD and SUDs. First-line FDA-approved medications for the treatment of OCD are clomipramine, fluoxetine, fluvoxamine, paroxetine, and sertraline. In individuals with SUDs, SSRIs are preferable to clomipramine because of more favorable side effect profiles; however in one study comparing clomipramine and fluvoxamine treatment, women exhibited a better overall treatment response and were more responsive to clomipramine (Mundo, Bareggi, Pirola, & Bellodi, 1999).

Researchers randomly assigned 60 individuals with substance abuse and OCD in a drug-free therapeutic community to combined OCD and SUD treatment, SUD treatment alone, or SUD treatment plus progressive muscle relaxation. At 12 months, the group receiving combined treatment had higher rates of abstinence, longer duration in treatment, and a greater reduction in OCD symptoms. No gender differences were reported (Fals-Stewart, Marks, & Schafer, 1993).

CONCLUSIONS

Anxiety, anxiety disorders, and SUDs commonly co-occur. Women have a greater risk for anxiety disorders, in general, and hence a greater risk of co-occurring anxiety and SUDs. Biological differences, including the influence of gonadal hormones on both anxiety disorders and SUDs, influence the presentation and course of illness for both anxiety and SUDS, and are therefore highly likely to influence their presentation and course when they co-occur. There has been little work focused on the treatment of co-occurring anxiety disorders and SUDs, in general, and no work specifically addressing gender differences in treatment. Future research could yield important findings with regard to gender-specific treatment that could improve treatment outcomes for both women and men with co-occurring anxiety and SUDs.

KEY POINTS

- In general, the prevalence rate of anxiety disorders is approximately two times higher in women as men.
- The prevalence of co-occurring anxiety disorders in individuals with SUDs follows this general pattern, with women with SUDs being twice as likely to have a co-occurring anxiety disorder, compared to men.

- There are gender differences in the course and presentation of anxiety disorders in women, with women presenting with more somatic symptoms and more comorbidity with other psychiatric disorders than their male counterparts.
- Gonadal hormones impact the course of illness in both SUDs and anxiety disorders in ways that are likely to account for some of the gender differences, but this area is currently underexplored.
- There is some evidence for gender differences in response to pharmacological treatments for anxiety disorders, but this area is also underexplored.
- There have been some investigations of psychotherapeutic treatments specifically targeting co-occurring SUDs and various anxiety disorders, but gender differences in response to these treatments have not been explored.

REFERENCES

Asterisks denote recommended readings.

Altshuler, L. L., Hendrick, V., & Cohen, L. S. (1998). Course of mood and anxiety disorders during pregnancy and the postpartum period. *Journal of Clinical Psychiatry*, 59(Suppl. 2), 29–33.

Andrade, L., Eaton, W. W., & Chilcoat, H. D. (1996). Lifetime co-morbidity of panic attacks and major depression in a population-based study: Age of onset. *Psychological Medicine*, 26, 991–996.

Ballenger, J. C., Davidson, J. R., Lecrubier, Y., Nutt, D. J., Borkovec, T. D., Rickels, K., et al. (2001). Consensus statement on generalized anxiety disorder from the International Consensus Group on Depression and Anxiety. *Journal of Clinical Psychiatry*, 62(Suppl. 11), 53–58.

Bonn-Miller, M. O., Zvolensky, M. J., Bernstein, A., & Stickle, T. R. (2007). Marijuana coping motives interact with marijuana use frequency to predict anxious arousal, panic-related catastrophic thinking, and worry among current marijuana users. *Depression and Anxiety*, 25, 862–873.

Book, S. W., Thomas, S. E., Randall, P. K., & Randall, C. L. (2008). Paroxetine reduces social anxiety in individuals with a co-occurring alcohol use disorder. *Journal of Anxiety Disorders*, 22(2), 310–318.

Bowen, R. C., D'Arcy, C., Keegan, D., & Senthilselvan, A. (2000). A controlled trial of cognitive behavioral treatment of panic in alcoholic inpatients with comorbid panic disorder. *Addictive Behaviors*, 25(4), 593–597.

Bruce, S. E., Yonkers, K. A., Otto, M. W., Eisen, J. L., Weisberg, R. B., Pagano, M., et al. (2005). Influence of psychiatric comorbidity on recovery and recurrence in generalized anxiety disorder, social phobia, and panic disorder: A 12-year prospective study. *American Journal of Psychiatry*, 162(6), 1179–1187.

Canadian Psychiatric Association. (2006). Clinical practice guidelines: Management of anxiety disorders. *Canadian Journal of Psychiatry*, 51(8 Suppl. 2), 9S–91S.

Carrigan, M. H., & Randall, C. L. (2003). Self-medication in social phobia: A review of the alcohol literature. *Addictive Behaviors*, 28(2), 269–284.

Cole, J. O., Orzack, M. H., Beake, B., Bird, M., & Bar-Tal, Y. (1982). Assessment of the abuse liability of buspirone in recreational sedative users. *Journal of Clinical Psychiatry*, 43(12 Pt. 2), 69–75.

Compton, W. M., 3rd, Cottler, L. B., Jacobs, J. L., Ben-Abdallah, A., & Spitznagel, E. L. (2003). The role of psychiatric disorders in predicting drug dependence treatment outcomes. *American Journal of Psychiatry*, 160(5), 890–895. (*)

Conway, K. P., Compton, W., Stinson, F. S., & Grant, B. F. (2006). Lifetime comorbidity of DSM-IV mood and anxiety disorders and specific drug use disorders: Results from the National Epidemiologic Survey on Alcohol and Related Conditions. *Journal of Clinical Psychiatry*, 67(2), 247–257. (*)

Cornelius, J. R., Salloum, I. M., Ehler, J. G., Jarrett, P. J., Cornelius, M. D., Perel, J. M., et al. (1997). Fluoxetine in depressed alcoholics: A double-blind, placebo-controlled trial. *Archives of General Psychiatry*, 54(8), 700–705.

Cosci, F., Schruers, K. R., Abrams, K., & Griez, E. J. (2007). Alcohol use disorders and panic disorder: A review of the evidence of a direct relationship. *Journal of Clinical Psychiatry, 68*(6), 874–880.

de Wit, H., Uhlenhuth, E. H., & Johanson, E. C. (1986). Individual differences in the reinforcing and subjective effects of amphetamine and diazepam. *Drug and Alcohol Dependence, 86,* 1625–1632.

Dick, C. L., Bland, R. C., & Newman, S. C. (1994). Epidemiology of psychiatric disorders in Edmonton: Panic disorder. *Acta Psychiatrica Scandinavica Supplement, 376,* 45–53.

DiFranza, J. R., Savageau, J. A., Rigotti, N. A., Ockene, J. K., McNeill, A. D., Coleman, M., et al. (2004). Trait anxiety and nicotine dependence in adolescents: A report from the DANDY study. *Addictive Behaviors, 29*(5), 911–919.

Fals-Stewart, W., Marks, A. P., & Schafer, J. (1993). A comparison of behavioral group therapy and individual behavior therapy in treating obsessive–compulsive disorder [see comments]. *Journal of Nervous and Mental Disease, 181*(3), 189–193.

Fink, G., Sumner, B. E., Rosie, R., Grace, O., & Quinn, J. P. (1996). Estrogen control of central neurotransmission: Effect on mood, mental state, and memory. *Cellular and Molecular Neurobiology, 16*(3), 325–344.

Fyer, A. J., Mannuzza, S., Chapman, T. F., Lipsitz, J., Martin, L. Y., & Klein, D. F. (1996). Panic disorder and social phobia: Effects of comorbidity on familial transmission. *Anxiety, 2*(4), 173–178.

Grant, B. F., Harford, T. C., Dawson, D. A., Chou, P., Dufour, M., & Pickering, R. (1994). Prevalence of DSM-IV alcohol abuse and dependence, United States, 1992. *NIAAA's Epidemiologic Bulletin, 35,* 243–248.

Grant, B. F., Hasin, D. S., Blanco, C., Stinson, F. S., Chou, S. P., Goldstein, R. B., et al. (2005). The epidemiology of social anxiety disorder in the United States: Results from the National Epidemiologic Survey on Alcohol and Related Conditions. *Journal of Clinical Psychiatry, 66*(11), 1351–1361.

Grant, B. F., Hasin, D. S., Chou, S. P., Stinson, F. S., & Dawson, D. A. (2004). Nicotine dependence and psychiatric disorders in the United States: Results from the National Epidemiologic Survey on Alcohol and Related Conditions. *Archives of General Psychiatry, 61*(11), 1107–1115.

Grant, B. F., Hasin, D. S., Stinson, F. S., Dawson, D. A., Goldstein, R. B., Smith, S., et al. (2006). The epidemiology of DSM-IV panic disorder and agoraphobia in the United States: Results from the National Epidemiologic Survey on Alcohol and Related Conditions. *Journal of Clinical Psychiatry, 67*(3), 363–374.

Grant, B. F., Stinson, F. S., Dawson, D. A., Chou, S. P., Dufour, M. C., Compton, W., et al. (2004). Prevalence and co-occurrence of substance use disorders and independent mood and anxiety disorders: Results from the National Epidemiologic Survey on Alcohol and Related Conditions. *Archives of General Psychiatry, 61*(8), 807–816. (*)

Halbreich, U. (1997). Hormonal interventions with psychopharmacological potential: An overview. *Psychopharmacology Bulletin, 33*(2), 281–286.

Hasin, D. S., Stinson, F. S., Ogburn, E., & Grant, B. F. (2007). Prevalence, correlates, disability, and comorbidity of DSM-IV alcohol abuse and dependence in the United States: Results from the National Epidemiologic Survey on Alcohol and Related Conditions. *Archives of General Psychiatry, 64*(7), 830–842.

Janowsky, D., Halbreich, U., & Rausch, J. (1996). Association between ovarian hormones, other hormones, emotional disorders, and neurotransmitters. In M. Jensvold, U. Halbreich, & J. Hamilton (Eds.), *Psychopharmacology and women: Sex, gender, and hormones* (pp. 85–106). Washington, DC: American Psychiatric Association.

Karno, M., Golding, J. M., Sorenson, S. B., & Burnam, M. A. (1988). The epidemiology of obsessive–compulsive disorder in five US communities. *Archives of General Psychiatry, 45*(12), 1094–1099.

Kendler, K. S., Walters, E. E., Neale, M. C., Kessler, R. C., Heath, A. C., & Eaves, L. J. (1995). The structure of the genetic and environmental risk factors for six major psychiatric disorders in women: Phobia, generalized anxiety disorder, panic disorder, bulimia, major depression, and alcoholism. *Archives of General Psychiatry, 52*(5), 374–383.

Kessler, R. C., Chiu, W. T., Demler, O., Merikangas, K. R., & Walters, E. E. (2005). Prevalence, sever-

ity, and comorbidity of 12-month DSM-IV disorders in the National Comorbidity Survey Replication. *Archives of General Psychiatry, 62*(6), 617–627.

Kessler, R. C., McGonagle, K. A., Zhao, S., Nelson, C. B., Hughes, M., Eshleman, S., et al. (1994).
Lifetime and 12-month prevalence of DSM-III-R psychiatric disorders in the United States: Results
from the National Comorbidity Survey. *Archives of General Psychiatry, 51*(1), 8–19.

Kirschbaum, C., Klauer, T., Filipp, S. H., & Hellhammer, D. H. (1995). Sex-specific effects of social
support on cortisol and subjective responses to acute psychological stress. *Psychosomatic Medicine, 57*(1), 23–31.

Koob, G. F., & Le Moal, M. (1997). Drug abuse: Hedonic homeostatic dysregulation. *Science,
278*(5335), 52–58.

Kornstein, S. G., Schatzberg, A. F., Thase, M. E., Yonkers, K. A., McCullough, J. P., Keitner, G. I., et
al. (2000). Gender differences in treatment response to sertraline versus imipramine in chronic
depression. *American Journal of Psychiatry, 157*(9), 1445–1452.

Kroboth, P. D., & McAuley, J. W. (1997). Progesterone: Does it affect response to drug? *Psychopharmacology Bulletin, 33*(2), 297–301.

Kushner, M. G., Abrams, K., & Borchardt, C. (2000). The relationship between anxiety disorders and
alcohol use disorders: A review of major perspectives and findings. *Clinical Psychology Review,
20*(2), 149–171. (*)

Kushner, M. G., Abrams, K., Thuras, P., Hanson, K. L., Brekke, M., & Sletten, S. (2005). Follow-up
study of anxiety disorder and alcohol dependence in comorbid alcoholism treatment patients.
Alcoholism: Clinical and Experimental Research, 29(8), 1432–1443.

Lindheim, S. R., Legro, R. S., Bernstein, L., Stanczyk, F. Z., Vijod, M. A., Presser, S. C., et al. (1992).
Behavioral stress responses in premenopausal and postmenopausal women and the effects of
estrogen. *American Journal of Obstetrics and Gynecology, 167*(6), 1831–1836.

Majewska, M. D. (1992). Neurosteroids: Endogenous bimodal modulators of the GABAA receptor: Mechanism of action and physiological significance. *Progress in Neurobiology, 38*(4),
379–395.

Markou, A., Kosten, T. R., & Koob, G. F. (1998). Neurobiological similarities in depression
and drug dependence: A self-medication hypothesis. *Neuropsychopharmacology, 18*(3),
135–174.

Marshall, J. R. (1996). Comorbidity and its effects on panic disorder. *Bulletin of the Menninger Clinic,
60*(2 Suppl. A), A39–53.

McEwen, B. S. (2000). Allostasis and allostatic load: Implications for neuropsychopharmacology. *Neuropsychopharmacology, 22*(2), 108–124.

McKeehan, M. B., & Martin, D. (2002). Assessment and treatment of anxiety disorders and co-morbid
alcohol/other drug dependency. *Alcoholism Treatment Quarterly, 20*, 45–59.

Meaney, M. J., Bhatnagar, S., Larocque, S., McCormick, C., Shanks, N., Sharma, S., et al. (1993). Individual differences in the hypothalamic–pituitary–adrenal stress response and the hypothalamic
CRF system. *Annals of the New York Academy of Sciences, 697*, 70–85.

Modell, J. G., Glaser, F. B., Cyr, L., & Mountz, J. M. (1992). Obsessive and compulsive characteristics
of craving for alcohol in alcohol abuse and dependence. *Alcoholism: Clinical and Experimental
Research, 16*(2), 272–274.

Moore, T. H., Zammit, S., Lingford-Hughes, A., Barnes, T. R., Jones, P. B., Burke, M., et al. (2007).
Cannabis use and risk of psychotic or affective mental health outcomes: A systematic review.
Lancet, 370(9584), 319–328.

Mundo, E., Bareggi, S. R., Pirola, R., & Bellodi, L. (1999). Effect of acute intravenous clomipramine
and antiobsessional response to proserotonergic drugs: Is gender a predictive variable? *Biological
Psychiatry, 45*(3), 290–294.

Nemeroff, C. B. (1996). The corticotropin-releasing factor (CRF) hypothesis of depression: New findings and new directions. *Molecular Psychiatry, 1*(4), 336–342.

Petrakis, I. L., Poling, J., Levinson, C., Nich, C., Carroll, K., Ralevski, E., & Rounsaville, B. (20060.
Naltrexone and disulfiram in patients with alcohol dependence and comorbid post-traumatic
stress disorder. *Biological Psychiatry, 60*(7), 777–783.

Pettinati, H. M., Dundon, W., & Lipkin, C. (2004). Gender differences in response to sertraline pharmacotherapy in type A alcohol dependence. *American Journal of the Addictions, 13*(3), 236–247. (*)

Pigott, T. A. (1999). Gender differences in the epidemiology and treatment of anxiety disorders. *Journal of Clinical Psychiatry, 60*(Suppl. 18), 4–5.

Pigott, T. A. (2003). Anxiety disorders in women. *Psychiatric Clinics of North America, 26*(3), 621–672, vi–vii.

Randall, C. L., Johnson, M. R., Thevos, A. K., Sonne, S. C., Thomas, S. E., Willard, S. L., et al. (2001). Paroxetine for social anxiety and alcohol use in dual-diagnosed patients. *Depression and Anxiety, 14*(4), 255–262.

Randall, C. L., Thomas, S., & Thevos, A. K. (2001). Concurrent alcoholism and social anxiety disorder: A first step toward developing effective treatments. *Alcoholism: Clinical and Experimental Research, 25*(2), 210–220.

Raphael, B., Wooding, S., Stevens, G., & Connor, J. (2005). Comorbidity: Cannabis and complexity. *Journal of Psychiatric Practice, 11*(3), 161–176.

Reiger, D. A., Farmer, M. E., Rae, D. S., Locke, B. Z., Keith, S. J., Judd, L. J., et al. (1990). Comorbidity of mental disorders with alcohol and other drug abuse. *Journal of the American Medical Association, 264*(19), 2511–2518.

Sapolsky, R. M., Alberts, S. C., & Altmann, J. (1997). Hypercortisolism associated with social subordinance or social isolation among wild baboons. *Archives of General Psychiatry, 54*(12), 1137–1143.

Schade, A., Marquenie, L. A., van Balkom, A. J., Koeter, M. W., de Beurs, E., van den Brink, W., et al. (2005). The effectiveness of anxiety treatment on alcohol-dependent patients with a comorbid phobic disorder: A randomized controlled trial. *Alcoholsim: Clinical and Experimental Research, 29*(5), 794–800.

Schuckit, M. A., Tipp, J. E., Bucholz, K. K., Nurnberger, J. I., Jr., Hesselbrock, V. M., Crowe, R. R., et al. (1997). The life-time rates of three major mood disorders and four major anxiety disorders in alcoholics and controls. *Addiction, 92*(10), 1289–1304.

Shalev, U., Grimm, J. W., & Shaham, Y. (2002). Neurobiology of relapse to heroin and cocaine: A review. *Pharmacology Review, 54*, 1–42.

Sherwin, B. B. (1991). The impact of different doses of estrogen and progestin on mood and sexual behavior in postmenopausal women. *Journal of Clinical Endocrinology and Metabolism, 72*(2), 336–343.

Sinha, R. (2001). How does stress increase risk of drug abuse and relapse? *Psychopharmacology (Berl), 158*(4), 343–359. (*)

Stein, M. B., Chartier, M. J., Hazen, A. L., Kozak, M. V., Tancer, M. E., Lander, S., et al. (1998). A direct-interview family study of generalized social phobia. *American Journal of Psychiatry, 155*(1), 90–97.

Steinberg, M. B., Akincigil, A., Delnevo, C. D., Crystal, S., & Carson, J. L. (2006). Gender and age disparities for smoking-cessation treatment. *American Journal of Preventive Medicine, 30*(5), 405–412.

Stewart, J. (2000). Pathways to relapse: The neurobiology of drug- and stress-induced relapse to drug-taking. *Journal of Psychiatry and Neuroscience, 25*(2), 125–136.

Substance Abuse and Mental Health Services Administration (SAMHSA). (2006). *National Survey on Drug Use and Health.* Retrieved from *http://www.oas.samhsa.gov/nsduh..htm.*

Terra, M. B., Barros, H. M., Stein, A. T., Figueira, I., Athayde, L. D., Spanemberg, L., et al. (2006). Does co-occurring social phobia interfere with alcoholism treatment adherence and relapse? *Journal of Substance Abuse Treatment, 31*(4), 403–409.

Vik, P. W. (2007). Methamphetamine use by incarcerated women: Comorbid mood and anxiety problems. *Women's Health Issues, 17*(4), 256–263.

Vincent, N., Schoobridge, J., Ask, A., Allsop, S., & Ali, R. (1998). Physical and mental health problems in amphetamine users from metropolitan Adelaide, Australia. *Drug and Alcohol Review, 17*(2), 187–195.

Williams, K. E., & Koran, L. M. (1997). Obsessive–compulsive disorder in pregnancy, the puerperium, and the premenstruum. *Journal of Clinical Psychiatry, 58*(7), 330–334; quiz 335–336.

Yonkers, K. A., Zlotnick, C., Allsworth, J., Warshaw, M., Shea, T., & Keller, M. B. (1998). Is the course of panic disorder the same in women and men? *American Journal of Psychiatry, 155*(5), 596–602.

Zweben, J. E., Cohen, J. B., Christian, D., Galloway, G. P., Salinardi, M., Parent, D., et al. (2004). Psychiatric symptoms in methamphetamine users. *American Journal of the Addictions, 13*(2), 181–190.

CHAPTER 13

Co-Occurring Eating and Substance Use Disorders

Lisa R. Cohen, PhD
Susan M. Gordon, PhD

This chapter focuses on eating disorders (EDs), a topic of special relevance to women in general and to women with substance use disorders (SUDs) in particular. The chapter is divided into three sections. The first section provides general information about ED diagnoses, associated characteristics, and cultural and ethnic issues. The second section focuses on the strong link between EDs and SUDs, with particular attention being paid to the association between bulimia and alcohol use disorders. The link between EDs and SUDs is also examined within the context of additional comorbidities and potential common factors in etiology. The third section reviews current treatments available for EDs and discusses treatment options for individuals with comorbid EDs and SUDs.

ED DIAGNOSES, ASSOCIATED CHARACTERISTICS, AND CULTURAL AND ETHNIC ISSUES

Female Gender as a Risk Factor for the Development of EDs

It is well-documented that EDs occur more frequently in women than in men, and that being female is a risk factor for the development of an ED. The lifetime prevalence of EDs in women is estimated at almost two to three times that of men (Hudson, Hiripi, Pope, & Kessler, 2007), with 90% of the cases of anorexia nervosa (AN) and bulimia nervosa (BN) occurring in females (American Psychiatric Association, 1994). Although EDs are also found in males, the disproportionate ratio of female-to-male sufferers is considerably greater than any other common psychiatric disorder.

ED Diagnoses

DSM-IV (American Psychiatric Association, 1994) classifies eating disorders into three categories: AN, BN, and eating disorder not otherwise specified (EDNOS). AN and BN are further divided into two subgroups each. AN includes restricting and binge–purge subtypes, and BN includes purging and nonpurging subtypes. EDNOS describes individuals with ED symptoms that do not meet the severity or number of criteria required for either an AN or BN diagnosis. The DSM-IV also includes a new eating disorder subtype, binge-eating disorder (BED), as a research category. In the current diagnostic system BED is classified under the EDNOS category.

Epidemiological studies have shown that EDs are relatively rare in the general female population. Lifetime prevalence of AN is estimated to be 0.5%, and lifetime prevalence of BN is estimated to be 1–3% (American Psychiatric Association, 1994). AN is the least common, and BED is the most common, of the three eating disorders (Nielsen, 2001; Striegel-Moore et al., 2003). There are specific subgroups of women in which EDs are considerably more prevalent; women with SUDs represent one such group.

The main features of AN are active maintenance of an extremely low body weight (less than 85% of what is considered normal for that person's age and height) and an intense fear of gaining weight. In childhood and early adolescence, the individual may not exhibit significant weight loss, but more commonly may fail to meet expected gains. Weight loss in individuals with AN is primarily achieved through a very restricted diet, at times coupled with purging (i.e., self-induced vomiting or the misuse of laxatives or diuretics) or excessive exercise. Even when dieting and exercise result in significant weight loss, the intense concern about weight gain does not diminish; in fact, it often increases, further fueling the disorder. For individuals with AN unremitting fear of becoming fat is tied to the belief that body weight and shape are primary determinants of self-evaluation. A host of physical consequences (e.g., amenorrhea in postmenarcheal females or a delay in menarche in prepubertal females) and medical complications (e.g., damage to vital organs) can occur, most of which is attributable to extreme weight loss and starvation.

There are two major patterns of eating behavior in AN. In the restrictive subtype, food restriction is utilized as the primary means of weight loss. These individuals do not exhibit binge–purge behavior and generally have less diffuse impulsivity. Individuals with the binge–purge subtype of AN appear to lack the more rigid discipline of those with the restrictive subtype. Whereas bingers–purgers may restrict food intake for periods of time, they also have powerful urges to binge, as the label of subtype denotes. Because of their fear of weight gain, individuals with AN engage in compensatory measures also found in those with BN (described below).

Like AN, one of the main criteria of BN is extreme preoccupation with body weight and shape, and the use of body weight and shape to determine, to a large degree, one's self-worth. Individuals with BN exhibit periods of binge eating followed by inappropriate compensatory behaviors to prevent weight gain. Unlike individuals with AN, individuals with BN typically maintain body weight that is at or above a normal level. A binge episode is classified as eating a larger amount of food than most people would eat within a similar period of time. A binge typically lasts less than 2 hours. A binge episode is commonly triggered by dysphoric mood states, and it is associated with an acute feeling of loss of control (e.g., a feeling that one cannot stop eating). Compensatory behaviors are used to control weight gain after binge episodes. More common behaviors include self-induced vomiting; misuse of laxatives, diuretics, or enemas; fasting; or excessive exercise. Exercise is considered excessive when it interferes with daily activities, occurs at inappropriate times or settings, or continues despite medical injury or complications. The severe and unrealistic dietary restriction, often used in the aftermath of a binge, ultimately triggers another binge episode, continuing the bulimic cycle.

Though research on BED is still in a relatively early stage, common features have been identified. Individuals with BED are in many ways similar to those diagnosed with BN. Individuals with BED experience frequent episodes of out-of-control eating, with the same binge-eating symptoms as those with BN. They also experience intense distress and concern about body shape and weight. Unlike individuals with BN, however, those with BED do not resort to compensatory behaviors, such as purging, to counteract excess calories consumed during a binge episode. Overall eating patterns of those with BED are also different. Whereas individuals with BN tend to fast or restrict eating between binge episodes, those with BED have lower restraint and tend to overeat in between binge episodes. As a result, many with the disorder are overweight. Thus, in addition to distress about out-of-control eating, those with BED also often contend with the shame and stigma of being overweight—which in turn can trigger additional binge episodes. BED seems to affect a somewhat older age group (e.g., onsets observed later than 21) than BN and AN, where the typical onset is late adolescence. BED also appears to have a less marked sex difference, with proportionally more male sufferers than other eating disorders.

It should be noted that some researchers have raised concerns about the validity and clinical usefulness of the existing classification system for EDs (Wonderlich, Joiner, Keel, Williamson, & Crosby, 2007). A number of the criteria for AN and BN have not been empirically validated. For example, the "fear of weight gain" criterion for AN may be culturally specific and not universally useful for diagnostic purposes. There is also little or conflicting evidence to support the subtypes for AN and BN, and investigations that attempt to distinguish between AN and BN diagnoses have also shown mixed results (Wonderlich et al., 2007). Furthermore, individuals with one ED often "migrate" from one category to another over time. In addition, rather than being a separate category, EDNOS appears to be a grouping of subthreshold symptoms of AN and BN. Individuals categorized with EDNOS may be clinically indistinguishable from those with the full diagnosis of AN or BN.

These limitations have led to suggestions for alternative approaches for ED diagnoses. One proposal is to create a single unitary diagnostic category "eating disorder," which would subsume all current ED diagnoses (Fairburn & Bohn, 2005). The rationale for this model is based on the view that the common characteristics of all EDs make them more similar than different.

Cultural Context

One way to understand the gender discrepancy and the nature of EDs in women is to examine the cultural context in which they tend to develop. In recent decades, Western cultures have promoted an increasingly thin beauty ideal for women (Katzmarzyk & Davis, 2001). Cultural idealization of, and consistent media exposure to, an ultra-slim body shape can negatively impact the development and perception of a young woman's body image. Not only does thinness in women signify attractiveness in contemporary Western culture, but it also has come to represent competence, success, and self-control. Given the high value that is placed on physical appearance in our society, individuals often use it as an important indicator of self-worth. Men are also increasingly exposed to unrealistic body ideals, and some are feeling pressure to conform, putting them at risk for developing EDs as well. However, women are more likely to be affected, since appearance is typically a more central component of their self-concept and an area in which they are more likely to be judged by others (Rodin, 1993).

According to Brownell (1991), the search for the perfect body is driven by two erroneous beliefs: (1) that the body is infinitely malleable and with hard work, the right diet, and exercise, anyone can achieve perfection; (2) that once this ideal is achieved, there will be substantial rewards, including happiness, wealth, and success in relationships and career. Because of genetic factors, the thin ideal body weight is unrealistically low for most women. This mismatch between cultural pressures and biological realities leads many adolescent and adult women to experience substantial discontent with their weight and shape. However, although a majority of women in Western culture report dissatisfaction with their bodies, only a small percentage of women go on to develop full-blown EDs.

Ethnicity and EDs

Though body dissatisfaction and EDs (AN and BN, in particular) occur most frequently in females of European origins in Western cultures, recent studies reveal a broader distribution among more ethnically diverse groups than previously suspected (Weiss, 1995). Research suggests that people of color and developing non-Western cultures that adopt values of Western culture are experiencing an increase in EDs and eating-related problems (Anderson-Fye & Becker, 2004; Becker, 2004; Striegel-Moore & Smolak, 1996). However, because studies of EDs in the United States have typically focused on European American women and girls, there is still relatively little information on the prevalence of eating disturbances and EDs in ethnic minority and non-Western groups in this country.

Studies that have examined eating-related pathology in minority populations have most often studied African American women. Reviews indicate that African American women diet less and experience less weight concern and body image dissatisfaction than European American women (Crago, Shisslak, & Estes, 1996). In a large-scale community study of young adult women, all EDs, especially AN and BN, were more common among European American women than African American women (Striegel-Moore et al., 2003). Researchers have suggested that this discrepancy may be related to greater weight tolerance, less body dissatisfaction, and less reliance on restrictive dieting for weight management in ethnic groups of people of color (Crago et al., 1996).

Although, on the whole, African American women appeared to have significantly less ED-related pathology than European American women, specific ED symptoms varied by race. African American women were less likely than European American women to report dieting and vomiting, but they reported binge eating at comparable levels (Striegel-Moore, Dohn, & Solomon, 2000). These results were in agreement with findings that BED seems to affect a broader racial distribution than other EDs (Marcus, Wing, & Fairburn, 1995).

In sum, African American women appear to have lower risk than European American women of developing an ED, characterized by body image disturbance and inappropriate compensatory behaviors, but equal risk of developing BED, which is characterized by binge episodes in the absence of compensatory behaviors (Striegel-Moore et al., 2003).

Since the current diagnostic criteria for EDs focuses on body image disturbances, and BED is a provisional diagnosis in the DSM-IV, there is concern that current diagnostic practice may not sufficiently capture EDs in minority racial and ethnic populations (Wonderlich et al., 2007). As a result, African American women may be underdiagnosed for EDs and less likely to receive treatment (Striegel-Moore & Bulik, 2007; Wonderlich et al., 2007). Expansion of the ED diagnoses might allow for more inclusion of clinically significant ED pathology experienced by individuals from other racial and ethnic minority groups (Wonderlich et al., 2007) and could help decrease the existing gap between European American and minority groups in terms of seeking and receiving ED treatment (Cachelin, Rebeck, Veisel, & Striegel-Moore, 2001; Striegel-Moore et al., 2003).

Some experts (King, 1993; Mumford, 1993) feel that racial differences in eating disorders have been overemphasized, noting that AN and BN rates have risen among African American women. Also, differences found among ethnic groups may be related to culturally inappropriate definitions of EDs and assessment measures, which have been developed in European American samples. Finally, all ethnic minorities cannot be lumped together into a single group. For example, whereas African American women appear less likely to develop EDs, Hispanic women may be as likely to develop them as European American women (Crago, Shisslak, & Estes, 1996).

THE ASSOCIATION BETWEEN EDs AND SUDs

Co-Occurrence of EDs and SUDs in Women

Over the past decade it has become increasingly clear that there is a significant relationship between EDs and SUDs in women. Numerous studies have demonstrated this association in both clinical and community samples. Women receiving treatment for EDs frequently report alcohol and other drug use and abuse (Evans & Lacey, 1992; Holderness, Brooks-Gunn, & Warren, 1994; Schuckit et al., 1996), and individuals entering treatment for SUDs often report disordered eating and compensatory behaviors, as well as preoccupation with food and body image (Bulik, Sullivan, Carter, & Joyce, 1997; Franko et al., 2005; Holderness et al., 1994).

In their review, Holderness and colleagues (1994) found rates of SUDs with co-occurring lifetime ED behaviors to range from 2 to 40% in clinical populations, with a median of 20% prevalence for bulimic symptoms. Most recently, the National Comorbidity Survey Replication Study found that the lifetime co-occurrence of alcohol abuse or dependence and EDs was between 25 and 34%, depending on the specific ED. Lifetime prevalence of illicit drug abuse or dependence in conjunction with EDs was somewhat lower, with a range from 8 to 26% (Hudson et al., 2007). These variations in prevalence rates are, in part, due to methodological issues, such as differing recruitment and assessment methods. Nonetheless, these rates are much higher than those found in the general population.

Though the robust relationship between SUDs and EDs is indisputable, questions have been raised as to whether or not this link is a unique one. Some studies with relevant comparison groups have indicated that it may not be unique. For example, high rates of SUDs were found in a sample of patients with BED, but these rates were not higher than those found in a psychiatric comparison group (Wilfley, Schwartz, Spurrell, & Fairburn, 2000). Similarly, EDs were frequently diagnosed in a sample of inpatients with SUDs, but they were also diagnosed at comparable levels in non-substance-abusing psychiatric inpatients (Grilo, Levy, Becker, Edell, & McGlashan, 1995). In a community sample, Dansky and colleagues (Dansky, Brewerton, & Kilpatrick, 2000) reported that prevalence rates of alcohol use disorders in women with BN were similar to those found in nonbulimic women with depressive disorder or PTSD.

Findings from other studies, however, have supported a specific relationship between EDs and SUDs. For example, Hudson and et al. found significantly higher rates of alcohol misuse in women diagnosed with BN, as compared to women diagnosed with depression (Hudson, Pope, Yurgelun-Todd, Jona, & Frankenberg, 1987). In a community-based study with four conditions (alcohol dependence, alcohol dependence with anxiety disorders, anxiety disorders only, and neither alcohol nor anxiety disorders), women with alcohol dependence had significantly higher levels of behavioral and attitudinal features of EDs and were more likely to meet criteria for BN or EDNOS than women in groups without alcohol dependence (Sinha et al., 1996).

Link between BN and Alcohol Use Disorders

Though EDs and SUDs frequently co-occur, comorbidity rates vary depending on type of ED diagnosis. Holderness and colleagues (1994) found that the strongest associations between

SUDs and EDs involved subtypes characterized by bulimic behaviors (e.g., binge–purge sub-type of AN and BN), rather than the restricting subtypes. Multiple other studies have also found that BN is the most common co-occurring ED diagnosis. Relatively less is known about the relationship between BED and SUDs, though studies have reported that the diag-nosis of EDNOS, including BED, was more likely to be made in individuals with SUDs than those without an SUD (Grilo et al., 1995; Grilo, Sinha, & O'Malley, 2002).

Likewise, certain substances of abuse, namely alcohol, are more highly correlated with the presence of EDs. A large study from Japan examined rates of EDs in women with alcohol dependence. The prevalence of EDs in women under 30 years of age was 72%, approximately 24 times the prevalence in the general Japanese population, with BN being the most common problem (Higuchi, Suzuki, Yamada, Parish, & Kono, 1993). Goldbloom et al. studied two different populations of women: those receiving treatment for alcohol use and those receiv-ing treatment for an ED. In women presenting for treatment of alcohol problems, 30.1% met criteria for EDs, and 26.9% of women seeking outpatient treatment for EDs met criteria for alcohol dependence (Goldbloom, Naranjo Bremner, & Hicks, 1992). In a population-based study, 22.9% of women with BN had alcohol dependence and 48.6% had co-occurring alco-hol abuse, as compared to controls who had prevalence rates of 8.6% and 0%, respectively, for alcohol abuse and dependence (Bulik, 1987). Another study reported that, by the age of 35, 50% of individuals with BN had met lifetime criteria for alcohol abuse or dependence (Beary, Lacey, & Merry, 1986).

Research has pointed toward possible factors that might heighten the vulnerability that alcohol use disorders and BN each poses for the development or worsening of the other disorder. For example, women with an ED may use alcohol and other substances to enhance dietary restraint/avoidance, appetite suppression, and compensatory behaviors (Gadalla & Piran, 2007). There is also evidence suggesting that individuals with EDs develop problem-atic drinking patterns at a more rapid rate than individuals without EDs. Finally, substance abuse has also been shown to increase the likelihood of crossover from BN to AN—a cross-over that increases the rates of morbidity and mortality (Tozzi et al., 2005).

Additional Psychiatric Comorbidity

SUDs and EDs often co-occur in the presence of additional psychiatric disorders. Co-occur-ring depressive disorder, posttraumatic stress disorder (PTSD), and other anxiety disorders are the most common Axis I diagnoses (Johnson, Cohen, Kasen, & Brook, 2002). Individuals with SUDs and EDs also tend to be diagnosed with borderline personality disorder, as they report affective instability and impulsivity (Sansone, Fine, & Nunn, 1994). Other person-ality disorders—antisocial, histrionic, obsessive–compulsive, and avoidant—also frequently co-occur.

Certain types of individuals are more likely to struggle with both EDs and SUDs. Studies on women with BN have repeatedly differentiated two distinct subgroups: those with comor-bid SUDs and those without comorbid SUDs. Findings have consistently shown that women with BN and a SUD have higher rates of psychiatric co-occurrence, impulsivity (e.g., cutting, stealing, suicide attempts), and cluster B personality disorders (particularly borderline per-sonality disorder) than women with BN but without an SUD (e.g., Bulik et al., 1997; Grilo et al., 1995; Lilenfeld, 1997; Suzuki, Higuchi, Yamada, Mitzutani, & Kono, 1993).

Additionally, some studies have found that the subgroup of women with BN and an SUD have higher rates of certain ED symptoms—specifically, more severe laxative use and food restriction—than those without an SUD (Bulik et al., 1997; Mitchell, Pyle, Eckert, & Hatsukami, 1990). Observations made in a study of women with alcohol dependence, both with and without EDs (primarily BN), are consistent with this literature. Specifically, women with alcohol dependence and an ED were found to have lower body weights and higher rates of borderline personality or depressive disorder diagnoses than women with alcohol dependence but without an ED (Suzuki et al., 1993).

Women with BN and an SUD have also been shown to have the highest rates of severe sexual abuse history compared to AN and BN groups without an SUD (Deep, Lilenfeld, Plotnicov, Pollice, & Kaye, 1999). Relatedly, rates of substance abuse are elevated in women with BN and BED for those who report a history of sexual or physical abuse (Dohm et al., 2002). Women who have been abused are at a greater risk of developing PTSD, which in turn increases the risk of developing both EDs and SUDs (Dansky et al., 2000). More recently, Corstorphine and colleagues (Corstorphine, Waller, Lawson, & Ganis, 2007) found associations between a history of childhood sexual abuse; high levels of alcohol, amphetamine, cocaine, and cannabis abuse; and impulsive behaviors such as self-cutting.

From these studies, as well as from clinical observations, a distinct profile of women with comorbid BN and SUDs emerges. This complicated subgroup, which has been labeled by some as the multi-impulsive category (Lacey & Evans, 1986), is characterized by multiple psychiatric and personality problems and a history of interpersonal trauma. Women in this group generally have poorer social, interpersonal and occupational functioning. The delineation of subgroups has important implications for treatment, as women with BN and an SUD may respond differently to interventions and are more likely to need comprehensive treatment services than women with BN but without an SUD.

Common Factors/Etiology

The co-occurrence of EDs and SUDs indicates the possibility of common or shared etiological factors. Though no specific links have been established, to date, several theories have been proposed to explain the relationship of these two disorders. These theories, however, are not exhaustive, nor are they mutually exclusive.

Some have speculated that the relationship between EDs and SUDs may be a result of their associations with other disorders. In the National Women's study (Dansky et al., 2000), alcohol abuse was higher in women with BN, as compared to women without BN, only when the influence of depressive disorder and PTSD was controlled. Thus, alcohol use disorders were indirectly related to BN, with the presence of posttraumatic stress and depressive disorders significantly impacting this relationship. These results led investigators to conclude that associations between BN and SUDs are due, at least partly, to their strong relationships with major depressive and posttraumatic stress disorders.

Other theories have posited that, irrespective of specific shared diagnoses, a common constellation of personality traits, characterized by poor impulse control and affective instability, predisposes individuals to develop both SUDs and EDs (Evans & Lacey, 1992). This theory has emerged based on the multiple studies discussed previously, which have identified a subtype of women with EDs and SUDs who exhibit multiple types of impulsive behaviors and deficits in emotion regulation. From this standpoint, both ED and SUD symptoms may represent different manifestations of self-regulatory behaviors (Beary et al., 1986; Holderness et al., 1994). This view is in line with the self-medication model, which has been applied to both EDs (Shoemaker, Smit, Biji, & Vollebergh, 2002) and SUDs (Khantzian, 1997). This model hypothesizes that some individuals, particularly those with trauma histories, use food and substances in an effort to manage or avoid distressing emotional and physical states.

Other researchers have examined biological findings for a potential common underlying factor. For example, research suggests that both EDs and alcohol use disorders may be related to atypical endogenous opioid peptide (EOP) activity (Grilo et al., 2002; Wolfe & Maisto, 2000). EOP activity has been found to have effects on both food and alcohol consumption. Other research suggests that both psychoactive drugs and overeating operate on neurotransmitters (i.e., serotonin, dopamine, and gamma-aminobutyric acid [GABA]) in similar ways. Volkow and O'Brien (2007) reported that dopamine receptor availability was lower in a group of individuals with compulsive overeating, which is also often found in individuals addicted to drugs and alcohol. As a result, they have proposed that some types of obesity may be related to excessive urges for food and suggest that the underlying brain mechanisms in compulsive overeating are similar to compulsive drug use found in addiction. For example, food-craving-related changes have been found in functional magnetic resonance imaging (fMRI) signals for three areas of the brain (the hippocampus, insula, and caudate) also involved in drug cravings (Pelchat Johnson, Chan, Valdez, & Ragland, 2004).

Compulsive overeating often results in obesity and chemical addictions, which are both characterized by the inability to refrain from the substance despite negative consequences. Food and drug consumption are both motivated by their rewarding properties, which are linked to dopaminergic activity (Volkow & O'Brien, 2007). Similar to repeated drug use, repeated consumption of foods high in sugars and fats may result in compulsive food consumption and poor food intake control for some vulnerable individuals (Pelchat, 2002; Volkow & O'Brien, 2007).

Not all investigators have embraced the addiction model of EDs (Wilson, 1991). The addiction model seems to fit best for EDs characterized by binge eating, such as BN, BED, and the binge type of AN, but does not explain the restricting type of AN. More research is necessary to demonstrate a strong link between biological processes and specific food groups and to explain the higher prevalence of EDs in cultures, ethnicities, and socioeconomic groups that prize thinness, as well as the co-occurrence of EDs and SUDs with other psychiatric disorders.

TREATMENT OF EDs AND TREATMENT OPTIONS FOR CO-OCCURRING EDs AND SUDs

Though debate continues on the exact meaning and cause of the co-occurrence of EDs and SUDs, the fact that they co-occur so frequently has major implications for assessment and treatment. Despite this strong association between the two disorders, and their clinical similarities, treatments for each disorder have been developed separately. This section identifies current evidence-based treatments for EDs and suggests ways in which to integrate SUD and ED treatment.

Treatments for EDs

Research has validated behavioral treatments for BN and BED, as well as pharmacological treatment for BN. Evidence-based behavioral treatments include cognitive-behavioral therapy and interpersonal psychotherapy. Psychopharmacology has focused on antidepressant medications.

Cognitive-Behavioral Therapy

Cognitive-behavioral therapy (CBT) is a short-term (approximately 20 weeks) structured, problem-oriented therapy. It is designed to help individuals identify and modify current behaviors and cognitive distortions associated with the disorder being treated. Over the course of treatment new techniques are added to previous ones in order to broaden the person's repertoire of coping skills and range of healthy cognitions.

CBT has been identified as the behavioral treatment of choice for EDs (American Psychiatric Association, 2006). CBT for an ED is focused on the processes that maintain binge-eating and purging behaviors, with a goal of disrupting these processes and developing more positive cognitions and healthier eating habits. The first stage of treatment primarily uses behavioral techniques, such as monitoring eating habits, weekly weighing, restricting food intake to preplanned meals and snacks, use of alternative pleasant behaviors to replace binge eating, and stimulus-control techniques to restrict overeating. The second stage of treatment continues the behavioral emphasis of establishing stable eating habits and introduces cognitive restructuring focused on the person's thoughts, beliefs, and values in relation to body image and weight; these are believed to maintain symptomatic behaviors. Problem-solving skills are also targeted and improved. Treatment concludes with a focus on maintaining the newly developed behaviors and cognitions following treatment completion. Unrealistic expectations about never again engaging in binge-eating or purging behaviors are addressed through relapse prevention interventions that predict a "lapse" and introduce interventions to prevent a "relapse."

CBT is the most extensively researched psychological intervention for BN, and many of the clinical trials have utilized a version of Fairburn's manual (Fairburn, Marcus, & Wilson, 1993). Although designed as an individual treatment approach, the manual has successfully been adapted for a group therapy format. Evaluations of its effectiveness for BN show that purging and dietary restraint behaviors and depression decrease as a result of treatment, whereas positive attitudes toward body shape, self-esteem, and social functioning increase. Although CBT is an effective treatment for BN, only 50% of individuals in CBT treatment completely cease their binge and purge behaviors (Wilson, 1996). Positive changes are more likely to occur in behaviors regarding food consumption, rather than in the underlying attitudes about weight or cognitions concerning body image.

Less research has been conducted on the use of CBT for BED, but results suggest that it is also effective for individuals with this diagnosis (Wilfley at al., 2002). Weight seems to decrease for patients with BED who abstain from binge eating, although the long-term effects of weight loss vary. CBT has not, however, been shown to be effective for reduction of anorexic symptoms.

Interpersonal Psychotherapy

Interpersonal psychotherapy (IPT) is a short-term (usually 15–20 sessions) and structured psychotherapy designed to help patients identify and modify problems in social functioning. IPT makes no assumptions about the cause of a psychiatric disorder. Rather, symptoms are examined and addressed within an interpersonal context. IPT focuses on current relationships that lead to, exacerbate, and/or maintain psychological symptoms, with the goal of helping patients develop greater mastery in interpersonal situations—which, in turn, is believed to bring about symptom change.

IPT was originally developed for the treatment of depression but has since been expanded to treat other populations and disorders, including EDs (Klerman & Weissman, 1993). The rationale for applying the IPT model to EDs is the interrelationship among interpersonal functioning, low self-esteem, negative mood, traumatic life events, and eating behavior (Fairburn et al., 1991). The treatment has three stages. The initial phase involves examination of a patient's interpersonal history to identify the problem area(s) associated with ED onset and maintenance; a plan is then provided to guide the patient in working on specified problem area(s). During the intermediate phase of treatment, strategies are implemented to help patients make changes in identified problem areas. In the termination phase, patients evaluate and consolidate gains and detail their plans for maintaining improvements.

IPT was applied to BN by Fairburn and colleagues (Fairburn et al., 1991); it was initially intended as a credible alternative to CBT. Results of a large-scale trial showed that IPT was equally as effective as CBT, although IPT took longer to produce effects. Patients in both treatment conditions improved substantially, with the changes being maintained over a 12-month follow-up period, and both were superior to behavioral therapy for BN (Fairburn, Jones, Peveler, Hope, & O'Connor, 1993; Fairburn et al., 1995). These findings were initially surprising considering that, unlike CBT, IPT does not directly address dietary issues or attitudes toward shape and weight. The researchers concluded that BN can be treated successfully without focusing upon the individual's eating habits and cognitions concerning shape and weight.

A group version of IPT has been used by Wilfley and colleagues to treat obese patients who binge eat (Wilfley et al., 1993). Findings from a large-scale controlled treatment trial comparing group IPT to group CBT showed similar results as those for BN (Wilfley et al., 2002). Both treatments showed initial and long-term efficacy for the core and related BED symptoms, indicating that group IPT is a viable alternative to group CBT for the treatment of overweight patients with BED. Based on these findings, IPT continues to gain recognition in the field of EDs and is considered an effective treatment for BN and BED. There is not, as of yet, empirical evidence supporting its role in the treatment of AN.

Pharmacotherapy

A number of pharmacotherapies are used in the treatment of EDs, especially BN. Antidepressant medications, specifically, have proven effective in reducing both binge-eating and purging symptoms (see Peterson & Mitchell, 1999, and Wilson & Fairburn, 1998 for reviews). In particular, selective serotonin reuptake inhibitors (SSRIs), such as fluoxetine, have been helpful in treating these symptoms, as evidenced by a number of randomized clinical trials (e.g., Fichter et al., 1991; Fluoxetine Bulimia Nervosa Collaborative Study Group, 1992; Goldstein, Wilson, Thompson, Potvin, & Rampey, 1995). EDs are characterized by alterations in serotonin activity in the brain, and these changes are modified by SSRI medication. Across studies, the effectiveness of SSRIs in reducing binge eating and vomiting ranges from 50 to 75%. In addition to reducing symptoms of bingeing and purging, SSRIs can reduce co-occurring symptoms of depression and anxiety that are common in patients with EDs as well as those with SUDs.

Other antidepressant agents that have been demonstrated as effective in clinical trials for the treatment of BN include tricyclic antidepressants (Agras, Dorian Kirkley, Arnow, & Bachman, 1987; Barlow, Blouin, Blouin, & Perez, 1988; Walsh, Hadigan, Devlin, Gladis, & Roose, 1991), monoamine oxidase inhibitors (Kennedy et al., 1988; Walsh, Stewart, Roose, Gladis, & Glassman, 1984), and trazodone (Pope, Keck McElroy, & Hudson, 1989).

Among patients with AN, pharmacotherapy is often helpful as a component of treatment following acute treatment to restore weight. SSRIs have been demonstrated to help alleviate depression and promote weight maintenance (Kaye, Weltzin, Hsu, & Bulik, 1991; American Psychiatric Association Work Group on Eating Disorders, 2000).

Combination Treatments

In clinical practice it is most common that patients with EDs are treated using a combination of approaches that is tailored to specific clinical needs. Because EDs are considered biopsychosocial disorders, treatment is complex and often requires a multidisciplinary approach. In addition to behavioral and pharmacological treatment, nutritional and medical supervision are also often indicated (Bowers, Andersen, & Evans, 2004). Multiple modalities, such as individual, group, and family treatments, are also often utilized. It appears that treatment is most effective within the context of a program that specializes in treating EDs (Wonderlich, Connolly, & Stice, 2004). However, most EDs, particularly AN and BED, are more often treated in a general medical setting (Hudson et al., 2007).

A number of studies has examined the efficacy of combining medication and individual psychotherapy in the treatment of BN (American Psychiatric Association Work Group on Eating Disorders, 2000). One study found that combining CBT and active medication was more effective than either intervention alone in reducing ED behaviors (Walsh et al., 1997), but other studies have not found the same results (e.g., Kaye et al., 1991).

Treatment of Co-Occurring EDs and SUDs

Although the literature is sparse, it appears that SUDs have not been found to negatively influence recovery from AN or BN (Franko et al., 2005; Mitchell et al., 1990; Strasser, Pike, & Walsh, 1992). Overall strategies for treatment of co-occurring SUDs and other psychiatric disorders have been described as integrated, sequential, and parallel (Busch, Weiss, & Najavits, 2005; Mueser, Noordsy, Drake, & Fox, 2003). *Integrated treatment* means that the treatment of both disorders is delivered at the same time by the same clinician or within the same treatment program. As we will see, integrated treatment is both rare and difficult to provide for EDs and SUDs. Sequential and parallel treatments are the more common approaches when SUDs and psychiatric disorders co-occur. In a *sequential treatment* model, patients first obtain treatment for one disorder, and then subsequent treatment of the other disorder. In a *parallel treatment* model, patients receive treatment for both disorders simultaneously but in two separate service settings, or with two clinicians who each specializes in the treatment of one of the disorders.

Integrated Treatment

Currently there is no evidence-based treatment that integrates SUD and ED treatment. Also, no research, to date, has been done comparing integrated versus sequential or parallel approaches to the treatment of these co-occurring disorders. It is rare to find programs that provide integrated treatment for EDs and SUDs. As a result, these co-occurring disorders are most often treated in programs that address either SUDs or EDs, but do not offer services for both disorders. For example, a recent national survey of publicly funded SUD treatment programs found that they inconsistently screen admissions for EDs and rarely use standard diagnostic instruments. Less than one in five publicly funded addiction treatment programs attempts to treat patients' EDs (Gordon et al., 2008).

Integration of SUD and ED treatment is challenging. Less than 60% of addiction treatment programs provide integrated care for any co-occurring psychiatric condition (Ducharme, Knudsen, & Roman, 2006). Although many patients with a co-occurring SUD and ED would most likely benefit from integrated treatment of their disorders, the service systems for accomplishing this goal generally do not currently exist in substance abuse treatment settings (Sinha & O'Malley, 2000). This may largely be due to the lack of expertise for managing EDs in addiction programs, where clinicians with expertise in treating both disorders are rare (National Center on Addiction and Substance Abuse at Columbia University [CASA], 2003).

In addition, basic goals of treatment for each disorder may create difficulties in integrating SUD and ED treatment. Many addiction treatment programs are based in 12-step philosophy, in which abstinence from addictive substances is the primary goal of treatment. These programs may prefer the abstinence-based Overeaters Anonymous approach (in which the emphasis is on abstaining from foods that may trigger binge eating episodes) to evidence-based behavioral and pharmacological treatments, which emphasizes moderation in food consumption as a treatment goal. It could also be difficult for patients to work toward the goal of abstinence from addictive substances at the same time as they are working toward the goal of moderation in food consumption.

Although it may be too difficult for providers who specialize either in SUD or ED treatment to offer truly integrated care, they can still provide an integrated foundation for care. First, providers should screen patients for EDs and SUDs. There are a number of relatively simple screening and assessment tools for EDs that can be administered by nonspecialists, including the Eating Disorder Examination-Questionnaire (Fairburn & Beglin, 1994). Second, clinicians can help motivate their patients to receive treatment by helping them to identify the mechanisms in which one disorder triggers the other. Providers can educate their patients about ED and SUD symptoms and consequences, as well as potential treatment outcomes. Finally, clinicians can develop a list of referrals for treating the other disorder and can cultivate professional relationships with these providers. These basic steps become the building blocks for successful sequential and parallel treatment.

Sequential Treatment

Though there are currently no accepted guidelines regarding the sequencing of treatments for co-occurring EDs and SUDs, one important consideration in determining the appropriate organization of services and treatment plan for an individual patient is to determine the severity of each disorder. Patients may meet diagnostic criteria for both disorders, but they will likely differ in severity or vary as to whether they are currently active or in remission. Other considerations for sequencing involve motivation for treatment, the patient's perception of which disorder is more distressing or impairing of functioning, and time of onset of each disorder.

Sequential treatment providers may falsely assume that one disorder is in remission when treatment for it concludes and the patient is transferred to a program for the other disorder. However, EDs and SUDs are both chronic disorders marked by relapse. It is important for clinicians to monitor the status of the disorder not currently being treated for signs of relapse. For example, a psychiatrist who referred a patient from an addiction program would, of course, monitor the patient's alcohol and drug use, while treating her ED. As patients decrease one set of symptomatic behaviors, they may increase the other behaviors as compensatory ways of handling stress. Emerging symptoms of the condition not being treated may become an opportunity for the clinician and patient to understand the common triggers for both sets of behaviors and to develop strategies to decrease both substance abuse and eating-disordered behaviors. It also is important for clinicians to recognize the limitations of their practice and to refer patients to continued treatment for relapse of the other disorder, as necessary.

Parallel Treatment

Parallel treatment for ED and SUD involves more than one treatment provider. Often a patient with co-occurring ED and SUD will be treated by a eating disorder specialist, certified addiction treatment counselor, psychiatrist or other physician, and nutritionist. In these cases it is very important that the multiple providers develop shared treatment goals and communicate frequently with each other.

FUTURE DIRECTIONS

The scientific study of EDs is in its infancy. The current diagnostic classification of EDs is questionable and may need revision to increase its clinical and scientific usefulness. Better diagnostic tools may increase the validity of epidemiological studies to determine prevalence and relationship of EDs to SUDs and other psychiatric disorders. The apparent relationship and prevalence of SUDs and EDs may become better understood through research into shared etiology, such as cravings. Finally, the needs of individuals who suffer from SUDs and EDs may be addressed through the development of specialized treatments. Clinical trials of new integrated treatment models may then be compared to parallel and sequential models to improve treatment protocols.

KEY POINTS

- Women have significantly higher rates of EDs than men, which is due in part to increasingly thin body ideals for women in Western culture.
- There appear to be ethnic differences in prevalence and type of ED symptoms, and minority women are less likely to receive ED treatment.
- There is a strong co-occurrence of EDs and SUDs, particularly between bulimic behaviors and alcohol use disorders.
- SUDs and EDs often co-occur in the context of other disorders such as depression, anxiety, PTSD, and borderline personality disorder.
- A subgroup of patients characterized by high levels of psychiatric comorbidity, impulsivity, dysregulated affect, and childhood abuse appears more likely to develop both EDs and SUDs.
- Recent biochemical evidence suggests commonality between addiction to substances and ED symptoms, lending support for an addiction model of EDs.
- Empirically validated treatments are available for EDs, but no evidence-based integrated treatment is available for co-occurring EDs and SUDs.
- SUD treatment programs rarely provide ED screening, assessment, or treatment.
- Clinicians not experienced in the treatment of co-occurring EDs and SUDs can screen for both conditions, educate their patients about the impact of one disorder on the other one, and design a treatment plan to address both conditions, either sequentially or in parallel.

REFERENCES

Asterisks denote recommended readings.

Agras, W. S., & Apple, R. F. (1997). *Overcoming eating disorders: A cognitive-behavioral therapy approach for bulimia nervosa and binge-eating disorder—therapist guide* (2nd ed.). New York: Oxford University Press. (*)

Agras, W. S., Dorian, B., Kirkley, B. G., Arnow, B., & Bachman, J. (1987). Imipramine in the treatment of bulimia: A double-blind controlled study. *International Journal of Eating Disorders, 6,* 29–38.

American Psychiatric Association. (1994). *Diagnostic and statistical manual of mental disorders* (4th ed.). Washington, DC: Author.

American Psychiatric Association. (2006). *Practice guidelines for the treatment of psychiatric disorders: Compendium 2006*. Washington, DC: Author.

American Psychiatric Association Work Group on Eating Disorders. (2000). Practice guideline for the treatment of patients with eating disorders. *American Journal of Psychiatry, 157,* 1–39.

Anderson-Fye, E., & Becker, A. E. (2004). Socio-cultural aspects of eating disorders. In J. K. Thompson (Ed.), *Handbook of eating disorders and obesity* (pp. 565–589). New York: Wiley.

Barlow, J., Blouin, J., Blouin, A., & Perez, E. (1988). Treatment of bulimia with desipramine: A double-blind crossover study. *Canadian Journal of Psychiatry, 33,* 129–133.

Beary, M. D., Lacey, J. H., & Merry, J. (1986). Alcoholism and eating disorders in women of fertile age. *British Journal of Addictions, 81,* 685–689.

Becker, A. E. (2004). Television, disordered eating, and young women in Fiji: Negotiating body image and identity during rapid social change. *Culture, Medicine, and Psychiatry, 28,* 533–559.

Bowers, W. A., Andersen, A. E., & Evans, K. (2004). Management of eating disorders: Inpatient and partial hospital programs. In T. D. Brewerton (Ed.), *Clinical handbook of eating disorders: An integrated approach* (pp. 349–376). New York: Marcel Dekker.

Brownell, K. D. (1991). Dieting and the search for the perfect body: Where physiology and culture collide. *Behavior Therapy, 22,* 1–12.

Bulik, C. M. (1987). Drug and alcohol abuse by bulimic women and their families. *American Journal of Psychiatry, 144,* 1604–1606.

Bulik, C. M., Sullivan, P. F., Carter, F. A., & Joyce, P. R. (1997). Lifetime comorbidity of alcohol dependence in women with bulimia nervosa. *Addictive Behaviors, 22,* 437–446.

Busch, A. B., Weiss, R. D., & Najavits, L. M. (2005). Co-occurring substance use disorders and other psychiatric disorders. In R. J. Frances, S. I. Miller, & A. H. Mack (Eds.), *Clinical textbook of addictive disorders* (3rd ed., pp. 271–302). New York: Guilford Press.

Cachelin, F. M., Rebeck, R., Veisel, C., & Striegel-Moore, R. H. (2001). Barriers to treatment for eating disorders among ethnically diverse women. *International Journal of Eating Disorders, 30*(3), 269–278.

Corstorphine, E., Waller, G., Lawson, R., & Ganis, C. (2007). Trauma and multi-impulsivity in the eating disorders. *Eating Behaviors, 8*(1), 23–30.

Crago, M., Shisslak, C. M., & Estes, L. S. (1996). Eating disturbances among American minority groups: A review. *International Journal of Eating Disorders, 19,* 239–248.

Dansky, B. S., Brewerton, T. D., & Kilpatrick, D. G. (2000). Comorbidity of bulimia nervosa and alcohol use disorders: Results from the National Women's Study. *International Journal of Eating Disorders, 27,* 180–190.

Deep, A. L., Lilenfeld, L. R., Plotnicov, K. H., Pollice, C., & Kaye, W. H. (1999) Sexual abuse in eating disorder subtypes and control women: The role of comorbid substance dependence in bulimia nervosa. *International Journal of Eating Disorders, 25,* 1–10.

Dohm, F. A., Striegel-Moore, R., Wilfley, D. E., Pike, K. M., Hook, J., & Fairburn, C. G. (2002). Self harm and substance use in a community sample of black and white women with binge eating disorders or bulimia nervosa. *International Journal of Eating Disorders, 32,* 389–400.

Ducharme, L. J., Knudsen, H. K., & Roman, P. M. (2006). Availability of integrated care for co-occurring substance abuse and psychiatric conditions. *Community Mental Health Journal, 42*(4), 363–375.

Evans, C., & Lacey, H. (1992). Multiple self-damaging behaviour among alcoholic women: A prevalence study. *British Journal of Psychiatry, 161,* 643–647.

Fairburn, C. G., & Beglin, S. J. (1994). Assessment of eating disorders: Interview or self-report questionnaire. *International Journal of Eating Disorders, 16,* 363–370.

Fairburn, C. G., & Bohn, K. (2005). Eating disorder NOS (EDNOS): An example of the troublesome "not otherwise specified" (NOS) category in DSM-IV. *Behavior Research and Therapy, 43*(6), 691–701.

Fairburn, C. G., Jones, R., Peveler, R. C., Carr, S. J., Solomon, R. A., O'Conner, M., et al. (1991).

Three psychological treatments for bulimia nervosa: A comparative trial. *Archives of General Psychiatry*, 48, 463–469.

Fairburn, C. G., Jones, R., Peveler, R. C., Hope, R. A., & O'Connor, M. (1993). Psychotherapy and bulimia nervosa: The longer term effects of interpersonal psychotherapy, behaviour therapy, and cognitive behaviour therapy. *Archives of General Psychiatry*, 50, 419–428.

Fairburn, C. G., Marcus, M. D., & Wilson, G. T. (1993). Cognitive behavior therapy for binge eating and bulimia nervosa: A comprehensive treatment manual. In C. G. Fairburn & G. T. Wilson (Eds.), *Binge eating: Nature, assessment, and treatment* (pp. 361–404). New York: Guilford Press.

Fairburn, C. G., Norman, P. A., Welch, S. L., O'Connor, M. E., Doll, H. A., & Peveler, R. C. (1995). A prospective study of outcome in bulimia nervosa and the long-term effects of three psychological treatments. *Archives of General Psychiatry*, 52, 304–312.

Fichter, M. M., Leibl, K., Rief, W., Brunner, E., Schmidt-Auberger, & Engel, R. R. (1991). Fluoxetine versus placebo: A double-blind study with bulimic inpatients undergoing intensive psychotherapy. *Pharmacopsychiatry*, 24, 1–7.

Fluoxetine Bulimia Nervosa Collaborative Study Group. (1992). Fluoxetine in the treatment of bulimia nervosa: A multicenter, placebo-controlled, double-blind trial. *Archives of General Psychiatry*, 49, 139–147.

Franko, D. L., Dorer, D. J., Keel, P. K., Jackson, S., Manzo, M. P., & Herzog, D. B. (2005). How do eating disorders and alcohol use disorder influence each other? *International Journal of Eating Disorders*, 38(3), 200–207.

Gadalla, T., & Piron, N. (2007). Co-occurrence of eating disorders and alcohol use disorders in women: A meta analysis. *Archives of Women's Mental Health*, 10(4), 133–140.

Goldbloom, D. S., Naranjo, C. A., Bremner, K. E., & Hicks, L. K. (1992). Eating disorders and alcohol abuse in women. *British Journal of Addiction*, 87, 913–919.

Goldstein, D. J., Wilson, M. G., Thompson, V. L., Potvin, J. H., & Rampey, A. H. (1995). Long-term fluoxetine treatment of bulimia nervosa. *British Journal of Psychiatry*, 166, 660–666.

Gordon, S., Johnson, A., Cohen, L., Killeen, T., Greenfield, S., & Roman, P. (2008). Assessment and treatment of co-occurring eating disorders in publicly funded addiction treatment programs. *Psychiatric Services*, 59(9), 1056–1059.

Grilo, C. M., Levy, K. N., Becker, D. F., Edell, W. S., & McGlashan, T. H. (1995). Eating disorders in female inpatients with versus without substance use disorders. *Addictive Behaviors*, 20(2), 255–260.

Grilo, C. M., Sinha, R., & O'Malley, S. S. (2002). Eating disorders and alcohol use disorders. *Alcohol Research and Health*, 26(2), 151–160.

Higuchi, S., Suzuki, K., Yanada, K., Parish, K., & Kono, H. (1993). Alcoholics with eating disorders: Prevalence and clinical course. *British Journal of Psychiatry*, 162, 403–406.

Holderness, C. C., Brooks-Gunn, J., & Warren, M. P. (1994). Co-morbidity of eating disorders and substance abuse: Review of the literature. *International Journal of Eating Disorders*, 16, 1–34.

Hudson, J. I., Hiripi, E., Pope, H. G., & Kessler, R. C. (2007). The prevalence and correlation of eating disorders in the National Comorbidity Survey Replication Study. *Biological Psychiatry*, 61, 348–358.

Hudson, J. I., Pope, H. G., Yurgelun-Todd, D., Jona, J. M., & Frankenberg, F. R. (1987). A controlled study of lifetime prevalence of affective and other psychiatric disorders in bulimic outpatients. *American Journal of Psychiatry*, 144, 1238–1287.

Johnson, J. G., Cohen, L. K., Kasen, S., & Brook, J. S. (2002). Psychiatric disorders associated with risk for the development of eating disorders during adolescence and early adulthood. *Journal of Consulting and Clinical Psychology*, 70, 1119–1128.

Katzmarzyk, P. T., & Davis, C. (2001). Thinness and body shape of Playboy centerfolds from 1978–1998. *International Journal of Obesity*, 25, 590–592.

Kaye, W. H., Weltzin, T. E., Hsu, L. K., & Bulik, C. (1991). An open trial of fluoxetine in patients with anorexia nervosa. *Journal of Clinical Psychiatry*, 52, 464–471.

Kennedy, S. H., Piran, N., Warsh, J., Prendergast, P., Mainprize, E., Whynot, C., et al. (1998). A trial of isocarboxazid in the treatment of bulimia nervosa. *Journal of Clinical Psychopharmacolology*, 8, 391–396.

Khantzian, E. (1997). The self-medication hypothesis of substance use disorders: A reconsideration and recent applications. *Harvard Review of Psychiatry, 4,* 231–244.

King, M. B. (1993). Cultural aspects of eating disorders. *International Review of Psychiatry, 5,* 205–216

Klerman, G., & Weissman, M. M. (1993). *New applications in interpersonal psychotherapy.* Washington, DC: American Psychiatric Association.

Lacey, J. H., & Evans, C. H. (1986). The impulsivist: A multi-impulsive personality disorder. *British Journal of Addiction, 81,* 641–649.

Lilenfeld, L., Kaye, W., Greeno, C., Merikangas, K. R., Plotnicov, K., Pollice, C., et al. (1997). Psychiatric disorders in women with bulimia nervosa and their first-degree relatives: Effects of comorbid substance dependence. *International Journal of Eating Disorders, 22,* 253–264.

Marcus, M. D., Wing, R. R., & Fairburn, C. G. (1995). Cognitive behavioral treatment of binge eating vs. behavioral weight control in the treatment of binge eating disorder. *Annals of Behavioral Medicine, 17,* S090.

Mitchell, J. E., Pyle, R., Eckert, E. D., & Hatsukami, D. (1990). The influence of prior alcohol and drug abuse problems on bulimia nervosa treatment outcome. *Addictive Behaviors, 15*(2), 169–173.

Mueser, K. T., Noordsy, D. L., Drake, R. E., & Fox, L. (2003). *Integrated treatment for dual disorders: A guide to effective practice.* New York: Guilford Press.

Mumford, D. B. (1993). Eating disorders in different cultures. *International Review of Psychiatry, 5,* 109–114.

National Center on Addiction and Substance Abuse at Columbia University (CASA). (2003). *The formative years: Pathways to substance abuse among girls and young women ages 8–22.* Available at *www.casacolumbia.org./usr_doc/Formative_Years_Pathways_2003R.pdf.*

Nielsen, S. (2001). Epidemiology and mortality of eating disorders. *Psychiatric Clinics of North America, 24,* 201–214.

Pelchat, M. L. (2002). Of human bondage: Food craving, obsession, compulsion, and addiction. *Physiology and Behavior, 76,* 347–352.

Pelchat, M. L., Johnson, A., Chan, R., Valdez, J., & Ragland, J. D. (2004). Images of desire: Food-craving activation during fMRI. *NeuroImage, 23,* 1486–1493.

Peterson, C. B., & Mitchell, J. E. (1999). Psychosocial and pharmacological treatment of eating disorders: A review of research findings. *Journal of Clinical Psychology, 55*(6), 685–697.

Pope, H. G., Keck, P. E., McElroy, S. L., & Hudson, T. L. (1998). A placebo-controlled study of trazodone in bulimia nervosa. *Journal of Clinical Psychopharmacology, 9,* 254–259.

Rodin, J. (1993). Cultural and psychosocial determinants of weight concerns. *Annals of Internal Medicine, 119,* 643–645.

Sansone, R. A., Fine, M. A., & Nunn, J. L. (1994). A comparison of borderline personality symptomatology and self-destructive behavior in women with eating, substance abuse, and both eating and substance abuse disorders. *Journal of Personality Disorders, 8*(3), 219–228.

Schuckit, M. A., Tipp, J. E., Anthenelli, R. M., Bucholz, K. K., Hesselbrock, V., & Nurnberger, J. I., Jr. (1996). Anorexia nervosa and bulimia nervosa in alcohol-dependent men and women and their relatives. *American Journal of Psychiatry, 153,* 74–82.

Shoemaker, C., Smit, F., Biji, R. V., & Vollebergh, W. A. (2002). Bulimia nervosa following psychological and multiple child abuse: Support for the self medication hypothesis in a population based cohort study. *International Journal of Eating Disorders, 32*(4), 381–388.

Sinha, R., & O'Malley, S. S. (2000). Alcohol and eating disorders: Implications for alcohol treatment and health services research. *Alcoholism: Clinical and Experimental Research, 24,* 1312–1319.

Sinha, R., Robinson, J., Merikangas, K., Wilson, G. T., Rodin, J., & O'Malley, S. S. (1996). Eating pathology among women with alcoholism and/or anxiety disorders. *Alcoholism: Clinical and Experimental Research, 20*(7), 1184–1191.

Strasser, T. J., Pike, K. M., & Walsh, B. T. (1992). The impact of prior substance abuse on treatment outcome for bulimia nervosa. *Addictive Behaviors, 17*(4), 387–395.

Striegel-Moore, R. H., & Bulik, C. M. (2007). Risk factors for eating disorders. *American Psychologist, 62*(3), 181–198.

Striegel-Moore, R. H., Dohm, F. A., Kraemer, H. C., Taylor, C. B., Daniels, S., Crawford, P. B., et al. (2003). Eating disorders in white and black women. *American Journal of Psychiatry*, *160*, 1326–1331.

Striegel-Moore, R. H., Dohm, F. A., & Solomon, E. E. (2000). Subthreshhold binge eating disorder. *International Journal of Eating Disorders*, *27*, 270–278.

Striegel-Moore, R. H., & Smolak, L. (1996). The role of race in the development of eating disorders. In L. Smolak, M. Levine, & R. H. Striegel-Moore (Eds.), *The developmental psychopathology of eating disorders* (pp. 259–284). Hillsdale, NJ: Erlbaum.

Suzuki, K., Higuchi, S., Yamada, K., Mitzutani, Y., & Kono, H. (1993). Young female alcoholics with and without eating disorders: A comparative study in Japan. *American Journal of Psychiatry*, *150*(7), 1053–1058.

Tozzi, F., Thornton, L. M., Klump, K. L., Fichter, M. M., Halmi, K. A., Kaplan, A. S., et al. (2005). Symptom fluctuation in eating disorders: Correlates of diagnostic crossover. *American Journal of Psychiatry*, *162*, 732–740.

Volkow, N. D., & O'Brien, C. P. (2007). Issues for DSM-V: Should obesity be included as a brain disorder? *American Journal of Psychiatry*, *164*(5), 708–710.

Walsh, B. T., Hadigan, C. M., Devlin, M. J., Gladis, M., & Roose, S. P. (1991). Long-term outcome of antidepressant treatment for bulimia nervosa. *American Journal of Psychiatry*, *148*, 1206–1212.

Walsh, B. T., Stewart, J. W., Roose, S. P., Gladis, M., & Glassman, A. H. (1984). Treatment of bulimia with phenelzine: A double-blind, placebo-controlled study. *Archives of General Psychiatry*, *41*, 1105–1109.

Walsh, B. T., Wilson, G. T., Loeb, K. L., Devlin, M. J., Pike, K. M., Roose, S. P., et al. (1997). Medication and psychotherapy in the treatment of bulimia nervosa. *American Journal of Psychiatry*, *154*, 523–531.

Weiss, M. G. (1995). Eating disorders and disordered eating in different cultures. *Cultural Psychiatry*, *18*, 537–551.

Wilfley, D. E., Agras, W. S., Telch, C. F., Rossiter, E. M., Schneider, J. A., Cole, A. G., et al. (1993). Group cognitive-behavioral therapy and group interpersonal psychotherapy for the nonpurging bulimic individual: A controlled comparison. *Journal of Consulting and Clinical Psychology*, *61*, 296–305.

Wilfley, D. E., Schwartz, M. H., Spurrell, E. B., & Fairburn, C. G. (2000). Using the Eating Disorder Examination to identify specific psychopathology of binge eating disorder. *International Journal of Eating Disorders*, *27*, 259–269.

Wilfley, D. E., Welch, R. R., Stein, R. I., Spurrell, E. B., Cohen, L. R., Saelens, B. E., et al. (2002). A randomized comparison of group cognitive behavior therapy and group interpersonal psychotherapy for the treatment of overweight individuals with binge eating disorder. *Archives of General Psychiatry*, *59*, 713–721.

Wilson, G. T. (1991). The addiction model of eating disorders: A critical analysis. *Advances in Behavior Therapy*, *12*, 27–72.

Wilson, G. T. (1996). Treatment of bulimia nervosa: When CBT fails. *Behavior Research Therapy*, *34*, 197–212.

Wilson, G. T., & Fairburn, C. G. (1998). Treatments for eating disorders. In P. E. Nathan, & J. M. Gorman (Eds.), *A guide to treatments that work* (2nd ed., pp. 501–530). New York: Oxford University Press. (*)

Wolfe, W. L., & Maisto, S. A. (2000). The relationship between eating disorders and substance use: Moving beyond co-prevalence research. *Clinical Psychology Review*, *20*, 617–631.

Wonderlich, S. A., Connolly, K. M., & Stice, E. (2004). Impulsivity as a risk factor for eating disorder behavior: Assessment implications with adolescents. *International Journal of Eating Disorders*, *36*(2), 172–182.

Wonderlich, S. A., Joiner, T., Keel, P., Williamson, D., & Crosby, R. (2007). Eating disorder diagnoses: Empirical approaches to classification. *American Psychologist*, *62*, 167–180.

CHAPTER 14

Trauma, Posttraumatic Stress Disorder, and Addiction among Women

Denise Hien, PhD

Recognition of the high rates of traumatic stress and related comorbidity among women in treatment for addictions has led to significant advances in the fields of epidemiology, assessment, and treatment of substance use disorders (SUDs) and trauma-related disorders. This chapter provides a summary of the prevalence findings of posttraumatic stress disorder (PTSD) and other comorbidity among substance users, and it presents widely accepted models for understanding the causal pathways between traumatic stress exposure and psychiatric consequences. Current knowledge of assessment and evidence- based practices for the treatment of PTSD and associated psychiatric comorbidity among female substance users are also reviewed. The chapter further aims to provide an understanding of the barriers that continue to exist regarding the implementation of these promising evidence-based approaches in community treatment programs.

EPIDEMIOLOGY OF PTSD AMONG TRAUMA-EXPOSED PERSONS

Histories of traumatic stress exposures have been documented in as many as 95% of people seeking or attending substance use treatment (Brown, 1989; Brown, Recupero, & Stout, 1995; Brown & Wolfe, 1994; Fullilove et al., 1993; Read, Brown, & Kahler, 2004). One of the most significant and common psychiatric consequences of traumatic exposure is the development of PTSD, a syndrome marked by symptoms of intense horror or fear following a psychologically distressing event involving a real or perceived threat to physical integrity. This disorder typically results from an extreme, catastrophic, or overwhelming experience and is typically accompanied by the following symptoms: reexperiencing of the event through flashbacks, nightmares, and intrusive memories; avoidance of stimuli associated with the event; and increased arousal (Amdur, Larsen, & Liberzon, 2000; American Psychiatric Association, 1994).

Although some studies of the general population have yielded estimates of PTSD as low as 0.4–3.1% (Davidson, Hughes, Blazer, & George, 1991; Helzer, Robins, & McEvoy, 1987; Schore, 2001), failure to ask specific questions concerning criminal victimization and childhood abuse may account for these low estimates. In studies that have used specific questions about victimization and child abuse, prevalence rates of PTSD in community samples have ranged from 13 to 36% (Breslau, Davis, Andreski, & Peterson, 1991; Kilpatrick, Saunders, Veronen, Best, & Von, 1987; Norris, 1992; Resnick, Kilpatrick, Dansky, Saunders, & Best, 1993). In a large epidemiological survey, 61% of men and 51% of women reported being exposed to trauma, with 5% of men and 10% of women developing PTSD (Kessler, Sonnega, Bromet, Hughes, & Nelson, 1995). There is evidence that the risk for developing PTSD is particularly high among victims of violent crime. Prevalence estimates of PTSD range from 14 to 80% among victims of sexual assault and from 13 to 23% among victims of physical assault (Breslau et al., 1991; Kilpatrick et al., 1987; Norris, 1992). In contrast to interpersonal victimization, accidents not involving injury and natural disasters are not associated with a high risk for developing PTSD (Freedy, Kilpatrick, & Resnick, 1993; Green et al., 1990; Resnick et al., 1993; Shore, Tatum, & Vollmer, 1986; Steinglass & Gerrity, 1990).

EPIDEMIOLOGY OF PTSD AMONG SUBSTANCE USERS

Prevalence of Comorbid PTSD and SUDs

Although traumatic exposure itself has not been shown to lead to an increased risk of SUD comorbidity for men or for women (Chilcoat & Breslau, 1998b), rates of PTSD in substance abuse populations are 1.4 to 5 times higher than among those without SUDs (Cottler, Compton, Mager, Spitznagel, & Janca, 1992). The prevalence of comorbid PTSD and SUD has been examined in two main ways from a host of cross-sectional and a few prospective studies, which I summarize below: One approach involves examining the frequency of PTSD among those presenting with SUDs; another involves examining the frequency of SUDs in those presenting with PTSD. Regardless of the approach used, nearly all studies indicate that these disorders co-occur more commonly than would be expected by chance alone.

SUDs in Individuals with Victimization and PTSD

An epidemiological survey (Helzer et al., 1987) of psychiatric illness in the general population revealed that men with PTSD were 5 times as likely to have a drug abuse or dependence disorder when compared with men without PTSD, and women with PTSD were 1.4 times as likely to have drug abuse or dependence as women without PTSD. More recent data from a longitudinal epidemiologic study of young adults (Breslau, Davis, & Schulz, 2003) indicated that exposure to trauma predicted drug abuse and dependence in those with PTSD (odds ratio, 4.3). In a cross-sectional survey of 3,132 adults, sexual assault was found to be a risk factor for the development of an SUD, and drug abuse/dependence was associated with a high risk of sexual assault subsequent to the development of the SUD (Burnam et al., 1988). In the Duke University Epidemiologic Catchment Area (ECA) Project (Winfield, George, Swartz, & Blazer, 1990), a history of sexual abuse was significantly related to both alcohol and drug abuse/dependence.

PTSD and Victimization in Individuals with SUDs

Reports from treatment-seeking samples of substance users have revealed a high prevalence of sexual and physical assault 20–65% of individuals in treatment for SUD reporting assault histories (Brown & Anderson, 1991; Brown et al., 1995; Grice, Dustan, & Brady, 1992; Ouimette, Read, & Brown, 2005; Rohsenow, Corbett, & Devine, 1988; Rounsaville, Weissman, Wilber, & Kleber, 1982; Simpson, Westerberg, Little, & Trujillo, 1994; Triffleman, Marmar, Delucchi, & Ronfeldt, 1995). Studies have documented PTSD rates among substance-using populations to be between 14 and 60% (Brady, Dansky, Back, Foa, & Carroll, 2001; Donovan, Padin-Rivera, & Kowaliw, 2001; Najavits, Weiss, & Shaw, 1997; Triffleman, 2003). In studies of individuals receiving treatment for an SUD, the prevalence of lifetime PTSD was reported to be as high as 80% (Brady, Killeen, Saladin, Dansky, & Becker, 1994; Dansky, Saladin, Brady, Kilpatrick, & Resnick, 1995; Fullilove et al., 1993; Hien & Scheier, 1996; Miller, Downs, & Testa, 1993), and the prevalence of current PTSD was between 30 and 59% (Dansky et al., 1995; Najavits et al., 1997). Additionally, studies report high rates of revictimization among those with childhood abuse histories, including intimate partner violence, stranger rape, and physical assault in adulthood (Hien, Nunes, & Levin, 1995; Hien & Scheier, 1996).

Individuals with comorbid SUD and PTSD typically have a more severe clinical profile than those with only one disorder (Najavits, Weiss, & Shaw, 1999). They tend to abuse more severe substances (e.g., cocaine; Cottler, Nishith, & Compton, 2001; Najavits et al., 1997); have high rates of psychiatric comorbidity, including depression (Brady, 1997); and have poorer treatment outcomes (Zweben, Clark, & Smith, 1994). A series of additional problems are often common, including problems related to interpersonal deficits, physical health issues, difficulty coping with parental responsibilities, homelessness, HIV/sexually transmitted infections risk behavior, and intimate partner violence (Brady, Dansky, Sonne, & Saladin, 1988; Triffleman, Marmar, Delucchi, & Ronfeldt, 1995).

Gender Differences in Rates of PTSD and Types of Trauma Exposure among Substance Users

We can conclude from the aforementioned research that those with SUDs have higher rates of traumatic exposures and that among those in SUD treatment, rates of PTSD exceed estimates for those without SUDs. Although these findings apply to both men and women, there are some gender-specific differences in prevalence that should be underscored. For example, as we noted above, in a general population men report higher rates of exposure to violence than do women, yet in terms of psychiatric consequences, men report lower rates of PTSD and depression than women, suggesting that men may be *less* likely to suffer psychiatric consequences or to report them, due to their exposure to trauma. Indeed, this is supported by the fact that the rate of comorbid PTSD in females with SUDs is two to three times higher than for males with SUDs. Also, whereas for men PTSD typically stems from combat or crime trauma, for women it most commonly derives from a history of repetitive childhood physical and/or sexual assault (Brown & Wolfe, 1994; De Young, 1982; Dohrenwend & Dohrenwend, 1976; Greenfeld, 1998). Finally, there is also evidence that women are more likely to have experienced a traumatic stressful event prior to the development of an SUD, whereas for men their trauma is more likely to follow their substance use involvement (e.g., Sonne, Back, Zuniga, Randall, & Brady, 2003).

Depending upon definition of *substance use* versus *substance use disorder* and control for type of traumatic event, the collective findings do suggest that for women, PTSD is more likely to be primary to the development of an SUD (e.g., Compton, Cottler, Phelps, Abdallah, & Spitznagel, 2000; Zilberman, Tavares, Blume, & el-Guebaly, 2003). The findings of gender differences may not, however, apply in all cases. For example, in a large ($n = 4,023$) national probability sample of adolescents, no gender differences in rates of comorbid PTSD and substance use following exposure to interpersonal violence were found, suggesting that it may be equally important to assess for substance use among adolescent girls as it is for the boys (Kilpatrick, Ruggiero, Acierno, Saunders, Resnick, & Best, 2003).

Nonetheless, as many as 80% of women seeking treatment for chemical dependency report lifetime histories of sexual and/or physical assault (Dansky et al., 1995; Dohrenwend & Dohrenwend, 1976; Dohrenwend et al., 1992; Fullilove et al., 1993; Fullilove, Lown, & Fullilove, 1992; Kalichman, Williams, Cherry, Belcher, & Nachimson, 1998; Murphy, Olivier, Monson, & Sobol, 1991). A substantial subgroup of women with SUDs exposed to violence suffer from the psychological sequelae of trauma, including PTSD *and* depressive disorders (Budd, 1989; Dohrenwend et al., 1992; Hien et al., 1995; Kalichman et al., 1998). Childhood abuse is an especially damaging type of trauma because it occurs early in life during crucial developmental years; such trauma often leads to significant and sustained psychiatric and physical impairments in adulthood. Trauma that occurs in childhood years is believed to disrupt affect regulation and interpersonal relatedness leading to long-term difficulties in these areas (Collins & Messerschmidt, 1993). Childhood sexual abuse is also a risk factor for subsequent victimization in various forms, including sexual assault, physical assault, and domestic violence. The findings of high rates of early child maltreatment and repeat victimization among females with SUDs are suggestive of a potentially gender-specific explanatory model for the development of addictive disorders among a subgroup of women.

PATHWAYS BETWEEN PTSD AND SUDs FOR WOMEN

The model that is most commonly cited and applied to understanding the pathways between addictive behavior and traumatic stress exposure is Khantzian's (1997) self-medication model. This model posits that some individuals use substances in an effort to manage or avoid distressing symptoms and to relieve painful emotions or physical sensations. In this model SUDs develop as a result of attempts to self-medicate negative affect. When applied to the specific case of PTSD and SUD comorbidity, self-medicating with alcohol and drugs is thought to lessen the effects of hyperarousal and numbing symptoms in individuals with posttraumatic stress. The hyperarousal symptoms would be diminished or masked by alcohol or other depressants, thereby providing temporary relief from the dysregulated feeling states that accompany PTSD.

Other potential pathways between PTSD and SUDs have been proposed, including the high-risk and susceptibility hypotheses (Chilcoat & Breslau, 1998a, 1998b). The high-risk hypothesis proposes that substance use and associated high-risk activities increase the risk of traumatic exposure, thereby indirectly increasing the likelihood of PTSD. Alternatively, the susceptibility hypothesis posits that substance use may play a causal role, in that people who use substances may be more susceptible to PTSD following a traumatic event due to impaired psychological or neurochemical systems resulting from extensive substance use.

Chilcoat and Breslau (1998a, 1998b) conducted a study testing causal pathways between PTSD and SUDs in a random sample of 1,007 adults (ages 21–30) who were members of a large health management organization (HMO). Participants completed baseline interviews and two follow-up interviews over a 5-year period. Using this prospective design and analytical strategies testing for causal inference, those with PTSD were found to have a fourfold increase in the likelihood of developing an SUD. Accordingly, the authors suggested that their findings provide most support for the self-medication model and least support for the high-risk model. However, they could not eliminate the susceptibility model as a possibility that some shared underlying factors also contribute to the development of PTSD. Notably, and in contrast to other reports (i.e., Cottler et al., 1992), in this large, prospective analysis, although gender was adjusted for in the analyses, no gender differences were reported in the causal pathways tested, nor in the rates of development of SUDs among those diagnosed with PTSD. Whether there are differences between causal pathways for men and women, such that, for example, the self-medication model is more applicable for women with PTSD and SUD, whereas the susceptibility model is more relevant for men with PTSD and SUDs, remains an untested empirical question.

AXIS I AND II COMORBIDITY WITH PTSD/SUDs

More often than not, individuals with PTSD have at least one additional psychiatric diagnosis. Based upon findings from the National Comorbidity Survey (Kessler et al., 1995), approximately 80% of women with PTSD meet criteria for at least one other psychiatric diagnosis, with 17% having one other diagnosis, 18% having two other diagnoses, and 44% having three or more additional diagnoses. The most common comorbid conditions with PTSD are SUDs (28% alcohol use disorders, 27% SUDs), affective disorders (49% major depression, 23% dysthymia, and 6% mania), and other anxiety disorders (15% with generalized anxiety, 28% with social phobia, and 29% with simple phobia). Patients with chronic trauma beginning in childhood are also likely to have a variety of additional psychiatric problems, including dissociation, poor impulse control, and personality-related disturbances. See Table 14.1 for information on PTSD/SUDs comorbidity and its consequences.

Although overall comorbidity rates do not differ for men and women, the types of associated disorders do. For example, in contrast to national epidemiology findings among those *without* PTSD, women are two times more likely than men to meet criteria for a depressive disorder, whereas for those *with* PTSD, women have concurrent depressive disorders at equal rates to men (Kessler et al., 1995). In line with national epidemiology estimates, women with PTSD are less likely to be diagnosed with antisocial personality disorder and more likely to be diagnosed with borderline personality and panic disorders (Kessler et al., 1995).

It bears noting that the relationship between PTSD and other associated disorders is often quite complex. The extent to which associated disorders typically follow the onset of PTSD remains unclear. There appear to be multiple pathways resulting in several different subtypes of patients with PTSD, rather than generalizable patterns of cause and effect. For example, whereas some individuals presenting with PTSD had preexisting psychological problems prior to trauma exposure, others developed additional disorders secondary to the onset of PTSD and its often-debilitating symptoms. There are also those for whom PTSD and related psychiatric conditions developed simultaneously, at the time of trauma exposure.

The substantial degree of overlap between PTSD symptoms and many other psychiatric disorders, most notably depression (i.e., sleep disturbance and social withdrawal) and other anxiety disorders (i.e., panic attacks and avoidance) has led some experts to believe that the PTSD diagnosis is flawed in that it fails to take into account the complexity of adaptation to trauma. This argument has led to the proposal that many conditions classified as comorbid disorders should instead be recognized as part of a complex range of trauma-related problems, rather than as separate and discrete disorders (van der Kolk, McFarlene, & Weisaeth, 1996).

Although future investigation is needed to clarify these issues, at present we do know that exposure to early, severe, and chronic trauma is associated with more complex adaptations to trauma, often characterized by impulse control deficits; unstable emotions and relationships; and disruptions in consciousness, memory, identity, and/or perception of the environment. The presence of other psychiatric disorders typically worsens and prolongs the

TABLE 14.1. PTSD Comorbidity and Consequences among Women

- PTSD is two to three times more common in women than in men.
- Among substance-using, treatment-seeking women, 55–99% report a history of physical and/or sexual abuse.
- Most women with this co-occurring disorder experienced childhood physical and/or sexual abuse; men with both disorders typically experienced crime victimization or war trauma.
- Women with PTSD and SUDs have a more severe clinical profile than those with just one of these disorders.
- Women with PTSD and SUDs are more likely to experience further trauma than women with substance abuse alone.
- Exposure to ongoing trauma is common in domestic violence, child abuse, and some substance-using lifestyles (e.g., the drug trade).
- While under the influence of substances, a woman may be more vulnerable to trauma (e.g., be less able to defend herself physically and more likely to have impaired cognitive faculties).
- Perpetrators of violent assault against women often use substances at the time of the assault.
- Helping the patient protect against future trauma is likely to be an important part of work in treatment.
- Becoming abstinent from substances does not resolve PTSD. Both disorders must be addressed in treatment.

course of PTSD and also complicates clinical assessment and diagnosis. In addition, the presence of additional psychiatric disorders often exacerbates PTSD symptoms and can prolong the course of the disorder.

DIAGNOSING PTSD IN PATIENTS WHO ARE SUBSTANCE-DEPENDENT

As discussed above, individuals with histories of traumatic stress exposures present for addiction treatment with a complex diagnostic picture and the possibility of at least one, if not more, psychiatric comorbidities. In the text revision of the fourth edition of the *Diagnostic and Statistical Manual of Mental Disorders* (DSM-IV-TR; American Psychiatric Association, 2000), an event or series of events is considered traumatic if the person experienced, witnessed, or was confronted with actual or threatened death or serious injury, or threat to the physical integrity of self or others, *and* if the person's response to the traumatic event involved fear, helplessness, or horror (Criterion A).

Symptoms that characterize PTSD usually begin within 3 months following the trauma, although symptom development may be delayed for weeks and even years. In order to meet the diagnosis, symptoms must be present for more than 1 month and must cause significant distress or impairment in social and/or occupational functioning. Kessler et al. (1995) estimated that, on average, a person with PTSD might endure 20 years of active symptoms and will experience almost 1 day per week of work impairment—which speaks to the huge toll of PTSD on the individual and on society. The characteristic symptoms of PTSD occur in three clusters. These clusters include (1) *reexperiencing* (e.g., intrusive and recurrent thoughts, images, perceptions, flashbacks of the traumatic experience, nightmares); (2) *avoidance and numbing* (e.g., feelings of detachment, persistent avoidance of memories, feelings, people, places, or situations that arouse recollection of the trauma); and (3) *increased arousal* (e.g., difficulty sleeping or concentrating, irritability/anger, exaggerated startle response, and a hyperalertness not present prior to traumatic exposure). Individuals with PTSD also often report associated features such as intense guilt about surviving if others did not, decreased awareness of their surroundings, forgetfulness/amnesia, feeling that things are unreal or strange, or feeling detached from their bodies. The course of the disorder is variable, with approximately half of the cases recovering in 3 months (termed acute PTSD) and others experiencing chronic PTSD (symptoms persist for over 3 months and often much longer). Studies have shown that over longer-term follow-up (1–2 years), women tend to have significantly longer duration of illness and more adverse consequences of PTSD than do men (e.g., Holbrook, Hoyt, Stein, & Sieber, 2002).

There are a number of issues that may make diagnosis of PTSD challenging among patients with SUDs, including symptom overlap, such as hyperarousal and psychostimulant effects, or numbing and depressant effects. These, however, may be readily "teased apart" once consideration is given to the Criterion A event—a traumatic event as defined by the DSM-IV involving specific threats to oneself or others (Criterion A1) and one or more identified emotional responses (Criterion A2) and time course in the development of symptoms. Or, an individual exposed to a Criterion A traumatic event may not meet the necessary criteria for all three PTSD symptom clusters, but still exhibit a clinically significant syndrome that is, in many ways, indistinguishable from PTSD. Examples may include partial or subthreshold PTSD (Marshall et al., 2001; Schutzwohl & Maercker, 1999). Dissociative symptoms, which can be evaluated as disruptions in functions of consciousness, memory, identity, or perception of the trauma, can make self-report of PTSD symptoms a challenge, as the patient may not have the ability to fully identify his or her symptoms with accuracy.

PSYCHOLOGICAL AND PHARMACOLOGICAL TREATMENTS FOR TRAUMA-RELATED COMORBIDITY WITH ADDICTION

Epidemiological studies of women's exposure to traumatic stress and its overlap with addictive disorders have underscored the continuing and urgent need for women's services that can address interpersonal violence and related psychological consequences. An emerging body of clinical treatment research reveals that women can benefit from trauma-related services in the context of addiction recovery. These findings directly countermand the positions of many substance use treatment providers who have contended that treating trauma was not possible until sobriety had been achieved. Indeed, the field has produced a growing body of manualized treatment approaches that promote psychological growth and recovery and minimize risks for relapse. Many of these approaches, however, have yet to be widely adopted in community treatment settings due to a number of barriers, including staff and client attitudes, lack of training and supervision, staffing challenges, and limited resources. In this section treatment considerations for addressing PTSD and SUD comorbidity are presented, highlighting empirical findings that support a consideration of these models as additions to addiction treatment for women. A review of contemporary approaches for the treatment of comorbid PTSD and SUD yields a host of psychotherapeutic and pharmacological options, the majority of which have some evidence of clinical efficacy in addition to more anecdotal, practice-based promise.

Psychotherapies

There are three basic models for addressing substance use and PTSD comorbidity: parallel, sequential, and integrated. Most treatments of choice, regardless of the model, include cognitive-behavioral therapy (CBT) for relapse prevention and some form of cognitive therapy for PTSD. *Parallel models* involve separate but simultaneous treatment of each disorder within its respective treatment system (by different providers and or programs). *Sequential models* provide treatment in stages so that, typically, addictive problems are addressed first; coping skills and other relapse prevention (Marlatt & Gordon, 1985) techniques are taught in preparation for working on trauma-related symptoms later in treatment. The rationale for the sequential therapy approaches includes the premise that unchecked substance abuse will impede therapeutic efforts directed at other problems (Nace, 1988) and that some of the behavioral therapies known to be effective in the treatment of PTSD, particularly exposure-based therapies that involve an element of imaginal re-experiencing of the trauma(s), can be stressful and therefore may interfere with early addiction recovery (Pitman et al., 1991).

In contrast, *integrated models* provide cognitive therapy for addictions side by side with cognitive therapy and psychoeducation for trauma-related disorders or PTSD. This approach underscores the importance of addressing trauma symptoms in tandem with SUDs. Within a psychoeducational framework, integrated treatments emphasize the links between trauma and addiction. Insofar as substance abuse represents self-medication of anxiety/PTSD symptoms, addressing the trauma first, or early in treatment, and providing some concurrent relief from PTSD symptoms may improve the chances of recovery from substance abuse (Back, Brady, Sonne, & Verduin, 2006; Brown et al., 1995; Ouimette, Ahrens, Moss, & Finney, 1997). A number of case studies in which successful treatment of anxiety symptoms of PTSD led to reductions in alcohol and drug abuse lends support to this idea (Fairbank, Gross, & Jeane, 1983; Keane & Kaloupek, 1982; Kilpatrick & Amick, 1985; Polles & Smith, 1995).

Integrated therapies often include prolonged exposure (PE), a technique that utilizes exposure-based methods for PTSD. PE has been widely used and is highly effective for PTSD and related pathology, such as depression and anxiety (Foa & Rothbaum, 1998). Based on its established efficacy in well-controlled trials, exposure has been chosen as the most appropriate form of psychotherapy for PTSD by the International Consensus Group on Depression and Anxiety (Ballenger et al., 2000) and is recommended as the most effective and rapidly acting nonpharmacological treatment for PTSD in the Expert Consensus Guidelines (Foa, Davidson, & Frances, 1999).

While exposure-based treatment has gained strong empirical support for efficacy and durability in treating PTSD symptoms, questions have been raised about its tolerability in the context of substance abuse. Exposure therapy had previously been considered contraindicated for patients with SUDs based largely on anecdotal concerns that these patients are too cognitively impaired for imagery procedures (Pitman et al., 1991), or that the intervention would be too emotionally distressing and could trigger a relapse (Coffey et al., 2002; Triffleman, Carroll, & Kellogg, 1999).

Despite these concerns, experts in the field of substance abuse treatment have begun to consider how patients with dual diagnoses could be safely and effectively treated with PE. The literature lends support to treatment approaches that combine exposure and more user-friendly forms of therapy, such as coping skills training, and that address both PTSD and SUDs concurrently in an integrated model. (See Table 14.2 for examples of exposure-based and other manual-based and empirically supported sequential or integrated PTSD/SUDs therapies.)

Pharmacotherapy for PTSD Comorbidity

There is increasing evidence to support the use of antidepressants, particularly selective serotonin reuptake inhibitors (SSRIs), as first-line therapy for individuals with PTSD (Conner, Sutherland, & Tupler, 1999; Marshall & Pierce, 2000; Pearlstein, 2000; van der Kolk, Dreyfuss, & Michaels, 1994). The most compelling evidence, to date, comes from two large

TABLE 14.2. Manualized Sequential and Integrated PTSD/SUDs Psychotherapy

- The *Addictions and Trauma Recovery Integrated Model* (ATRIUM; Miller & Guidry, 2001) is a 12-week model for individuals and groups that, in addition to standard CBT, uses a relationship focus to examine mental, physical, and spiritual domains. This treatment also addresses somatic symptoms through expressive therapy approaches.
- *Concurrent Treatment of PTSD and Cocaine Dependence* (CTPSD; Brady et al., 2001) is a sequential manualized treatment consisting of combined imaginal and *in vivo* exposure therapy for PTSD and cognitive-behavioral relapse prevention techniques for individuals with comorbid PTSD and cocaine dependence. CTPSD includes 16 individual 90-minute psychotherapy sessions delivered one to two times per week. Approximately six to nine of those sessions include imaginal exposure.
- *Substance Dependency–Post-Traumatic Stress Disorder Therapy* (SDTP; Triffleman et al., 1999) is a 20-week, twice-weekly, two-phase sequential manualized outpatient treatment that also utilizes relapse prevention, coping skills, psychoeducation, and *in vivo* exposure for individuals with civilian-related PTSD.
- *Seeking Safety* (SS; Najavits, 2002) is the most widely used and best known integrated therapy. SS is a manualized treatment specifically designed to integrate treatments for to both PTSD and substance use (Najavits, Weiss, Shaw, & Muenz, 1998; Najavits, Weiss, & Liese, 1996). It is a 25-session structured, problem-oriented psychotherapy that adapts cognitive-behavioral techniques to help patients attain abstinence from substances, decrease PTSD symptoms, and decrease high-risk behaviors.
- *Transcend* (Donovan et al., 2001) is a 12-session weekly sequential group therapy that was tested with men in a partial hospitalization treatment program. The first six sessions consist of skill development (problem solving, anger management, emotional awareness), and the second six sessions are devoted to trauma processing (presentations of traumatic events with group feedback and nightmare resolution techniques). Substance abuse education, relapse prevention techniques, peer support, and 12-step attendance are encouraged throughout.
- *Trauma Recovery and Empowerment* (TREM; Fallot & Harris, 2002) is a manualized group psychotherapy originally designed for women with severe mental disorders and trauma histories that has been used in SAMSHA's Women, Co-Occurring Disorders and Violence project. Using a structured approach, TREM works with a skills-based model that also addresses long-term effects of trauma and histories of childhood exposures to physical and sexual abuse. There are 33 topics with relevant workbooks.

double-blind controlled trials that compared the use of sertraline to a placebo in approximately 400 subjects combined (Brady et al., 2000; Davidson, van der Kolk, & Brady, 1997). In both studies samples were comprised of approximately 75% women, and more than 60% of the women in the two samples identified a physical or sexual assault as the primary trauma. Findings from both large studies demonstrated that overall, sertraline was well tolerated and showed a significantly greater response rate than placebo. In both studies sertraline was superior to placebo in reducing the three symptom clusters of PTSD, particularly the cluster of avoidance and numbing.

Brady and colleagues (Brady, Sonne, & Roberts, 1995) are the first group to investigate the use of sertraline in a PTSD population with a dual diagnosis of alcohol dependence (Brady et al., 2005). The findings revealed that although sertraline, as compared to placebo, has some beneficial impact upon PTSD symptoms among patients with alcohol dependence, there was no impact on alcohol use until a cluster analysis was undertaken. The cluster that was significantly more responsive to sertraline for the alcohol outcomes was characterized as having *less severe* alcohol use and earlier-onset PTSD (i.e., PTSD *preceded* the onset of alcohol dependence). These findings are also in line with findings from psychopharmacological treatment of depression–alcohol comorbidity treatment with sertraline. Collectively, these findings provide a rationale for sertraline treatment of women with PTSD, especially in earlier stages of harmful drinking potentially prior to the development of a diagnosable alcohol disorder, as they may be the group most responsive to combined psychosocial and medication treatments.

Few other trials have addressed medication treatment for PTSD and SUD comorbidity, although one promising though small trial reported that the anticonvulsant lamotrigine could be efficacious with simple PTSD (without substance abuse) (Brady & Verduin, 2005). However, pharmacotherapy is often an essential component of treatment for those with PTSD, SUD and other psychiatric comorbidities such as depression. Moreover, since sleeping problems are hallmark symptoms for those with trauma histories and PTSD, a variety of nonaddictive sleeping medications (e.g., trazedone, Lunesta) to aid insomnia may be considered carefully for short-term usage.

BARRIERS TO APPLYING TRAUMA-FOCUSED METHODS IN COMMUNITY SUBSTANCE ABUSE PROGRAMS

Our review of the literature on epidemiology, pathways, assessment and empirically supported treatment models for traumatic exposure, PTSD and related psychiatric comorbidities among women who use substances reflects the wealth and breadth of advances that have been made in the past 20 years. Nonetheless, a prevailing concern within the treatment community exists regarding how and when to intervene with respect to trauma models; fewer treatment programs include trauma-specific programming than should be the case, given the fact that the majority of women in substance abuse treatment do have trauma-related problems and comorbidities. One of the main reasons for this omission, despite all the treatment advances, as we have referred to extensively elsewhere (Hien, Litt, Cohen, Miele, & Campbell, 2009), is the fear of opening "Pandora's box"—that is, causing a substance-using woman with PTSD to relapse more quickly than she would if the trauma material had not been addressed. Resistance can come from the patient who has built a lifetime of methods for dissociating from triggering material; likewise, many providers of substance abuse treatment have their own fears and may avoid encouraging disclosure even when the patient is willing and able to talk.

FUTURE DIRECTIONS

The field of treatment for women with addictions and trauma-related comorbidity has advanced tremendously over the past 15 years. We now have an encouraging evidence base of psychological and psychopharmcological interventions that show promise in helping women with addictions and trauma increase their quality of life, live with their symptoms in recovery, and transcend their past interpersonal violence. Future directions include further study of combination approaches and adjunctive therapies that can focus not only on mental but also on physical health concerns, improving outcomes for this vulnerable population. Integrating trauma treatment into community-based substance abuse services continues to be a challenge for the field and should involve considerations around course of illness and program resources, such as availability of medication/psychiatric support, domestic violence services, and medical case management.

KEY POINTS

- Many women in treatment for substance use have a history of interpersonal violence and trauma exposure that began in childhood and is repeated in adulthood revictimization.
- Posttraumatic stress often precedes the SUD, supporting a self-medication model in this

special population. There are also clear neurobiological underpinnings to the comorbidity of PTSD and SUDs.

• A review of contemporary approaches for the treatment of comorbid PTSD and SUDs yields a host of psychotherapeutic and pharmacological options, the majority of which have some evidence of clinical efficacy in addition to more anecdotal, practice-based promise.

• Trauma may be safely treated in the context of substance use treatment, but specialized approaches must be used.

REFERENCES

Asterisks denote recommended readings.

Amdur, R. L., Larsen, R. L., & Liberzon, I. (2000). Emotional processing in combat-related posttraumatic stress disorder: A comparison with traumatized and normal controls. *Journal of Anxiety Disorders, 14*(3), 219–238.

American Psychiatric Association. (1994). *Diagnostic and statistical manual of mental disorders* (4th ed.). Washington, DC: Author.

American Psychiatric Association. (2000). *Diagnostic and statistical manual of mental disorders* (4th ed., text rev.). Washington, DC: Author.

Back, S. E., Brady, K. T., Sonne, S. C., & Verduin, M. L. (2006). Symptom improvement in co-occurring PTSD and alcohol dependence. *Journal of Nervous and Mental Disease, 194*(9), 690–696.

Ballenger, J. C., Davidson, J. R. T., Lecrubier, Y., Nutt, D. J., Foa, E. B., Kessler, R. C., et al. (2000). Consensus statement on posttraumatic stress disorder from the International Consensus Group on Depression and Anxiety. *Journal of Clinical Psychiatry, 61*(Suppl. 5), 60–66.

Brady, K. T. (1997). Posttraumatic stress disorder and comorbidity: Recognizing the many faces of PTSD. *Journal of Clinical Psychiatry, 58*(12–15). (*)

Brady, K. T., Dansky, B. S., Back, S. E., Foa, E. B., & Carroll, K. M. (2001). Exposure therapy in the treatment of PSTD among cocaine-dependent individuals: Preliminary findings. *Journal of Substance Abuse Treatment, 21,* 47–54.

Brady, K. T., Dansky, B. S., Sonne, S. C., & Saladin, M. E. (1988). Posttraumatic stress disorder and cocaine dependence: Order of onset. *American Journal on Addictions, 7,* 128–135.

Brady, K. T., Killeen, T., Saladin, M. E., Dansky, B. S., & Becker, S. (1994). Comorbid substance use and posttraumatic stress disorder: Characteristics of women in treatment. *American Journal on Addictions, 3*(2), 160–164.

Brady, K. T., Pearlstein, T., Asnis, G. M., Baker, D., Rothbaum, B., Sikes, C. R., et al. (2000). Efficacy and safety of sertraline treatment of posttraumatic stress disorder: A randomized controlled trial. *Journal of the American Medical Association, 283*(4), 1837–1844.

Brady, K. T., Sonne, S., Anton, R. F., Randall, C. L., Back, S. E., & Simpson, K. (2005). Sertraline in the treatment of co-occurring alcohol dependence and posttraumatic stress disorder. *Alcoholism: Clinical and Experimental Research, 29*(3), 395–401. (*)

Brady, K. T., Sonne, S. C., & Roberts, J. M. (1995). Sertraline treatment of comorbid posttraumatic stress disorder and alcohol dependence. *Journal of Clinical Psychiatry, 56,* 502–505.

Brady, K. T., & Verduin, M. L. (2005). Pharmacotherapy of comorbid mood, anxiety, and substance use disorders. *Substance Use and Misuse, 40*(13), 2021–2041.

Breslau, N., Davis, G., Andreski, P., & Peterson, E. L. (1991). Traumatic events and posttraumatic stress disorder in an urban population of young adults. *Archives of General Psychiatry, 48,* 216–222.

Brown, G. R., & Anderson, B. (1991). Psychiatric morbidity in adult inpatients with childhood histories of sexual and physical abuse. *American Journal of Psychiatry, 148*(1), 55–61.

Brown, P. J., Recupero, P. R., & Stout, R. (1995). PTSD substance abuse comorbidity and treatment utilization. *Addictive Behaviors, 20*(2), 251–254.

Brown, P. J., & Wolfe, J. (1994). Substance abuse and post-traumatic stress disorder comorbidity. *Drug and Alcohol Dependence, 35,* 51–59.

Brown, S. A. (1989). Life events of adolescents in relation to personal and parental substance abuse. *American Journal of Psychiatry, 146*, 484–489.

Budd, R. D. (1989). Cocaine abuse and violent death. *American Journal of Drug and Alcohol Abuse, 15*(4), 375–382.

Burnam, M. A., Stein, J. A., Golding, J. M., Siegel, J. M., Sorenson, S. B., Forsythe, A. B., et al. (1988). Sexual assault and mental disorders in a community population. *Journal of Consulting and Clinical Psychology, 56*, 843–850.

Chilcoat, H. D., & Breslau, N. (1998a). Investigations of causal pathways between PTSD and drug use disorders. *Addictive Behaviors, 23*, 827–840.

Chilcoat, H. D., & Breslau, N. (1998b). Posttraumatic stress disorder and drug disorders: Testing causal pathways. *Archives of General Psychiatry, 55*, 913–917.

Coffey, S. F., Saladin, M. E., Drobes, D. J., Brady, K., Dansky, B. S., & Kilpatrick, D. G. (2002). Trauma and substance cue reactivity in individuals with comorbid posttraumatic stress disorder and cocaine or alcohol dependence. *Drug and Alcohol Dependence, 65*, 115–127.

Collins, J. J., & Messerschmidt, P. M. (1993). Epidemiology in alcohol-related violence. *Alcohol Health and Research World, 17*(2), 93–100.

Compton, W. M., III, Cottler, L. B., Phelps, D. L., Abdallah, A. B., & Spitznagel, E. L. (2000). Psychiatric disorders among drug dependent subjects: Are they primary or secondary? *American Journal on Addictions, 9*(2), 126–134.

Conner, K. M., Sutherland, S. M., & Tupler, L. A. (1999). Fluoxetine in posttraumatic stress disorder: Randomized, double-blind study. *British Journal of Psychiatry, 175*, 17–22.

Cottler, L. B., Compton, W. M., Mager, D., Spitznagel, E. L., & Janca, A. (1992). Post-traumatic stress disorder among substance users from the general population. *American Journal of Psychiatry, 149*, 664–670.

Cottler, L. B., Nishith, P., & Compton, W. M. (2001). Gender differences in risk factors for trauma exposure and post-traumatic stress disorder among inner-city drug abusers in and out of treatment. *Comprehensive Psychiatry, 42*(2), 111–117.

Dansky, B. S., Saladin, M. E., Brady, K. T., Kilpatrick, D. G., & Resnick, H. S. (1995). Prevalence of victimization and posttraumatic stress disorder among women with substance use disorders: Comparison of telephone and in-person assessment samples. *International Journal of the Addictions, 30*(9), 1079–1099.

Davidson, J. R. T., Hughes, D., Blazer, D. G., & George, L. K. (1991). Post-traumatic stress disorder in the community: An epidemiological study. *Psychological Medicine, 21*, 713–721.

Davidson, J. R. T., van der Kolk, B. A., & Brady, K. (1997, September). *Double-blind comparison of sertraline and placebo in patients with posttraumatic stress disorder.* Paper presented at the 10th annual meeting of the European College of Neuropharmacology.

De Young, M. (1982). *The sexual victimization of children.* Jefferson, NC: McFarland.

Dohrenwend, B. P., & Dohrenwend, S. (1976). Sex differences and psychiatric disorders. *American Journal of Sociology, 81*, 1447–1454.

Dohrenwend, B. P., Levav, I., Shrout, P. E., Schwartz, S., Naveh, G., Link, B. G., et al. (1992). Socioeconomic status and psychiatric disorders: The causation–selection issue. *Science, 255*, 946–952.

Donovan, B., Padin-Rivera, E., & Kowaliw, S. (2001). "Transcend": Initial outcomes from a posttraumatic stress disorder/substance abuse treatment program. *Journal of Traumatic Stress, 14*(4), 757–772.

Fairbank, J. A., Gross, R. T., & Jeane, T. M. (1983). Treatment of posttraumatic stress disorder: Evaluating outcome with a behavioral code. *Behavioral Modification, 7*, 557–568.

Fallot, R. D., & Harris, M. (2002). The trauma recovery and empowerment model (TREM): Conceptual and practical issues in a group intervention for women. *Community Mental Health Journal, 38*(6), 475–485.

Foa, E., Davidson, J. R., & Frances, A. (1999). The expert consensus guideline series: Treatment of posttraumatic stress disorder. *Journal of Clinical Psychiatry, 60*(Suppl. 16), 1–79.

Foa, E., & Rothbaum, B. O. (1998). *Treating the trauma of rape: Cognitive-behavioral therapy for PTSD.* New York: Guilford Press.

Freedy, J. R., Kilpatrick, D. G., & Resnick, H. S. (1993). Natural disasters and mental health: Theory, assessment, and intervention. *Journal of Social Behavioral and Personality, 8,* 49–103.

Fullilove, M. T., Fullilove, R. E., Smith, M., Winkler, K., Michael, C., Panzer, P. G., et al. (1993). Violence, trauma, and post-traumatic stress disorder among women drug users. *Journal of Traumatic Stress, 6*(4), 533–543.

Fullilove, M. T., Lown, E. A., & Fullilove, R. E. (1992). Crack 'hos and skeezers: Traumatic experiences of women crack users. *Journal of Sex Research, 29*(2), 275–287.

Green, B. L., Lindy, J. D., Grace, M. C., Gleser, G. C., Leonard, A. C., Korol, M., et al. (1990). Buffalo Creek survivors in the second decade: Stability of stress symptoms. *American Journal of Orthopsychiatry, 60,* 43–54.

Greenfeld, L. A. (1998). *Alcohol and crime: An analysis of national data on the prevalence of alcohol involvement in crime.* Retrieved December 13, 2007, from *www.ojp.usdoj.gov/bjs/pub/pdf/ac.pdf.*

Greenfield, S. F., Brooks, A. J., Gordon, S., Green, C. A., Hegedus, A., Kropp, F., et al. (2007). Substance abuse treatment entry, retention, and outcomes in women: A review of the literature. *Drug and Alcohol Dependence, 86,* 1–21. (*)

Grice, D. E., Dustan, L. R., & Brady, K. T. (1992, May). *Assault, substance abuse, and Axis I comorbidity.* Paper presented at the 145th anniversary meeting of the American Psychiatric Association.

Helzer, J. E., Robins, L. N., & McEvoy, L. (1987). Posttraumatic stress disorder in the general population: Findings from the Epidemiologic Catchment Area Study. *New England Journal of Medicine, 387,* 1630–1634.

Hien, D. A., Cohen, L. R., & Campbell, A. (2005). Is traumatic stress a vulnerability factor for development of substance use disorders in women? *Special Issue of Clinical Psychology Review, 25*(6), 813–823. (*)

Hien, D. A., Cohen, L. R., Miele, G. M., Litt, L. C., & Capstick, C. (2004). Promising treatments for women with comorbid PTSD and substance use disorders. *American Journal of Psychiatry, 161,* 1426–1432. (*)

Hien, D. A., Litt, L., Cohen, L. C., Miele, G. M., & Campbell, A. N. (2009). *Integrating trauma services for women in addictions treatment.* New York: American Psychological Association.

Hien, D. A., Nunes, E. V., & Levin, F. B. (1995, June). *Violence, psychiatric comorbidity, and gender: Predictors of outcome in methadone patients.* Paper presented at the 57th annual College on Problems of Drug Dependence.

Hien, D. A., & Scheier, J. (1996). Short term predictors of outcome for drug-abusing women in detox: A follow-up study. *Journal of Substance Abuse Treatment, 13,* 227–231.

Holbrook, T. L., Hoyt, D. B., Stein, M. B., & Sieber, W. J. (2002). Gender differences in long-term posttraumatic stress disorder outcomes after major trauma: Women are at higher risk of adverse outcomes than men. *Journal of Trauma, Injury, Infection, and Critical Care, 53*(5), 882–888.

Kalichman, S., Williams, E., Cherry, C., Belcher, L., & Nachimson, D. (1998). Sexual coercion, domestic violence, and negotiating condom use among low-income African American women. *Journal of Women's Health, 7*(3), 371–378.

Keane, T. M., & Kaloupek, D. G. (1982). Imaginal flooding in the treatment of a posttraumatic stress disorder. *Journal of Clinical and Consulting Psychology, 50*(1), 138–140.

Kessler, R., Sonnega, A., Bromet, E., Hughes, M., & Nelson, C. (1995). Posttraumatic stress disorder in the National Comorbidity Study. *Archives of General Psychiatry, 52,* 1048–1060. (*)

Khantzian, E. (1997). The self-medication hypothesis of substance use disorders: A reconsideration and recent applications. *Harvard Review of Psychiatry, 4,* 231–244.

Kilpatrick, D. G., & Amick, A. E. (1985). Rape trauma. In M. Herson & C. G. Last (Eds.), *Behavior therapy case book* (pp. 86–103). New York: Springer.

Kilpatrick, D. G., Ruggiero, K. J., Acierno, R., Saunders, B. E., Resnick, H. S., & Best, C. L. (2003). Violence and risk of PTSD, major depression, substance abuse/dependence, and comorbidity: Results from the National Survey of Adolescents. *Journal of Consulting and Clinical Psychology, 71*(4), 692–700.

Kilpatrick, D. G., Saunders, B. E., Veronen, L. J., Best, C. L., & Von, J. M. (1987). Criminal victimization: Lifetime prevalence, reporting to police, and psychological impact. *Crime and Delinquency, 33*, 479–489.

Marlatt, G., & Gordon, J. (1985). *Relapse prevention: Maintenance strategies in the treatment of addictive behaviors*. New York: Guilford Press.

Marshall, R. D., Olfson, M., Hellman, F., Blanco, C., Guardino, M., & Struening, E. L. (2001). Comorbidity, impairment, and suicidality in subthreshold PTSD. *American Journal of Psychiatry, 158*(9), 1467–1473.

Marshall, R. D., & Pierce, D. (2000). Implications of recent findings in posttraumatic stress disorder and the role of pharmacotherapy. *Harvard Review of Psychiatry, 7*(5), 247–256.

Miller, B., Downs, W., & Testa, M. (1993). Interrelationships between victimization experiences and women's alcohol use. *Journal of Studies on Alcohol, 11*, 109–117.

Miller, D., & Guidry, L. (2001). *Addictions and trauma recovery healing the body, mind and spirit*. New York: Norton.

Murphy, J. M., Olivier, D. C., Monson, R. R., & Sobol, A. M. (1991). Depression and anxiety in relation to social status: A prospective epidemiologic study. *Archives of General Psychiatry, 48*(3), 223–229.

Nace, E. P. (1988). Posttraumatic stress disorder and substance abuse: Clinical issues. *Recent Developments in Alcoholism, 6*, 9–26.

Najavits, L. M. (2002). *Seeking safety: A treatment manual for PTSD and substance abuse*. New York: Guilford Press. (*)

Najavits, L. M., Weiss, R., & Liese, B. S. (1996). Group cognitive-behavioral therapy for women with PTSD and substance use disorder. *Journal of Substance Abuse Treatment, 13*, 13–22.

Najavits, L. M., Weiss, R., & Shaw, S. (1997). The link between substance abuse and posttraumatic stress disorder in women: A research review. *American Journal on Addictions, 6*(4), 237–283.

Najavits, L. M., Weiss, R., & Shaw, S. (1999). A clinical profile of women with PTSD and substance dependence. *Psychology of Addictive Behaviors, 13*, 98–104.

Najavits, L. M., Weiss, R. D., Shaw, S. R., & Muenz, L. (1998). "Seeking safety": Outcome of a new cognitive-behavioral psychotherapy for women with posttraumatic stress disorder and substance dependence. *Journal of Trauma and Stress, 11*, 437–456.

Norris, F. H. (1992). Epidemiology of trauma: Frequency and impact of different potentially traumatic events on different demographic groups. *Journal of Consulting and Clinical Psychology, 60*, 409–418.

Ouimette, P. C., Ahrens, C., Moss, R. H., & Finney, J. W. (1997). Posttraumatic stress disorder in substance abuse patients: Relationship to one-year posttreatment outcomes. *Psychology of Addictive Behaviors, 11*, 34–47.

Pearlstein, T. (2000). Antidepressant treatment of posttraumatic stress disorders. *Journal of Clinical Psychiatry, 61*, 40–53.

Pitman, R. K., Altman, B., Greenwald, E., Longpre, R. E., Macklin, M. L., Poire, R. E., et al. (1991). Psychiatric complications during flooding therapy for posttraumatic stress disorder. *Journal of Clinical Psychiatry, 52*(1), 17–20.

Polles, A. G., & Smith, P. O. (1995). Treatment of coexisting substance dependence and posttraumatic stress disorder. *Psychiatric Services, 46*(7), 729–730.

Read, J. P., Brown, P. J., & Kahler, C. W. (2004). Substance use and posttraumatic stress disorders: Symptom interplay and effects on outcome. *Addictive Behaviors, 20*, 1–8.

Resnick, H. S., Kilpatrick, D. G., Dansky, B. S., Saunders, B. E., & Best, C. L. (1993). Prevalence of civilian trauma and posttraumatic stress disorder in a representative national sample of women. *Journal of Consulting and Clinical Psychology, 61*(6), 984–991.

Rohsenow, D. J., Corbett, R., & Devine, D. (1988). Molested as children: A hidden contribution to substance abuse? *Journal of Substance Abuse Treatment, 5*, 13–18.

Rounsaville, B. J., Weissman, M. M., Wilber, C. H., & Kleber, H. D. (1982). Pathways to opiate addiction: An evaluation of differing antecedents. *British Journal of Psychiatry, 141*, 437–446.

Schore, A. N. (2001). Effects of a secure attachment relationship on right brain development, affect regulation, and infant mental health. *Infant Mental Health Journal, 22*(1–2), 7–66.

Schutzwohl, M., & Maercker, A. (1999). Effects of varying diagnostic criteria for posttraumatic stress disorder are endorsing the concept of partial PTSD. *Journal of Traumatic Stress, 12*(1), 155–165.

Shore, J. H., Tatum, E. L., & Vollmer, W. M. (1986). Psychiatric reactions to disaster: The Mt. St. Helens experience. *American Journal of Psychiatry, 143*, 590–595.

Simpson, T. L., Westerberg, V. S., Little, L. M., & Trujillo, M. (1994). Screening for childhood physical and sexual abuse among outpatient substance abusers. *Journal of Substance Abuse Treatment, 11*(4), 347–358.

Sonne, S. C., Back, S. E., Zuniga, D. C., Randall, C. L., & Brady, K. T. (2003). Gender differences in individuals with comorbid alcohol dependence and post-traumatic stress disorder. *American Journal on Addictions, 12*, 412–423. (*)

Steinglass, P., & Gerrity, E. (1990). Natural disasters and post-traumatic stress disorder: Short-term versus long-term recovery in two disaster-affected communities. *Journal of Applied Social Psychology, 20*, 1746–1765.

Triffleman, E. (2003). Issues in implementing posttraumatic stress disorder treatment outcome research in community-based treatment program. In J. L. Sorensen, R. A. Rawson, J. Guydish, & J. E. Zweben (Eds.), *Drug abuse treatment through collaboration: Practice and research partnerships that work* (pp. 227–247). Washington, DC: American Psychological Association.

Triffleman, E., Carroll, K. M., & Kellogg, S. (1999). Substance dependence posttraumatic stress disorder therapy: An integrated cognitive-behavioral approach. *Journal of Substance Abuse Treatment, 17*, 3–14.

Triffleman, E., Marmar, C. R., Delucchi, K. L., & Ronfeldt, H. (1995). Childhood trauma and PTSD in substance abuse inpatients. *Journal of Nervous and Mental Disease, 183*(3), 172–176.

van der Kolk, B. A., Dreyfuss, D., & Michaels, M. (1994). Fluoxetine in posttraumatic stress disorder. *Journal of Clinical Psychiatry, 55*, 517–522.

van der Kolk, B. A., McFarlene, A., & Weisaeth, L. (1996). *Traumatic stress: The effects of overwhelming experience on mind, body, and society.* New York: Guilford Press.

Winfield, I., George, L. K., Swartz, M., & Blazer, D. G. (1990). Sexual assault and psychiatric disorders among a community sample of women. *American Journal of Psychiatry, 147*(3), 335–341.

Zilberman, M. L., Tavares, H., Blume, S. B., & el-Guebaly, N. (2003). Substance use disorders: Sex differences and psychiatric comorbidities. *Canadian Journal of Psychiatry, 48*(1), 5–13.

Zweben, J. E., Clark, W. H., & Smith, D. E. (1994). Traumatic experiences and substance abuse: Mapping the territory. *Journal of Psychoactive Drugs, 26*(4), 327–344.

CHAPTER 15

Psychotic Disorders in Women with Substance Abuse

Kim-Chi Nguyen, BS, BA
E. Sherwood Brown, MD, PhD

SCHIZOPHRENIA AND COMORBIDITY

Overview

Psychosis occurs when reality testing is impaired. Symptoms of psychosis include seeing, hearing, tasting, or smelling things that other people cannot detect; fixed false beliefs; and disorganized thoughts or behaviors. Psychosis is a defining symptom of schizophrenia and related disorders but can also occur with mood disorders or in response to prescription or illicit drugs or medical illness. The symptoms of psychosis in patients with schizophrenia can be chronic, whereas as part of other conditions, they may be more transient or recurrent in nature. Treatment of psychosis generally involves the use of antipsychotics such as risperidone or haloperidol and occasionally electroconvulsive therapy.

The diagnosis of schizophrenia is made according to DSM-IV-TR Criteria A, B, and C (American Psychiatric Association, 2000). Criterion A requires the manifestation of two or more symptoms that include positive symptoms (e.g., hallucinations, delusions, disorganized speech, catatonic behavior) and negative symptoms (e.g., alogia, avolition, blunted or flat affect). Criterion B refers to the interpersonal or occupational dysfunction that results from the disease. Criterion C requires at least 6 months' duration of symptoms, including at least 1 month of Criterion A symptoms. The diagnoses of schizophreniform disorder and brief psychotic disorder are based on similar symptoms as schizophrenia, but the required time course of symptoms differs. The symptoms of schizophreniform disorder must be present for 1–6 months, and for brief psychotic disorder, for 1 month or less. Delusional disorder refers to the presence of fixed, false beliefs that are not accompanied by other psychotic symptoms. Schizoaffective disorder differs from schizophrenia in that there are symptoms of mania and depression during much of the illness.

Sex Differences in Schizophrenia

Sex differences are prominent in schizophrenia. Women have a later onset, are more receptive to antipsychotic medication, and generally experience a more benign course than men. A long-term study of 163 inpatients with chronic schizophrenia found that women at baseline were more often married than men, and had better sexual and social premorbid function (McGlashan & Bardenstein, 1990). A follow-up study 15 years later revealed that women again were more often married, more often had children, were better able to sustain employment, and had higher social and global functioning. While at baseline there was no correlation between sex and substance abuse or aggression, at follow-up, a significantly greater number of men had substance use disorders (SUDs), as compared to women. Sex differences in symptoms and general function decrease with age, and those of both sexes older than 50 years show much improvement in both areas (Childers & Harding, 1990).

Szymanski et al. (1995) followed patients with first-break schizophrenia and found that women were older at first onset of psychotic symptoms and at first hospitalization than men and had better premorbid function. At onset, more men than women exhibited primarily negative symptoms. Although there were no differences in global symptom levels at first hospitalization, women exhibited fewer symptoms after treatment with typical antipsychotic medications, which included fluphenazine hydrochloride, haloperidol, and molindone. Moreover, more women achieved full symptom remission than did men (87 vs. 55%). The typical antipsychotics inhibit dopamine action, and dopamine decreases prolactin release. Prolactin levels were significantly higher in females, suggesting that the medications were more effective in women. Measurements of plasma fluphenazine levels did not differ between males and females and could not account for the differential treatment response.

The relatively more benign course that women with schizophrenia experience may be due to the protective effects of estrogen (Lindamer, Buse, Lohr, & Jeste, 2001). A study comparing 52 postmenopausal women with and without hormone replacement therapy (HRT) found that HRT was associated with fewer negative symptoms on the Brief Psychiatric Rating Scale. No difference in general psychopathology was found between the groups; however, those with HRT were on lower daily doses of antipsychotic medication. The estrogen given in HRT may abate the psychopathology of schizophrenia so that smaller doses of medication are required for equal effectiveness.

SUDs AND PSYCHOTIC DISORDERS

Overview

SUDs co-occur with bipolar, depressive, and anxiety disorders as well as with psychotic disorders such as schizophrenia. Indeed, schizophrenia is associated with increased risk of SUDs (Regier et al., 1990). Problems with concurrent diagnoses include the masking of the mental illness by drug use and the possibility of a drug-induced psychosis that mimics psychiatric illness. Untreated mental illness may lead to substance use, and untreated SUDs can result in the recurrence or exacerbation of psychotic symptoms. The association between SUDs and mental illness requires that both disorders be treated concurrently, because failure to manage either disorder can contribute to a more difficult course of illness and poor prognosis for both illnesses.

Much research has been conducted on co-occurring SUDs and schizophrenia, but few studies have examined sex differences. The sections that follow examine psychotic disorders in women with concurrent SUDs. Models for the development of comorbid schizophrenia and SUDs as well as treatment options are discussed.

Prevalence

De Leon and Diaz (2005) performed a meta-analysis of 49 studies conducted worldwide to examine the relationship between cigarette smoking and schizophrenia. Of a total of 7,593 schizophrenia patients, 62% smoked. Patients with schizophrenia were 5.3 times more likely to smoke than the general population. The 71% prevalence of smoking in men with schizophrenia was significantly higher than that of women at 44%. Importantly, patients with schizophrenia had 1.9 times higher odds of smoking than did the population of patients with other mental illnesses, such as mood disorders. Indeed, a number of other studies has found a relationship between smoking and schizophrenia. As a follow-up to the British National Survey of Psychiatric Morbidity, Wiles et al. (2006) examined a nationally representative group of people for incident psychotic symptoms, including hypomania, thought insertion, paranoia, strange experiences, and hallucinations. Of the 2,406 subjects who completed the baseline and the follow-up study 18 months later, those who smoked were found to be 70% more likely to exhibit incident psychotic symptoms that occurred after the baseline and before the follow-up.

Regier and colleagues (1990) examined data from the Wave 1 survey (1980–1984) of the Epidemiologic Catchment Area (ECA) study of the National Institute of Mental Health (NIMH) to find prevalence rates for schizophrenia and SUDs in the general U.S. population. Interviews with 20,291 subjects, representative of the U.S. population based on age, sex, and race according to the U.S. census, were conducted using DSM-III criteria. One-month, 6-month, and lifetime prevalence rates for schizophrenia and schizophreniform disorders together were 0.7%, 0.9%, and 1.5%, respectively. The lifetime occurrence of schizophrenia in the population was 1.4%. Data analysis showed an increased prevalence of comorbidity in persons with schizophrenia. Persons with schizophrenia had a 4.6 times greater chance of having an SUD than the general population. Odds of people with schizophrenia having an alcohol disorder or another drug disorder were 3.3 and 6.2 times higher, respectively, than that of the general population. SUDs that include abuse and dependence occurred in 47.0% of respondents with schizophrenia. Of those with schizophrenia, 33.7% had an alcohol use disorder, and 27.5% had a substance use disorder other than alcohol.

A study conducted in Germany found similar results for comorbidity (Soyka et al., 1993). Patients with chronic schizophrenia (n = 447) admitted to a state psychiatric hospital had a lifetime SUD prevalence of 42.9%, with alcohol use disorders occurring in 34.6% of patients. Marijuana was the most commonly abused illicit drug. No sex differences in predilection for specific drugs were found. A different study found marijuana, psychostimulants, and hallucinogens to be the most common drugs of abuse (Mueser et al., 1990). Compared with the results of the above ECA study, people with schizophrenia were found to differ slightly from the general population in the choice drugs of abuse (Regier et al., 1990). Opiates were much less preferred by people with schizophrenia than by the general population.

Comorbidity

Characteristics

Concurrent SUDs and schizophrenia are reported at a higher prevalence in men than women. Van Mastrigt, Addington, and Addington (2004) found concurrent drug use to be associated with the male sex in subjects with first-episode psychoses. Of the 357 patients with psychotic disorders that included schizophrenia (37%) and schizophreniform disorder (37%), 45% had an SUD, and men had higher levels of alcohol and cannabis use, as compared to women. Mueser and colleagues (1990) found sex differences in a sample of acute-care patients with schizophrenia spectrum disorders. Of the 149 patients, 36% were female. A greater percentage of males than females abused alcohol and cannabis. At 57%, twice as many males than females had an alcohol use disorder. At 55%, a cannabis use disorder was reported by males at three times the rate reported by females.

While there appear to be sex differences in the prevalence of SUDs, there may not be sex differences in severity of drug use. Gearon and Bellack (2000) studied a group of men and women with schizophrenia spectrum disorders who were also diagnosed with concurrent drug abuse or dependence disorders and found no sex differences in drug preference or the severity or duration of drug use. A different study found that women had a less severe drinking history than men, but they were equally impaired in learning and memory, abstract problem solving, visuospatial processing, and perceptual–motor skills (Glenn & Parsons, 1992). The increased impairments with lesser amounts of alcohol led the authors to hypothesize that women with schizophrenia who abused substances are especially vulnerable to becoming victims of violence because they are less able to assess the dangers in their environment.

As was discussed, Gearon and Bellack (2000) found that drug use severity did not differ between men and women. In the same study, they discovered differential effects of drug use in women. Women with SUDs had higher numbers of previous hospitalizations and greater positive and general symptoms then their male counterparts. In addition, they had an earlier age of diagnosis of schizophrenia and a lower level of general functioning than women without an SUD. Effect sizes for factors, including age at onset, general level of functioning, number of positive symptoms, and total number of symptoms in general, were calculated by comparing women who abused drugs with those who abstained, with a parallel comparison conducted in men. For these factors the effect sizes in the female group were at least twice greater than that of the male group, indicating that a greater difference exists between women than men. This finding implies that substance use may have a greater negative effect on course of illness in women than men.

Another study of 92 inpatients with schizophrenia, with equal representation of men and women, sought to explain why men more frequently used illicit drugs than women (Haas, Glick, Clarkin, Spencer, & Lewis, 1990). Women were at least three times more likely to be married or to have been previously married than men. Before treatment, there were no sex differences in symptomatology or general functioning (including social and occupational functioning). Treatment with inpatient family intervention stressing education on all aspects of schizophrenia, including stressors and the need for continued treatment improved the clinical outcome in females more than males. Families of male patients more frequently canceled sessions and were more often late than those of female patients while families of female patients treated with inpatient family intervention had a greater reduction in rejecting attitudes toward the patient than did those of males. Although there were no sex differences in length of hospital stay or number of readmissions, the composite of symptomatology and functioning was worse in men at the 18-month follow-up. Men were worse at maintaining a daily routine and had lower levels of functioning at work. At 18 months, men continued to abuse narcotics more and reported more severe levels of abuse. Haas and colleagues hypothesized that men with schizophrenia have self-imposed as well as family and social expectations that are less realistic than those of women; in turn, these overreaching expectations make it harder for them to adjust to living with a mental disorder.

Increased aggression in subjects with dual diagnoses was shown in a 6-month study of 89 outpatients with schizophrenia, schizoaffective disorder, or schizophreniform disorder (Cuffel, Shumway, Chouljian, & MacDonald, 1994). Patients who used multiple substances were 12 times more likely to be violent. Violence was defined as verbal and nonverbal threats to harm others as well as physical fights and use of a weapon. Soyka, Albus, Immler, Kathmann, and Hippius (2001) studied patients with schizophrenia admitted to a state psychiatric hospital (1989–1990). At discharge, patients with concurrent SUDs were more aggressive and showed less insight into the disease than patients without SUDs. The frequency of delinquency and suicide attempts was higher in patients with a lifetime prevalence of SUDs.

The existence of co-occurring SUDs complicates the treatment of any mental illness. Medication nonadherence is one of the greatest challenges facing mental health care providers who treat patients with co-occurring substance use and psychiatric disorders. There is much evidence supporting a correlation between SUDs and medication nonadherence, but a causal relationship has not been established. A study measuring medication nonadherence in 135 subjects with either dual or single diagnosis found that the former were eight times more likely than the latter to be nonadherent (Owen, Fischer, Booth, & Cuffel, 1996). Nonadherence decreased from 40% at baseline to 15% at follow-up after the prescription of medication. The 29 individuals with SUDs reported a much higher nonadherence rate than those who did not use drugs: 41% vs. 8%. A consequence of nonadherence was greater symptom severity. Olfson et al. (2000) explored predictors of medication nonadherence in 316 patients with schizophrenia or schizoaffective disorder. At baseline, 42% of the patients were actively using drugs, and 38% were abusing alcohol. At 3-month follow-up, nearly 20% of baseline subjects were nonadherent, as defined by a week or more of not taking medication. The nonadherent subjects were more likely to meet the 6-month SUD diagnosis than the adherent subjects. The former were also twice as likely to be admitted to psychiatric hospitals and emergency rooms. At follow-up, the noncompliant patients were more likely to drop out of treatment when admitted to day hospitals or mental health clinics. Factors affecting nonadherence included a history of medication noncompliance, family refusal to participate in treatment, and an SUD.

Hunt, Bergen, and Bashir (2002) conducted a 4-year study of 99 patients recruited from acute care hospitals and crisis clinics to examine the negative consequences of SUDs and medication nonadherence. Those with SUDs were more likely male and of a younger age. Subjects with a history of SUDs were admitted to the hospital three times more often in the follow-up period and were twice as likely to be medication nonadherent than those without SUDs. Treatment adherence and lack of substance abuse were factors that increased community survival time (i.e., time between hospital readmissions). Median survival time before first hospital readmission for those with neither an SUD nor nonadherence was seven times that of those with both.

Substance use may also decrease the efficacy of antipsychotic drugs. A study of 35 males with acute psychosis and various diagnoses, including schizophrenia, schizophreniform, and mania, found that drug use resulted in a reduced early response to antipsychotic medication (Bowers, Mazure, Nelson, & Jatlow, 1990). Over 50% of the group of drug users had a poor response, compared to only 10% of those who did not use drugs.

Co-occurring disorders with schizophrenia are associated with a greater rate of hospitalization, possibly as a result of medication nonadherence. Gupta, Hendricks, Kenkel, Bhatia, and Haffke (1996) studied relapse in 22 male patients with schizophrenia for 2 years and found that the half with SUDs were readmitted to the hospital five times more often than those without SUDs. They found a relationship between number of hospital admissions and number of positive symptoms, such as delusions and hallucinations, exhibited by those with SUDs. Another small study found that, in a 2-year span, 86% of subjects dependent on alcohol received care in a hospital, compared to half that number in the nondependent group (Gerding, Labbate, Measom, Santos, & Arana, 1999). The alcohol-dependent group was also admitted to the hospital more than twice as often and had average hospital stays that were over twice as long as those without alcohol dependence.

Pristach and Smith (1990) studied a group of 28 male and 14 female inpatients diagnosed with schizophrenia to explore reasons for nonadherence in those with psychotic disorders who also abused substances. They found that patients often discontinued medication because they feared a negative interaction between the medication and alcohol. The fear may stem from doctors' warnings not to mix medications with alcohol.

Homelessness

Schizophrenia is associated with a high rate of homelessness. An association between homelessness and substance use was found in a group of chronically ill outpatients receiving continuing care from ambulatory community services, with equal male and female representation (Drake, Wallach, & Hoffman, 1989). Subjects suffered from schizophrenia, schizoaffective disorder (71% of study population), bipolar disorder, or personality disorders. Of those with schizophrenia, 14% were predominantly homeless and 10% were occasionally homeless. Among those with schizoaffective disorder, 33% were predominantly homeless and 11% occasionally homeless. The rate of alcohol use disorders in the predominantly homeless population was 59%, four times greater than in the stable housing group. Drug use disorders were also four times as prevalent in the homeless group. Hospitalizations occurred in 75% of the predominantly homeless compared to 35% of those with stable housing. Medication nonadherence in the predominantly homeless population occurred in 63%, whereas only 18% of those with stable housing were nonadherent. The data support a relationship between substance use and nonadherence, but homelessness is associated with medication noncompliance (independent of substance use) as well (Opler et al., 2001).

Caton et al. (1995) studied schizophrenia in 100 homeless women and an equal number of their counterparts who had never been homeless. They found that homelessness in women is associated with an increased rate of SUDs. The homeless group had a 30% prevalence of alcohol use disorders and an equal prevalence of illicit drug use disorders, whereas the never-homeless group abused alcohol and illicit drugs at about half those rates. A parallel study in men found no difference in the prevalence of alcohol use disorders in the homeless and never-homeless men (Caton et al., 1994). Illicit drug use disorders were nearly twice as common in homeless as in never-homeless men (77 vs. 44%). Homelessness was also found to be associated with increased incarceration. Homeless men were three times more likely to have a history of incarceration than never homeless men (72 vs. 25%). A comparison of the results of the two studies found significant sex differences. These studies reiterate the finding that SUDs are more prevalent in men than in women. In men, alcohol and drug use disorders were respectively 1.5–2.5 and 3–5 times greater than in women. Antisocial personality disorder (ASPD) was found at 5–10 times the rate in men as in women, and it was found in 42% of the homeless men compared to 9% of the never-homeless men (Caton et al., 1994). The likelihood of homelessness was increased tenfold in women with ASPD (Caton et al., 1995).

ASPD is linked to an increased severity of substance abuse in patients with schizophrenia and comorbid SUDs (Mueser et al., 1997). A study of 156 patients found that subjects with a dual diagnosis (i.e., ASPD and an SUD) abused drugs at an earlier age and in greater quantity. A greater number of those with ASPD had a history of drug abuse and drug abuse treatment. Substance abuse is highly prevalent in people with ASPD: 84% of people with ASPD have a concurrent SUD (Regier et al., 1990).

An important consequence of homelessness in women with schizophrenia is an increased risk of becoming a victim of violence (Goodman, Dutton, & Harris, 1995). About half of the women in the study also had a concurrent SUD. Although the researchers do not directly compare those with and without SUDs, the data suggest an association between increased risk for violence and an SUD. Homelessness resulting from SUDs may be a mediating factor in the increased risk for assault and trauma.

Models

Several mechanisms have been proposed to explain the association of SUDs and schizophrenia (Mueser, Drake, & Wallach, 1998). Few studies on comorbidity models examine sex differences. The self-medication hypothesis postulates that specific substances are used in an attempt to relieve specific psychiatric symptoms such as dysphoria, anxiety, or negative symptoms. A limitation of this hypothesis is that polysubstance abuse is common in patients with comorbidity. The supersensitivity model suggests that those with mental illness are more sensitive to the negative effects of drugs and alcohol, which increases their vulnerability to the negative consequences of substance use that includes relapse and rehospitalization. Studies have shown that people with schizophrenia, when challenged with amphetamine, required less of the drug to feel its negative effects than do control groups without mental illness (Lieberman, Kane, & Alvir, 1987).

Schizophrenia and SUDs may share common genetic vulnerabilities, as is explained by the common factor model. A genetic link between schizophrenia and SUDs is supported by data from a US study on the heritability of schizophrenia and alcoholism (Kendler, 1985). Schizophrenia and substance use disorders may share common genetic vulnerabilities as is explained by the common factor model. A genetic link between schizophrenia and substance use disorders is supported by data from a U.S. study on the heritability of schizophrenia and alcoholism (Kendler, 1985). Monozygotic (MZ) and dizygotic (DZ) index twins with comorbid schizophrenia and alcoholism were found from 15,924 pairs of Caucasian male twins. The co-twins of these 81 index twins were evaluated for schizophrenia and alcohol use disorders. Results showed significantly more MZ than DZ co-twins had schizophrenia, alcoholism, or both, implying that there exists a genetic predisposition to both alcoholism and schizophrenia. Further evidence comes from a study conducted by Chen et al. (2005) on subjects with psychosis induced by methamphetamine (MAMP). Drug-induced psychosis manifests with symptoms similar to schizophrenia, such as auditory and visual hallucinations and delusions of persecution and reference. Users of MAMP who experienced drug-induced psychosis had more schizoid/schizotypal traits in childhood than those who did not experience psychosis. A subsequent study examined the family members of the above subjects, with and without a lifetime diagnosis of MAMP-induced psychosis. Family members of subjects exhibiting psychosis had a higher morbid risk of schizophrenia than those in the nonpsychosis group. Furthermore, morbid risk was higher in family members of subjects who had prolonged MAMP-induced psychosis than in those with brief psychosis. The data from this study suggest that users of MAMP with a genetic predisposition to schizophrenia are more likely to experience drug-induced psychosis. The common factor model is also supported by results of a study on the effects of alcohol and cocaine on rats with neonatal ventral hippocampal lesions (NVHLs), an animal model of schizophrenia (Conroy, Rodd, & Chambers, 2007). Ethanol and cocaine increased locomotor activation in NVHL rats but not in placebo rats that did not have the lesion. These behavioral changes may be linked to the process of addiction and suggest that schizophrenia may increase vulnerability to substance abuse.

A different theory suggests that substance use may precede and facilitate the development of schizophrenia. This model postulates that drug abuse can induce a chronic psychosis that is similar to schizophrenia. Andréasson, Allebeck, Engstrom, and Rydberg (1987) followed 45,570 Swedish conscripts in the national register of psychiatric care for 15 years. Of the 752 subjects who had used cannabis more than 50 times at conscription, 2.8% subsequently developed schizophrenia. Of those who had never used cannabis at conscription, less than 0.5% were later diagnosed with schizophrenia. The odds of developing schizophrenia increased with increasing cannabis use. Schizophrenia with prior cannabis use was characterized by positive symptoms and an earlier onset (Andréasson, Allebeck, & Rydberg, 1989). An alternative explanation for these data is that latent schizophrenia may cause increased cannabis use.

Studies conducted in the past decade closely examined the neurological relationship between drug abuse and schizophrenia. Green, Zimmet, Strous, and Schildkraut (1999) proposed the brain reward dysfunction model that posits that dopamine-mediated mesocorticolimbic circuits implicated in responses to reward stimuli, are dysfunctional in people with schizophrenia. This primary mesocorticolimbic dysfunction results in a decreased ability to feel pleasure from naturally rewarding stimuli, and thereby causes an increased biologic vulnerability to the development of SUDs. Chambers, Krystal, and Self (2001) added that substance use is the direct result of schizophrenia, which alters neurodevelopment in the mesocorticolimbic dopamine system. The psychotic disorder pathologically changes brain development in such a way that it increases vulnerability to addiction even before the outward manifestations of the psychotic disease lead to the diagnosis of schizophrenia. Little research has been conducted on sex differences in biological models of comorbidity.

Treatment

Treatment for psychotic disorders involves the use of typical (i.e., first-generation) antipsychotic medications that have not been shown to be effective in treating SUDs. Typical antipsychotics do not improve the functioning of the mesolimbic reward circuit that regulates addiction and may even worsen the dysfunction by blocking the D_2 dopamine receptors (Green et al., 1999). However, some medications have been shown to be effective in treating dual-diagnosis patients, although no sex differences in effectiveness specific to these drugs have been documented. Use of clozapine, an atypical (second-generation) antipsychotic, shows more promise in the treatment of comorbid disorders, possibly as a result of its weak D_2 blockade activity and its effects on both dopaminergic and noradrenergic systems. Zimmet, Strous, Burgess, Kohnstamm, and Green (2000) studied 43 patients with comorbid schizophrenia or schizoaffective disorder and an SUD who were treated with clozapine. No subject who was actively using substances increased his or her use while on clozapine, and no subject initiated drug use. Moreover, 83% of alcohol users achieved abstinence. Data showed a significant correlation between decreased substance use and decreased global clinical symptoms. Drake, Xie, McHugo, and Green (2000) examined the effects of clozapine compared to typical antipsychotics in the treatment of comorbid schizophrenia or schizoaffective disorder and an SUD. After 6 months the clozapine group showed improvement in severity of alcohol and cannabis use as well as stage of substance abuse treatment. Improvements continued after patients were discharged from the hospitals. The clozapine group averaged 12.5 drinking days versus 54 days in the group taking typical antipsychotics. Remission was achieved in 79% of the former and in 35% of the latter group. Cannabis users on clozapine showed similar results, with 64% attaining abstinence, as compared to 32% in the group taking typical antipsychotics.

Among patients with co-occurring schizophrenia and cocaine dependence, risperidone-treated patients showed greater improvement than those in the typical antipsychotic group (Smelson et al., 2002). Data demonstrated cocaine relapse in 70% of those on typical antipsychotics but only 12.5% of those on risperidone. Furthermore, patients taking risperidone exhibited less cue reactivity to craving intensity and depression.

Petrakis et al. (2004) added naltrexone to the treatment regime of patients with schizophrenia and alcohol dependence, already being treated with antipsychotics. Patients who received naltrexone treatment had significantly fewer drinking days, fewer heavy drinking days, fewer drinks, and decreased craving as compared to the group without naltrexone. Positive and Negative Scale (PANSS) scores used to measure severity of schizophrenia were similar in both groups. The use of naltrexone decreased alcohol dependence and did not exacerbate symptoms of schizophrenia.

The program for assertive community treatment (PACT) utilizes available tools such as case management of patients and delivers services directly to patients in their environment. Clinical teams working with small, shared caseloads engage patients in their treatment regime and provide more convenience for them. Herinckx, Kinney, Clarke, and Paulson (1997) studied attrition rates in patients with chronic mental illness randomly assigned to usual care or PACT treatment programs. Mental illness included affective disorders or schizophrenia (60% of patients). An SUD was diagnosed in about 30% of subjects in each group. Attrition or drop-out rate was high in all treatment programs within the first 9 months. Subsequently, patients continued to drop out of the usual-care group at steady rates not seen in the PACT groups. The PACT groups retained 70% of patients—20% more than the usual-care group. Predictors of survival time in treatment programs included type of treatment program, number of nights spent homeless, diagnosis of a psychotic disorder, and substance use but not sex. Other studies have shown that PACT successfully engages patients in treatment, improves housing stability, and reduces negative outcomes such as hospital use (Mueser, Bond, Drake, & Resnick, 1998).

Co-occurring substance use results in poorer prognoses for patients with psychotic disorders, yet treatment of SUDs is often ignored when treating mental health illnesses. Harris and Edlund (2005) examined data from the 2001 and 2002 National Survey on Drug Use and Health (NSDUH, 2002, 2003; Substance Abuse and Mental Health Services Administration, 2002, 2003) to find the relationships between substance abuse, mental illnesses, and mental health care. These surveys, conducted yearly on a large group of people, are nationally representative. Among people with an SUD, only 20% received any treatment; however, comorbidity with a mental illness increased the treatment rate to 54%. Nevertheless, the majority of those with comorbid disorders who received mental health care were treated only for the mental illness, and only 30% received any treatment for substance abuse.

CONCLUSIONS

A clear relationship between schizophrenia and an increased prevalence of SUDs has been documented, yet inadequate attention is paid to treating the SUD—a lacuna that likely complicates the prognosis. Mental health care providers should screen for and treat SUDs in patients with psychotic disorders and this treatment should include PACT. The treatment regime should also address the attitudes of family members toward the patient and the disease. In addition, psychoeducational strategies to teach them how to recognize their psychotic symptoms can help patients assess their health more accurately. Longitudinal studies on the long-term efficacy of atypicals in decreasing drug relapse are needed. Further studies may elucidate the neurobiological model of schizophrenia and substance use in order for more effective drugs that treat both disorders to be produced. More data is needed on the efficacy of treating comorbid disorders with a combination of antipsychotics and newer drugs such as acamprosate and buproprion that are used independently for alcohol and smoking cessation, respectively.

KEY POINTS

- Schizophrenia frequently has a more benign course in women, but sex differences disappear with increasing age and concurrent substance use.
- Concurrent SUDs are found more commonly in men than in women with schizophrenia.

However, women may be more vulnerable than men to the adverse consequences of substance use.
- Substance use is associated with increased homelessness, symptom severity, and medication nonadherence.
- Greater hospitalizations and psychotic relapses are seen in patients with dual diagnosis.
- Schizophrenia may alter the mesocorticolimbic system, thereby increasing patient vulnerability to SUDs.
- Medications such as clozapine, risperidone, and naltrexone may be effective in treating concurrent SUDs and schizophrenia.

REFERENCES

Asterisks denote recommended readings.

American Psychiatric Association. (2000). *Diagnostic and statistical manual of mental disorders* (4th ed., text rev.). Washington, DC: Author.

Andréasson, S., Allebeck, P., Engstrom, A., & Rydberg, U. (1987). Cannabis and schizophrenia: A longitudinal study of Swedish conscripts. *Lancet, 2,* 1483–1486.

Andréasson, S., Allebeck, P., & Rydberg, U. (1989). Schizophrenia in users and nonusers of cannabis: A longitudinal study in Stockholm County. *Acta Psychiatrica Scandinavica, 79,* 505–510.

Bowers, M. B., Mazure, C. M., Nelson, J. C., & Jatlow, P. I. (1990). Psychotogenic drug use and neuroleptic response. *Schizophrenia Bulletin, 16,* 81–5.

Caton, C. L. M., Shrout, P. E., Dominguez, B., Eagle, P. F., Opler, L. A., & Cournos, F. (1995). Risk factors for homelessness among women with schizophrenia. *American Journal of Public Health, 85,* 1153–1156.

Caton, C. L. M., Shrout, P. E., Eagle, P. F., Opler, L. A., Felix, A., & Dominguez, B. (1994). Risk factors for homelessness among schizophrenic men. *American Journal of Public Health, 84,* 265–270.

Chambers, R. A., Krystal, J. H., & Self, D. W. (2001). A neurobiological basis for substance abuse comorbidity in schizophrenia. *Biological Psychiatry, 50,* 71–83. (*)

Chen, C., Lin, S., Sham, P. C., Ball, D., Loh, el-W., & Murray, R. M. (2005). Morbid risk for psychiatric disorder among the relatives of methamphetamine users with and without psychosis. *American Journal of Medical Genetics: Part B, Neuropsychiatric Genetics, 136*(1), 87–91.

Childers, S. E., & Harding, C. M. (1990). Gender, premorbid social functioning, and long-term outcome in DSM-III schizophrenia. *Schizophrenia Bulletin, 16,* 309–318.

Conroy, S. K., Rodd, Z., & Chambers, R. A. (2007). Ethanol sensitization in a neurodevelopmental lesion model of schizophrenia in rats. *Pharmocology, Biochemistry and Behavior, 86,* 386–394.

Cuffel, B. J., Shumway, M., Chouljian, T. L., & MacDonald, T. A. (1994). A longitudinal study of substance use and community violence in schizophrenia. *Journal of Nervous and Mental Disease, 182,* 704–708.

De Leon, J., & Diaz, F. J. (2005). A meta-analysis of worldwide studies demonstrates an association between schizophrenia and tobacco smoking behaviors. *Schizophrenia Research, 76,* 135–157. (*)

Drake, R. E., Wallach, M. A., & Hoffman, J. S. (1989). Housing instability and homelessness among aftercare patients of an urban state hospital. *Hospital and Community Psychiatry, 40*(1), 46–51.

Drake, R. E., Xie, H., McHugo, G. J., & Green, A. I. (2000). The effects of clozapine on alcohol and drug use disorders among patients with schizophrenia. *Schizophrenia Bulletin, 26,* 441–449.

Gearon, J. S., & Bellack, A. S. (2000). Sex differences in illness presentation, course and level of functioning in substance-abusing schizophrenia patients. *Schizophrenia Research, 43*(1), 65–70. (*)

Gerding, L. B., Labbate, L. A., Measom, M. O., Santos, A. B., & Arana, G. W. (1999). Alcohol dependence and hospitalization in schizophrenia. *Schizophrenia Research, 38,* 71–75.

Glenn, S. W., & Parsons, O. A. (1992). Neuropsychological efficiency measures in male and female alcoholics. *Journal of Studies on Alcohol, 53,* 546–552.

Goodman, L. A., Dutton, M. A., & Harris, M. (1995). Episodically homeless women with serious mental illness: Prevalence of physical and sexual assault. *American Journal of Orthopsychiatry*, 65(4), 468–479.

Green, A. I., Zimmet, S. V., Strous, R. D., & Schildkraut, J. J. (1999). Clozapine for comorbid substance use disorder and schizophrenia: Do patients with schizophrenia have a reward-deficiency syndrome that can be ameliorated by clozapine? *Harvard Review of Psychiatry*, 6, 287–296. (*)

Gupta, S., Hendricks, S., Kenkel, A. M., Bhatia, S. C., & Haffke, E. A. (1996). Relapse in schizophrenia: Is there a relationship to substance abuse? *Schizophrenia Research*, 20, 153–156.

Haas, G. L., Glick, I. D., Clarkin, J. F., Spencer, J. H., & Lewis, A. B. (1990). Gender and schizophrenia outcome: A clinical trial of an inpatient family intervention. *Schizophrenia Bulletin*, 16, 277–292. (*)

Harris, K. M., & Edlund, M. J. (2005). Use of mental health care and substance abuse treatment among adults with co-occurring disorders. *Psychiatric Services*, 56, 954–959.

Herinckx, H. A., Kinney, R. F., Clarke, G. N., & Paulson, R. I. (1997). Assertive community treatment versus usual care in engaging and retaining clients with severe mental illness. *Psychiatric Services*, 48, 1297–1306.

Hunt, G. E., Bergen, J., & Bashir, M. (2002). Medication compliance and comorbid substance abuse in schizophrenia: Impact on community survival 4 years after a relapse. *Schizophrenia Research*, 54, 253–264.

Kay, S. R., Opler, L. A., & Fiszbein, A. (2000). *The Positive and Negative Syndrome Scale (PANSS) manual*. Toronto: Multi-Health Systems.

Kendler, K. S. (1985). A twin study of individuals with both schizophrenia and alcoholism. *British Journal of Psychiatry*, 147, 48–53.

Lieberman, J. A., Kane, J. M., & Alvir, J. (1987). Provocative tests with psychostimulant drugs in schizophrenia. *Psychopharmacology*, 91, 415–433.

Lindamer, L. A., Buse, D. C., Lohr, J. B., & Jeste, D. B. (2001). Hormone replacement therapy in postmenopausal women with schizophrenia: Positive effect on negative symptoms? *Biological Psychiatry*, 49, 47–51.

McGlashan, T. H., & Bardenstein, K. K. (1990). Gender differences in affective, schizoaffective, and schizophrenic disorders. *Schizophrenia Bulletin*, 16, 319–329.

Mueser, K. T., Bond, G. R., Drake, R. E., & Resnick, S. G. (1998). Models of community care for severe illness: A review of research on case management. *Schizophrenia Bulletin*, 24, 37–74.

Mueser, K. T., Drake, R. E., Ackerson, T. H., Alterman, A. I., Miles, K. M., & Noordsy, D. L. (1997). Antisocial personality disorder, conduct disorder, and substance abuse in schizophrenia. *Journal of Abnormal Psychology*, 106, 473–477.

Mueser, K. T., Drake, R. E., & Wallach, M. A. (1998). Dual diagnosis: A review of etiological theories. *Addictive Behaviors*, 23(6), 717–734.

Mueser, K. T., Yarnold, P. R., Levinson, D. F., Singh, H., Bellack, A. S., Kee, K., et al. (1990). Prevalence of substance abuse in schizophrenia: Demographic and clinical correlates. *Schizophrenia Bulletin*, 16, 31–56. (*)

Olfson, M., Mechanic, D., Hansell, S., Boyer, C. A., Walkup, J., & Weiden, P. J. (2000). Predicting medication noncompliance after hospital discharge among patients with schizophrenia. *Psychiatric Services*, 51, 216–222.

Opler, L. A., White, L., Caton, C. L. M., Dominguez, B., Hirshfield, S., & Shrout, P. E. (2001). Gender differences in the relationship of homelessness to symptom severity, substance abuse, and neuroleptic noncompliance in schizophrenia. *Journal of Nervous and Mental Disease*, 189, 449–456.

Owen, R. R., Fischer, E. P., Booth, B. M., & Cuffel, B. J. (1996). Medication noncompliance and substance abuse among patients with schizophrenia. *Journal of Psychiatric Services*, 47, 853–858.

Petrakis, I. L., O'Malley, S., Rounsaville, B., Poling, J., McHugh-Strong, C., & Krystal, J. H. (2004). Naltrexone augmentation of neuroleptic treatment in alcohol abusing patients with schizophrenia. *Psychopharmacology*, 172, 291–297.

Pristach, C. E., & Smith, C. M. (1990). Medication compliance and substance abuse among schizophrenic patients. *Hospital and Community Psychiatry*, 41, 1345–1348.

Regier, M. D., Farmer, M. E., Rae, D. S., Locke, B. Z., Keith, S. J., Judd, L. L., et al. (1990). Comorbidity of mental disorders with alcohol and other drug abuse: Results from the Epidemiologic Catchment Area (ECA) study. *Journal of the American Medical Association, 264,* 2511–2518. (*)

Smelson, D. A., Losonczy, M. F., Davis, C. W., Kaune, M., Williams, J., & Ziedonis, D. (2002). Risperidone decreases craving and relapse in individuals with schizophrenia and cocaine dependence. *Canadian Journal of Psychiatry, 47,* 671–675.

Soyka, M., Albus, M., Immler, B., Kathmann, N., & Hippius, H. (2001). Psychopathology in dual diagnosis and non-addicted schizophrenics: Are there differences? *European Archives of Psychiatry and Clinical Neuroscience, 251*(5), 232–238.

Soyka, M., Albus, M., Kathmann, N., Finelli, A., Hofstetter, S., Holzbach, R., et al. (1993). Prevalence of alcohol and drug abuse in schizophrenic inpatients. *European Archives of Psychiatry and Clinical Neuroscience, 242*(6), 362–372.

Substance Abuse and Mental Health Services Administration. (2002). *Results from the 2001 National Household Survey on Drug Use and Health: National Findings.* (DHHS Publication No. SMA-02-3759). Rockville, MD: Author.

Substance Abuse and Mental Health Services Administration. (2003). *Results from the 2002 National Household Survey on Drug Use and Health: National Findings.* (DHHS Publication No. SMA-03-3836). Rockville, MD: Author.

Szymanski, S., Lieberman, J. A., Alvir, J. M., Mayerhoff, D., Loebel, A., Geisler, S., et al. (1995). Gender differences in onset of illness, treatment response, course, and biologic indexes in first-episode schizophrenic patients. *American Journal of Psychiatry, 152,* 698–703. (*)

Van Mastrigt, S., Addington, J., & Addington, D. (2004). Substance misuse at presentation to an early psychosis program. *Social Psychiatry and Psychiatric Epidemiology, 39,* 69–72.

Wiles, N. J., Zammit, S., Bebbington, P., Singleton, N., Meltzer, H., & Lewis, G. (2006). Self-reported psychotic symptoms in the general population: Results from the longitudinal study of the British National Psychiatric Morbidity Survey. *British Journal of Psychiatry, 188,* 519–526.

Zimmet, S. V., Strous, R. D., Burgess, E. S., Kohnstamm, S., & Green, A. I. (2000). Effects of clozapine on substance use in patients with schizophrenia and schizoaffective disorder: A retrospective survey. *Journal of Clinical Psychopharmacology, 20,* 94–98.

CHAPTER 16

Concurrent Personality Disorders and Substance Use Disorders in Women

Lisa A. Burckell, PhD
Shelley McMain, PhD

Over the past two decades, the rapidly growing research on personality disorders (PDs) has included attention to the treatment of comorbid PDs and substance use disorders (SUDs). Interest in the relationship between these disorders has focused historically on males diagnosed with antisocial personality disorder (ASPD). While the majority of research in this area has disregarded gender differences, some recent studies have addressed the unique issues related to the co-occurrence of PDs and SUDs in women. This chapter reviews the prevalence of concurrent PDs and SUDs in women, highlighting important gender differences. We discuss the explanations for this co-occurrence and subsequent implications for assessment and treatment. Finally, we examine new integrated treatment models tailored to address the needs of this group, highlighting empirical evidence where available.

PERSONALITY DISORDERS

PDs are serious mental disorders characterized by inflexible patterns of thoughts and actions that are pervasive across situations and that deviate markedly from cultural norms (American Psychiatric Association, 2000). Individuals meeting criteria for a PD diagnosis are characterized by impaired functioning in at least two areas, such as impulsivity, interpersonal functioning, affectivity, and cognition. A PD diagnosis commonly co-occurs with other PDs and Axis I disorders (Torgersen, Kringlen, & Cramer, 2001). The onset of personality-disordered symptoms occurs during adolescence or early adulthood. Recent evidence suggests that symptoms diminish with age, contrary to assumptions that they are stable over time (Lenzenweger, Lane, Loranger, & Kessler, 2007; Zanarini, Frankenburg, Hennen, Reich, & Silk, 2005). The fourth edition of the *Diagnostic and Statistical Manual of Mental Disorders* (American Psychiatric Association, 2000) identifies 10 categories of PDs, divided into three clusters:

- *Cluster A* (odd or eccentric): paranoid personality disorder, schizoid personality disorder, schizotypal personality disorder.
- *Cluster B* (dramatic, erratic, emotional): borderline personality disorder, antisocial personality disorder, narcissistic personality disorder, histrionic personality disorder.
- *Cluster C* (anxious and fearful): avoidant personality disorder, obsessive–compulsive personality disorder, dependent personality disorder.

One additional category of PD, designated "not otherwise specified" (NOS), is reserved for individuals who exhibit symptoms of a PD but do not meet the threshold for a specific one.

EPIDEMIOLOGY

Personality Disorders

Surveys of community samples estimate the prevalence rate across sexes for any PD to range from 3.4 to 14.8% (Coid, Yang, Tyrer, Roberts, & Ullrich, 2006; Grant et al., 2004b; Lenzenweger et al., 2007; Samuels, Nestadt, Romanoski, Folstein, & McHugh, 1994), with women reporting lower rates of PDs than men (3.4 versus 5.4%; Coid et al., 2006). The estimated prevalence of specific clusters of PDs in the general population is as follows: 5.7% Cluster A; 1.5% Cluster B; 6.0% Cluster C; and 9.1% for any PD (Lenzenweger et al., 2007). There are no apparent gender differences in prevalence rates across the three clusters of PDs (Torgersen et al., 2001). In contrast, studies based on clinical samples reveal different patterns of prevalence rates. Whereas Cluster B PDs are the least represented of the three clusters in general community samples, they are overrepresented in clinical samples across both genders. This overrepresentation is due to erratic and impulsive behaviors that prompt treatment, such as self-injurious actions and substance abuse. In women, the most commonly diagnosed PD is borderline personality disorder (BPD; Feske, Tarter, Kirisci, & Pilkonis, 2006).

Comorbid PDs and SUDs in Women

Several studies have confirmed high rates of overlap between PDs and SUDs (Grant et al., 2004a; Grant et al., 2004b; Lenzenweger et al., 2007). The vast majority of prevalence studies are based on samples of men and/or mixed-gender samples that include only a small proportion of women. Findings revealed that among individuals with a PD, 16.4% had a current alcohol use disorder and 6.5% had a current drug use disorder (Grant et al., 2004b). Conversely, among individuals with an alcohol use disorder, 28.6% had at least one PD, and among those with a drug use disorder, 47.7% had at least one PD. Surprisingly, ASPD was more strongly associated with alcohol and drug use disorders in women than in men in this community survey. The authors speculated that this was likely due to the fact that men with ASPD are underrepresented in community samples due to their higher rates of incarceration. Overall, although the rates of comorbid PDs and SUDs are higher in men, the presence of any PD is strongly associated with SUDs in both genders.

Studies based on clinical samples reveal rates of overlap between PDs and SUDs that far exceed those in the general population. The reported overlap between PDs and SUDs ranges from 2 to 84% (for reviews, see Sher & Trull, 2002; Verheul, van den Brink, & Hartgers, 1995). This considerable variability in reported rates is due to differences in assessment methods and samples.

SUDs are more strongly associated with Axis II disorders than with Axis I disorders

(Koenigsberg, Kaplan, Gilmore, & Cooper, 1985; Warshaw, Dolan, & Keller, 2000). Individuals with SUDs commonly meet the criteria for more than one PD (DeJong, van den Brink, Harteveld, & van der Wielen, 1993). Studies examining gender differences show a nonsignificant trend for females with SUDs to have more Axis II disorders than males (Verheul et al., 1995). The rates of PDs are higher in drug users than in alcohol users (Seivewright & Daly, 1997; Verheul et al., 1995). High rates of PDs are found among subgroups of females with SUDs, including those with alcohol or heroin dependence (Thevos, Brady, Grice, Dustan, & Malcolm, 1993), as well as those with cocaine dependence (Brooner, King, Kidorf, Schmidt, & Bigelow, 1997).

Cluster B and C PDs are most frequently associated with SUDs in both men and women (Rounsaville et al., 1998; Warshaw et al., 2000). The comorbidity of specific PDs and alcohol and drug use disorders differs between the sexes. In a review of the prevalence of PDs among patients who abuse alcohol or drugs, comorbid BPD and SUDs frequently are noted in men and women; however, the highest observed rates were found in a female sample (Verheul et al., 1995). BPD is a significant correlate of SUDs in women, even after controlling for the effects of other comorbid PDs (Feske et al., 2006; Trull, Sher, Minks-Brown, Durbin, & Burr, 2000; Vaglum & Vaglum, 1985). In a review of studies that examined the comorbidity of BPD and SUDs, Trull et al. (2000) found that an estimated 57.4% of individuals with BPD met the criteria for an SUD, and approximately one-third of patients with an SUD had a BPD diagnosis. While the rate of ASPD is estimated to be one and a half times more common among men than women, the presence of an ASPD diagnosis in women is also highly correlated with SUDs (Chapman & Cellucci, 2007; Ross, Glaser, & Stiasny, 1988; Verheul et al., 1995). Since Cluster B PDs, specifically BPD, are more strongly associated with alcohol and drug use disorders in women than are the other clusters, we focus primarily on this subgroup.

EXPLANATIONS FOR THE COMORBIDITY OF PDs AND SUDs IN WOMEN

The common co-occurrence of PDs and SUDs has fueled interest in understanding the reasons for the high rates. Theories advanced to explain this overlap are discussed briefly below.

Biological Factors

Some researchers speculate that the development of co-occurring PDs and SUDs results from inheritance. Evidence supports the familial transmission of SUDs (e.g., Merikangas et al., 1998; Prescott, Aggen, & Kendler, 1999) and PDs (e.g., Torgersen et al., 2000). Family studies reveal higher rates of substance problems and ASPD in the relatives of individuals diagnosed with alcohol dependence compared to nonalcoholics (e.g., Nurnberger et al., 2004). Finally, relatives of women diagnosed with PDs, particularly those with Cluster B PDs, have higher rates of SUDs compared to the general population (White, Gunderson, Zanarini, & Hudson, 2003).

Psychological Factors

Some women may have personality traits that create vulnerability for the co-occurrence of both disorders. The most commonly implicated traits are impulsivity and negative emotionality.

Impulsivity

A significant body of research supports the relationship of impulsivity to both SUDs (Caspi, Moffitt, Newman, & Silva, 1996; Elkins, King, McGue, & Iacono, 2006; Hopwood et al., 2007; Sher, Bartholow, & Wood, 2000; Slutske et al., 2002) and PDs, particularly the Cluster B PDs such as ASPD and BPD (e.g., Chapman & Cellucci, 2007), as well as to their co-occurrence (e.g., Stepp, Trull, & Sher, 2005).

Although men have been found to have higher levels of impulsivity and substance use than women, high levels of impulsivity are also commonly reported by women who abuse drugs and alcohol (e.g., Lejuez, Bornovalova, Reynolds, Daughters, & Curtain, 2007) and by women with comorbid PDs and SUDs (e.g., Chapman & Cellucci, 2007; Johnson et al., 2003). In one study, women who reported similar levels of impulsivity as men had levels of substance use that were comparable to, or surpassed, those of men (Lejuez et al., 2007). However, Johnson, Shea, Yen, Battle, Zlotnick, Sanislow, et al. (2003) found that males with BPD had higher rates of SUDs than females with BPD (94.6 vs. 58.3%), even though trait impulsivity did not differ by gender.

Negative Emotionality

Several theories support a link between negative emotionality and PDs and SUDs. Although the empirical evidence to support these theories is mixed, some studies support a strong association between alcohol use disorders and negative emotionality (Elkins et al., 2006; Jackson & Sher, 2003). The relationship between illicit substance abuse and negative emotionality, however, has been shown to be less robust than its link to impulsivity (Elkins et al., 2006). Women report higher levels of negative emotionality than men (e.g., Goodwin & Gotlib, 2004), and in turn, negative emotionality may be more salient to the onset of SUDs in women than in men. For example, in a matched sample of men and women in treatment for alcohol dependence, women scored higher on negative emotionality compared to men, whereas men scored higher on sensation seeking—an aspect of impulsivity. This finding suggests that the development of alcohol dependence may be more closely linked to negative emotionality in women and to impulsivity in men (Wiejers et al., 2003).

There is also evidence to support a link between negative emotionality and some specific PDs, particularly BPD. Negative emotionality and emotional dysregulation are theorized to be key factors in the development of BPD (Linehan, 1993; Skodol et al., 2002; Trull et al., 2000), and the association between negative emotionality and BPD is well supported (Bagge et al., 2004; Ball, Tennen, Poling, Kranzler, & Rounsaville, 1997; Taylor, Reeves, James, & Bobadilla, 2006). Some evidence indicates that negative emotionality is also associated, though indirectly, with ASPD (Miller, Lynam, & Leukefeld, 2003).

Combination of Impulsivity and Negative Emotionality

Many researchers speculate that both impulsivity and negative emotionality play a role in the co-occurrence of PDs and SUDs, particularly BPD (Trull et al., 2000). Girls who have higher levels of negative emotionality and impulsivity may place extra demands on their environments. For example, they may be more "emotional" and "reactant"; parents may not be equipped to respond effectively and may behave in ways that invalidate the child (e.g., "Stop being so emotional!"). These temperamentally sensitive girls may not have the skills to cope with intense affect, and their parents may fail to model effective coping strategies. As a result, these girls are vulnerable to developing maladaptive means to regulate their negative affect (e.g., self-harm or substance use) (Linehan, 1993). In a related finding, high negative emotionality coupled with higher impulsivity was strongly associated with BPD features and substance use among college students (Taylor et al., 2006), and this combination of high impulsivity and negative emotionality distinguished individuals with co-morbid BPD and SUDs from those with comorbid ASPD and SUDs (Ball et al., 1997).

Impulsivity may act as a vulnerability factor that moderates the association between affect lability and alcohol-related problems, and this association strengthens as impulsivity increases (Simons, Carey, & Gaher, 2004). Mood fluctuations experienced by women with BPD can lead to a search for "quick" solutions, such as substance use, to regulate their mood (Trull et al., 2000). The use of substances to regulate emotions is highly reinforcing because the substances work effectively in the moment. Individuals with higher levels of impulsivity report greater relief from substance use (e.g., Levenson, Oyama, & Meek, 1987). Therefore, impulsive women are particularly vulnerable to the effects of this negative reinforcement.

Social Factors

Various environmental factors can contribute to the development of PDs and SUDs. For example, factors such as lack of family support (e.g., Wills & Cleary, 1996), substance-using friends (Curran, Stice, & Chassin, 1997), and economically disadvantaged neighborhood contexts (e.g., Luthar & D'Avanzo, 1999) contribute to the development of these comorbid disorders. Research demonstrates that poorer neighborhoods (Lynman et al., 2000) and childhood physical abuse (Jaffee, Caspi, Moffitt, & Taylor, 2004) are related to the development of the antisocial behaviors linked to ASPD. Similarly, environmental factors are implicated in the onset of BPD (for a review, see Zanarini, 2000). For example, Zanarini et al. (1997) found that among inpatients, individuals with a BPD diagnosis reported higher rates of childhood abuse than individuals diagnosed with other PDs. Experiences such as abuse often lead individuals to discount their personal experiences. These invalidating experiences are thought to lead to emotional regulation problems that underlie the co-occurrence of PDs and SUDs. Linehan (1993) speculates that women with BPD have a higher risk of exposure to invalidating experiences than men due to the higher rates of sexual abuse and sexism among girls and females in our culture experience.

Interconnecting Pathways

Addiction problems and PD symptoms also interact to contribute to the development, maintenance, and course of each disorder. For example, substance abuse can heighten traits of impulsivity and negative affectivity, both core features of BPD. Conversely, individuals with high levels of impulsivity and negative affectivity are more likely than others to use substances to regulate their affect. The presence of BPD and conduct disorder features in early adolescence—precursors of ASPD—are risk factors for future substance abuse problems (Cohen, Chen, Crawford, Brook, & Gordon, 2007). In a related finding, the presence of BPD features was associated with earlier onset of substance use, though the presence of these features did not impact the chronicity of SUDs (Skodol, Oldham, & Gallaher, 1999). There is evidence that the presence of one disorder can extend or alter the course of the other. For example, individuals diagnosed with both BPD and SUDs have worse outcomes than those with BPD alone (Links et al., 1995).

CONSEQUENCES OF CO-OCCURRING
PDs AND SUDs IN WOMEN

The co-occurrence of PDs and SUDs predicts a more severe clinical profile than a diagnosis of either disorder alone (Kosten, Kosten, & Rounsaville, 1989; Skodol et al., 1999) and is associated with more extensive involvement in substance use, including earlier age of onset, greater severity of use, higher rates of polydrug use, and longer lifetime use of illicit drugs (e.g., Brooner et al., 1997; Darke, Williamson, Ross, Teesson, & Lynskey, 2003; Nace, Davis, & Gaspari, 1991). Conversely, compared to late-onset substance use, early onset use is associated with higher rates of ASPD, BPD, and passive–aggressive symptoms (Franken & Hendriks, 2000). Addiction to certain substances, such as cocaine, is associated with higher rates of Axis II pathology in women than is alcohol abuse (Thevos et al., 1993). Finally, women engaged in polydrug abuse have higher rates of ASPD than do those abusing one drug (Ross et al., 1988).

The overlap of PDs and SUDs is associated with higher levels of psychological distress and psychopathology than is either disorder alone (Brooner et al., 1997; Darke, Williamson, Ross, Teesson, & Lynskey, 2004; Nace et al., 1991). A comparison of patients with BPD, with and without substance abuse problems, revealed higher levels of psychopathology and impulsivity in the substance-abusing group (Links et al., 1995). Conversely, comparisons of individuals with both SUDs and BPD reveal higher levels of psychopathology and need for psychiatric services than those individuals with a BPD diagnosis only (Darke et al., 2003; Kosten et al., 1989; Nace et al., 1991). These findings highlight the likelihood that patients with comorbid PDs and SUDs will require additional psychiatric assessment and treatment.

High rates of self-harm, suicidal, and other risk behaviors are common in women with co-morbid PDs and SUDs (Darke et al., 2003; Inman, Bascue, & Skoloda, 1985; Links et al., 1995; Nace, Saxon, & Shore, 1983). Comorbid BPD and SUDs compared to BPD alone is related to higher rates of suicidal behaviors, including suicide attempts, nonsuicidal self-injurious behavior, and parasuicidal ideation (Darke et al., 2003; Inman et al., 1985; Links et al., 1995; Nace et al., 1983; Stone, 1989; van den Bosch, Verheul, & van den Brink, 2001). Substance abuse increases vulnerability to engage impulsively in suicidal behaviors as well as other high-risk behaviors (van den Bosch et al., 2001). For example, patients with BPD and SUDs, compared to those without SUDs, reported higher rates of sexual promiscuity and prostitution (Miller, Abrams, Dulit, & Minna, 1993). Individuals with a diagnosis of BPD who use heroin, compared to those without a BPD diagnosis, have an increased risk of overdose and participation in risky drug use behaviors such as needle sharing (Darke et al., 2004). Similarly, a diagnosis of ASPD in women who engage in intravenous drug use was associated with greater risk for HIV infection, compared to women without ASPD (Brooner, Herbst, Schmidt, Bigelow, & Costa, 1993), and the presence of ASPD increased the risk for heroin overdose (Darke et al., 2004). In sum, comprehensive treatment for PDs and SUDs may need to include education about sexually transmitted diseases, skills to reduce impulsive sex, and a focus on securing a safe means of employment (Chen, Brown, Lo, & Linehan, 2007), as well as suicide prevention strategies.

Several studies indicate that the co-occurrence of PDs and SUDs, compared to the presentation of either disorder alone, is associated with poorer general functioning and higher levels of psychosocial impairment (Brooner et al., 1997). The presence of ASPD in females who abuse drugs was associated with lower levels of education (Ross et al., 1988). Patients with BPD and SUDs have higher rates of unemployment and a greater likelihood of being underemployed, compared to their non-substance-abusing counterparts (Miller et al., 1993). Additionally, comparisons between patients with and without PD who abuse substances indicate that the former report less satisfaction with their lives, particularly in the areas of emotional health and relationships (Nace & Davis, 1993). For this subgroup of women, interventions directed at enhancing social supports may be a critical component of treatment success. However, the health care system can inadvertently be iatrogenic for these women if they come to depend on the social support provided, as this can act as a disincentive for them to develop other social networks that could assist in treatment progress.

ASSESSMENT CONSIDERATIONS

Given the overlap of co-occurring PDs and SUDs in women and the challenges associated with treating this population, clinicians should assess for the presence of both disorders as well as coexisting disorders. Two semistructured interviews, the Structured Clinical Interview for the DSM, or SCID (First, Spitzer, Gibbon, & Williams, 1995) and the International Personality Disorder Exam, or IPDE (Loranger, 1995), are widely recommended to conduct comprehensive diagnostic assessments. It is critical for therapists to obtain a complete diagnostic picture during treatment planning, since empirically supported PD treatments exist.

To acquire a comprehensive understanding of a patient, it is recommended that the clinician conduct a detailed assessment of level of functioning in multiple areas, including employment/productivity, financial support, social support, and legal status. This aspect of the assessment is critical, since level of functioning is one of the best predictors of treatment response (Shane, Jasiukaitis, & Green, 2003). The presence of suicidal and other high-risk, impulsive behaviors should also be evaluated, since they are associated with increased overall risk (Shane et al., 2003).

It is important to consider genetic and environmental factors that may have contributed to the development and maintenance of presenting problems. Specific questions about a patient's family history of mental health disorders, substance problems, or temperamental style will provide clues. For example, information about the patient's personality during early childhood and onward is relevant to conceptualizing the patient's problems and making a diagnosis. Pervasive invalidating experiences are also theorized to play an important role in the development of BPD and SUDs (Linehan, 1993). Thus, clinicians need to obtain information about childhood and adulthood traumatic experiences—emotional, physical, and sexual—that these women may have experienced or are continuing to encounter.

Several factors can complicate the diagnosing of co-occurring PDs and SUDs. First, women in an acute period of substance use often exhibit features of behavioral dyscontrol and emotional dysregulation that resemble symptoms of PDs, thereby making it difficult to distinguish a primary PD from an SUD (Brady, Grice, Dustan, & Randall, 1993). For example, cocaine intoxication can lead to emotional lability that mimics the symptoms of BPD. These "pseudo-PD" symptoms often abate once abstinence from substances is achieved. To distinguish addictive behaviors from PD symptoms, it is critical to consider the onset and duration of symptoms. Symptoms characteristic of an independent PD are longstanding and occur outside of acute periods of substance use, whereas behavior stemming from the misuse of substances is pronounced during periods of intoxication and withdrawal, yet will abate during periods of abstinence. Since many individuals have difficulty accurately recalling the onset of their symptoms, particularly if they are in an acute withdrawal state, it is often necessary to obtain corroborating information from their family members, friends, and previous health care providers.

Another complication is that patients can be reticent to disclose critical information that is relevant to their treatment. Based on our experience, women are particularly guarded about disclosing impulsive behaviors that are accompanied by intense feelings of shame, such as substance use, shoplifting, prostitution, sexual promiscuity, reckless driving, self-harm, and bingeing, and purging. It follows that, compared to men, women with SUDs are more likely to enter into treatment via the mental health system than via the addiction treatment system, since they view their problems as mental health issues rather than addiction problems and consider the latter to be indirectly related to their treatment goals (Greenfield et al., 2007). Thus, it is important for clinicians to inquire directly and nonjudgmentally about substance use behaviors and other impulsive problems.

TREATMENT CHALLENGES

The impact of co-occurring PDs and SUDs on women's response to treatment is not entirely clear. Some studies have found patients with co-occurring BPD and SUDs to have poorer treatment retention and treatment response and higher rates of premature withdrawal and discharge from treatment compared to their non-BPD counterparts (Cacciola, Rutherford, Alterman, McKay, & Snider, 1996; Kosten et al., 1989; McCann, Flynn, & Gersh, 1992). Furthermore, patients with BPD and SUDs are twice as likely to be diagnosed with BPD 7 years after their index admission, compared to their non-substance-abusing counterparts (Links et al., 1995). However, the results of other studies indicate that patients with PDs and SUDs benefit from treatment as well as their non-PD counterparts (Links et al., 1995). Although these women can benefit from treatment, the management of these patients is complicated by several factors.

Stigma

Women with comorbid PDs and SUDs are a doubly stigmatized group. Historically, substance abuse has been viewed as a moral, legal, or characterological problem, and these pejorative views have influenced how it is treated (Leshner, 1997). Discrimination can lead to treatment avoidance, failure to disclose substance use, and an increase in symptomatology (Vaillancourt & Keith, 2007). The stigma is particularly heightened for childbearing women and women belonging to certain cultural groups. These pervasive negative attitudes help to explain why women often fail to discontinue substance abuse during pregnancy, despite the incentives to do so (Leslie, 2007). Personality diagnoses—widely regarded as psychiatry's stepchildren—are also one of the most stigmatized of mental disorders (Paris, 2006). Individuals with BPD and ASPD are commonly described as "manipulative," and these descriptions persist even in the DSM-IV (American Psychiatric Association, 2000). Women are more likely to be subjected to these biases, given the high rates of BPD among females. Thus, women with co-occurring PDs and SUDs often face significant stigma that reduces the likelihood that they will seek treatment, disclose their substance use, or remain in treatment. Thus, positive therapist attitudes are critical to effective treatment (Penn, Brooks, & Worsham, 2002).

Issues Related to Treatment Engagement

Women with co-occurring PDs and SUDs experience pervasive emotional, interpersonal, and motivational impairments that impede their engagement in treatment services. Their significant interpersonal problems contribute to difficulties in forming a treatment alliance. Furthermore, these women are particularly impulsive and can make choices affected by their mood or substance use that can compromise treatment engagement. For example, use of substances can lead to poor attendance (e.g., failure to remember appointments); or a woman with BPD who is overwhelmed by anxiety might decide that she does not "feel" like attending a particular session, despite her commitment to treatment in general.

There may be ambivalence about addressing substance abuse, and it may not be viewed as the primary reason patients are seeking help: That is, they are likely to enter treatment to address other problems they are experiencing rather than to treat substance abuse (e.g., Greenfield et al., 2007). Also, some may feel forced to enter treatment for legal or personal consequences (e.g., the end of a relationship) that are related to their substance abuse. The therapist and treatment team may want the patient to abstain or to reduce her use; however, pushing for this when the patient does not agree may lead to dropout or poor engagement (e.g., Longabaugh et al., 1994). Therapists can implement strategies to minimize reactivity and to promote decreased substance use; specifically, they can explore how substance use impacts the patient's primary concerns (Linehan, 1993). Through this approach, patients are encouraged to assume an active role in their treatment and their lives—an opportunity that many have yet to experience.

Women with co-occurring PDs and SUDs often lack a social network that supports their treatment goals or reinforces their progress. For example, a woman may be involved with a substance-abusing partner who becomes threatened by her desire for change. Reported relationship quality is higher among couples where substance use is shared, and is lower when one partner is abstinent and the other continues use (Fals-Stewart, Birchler, & O'Farrell, 1999). In order to preserve their relationship or to avoid conflict or further abuse, women may resume substance use. Women with BPD, who often fear abandonment, are vulnerable to relapse and may drop out of treatment if their partners voice disapproval. If supportive partners exist, enlisting their participation can enhance treatment outcomes (Fals-Stewart, Birchler, & Kelley, 2006; Winters, Fals-Stewart, O'Farrell, Birchler, & Kelley, 2002).

Complexity of Problems in the Absence of Adequate Treatment Resources

Another clinical challenge related to the management of women with comorbid PDs and SUDs is the volume of complex problems these women experience. For example, therapists can be pulled into focusing on the "crisis of the day" and fail to adequately address the underlying issues that precipitate these crises. Based on her experiences in working with women with multiple, complex problems, Linehan (1993) proposed a specific treatment hierarchy to ensure that frequent crises do not undermine the larger treatment goals. In dialectical behavior therapy (DBT), treatment targets are hierarchically organized in the following order of priority (1) life-interfering behaviors, (2) treatment-interfering behaviors, and (3) quality-of-life-interfering behaviors. Substance abuse falls at the top of the quality-of-life-interfering behaviors. Application of this hierarchy provides a means for the therapist to navigate the crises and issues that these women bring to treatment.

The absence of specialized treatment resources presents an additional challenge. At present, programs that provide specialized integrated treatment for women with co-morbid PDs and SUDs are limited. Furthermore, given the overlap among PDs and Axis I disorders, it would be impractical to develop separate manuals to account for every possible combination of PD and SUD (Ball, 1998). Therapists are often faced with the question of how to tailor treatment plans to address the unique issues presented by patients. Many therapists and clinics lack the resources or expertise to provide comprehensive treatments that draw upon diverse strategies. Further, attempting to treat patients who have multiple, complex problems in the absence of adequate resources and effective treatment options can lead to clinician burnout. In the absence of specialized integrated programming, one option is for clinicians to build competence in the treatment of both personality and substance abuse problems. In addition, treatment can be enhanced if clinicians develop partnerships with other programs in order to execute an integrated treatment plan that addresses the diverse needs of these women.

TREATMENT APPROACHES

Historically, patients with PDs and addiction problems have been treated differently from those without addiction problems. The differential treatment is rooted in the well-established practice of excluding individuals with substance problems from treatment programs in the mental health system. The clinical and empirical research literature reveals a bias toward sequential or parallel treatment models—that is, treatments in which addiction problems and mental health problems are addressed separately by different clinicians. Much of the research designed to evaluate the efficacy of treatment for individuals with BPD excluded patients with comorbid SUDs (Bateman & Fonagy, 1999; Clarkin, Levy, Lenzenweger, & Kernberg, 2007; Linehan, Armstrong, Suarez, Allmon, & Heard, 1991; Munroe-Blum & Marziali, 1995; Stevenson & Meares, 1992).

Over the past two decades, there has been a growing interest in the development of integrated treatment models for individuals with concurrent Axis I and II disorders. This heightened interest is largely due to greater awareness of the perceived limitation of sequential or parallel treatment models—namely, the challenge of treating one disorder in the absence of attention to the other disorder. Recently, two cognitive therapy approaches for the treatment of comorbid PDs and SUDs have been described in the literature: DBT and schema-focused therapy. These treatment approaches are discussed briefly below.

DBT for Substance-Abusing Individuals with BPD

DBT, as mentioned, is a broad-based cognitive-behavioral approach originally developed in the early 1980s by Marsha Linehan for suicidal patients with BPD (Linehan, 1993). Over the past decade, it has been adapted to address problems associated with concurrent substance use and BPD (Linehan & Dimeff, 1997; McMain, Sayrs, Dimeff, & Linehan, 2007). The model is based on the premise that pervasive deficits in emotion regulation underlie the problems that beset patients with comorbid BPD and SUDs. Substance abuse, like other maladaptive problems (e.g., self-harm), functions to modulate dysregulated affect or is the consequence of it. To address the unique issues related to individuals who abuse substances, additional treatment elements were incorporated into the standard DBT protocol. Therapists utilize more active outreach because of the problems related to poorer treatment retention when patients with BPD also abuse substances. Other modifications include a dialectical approach to substance abuse goals—"dialectical abstinence." Therapists balance pushing patients to eliminate substances while simultaneously focusing on minimizing the harm associated with substance abuse. A basic premise is that the most realistic goal for a patient with BPD and an SUD is abstinence. However, if patients fail to achieve abstinence, a harm reduction approach can be critical to helping them reduce shame about the relapse or slip, so that they can return to abstinence.

All standard modes of DBT (individual therapy, skills group, telephone coaching, therapist consultation team) are delivered intact to patients with BPD and an SUD. Patients with BPD either with or without comorbid SUDs can participate successfully in the same DBT program. The four core DBT skills—mindfulness, distress tolerance, emotion regulation, and interpersonal effectiveness—are relevant to both substance abuse behaviors and to other problem behaviors. A few additional skills, such as the mindfulness skill of "urge surfing," are woven into the core skills modules to specifically address problems associated with coping with cravings, urges, and relapses. Supplementing treatment with case management can address the numerous life problems, such as unemployment or lack of housing, that some patients with BPD and an SUD experience.

DBT has garnered the most attention in the empirical literature, with several positive reports supporting its use in the treatment of women with BPD who also abuse substances. Four randomized controlled trials have evaluated its effectiveness when adapted for the treatment of concurrent BPD and SUDs. Linehan et al. (1999) evaluated 1 year of DBT compared to a treatment-as-usual for women with substance dependence and BPD, and found that DBT participants had superior outcomes on drug abuse at 1 year and 16-month follow-up as well as better treatment retention over the treatment year. In a second study, Linehan et al. (2002) evaluated the effectiveness of DBT for women with opiate dependence and BPD. Participants were randomly assigned to 1 year of either DBT or comprehensive validation therapy (CVT) with 12-step treatment. Results indicated that both groups showed significant reductions in drug use over the course of the treatment year, but the DBT group maintained their gains during the 1-year follow-up, whereas the CVT group showed an increase in their substance use. However, although DBT was superior with regard to substance use outcomes, the control condition showed better overall treatment retention (100 vs. 64%). Trials conducted independently of the treatment developer have also showed promise for DBT (McMain et al., 2004; Verheul et al., 2003).

Dual-Focused Schema Therapy

Dual-focused schema therapy (DFST; Ball, 1998) is an adaptation of Young's (1990) schema-focused therapy for the treatment of diverse PDs and substance abuse. Standard schema-focused cognitive therapy for the treatment of PDs targets core maladaptive cognitive schemas related to self, others, and events that are assumed to be learned in childhood and that organize a person's beliefs and behaviors. In addition to targeting the maladaptive schemas, DFST includes specific interventions that target maladaptive schemas and are integrated with specific relapse prevention techniques to address substance abuse. For example, traditional relapse prevention strategies are used to address cravings, urges, and interpersonal and affective factors. Addictive behaviors and personality-disordered symptoms are also addressed via common techniques, including functional analysis, cognitive restructuring techniques, and strategies to enhance lifestyle and increase coping with environmental and internal cues.

A recent randomized trial compared the efficacy of DFST with 12-step drug counseling (Ball, Cobb-Richardson, Connolly, Bujosa, & O'Neall, 2005). The study involved a predominantly (92%) male sample of 52 homeless patients with opioid dependence and co-occurring PDs. Patient were randomized to 24 weeks of either DFST or standard group substance abuse counseling. Individuals in both conditions received standard case management to supplement therapy. While there were no between-group differences in treatment retention, participants receiving DFST, compared to those receiving standard group treatment, utilized treatment better (e.g., attended more individual sessions, attended more weeks in therapy). Despite this finding, overall low retention rates across both groups (40%) made it impossible to compare other treatment outcomes.

CONCLUSIONS

In summary, the co-occurrence of addiction and PDs in women is common. Women with these co-occurring disorders have a more severe clinical profile than those with either disorder alone and consequently are less likely to respond favorably to standard addiction treatments. There is a need to modify assessments and treatments in order to address the unique needs of these women. A few cognitive-behavioral therapies, such as DBT and DFST, have been modified for the treatment of addiction-related problems in patients with PDs and show promise. However, more research is needed to enhance interventions to address the multiple, complex problems that these women experience. Despite the challenges that women with these diagnoses face and the complexity of treating their concerns, they can benefit from treatment and lead more fulfilling lives.

KEY POINTS

- PDs, in particular Cluster B (i.e., BPD), are prevalent among women who abuse substances.
- The presence of personality pathology among women with SUDs is associated with greater dysfunction and a more complicated clinical course. Consequently, clinicians should screen for and assess the presence of personality disorders. Assessments should extend beyond a diagnostic assessment to a consideration of the nature and severity of functioning across behavioral, emotional, interpersonal, and cognitive domains.
- Ongoing monitoring of suicide risk should not be overlooked in view of the heightened risk for suicide attempts among women with comorbid PDs and SUDs.
- Treatment should be individualized to address the unique problems experienced by women with comorbid PDs and SUDs. Clinicians need to gain a comprehensive understanding of the patient level of functioning, including strengths and areas of impairment, in order to determine an appropriate course of treatment.
- Some specific cognitive-behavioral treatments show promise for the treatment of women with comorbid PDs and SUDs (e.g., DBT for patients with BPD and an SUD). It is generally recommended that treatment be structured and focused on enhancing coping skills to address problems.
- Treatment for women with co-occurring PDs and SUDs is typically more extensive and longer in duration as compared to women with PDs or SUDs only.

REFERENCES

Asterisks denote recommended readings.

American Psychiatric Association. (2000). *Diagnostic and statistical manual of mental disorders* (4th ed.). Washington, DC: Author.

Bagge, C., Nickell, A., Stepp, S., Durrett, C., Jackson, K., & Trull, T. J. (2004). Borderline personality disorder features predict negative outcomes 2 years later. *Journal of Abnormal Psychology, 113,* 279–288.

Ball, S. A. (1998). Manualized treatment for substance abusers with personality disorders: Dual focus schema therapy. *Addictive Behaviors, 23,* 883–891.

Ball, S. A., Cobb-Richardson, P., Connolly, A., Bujosa, C. T., & O'Neall, T. W. (2005). Substance abuse and personality disorders in homeless drop-in center clients: Symptom severity and psychotherapy retention in a randomized clinical trial. *Comprehensive Psychiatry, 46,* 371–379.

Ball, S. A., Tennen, H., Poling, J., Kranzler, H. R., & Rounsaville, B. J. (1997). Personality, temperament, and character dimensions and the DSM-IV personality disorders in substance abusers. *Journal of Abnormal Psychology, 106,* 545–553.

Bateman, A., & Fonagy, P. (1999). Effectiveness of partial hospitalization in the treatment of borderline personality disorder: A randomized controlled trial. *American Journal of Psychiatry, 156,* 1563–1569.

Brady, K. T., Grice, D., Dustan, L., & Randall, C. (1993). Gender differences in substance use disorders. *American Journal of Psychiatry, 150,* 1707–1711.

Brooner, R. K., Herbst, J. H., Schmidt, C. W., Bigelow, G. E., & Costa, P. T. (1993). Antisocial personality disorder among drug abusers: Relations to other personality diagnoses and the five-factor model of personality. *Journal of Nervous and Mental Disease, 181,* 313–319.

Brooner, R. K., King, V. L., Kidorf, M., Schmidt, C. W., Jr., & Bigelow, G. E. (1997). Psychiatric and substance use comorbidity among treatment-seeking opioid abusers. *Archives of General Psychiatry, 54,* 71–80.

Cacciola, J. S., Rutherford, M. J., Alterman, A. I., McKay, J. R., & Snider, E. (1996). Personality disorders and treatment outcome in methadone maintenance patients. *Journal of Nervous and Mental Disease, 184,* 234–239.

Caspi, A., Moffitt, T., Newman, D., & Silva, P. (1996). Behavioral observations at age 3 predict adult psychiatric disorders: Longitudinal evidence from a birth cohort. *Archives of General Psychiatry, 53,* 1033–1039.

Chapman, A. L., & Cellucci, T. (2007). The role of antisocial and borderline personality features in substance dependence among incarcerated females. *Addictive Behaviors, 32,* 1131–1145.

Chen, E., Brown, M. Z., Lo, T. T. Y., & Linehan, M. M. (2007). Sexually transmitted disease rates and high-risk sexual behaviors in borderline personality disorder versus borderline personality disorder with substance use disorder. *Journal of Nervous and Mental Disease, 195,* 125–129.

Clarkin, J. F., Levy, K. N., Lenzenweger, M. F., & Kernberg, O. F. (2007). Evaluating three treatments for borderline personality disorder: A multiwave study. *Archives of General Psychiatry, 164,* 922–928.

Cohen, P., Chen, H., Crawford, T. N., Brook, J. S., & Gordon, K. (2007). Personality disorders in early adolescence and the development of later substance use disorders in the general population. *Drug and Alcohol Dependence, 88,* 71–84.

Coid, J., Yang, M., Tyrer, P., Roberts, A., & Ullrich, S. (2006). Prevalence and correlates of personality disorder in Great Britain. *British Journal of Psychiatry, 188,* 423–431.

Curran, P., Stice, E., & Chassin, L. (1997). The relationship between alcohol use and peer alcohol use: A longitudinal random coefficients model. *Journal of Consulting and Clinical Psychology, 65,* 130–140.

Darke, S., Williamson, A., Ross, J., Teesson, M., & Lynskey, M. (2004). Borderline personality disorder, antisocial personality disorder, and risk-taking among heroin users: Findings from the Australian Treatment Outcome Study (ATOS). *Drug and Alcohol Dependence, 74,* 77–83.

DeJong, C. A. J., van den Brink, W., Harteveld, F. M., & van der Wielen, E. G. M. (1993). Personality disorders in alcoholics and drug addicts. *Comprehensive Psychiatry, 34,* 87–94.

Elkins, I. J., King, S. M., McGue, M., & Iacono, W. G. (2006). Personality traits and the development of nicotine, alcohol, and illicit drug disorders: Prospective links from adolescence to young adulthood. *Journal of Abnormal Psychology, 115,* 26–39.

Fals-Stewart, W., Birchler, G., & Kelley, M. (2006). Learning sobriety together: A randomized clinical trial examining behavioral couples therapy with alcoholic female patients. *Journal of Consulting and Clinical Psychology, 74,* 579–591.

Fals-Stewart, W., Birchler, G. R., & O'Farrell, T. J. (1999). Drug-abusing patients and their intimate partners: Dyadic adjustment, relationship stability, and substance use. *Journal of Abnormal Psychology, 108,* 11–23.

Feske, U., Tarter, R., Kirisci, L., & Pilkonis, P. (2006). Borderline personality and substance use in women. *American Journal on Addictions, 15,* 131–137.

First, M. B., Spitzer, R. L., Gibbon, M., & Williams, J. B. W. (1995). *Structured Clinical Interview for*

Axis I DSM-IV Disorders—Patient Edition (SCID-I/P). New York: Biometrics Research Department, New York State Psychiatric Institute.

Franken, I., & Hendriks, V. (2000). Early onset of illicit substance use is associated with greater Axis-II comorbidity, not with Axis-I comorbidity. *Drug and Alcohol Dependence, 59,* 305–308.

Goodwin, R. D., & Gotlib, I. H. (2004). Gender differences in depression: The role of personality factors. *Psychiatry Research, 126,* 135–142.

Grant, B. F., Stinson, F., Dawson, D., Chou, S. P., Dufour, M. C., Compton, W. M., et al. (2004a). Prevalence and co-occurrence of substance use disorders and independent mood and anxiety disorders: Results from the National Epidemiologic Survey on Alcohol and Related Conditions (NESARC). *Archives of General Psychiatry, 61,* 807–816.

Grant, B. F., Stinson, F., Dawson, D., Chou, S. P., Ruan, J., & Pickering, R. (2004b). Co-occurrence of 12-month alcohol and drug use disorders and personality disorders in the United States. *Archives of General Psychiatry, 61,* 361–368. (*)

Greenfield, S., Brooks, A., Gordon, S., Green, C., Kropp, F., McHugh, R., et al. (2007). Substance abuse treatment entry, retention, and outcome in women: A review of the literature. *Drug and Alcohol Dependence, 86,* 1–21.

Hopwood, C., Morey, L., Shea, T., McGlashan, T., Sanislow, C., Grilo, C., et al. (2007). Personality traits predict current and future functioning comparably for individuals with major depressive and personality disorders. *Journal of Nervous and Mental Disease, 195,* 266–269.

Inman, D. J., Bascue, L. O., & Skoloda, T. (1985). Identification of borderline personality disorder among substance abuse inpatients. *Journal of Substance Abuse Treatment, 2,* 229–232.

Jackson, K., & Sher, K. (2003). Alcohol use disorders and psychological distress: A prospective state–trait analysis. *Journal of Abnormal Psychology, 112,* 599–613.

Jaffee, S., Caspi, A., Moffitt, T., & Taylor, A. (2004). Physical maltreatment victim to antisocial child: Evidence of an environmentally mediated process. *Journal of Abnormal Psychology, 113,* 44–55.

Johnson, D. M., Shea, M. T., Yen, S., Battle, C., Zlotnick, C., Sanislow, C. A., et al. (2003). Gender differences in borderline personality disorder: Findings from the Collaborative Longitudinal Personality Disorders Study. *Comprehensive Psychiatry, 44,* 284–292.

Koenigsberg, H., Kaplan, R., Gilmore, M., & Cooper, A. E. (1985). The relationship between syndrome and personality disorder in DSM-III: Experience with 2,462 patients. *American Journal of Psychiatry, 142,* 207–212.

Kosten, T. A., Kosten, T. R., & Rounsaville, B. J. (1989). Personality disorders in opiate addicts show prognostic specificity. *Journal of Substance Abuse Treatment, 6,* 163–168.

Lejuez, C. W., Bornovalova, M. A., Reynolds, E. K., Daughters, S. B., & Curtain, J. J. (2007). Risk factors in the relationship between gender and crack/cocaine. *Experimental and Clinical Psychopharmocology, 15,* 165–175.

Lenzenweger, M., Lane, M. C., Loranger, A. W., & Kessler, R. C. (2007). DSM-IV personality disorders in the national comorbidity survey replication. *Biological Psychiatry, 62,* 553–564.

Leshner, A. I. (1997). Addiction is a brain disease, and it matters. *Science, 278,* 45–47.

Leslie, M. (2007). Engaging pregnant women and mothers in services: A relational approach. In N. Poole & L. Greaves (Eds.), *Highs and lows: Canadian perspectives on women and substance use* (pp. 239–246). Toronto: Centre for Addiction and Mental Health.

Levenson, R., Oyama, O., & Meek, P. (1987). Greater reinforcement from alcohol for those at risk: Parental risk, personality risk, and sex. *Journal of Abnormal Psychology, 96,* 242–253.

Linehan, M. M. (1993). *Cognitive-behavioral treatment of borderline personality disorder.* New York: Guilford Press.

Linehan, M. M., Armstrong, H. E., Suarez, A., Allmon, D., & Heard, H. L. (1991). Cognitive-behavioral treatment of chronically parasuicidal borderline patients. *Archives of General Psychiatry, 48,* 1060–1064.

Linehan, M. M., & Dimeff, L. A. (1997). *Dialectical behavior therapy manual of treatment interventions for drug abusers with borderline personality disorder.* Seattle: University of Washington.

Linehan, M. M., Dimeff, L. A., Reynolds, S. K., Comtois, K. A., Welch, S. S., Heagerty, P., et al. (2002). Dialectical behavior therapy versus comprehensive validation therapy plus 12-step for the treatment of opioid dependent women meeting the criteria for borderline personality disorder. *Drug and Alcohol Dependence, 67,* 13–26.

Linehan, M. M., Schmidt, H., Dimeff, L. A., Craft, J. C., Kanter, J., & Comtois, K. A. (1999). Dialectical behavior therapy for patients with borderline personality disorder and drug-dependence. *American Journal on Addictions, 8,* 279–292.

Links, P. S., Heslegrave, R. J., Ronald, J., Mitton, J. E., van Reekum, R., & Patrick, J. (1995). Borderline personality disorder and substance abuse: Consequences of comorbidity. *Canadian Journal of Psychiatry, 40,* 9–14.

Longabaugh, R., Rubin, A., Malloy, P., Beattie, M., Clifford, P., & Noel, N. (1994). Drinking outcomes of alcohol abusers diagnosed as antisocial personality disorder. *Alcoholism: Clinical and Experimental Research, 18,* 785–788.

Loranger, A. W. (1995). *International Personality Disorder Examination (IPDE) manual.* White Plains, NY: Cornell Medical Center.

Luthar, S., & D'Avanzo, K. (1999). Contextual factors in substance abuse: A study of suburban and inner-city adolescents. *Development and Psychopathology, 11,* 845–867.

Lynman, D. R., Caspi, A., Moffitt, T. E., Wikstrom, P. H., Loeber, R., & Novak, S. (2000). The interaction between impulsivity and neighborhood context on offending: The effects of impulsivity are stronger in poorer neighborhoods. *Journal of Abnormal Psychology, 109,* 563–574.

McCann, J. T., Flynn, P. M., & Gersh, D. M. (1992). MCMI-II diagnosis of borderline personality disorder: Base rates versus protypic items. *Journal of Personality Assessment, 58,* 105–114.

McMain, S., Korman, L., Blak, T., Dimeff, L., Collis, R., & Beadnell, B. (2004, November). *Dialectical behavior therapy for substance users with borderline personality disorder: A randomized controlled trial in Canada.* Paper presented at the annual meeting of the Association for the Advancement of Behavior Therapy, New Orleans, LA.

McMain, S., Sayrs, J., Dimeff, L., & Linehan, M. (2007). Dialectical behavior therapy for individuals with BPD and substance dependence. In L. A. Dimeff & K. Koerner (Eds.), *Dialectical behavior therapy in clinical practice* (pp. 145–173). New York: Guilford Press. (*)

Merikangas, K., Stolar, M., Stevens, D., Goulet, J., Preisig, M., Fenton, B., et al. (1998). Familial transmission of substance use disorders. *Archives of General Psychiatry, 55,* 973–979.

Miller, F. T., Abrams, T., Dulit, R., & Minna, F. (1993). Substance abuse in borderline personality disorder. *American Journal of Drug and Alcohol Abuse, 19,* 491–497.

Miller, J. D., Lynam, D., & Leukefeld, C. (2003). Examining antisocial behavior through the use of the five factor model facets. *Aggressive Behavior, 29,* 497–514.

Munroe-Blum, H., & Marziali, E. (1995). A controlled trial of short-term group treatment for borderline personality disorder. *Journal of Personality Disorders, 9,* 190–198.

Nace, E. P., & Davis, C. W. (1993). Treatment outcome in substance-abusing patients with a personality disorder. *American Journal on Addictions, 2,* 26–33.

Nace, E. P., Davis, C. W., & Gaspari, J. P. (1991). Axis II comorbidity in substance abusers. *American Journal of Psychiatry, 148,* 120.

Nace, E. P., Saxon, J. J., & Shore, N. (1983). A comparison of borderline and nonborderline alcoholic patients. *Archives of General Psychiatry, 40,* 54–56.

Nurnberger, J., Wiegand, R., Bucholz, K., O'Connor, S., Meyer, E., Reich, T., et al. (2004). A family study of alcohol dependence: Coaggregation of multiple disorders in relatives of alcohol-dependent probands. *Archives of General Psychiatry, 61,* 1246–1256.

Paris, J. (2006). Personality disorders: Psychiatry's stepchildren come of age. *Psychiatric News, 41,* 33.

Penn, P., Brooks, A., & Worsham, B. (2002). Treatment concerns of women with co-occurring serious mental illness and substance abuse disorders. *Journal of Psychoactive Drugs, 34,* 355–362.

Prescott, C., Aggen, S., & Kendler, K. (1999). Sex differences in the sources of genetic liability to alcohol abuse and dependence in a population-based sample of U.S. twins. *Alcoholism: Clinical and Experimental Research, 23,* 1136–1144.

Ross, H., Glaser, F., & Stiasny, S. (1988). Sex differences in the prevalence of psychiatric disorders in patients with alcohol and drug problems. *British Journal of Addiction, 83,* 1179–1192.

Rounsaville, B. J., Kranzler, H. R., Ball, S., Tennen, H., Poling, J., & Triffleman, E. (1998). Personality disorders in substance abusers: Relation to substance use. *Journal of Nervous and Mental Disease, 186,* 87–95.

Samuels, J., Nestadt, G., Romanoski, A., Folstein, M., & McHugh, P. (1994). DSM-III personality disorders in the community. *American Journal of Psychiatry, 151,* 1055–1062.

Seivewright, N., & Daly, C. (1997). Personality disorder and drug use: A review. *Drug and Alcohol Review, 16,* 235–250. (*)

Shane, P. A., Jasiukaitis, P., & Green, R. S. (2003). Treatment outcomes among adolescents with substance abuse problems: The relationship between comorbidities and post-treatment substance involvement. *Evaluation and Program Planning, 26,* 393–402.

Sher, K. J., Bartholow, B. D., & Wood, M. D. (2000). *Journal of Consulting and Clinical Psychology, 68,* 818–829.

Sher, K. J., & Trull, T. J. (2002). Substance use disorder and personality disorder. *Current Psychiatry Reports, 4,* 25–29.

Simons, J. S., Carey, K. B., & Gaher, R. M. (2004). Liability and impulsivity synergistically increase risk for alcohol-related problems. *American Journal of Drug and Alcohol Abuse, 30,* 685–694.

Skodol, A. E., Guderson, J. G., Pfohl, B., Widiger, T. A., Livesley, W. J., & Siever, L. J. (2002). The borderline diagnosis: I. Psychopathology, comorbidity, and personality structure. *Biological Psychiatry, 51,* 936–950.

Skodol, A. E., Oldham, J. M., & Gallaher, P. E. (1999). Axis II comorbidity of substance use disorders among patients referred for treatment of personality disorders. *American Journal of Psychiatry, 156,* 733–738.

Slutske, W. S., Health, A. C., Madden, A. F., Bucholz, K. K., Statham, D. J., & Martin, N. G. (2002). Personality and the genetic risk for alcohol dependence. *Journal of Abnormal Psychology, 111,* 124–133.

Stepp, S. D., Trull, T. J., & Sher, K. J. (2005). Borderline personality features predict alcohol use problems. *Journal of Personality Disorders, 19,* 711–722.

Stevenson, J., & Meares, R. (1992). An outcome study of psychotherapy for patients with borderline personality disorder. *American Journal of Psychiatry, 149,* 358–362.

Stone, M. H. (1989). The course of borderline personality disorder. In A. Tasman, R. E. Hales, & A. J. Frances (Eds.), *American Psychiatric Press Review of Psychiatry* (pp. 103–122). Washington, DC: American Psychiatric Association.

Taylor, J., Reeves, M., James, L., & Bobadilla, L. (20060. Disinhibitory trait profile and its relation to cluster B personality disorder features and substance use problems. *European Journal of Personality, 20,* 271–284.

Thevos, A. K., Brady, K. T., Grice, D., Dustan, L., & Malcolm, R. (1993). A comparison of psychopathology in cocaine and alcohol dependence. *American Journal of Addiction, 2,* 279–286.

Torgersen, S., Kringlen, E., & Cramer, V. (2001). The prevalence of personality disorders in a community sample. *Archives of General Psychiatry, 58,* 590–596.

Torgersen, S., Lygren, S., Oien, P. A., Skre, I., Onstad, S., Edvardsen, K., et al. (2000). A twin study of personality disorders. *Comprehensive Psychiatry, 41,* 416–425.

Trull, T. T., Sher, K. J., Minks-Brown, C., Durbin, J., & Burr, R. (2000). Borderline personality disorder and substance use disorders: A review and integration. *Clinical Psychology Review, 20,* 235–253. (*)

Vaglum, S., & Vaglum, P. (1985). Borderline and other mental disorders in alcoholic female psychiatric patients: A case control study. *Journal of Psychopathology and Behavioral Assessment, 18,* 50–60.

Vaillancourt, A., & Keith, B. (2007). Substance use among women in "The Sticks": Northern perspectives. In N. Poole & L. Greaves (Eds.), *Highs and lows: Canadian perspectives on women and substance use* (pp. 37–50). Toronto: Centre for Addiction and Mental Health.

van den Bosch, L. M. C., Verheul, R., & van den Brink, W. (2001). Substance abuse in borderline personality disorder: Clinical and etiological correlates. *Journal of Personality Disorders, 15,* 416–424.

Verheul, R., van den Bosch, L. M. C., Koeter, M., de Ridder, M. A. J., Stijnen, T., & van den Brink, W.

(2003). Dialectical behaviour therapy for women with borderline personality disorder: 12-month randomised clinical trial in The Netherlands. *British Journal of Psychiatry*, *182*, 135–140.

Verheul, R., van den Brink, W., & Hartgers, C. (1995). Prevalence of personality disorders among alcoholics and drug addicts: An overview. *European Journal of Addiction Research*, *1*, 166–177. (*)

Warshaw, M. G., Dolan, R. T., & Keller, M. B. (2000). Suicidal behavior in patients with current or past panic disorder: Five years of prospective data from the Harvard/Brown Anxiety Research Program. *American Journal of Psychiatry*, *157*, 1876–1878.

Weiss, R. D., Mirin, S. M., Griffin, M. L., Gunderson, J. G., & Hufford, C. (1993). Personality disorders in cocaine dependence. *Comprehensive Psychiatry*, *34*, 145–149.

White, C., Gunderson, J., Zanarini, M., & Hudson, J. (2003). Family studies of borderline personality disorder: A review. *Harvard Review of Psychiatry*, *11*, 8–19.

Wiejers, H. G., Wiesbeck, G. A., Wodarz, N., Keller, H., Michel, T., & Boning, J. (2003). Gender and personality in alcoholism. *Archives of Women's Mental Health*, *6*, 245–252.

Wills, T., & Cleary, S. (1996). How are social support effects mediated? A test with parental support and adolescent substance use. *Journal of Personality and Social Psychology*, *71*, 937–952.

Winters, J., Fals-Stewart, W., O'Farrell, T., Birchler, G., & Kelley, M. (2002). Behavioral couples therapy for female substance-abusing patients: Effects on substance use and relationship adjustment. *Journal of Consulting and Clinical Psychology*, *70*, 344–355.

Zanarini, M. C. (2000). Childhood experiences associated with the development of borderline personality disorder. *Psychiatric Clinics of North America*, *23*, 89–101.

Zanarini, M. C., Frankenburg, F. R., Hennen, J., Reich, D. B., & Silk, K. R. (2005). Psychosocial functioning of borderline patients and Axis II comparison subjects followed prospectively for six years. *Journal of Personality Disorders*, *19*, 19–29.

Zanarini, M. C., Williams, A. A., Lewis, R. E., Reich, R. B., Vera, S. C., Marino, M. F., et al. (1997). Reported pathological childhood experiences associated with the development of borderline personality disorder. *American Journal of Psychiatry*, *154*, 1101–1106.

PART IV

TREATMENT OUTCOME

CHAPTER 17

Gender-Specific Treatment for Women with Substance Use Disorders

Shelly F. Greenfield, MD, MPH
Sandrine Pirard, MD, PhD

Differences between women and men with substance use disorders (SUDs) are well documented, and yet most of the traditional treatment models have been designed for men. More recently, however, gender-sensitive services have emerged and with them an increasing body of literature examining characteristics associated with treatment outcomes in women with SUDs. A recent review on the topic, searching the English literature from 1975 to 2005 using Medline and PsychInfo databases, found that 90% of the 280 selected articles were published since 1990, with over 40% of those since the year 2000 (Greenfield, Brooks, et al., 2007).

In this chapter we first discuss the rationale for gender-specific psychosocial treatments based on gender differences in the general population and in patients with SUDs. We refer to services that are *gender-sensitive* as those that may not have been designed specifically for women but take into account a range of issues for women's addiction and recovery. *Gender-specific* services and treatments are designed specifically for women and may provide information and treatment specific for women and/or services for women (e.g., prenatal care, child care). We then review the different types of services for women with SUDs (women-only programs vs. specific interventions in mixed-gender programs) and provide some data on their availability within the United States and other countries. Next, we review the literature on the effect of gender on substance abuse treatment outcomes before analyzing the outcome data in gender-specific versus mixed-gender programs. Finally, we discuss some factors that potentially mediate the effectiveness of gender-specific programs, and then summarize future directions and key points.

RATIONALE FOR GENDER-SPECIFIC TREATMENTS

Several arguments have been made to support the rationale for gender-specific treatments. For example, differences in interaction styles and the traditional societal dominance of men might negatively affect women attending mixed-gender programs (Hodgins, el-Guebaly, & Addington, 1997; LaFave & Echols, 1999; Nelson-Zlupko, Kauffman, & Dore, 1995; Schliebner, 1994; Welle, Falkin, & Jainchill, 1998; Wilke, 1994). Furthermore, women might not respond well to the use of a confrontational style (Kauffman, Dore, & Nelson-Zlupko, 1995), but may benefit from a style that is less structured and rigid (Hodgins et al., 1997). More specifically, females with SUDs differ significantly from their male counterparts in terms of risk factors, natural history, presenting problems, motivations for treatment, and reasons for relapse (Davis, 1994; Hodgins et al., 1997; Hughes et al., 1995; Pelissier, Camp, Gaes, Saylor, & Rhodes, 2003; Saunders, Baily, Phillips, & Allsop. 1993). Two significant predictive factors of treatment outcomes, in particular, are found more frequently in women than men with SUDs: psychiatric comorbidity (Alonso et al., 2004; Castel, Rush, Urbanoski, & Toneatto, 2006; Chander & McCaul, 2003; Lewis, 2006; Peles, Schreiber, Naumovsky, & Adelson, 2007) and history of trauma (Green, Polen, Dickinson, Lynch, & Bennett, 2002; Greenfield, 2002; O'Hare, 1995; Pirard, Sharon, Kang, Angarita, & Gastfriend, 2005; Wallen, 1992). Based on these differences, it is argued that gender-specific programs must address specific psychosocial issues affecting women, especially pregnant women and women with dependent children (Jansson et al., 1996; Knight, Hood, Logan, & Chatham, 1999; Nelson-Zlupko et al., 1995; Substance Abuse and Mental Health Services Administration [SAMHSA], 1993; Volpicelli, Markman, Monterosso, Filing, & O'Brien, 2000).

Over the lifetime, women are less likely than men to receive treatment for alcohol and drug use disorders in any treatment setting (Brady & Ashley, 2005; Dawson, 1996; Hansen et al., 2004). Women are also less likely than men to seek treatment in specific service settings for substance abuse, and the proportion of women in substance abuse treatment programs is lower than what would be expected, based on the prevalence of these disorders among women in the general population (Brady & Ashley, 2005; Pelissier & Jones, 2005; SAMHSA, 2004; Schober & Annis, 1996; Weisner, 1993; Weisner & Schmidt, 1992). Weisner and Schmidt (1992) found that women with problem drinking were more likely than men to seek care in non-alcohol-specific settings, especially mental health treatment services. On the other hand, Mojtabai (2005) found that men were less likely to use mental health, but not substance abuse, services than women. Those differences might account for the lower than expected ratio of women to men seeking treatment in specialized substance abuse programs (Greenfield, Brooks, et al., 2007).

These observations also underline differences in the way that men and women with SUDs perceive their needs. Along those lines, several authors have suggested that determining the most effective approach to women's treatment should take into account more than the issue of gender (Copeland, Wayne, Didcott, & Biggs, 1993; Nelson-Zlupko, Dore, Kauffman, & Kaltenbach, 1996; Swift & Copeland, 1996). Swift and Copeland (1996) found that women who attended women-only programs positively endorsed them, particularly for the increased understanding and ability to relate to other women (40%), and for the promotion of a feeling of safety (35%). Only 7% believed that there was no difference between mixed-gender and women-only programs, or had nothing positive to say about women-only services. Forty-two percent of the women surveyed did not have strong feelings for or against mixed-gender programs. However, 11% of the women surveyed felt uncomfortable or unsafe in mixed-gender programs, 10% perceived male clients to be arrogant or sexist, and 6% felt harassed or dominated in such programs (Swift & Copeland, 1996). Nelson-Zlupko et al. (1996) interviewed women attending a comprehensive gender-specific treatment program to gather information pertaining to their present and past experiences. Five major themes emerged: (1) individual counseling may be the most important factor in treatment retention among women; (2) sexual harassment was often present in mixed-gender programs; (3) child care was essential for recovery of women with children; (4) mixed-gender treatment groups were not conducive to the open expression of women's needs and experiences; and (5) the effectiveness of gender-specific services, such as child care and women-only therapy groups, was reduced in the context of traditional programs that might fail to support and promote women (Nelson-Zlupko et al., 1996).

Much of the research on gender-sensitive treatment has considered services intended to meet women's specific treatment needs, and theoretical models that focus on addiction and recovery for women have also emerged in recent years (Velasquez & Stotts, 2003). Such gender-sensitive models view substance abuse in the context of relationships, including broader relational and multigenerational systems. Indeed, women's addiction has been described as more "socially embedded" than men's (Saunders et al., 1993). Historically, programs have been designed predominantly based on "male cultural" norms (Hodgins et al., 1997; Saunders et al., 1993) and might not meet the needs of women.

Women entering substance abuse treatment have higher rates of trauma, are more likely to have partners who are using drugs or alcohol, have fewer friends than their male counterparts, and are more likely to have dependent children (McComish, Greenberg, Ager, Chruscial, & Laken, 2000; McComish et al., 2003). Therefore, recommendations have been made to include a continuum of coordinated and family-focused services and interventions guided by women-specific substance abuse models (McKay, Gutman, McLellan, Lynch, & Ketterlinus, 2003; Washington Sate Department of Social and Health Services and Department of Health, 1999). Focusing on repairing relationships with children and family members, enhancing the quality of the family/domestic environment, addressing trauma, as well as developing support systems to prevent relapse are all crucial for women with SUDs (Comfort & Kaltenbach, 2000; Finkelstein, 1994; Kearney, 1998; Lewis, 2004; Orwin, Francisco, & Bernichon, 2001; Washington Sate Department of Social and Health Services and Department of Health, 1999).

DESCRIPTION AND AVAILABILITY OF SERVICES FOR WOMEN

Gender-specific treatment for women may be organized as either female-only programs or female-only interventions within mixed-gender programs (Hodgins et al., 1997). Mixed-gender programs, however, are less likely to adequately address psychosocial needs that are more prevalent in women, as well as certain subpopulations, or to provide specialized intervention for particular subgroups of women. Mixed-gender programs, for example, are less likely to adequately address women's barriers to treatment, such as child care needs and financial concerns (Grella, Polinsky, Hser, & Perry, 1999; Hodgins et al., 1997). In a study of 161 drug treatment programs serving women in Los Angeles County, Grella et al. (1999) found that women-only programs (n = 31) were more likely than mixed-gender programs (n = 130) to have a treatment priority for pregnant women with SUDs; to provide prenatal, postpartum, and well-baby services; and to provide psychosocial services such as job training, life skills training, client advocacy, transportation, and assistance with housing. Special programming for pregnant women, Latinas, Native Americans, and women with heroin dependence were more frequently provided. Women-only programs also were more likely than mixed-gender programs to provide peer support groups, on-site 12-step meetings, and social outings (Grella et al., 1999). Another study comparing outcomes for women in specialized, women-only programs (n = 747) versus standard mixed-gender programs (n = 823) in Washington State showed that in addition to providing standard services, specialized agencies were required to address issues specific to women and their children, including same-gender services, substance abuse education tailored to women (e.g., relationship issues), specialized case management (e.g., interface between the criminal, juvenile justice system, and child welfare services), medical and mental health services with focus on specific issues (e.g., pregnancy, labor, delivery, lactation, fetal alcohol syndrome, adult and child nutrition, sexually transmitted diseases [STDs], and HIV), and specialized counseling for eating disorders, sexual assault, domestic violence, childhood abuse, and family dysfunction. These women-only programs also provided significantly more service referrals (e.g., referrals to another health provider and to self-help groups; referrals for medical or dental services, mental health services, vocational rehabilitation or job placement) after treatment completion than did standard mixed-gender programs (Claus et al., 2007).

According to the most recent National Survey of Substance Abuse Treatment Services (N-SSATS), which collects data on both public and private treatment centers, only 33% of facilities offered special programs for adult women and 14% offered programs or groups for pregnant/postpartum women (SAMHSA, 2005). The number of women-only programs peaked in the early-to-mid-1990s, in part triggered by the "crack babies" scare of the mid-1980s, but was in decline by the end of the century (Grella, 1999; Grella & Greenwell, 2004).

In the European Union (EU), it is estimated that nearly one in four (23%) women accessing drug outpatient treatment services is living with children, yet access to drug treatment units for women with children is limited. Gender-specific treatment is usually targeted at pregnant women with SUDs and those with children. In most, but not all, European countries there is at least one treatment unit for women only, and inmates with SUDs have access to gender-specific resources in only a few countries. However, harm reduction agencies in several EU countries are implementing interventions that specifically target females with SUDs, especially in the context of their involvement in sex work and related individual and public health risks (European Monitoring Center for Drugs and Drug Addiction [EMCDDA], 2006).

GENDER AND TREATMENT OUTCOMES

Longer substance abuse treatment episodes and successful completion are usually related to positive outcomes, but as many as 50% of patients in addiction treatment drop out of treatment within the first month (Stark, 1992). Treatment retention has been defined as a dichotomous variable, such as attendance of a specific number of treatment sessions (Brady, Killeen, Saladin, Dansky, & Becker, 1994; Green et al., 2002), specific treatment duration (Arfken, Klein, di Menza, & Schuster, 2001), or more recently as a continuous measure, such as length of stay (LOS) (Brady & Ashley, 2005; Comfort, Loverro, & Kaltenbach, 2000). Treatment completion is defined as having completed the designated treatment course (either predetermined length or completion of treatment goals) (Brady & Ashley, 2005). The results of clinical, non-population-based studies that have examined gender differences in substance abuse treatment retention and completion are inconsistent. Women were found to be more likely than men to drop out and not complete substance abuse treatment in five studies (Arfken et al., 2001; King & Canada, 2004; McCaul, Svikis, & Moore, 2001; Petry & Bickel, 2000; Sayre et al., 2002). However, two studies showed that women were less likely than men to drop out or not complete treatment (Hser, Huang, Teruya, & Anglin, 2004; Maglione, Chao, & Anglin, 2000). Four studies showed no gender difference in treatment retention or LOS (Fiorentine, Anglin, Gil-Rivas, & Taylor, 1997; Green et al., 2002; Mertens & Weisner, 2000; Veach, Remley, Kippers, & Sorg, 2000). In contrast to these smaller studies, evidence from larger, population-based studies provide a convergence of results showing few or no gender differences in treatment retention (Brady & Ashley, 2005; Hser et al., 2001; Joe, Simpson, & Broome, 1999; Simpson et al., 1997). Of particular interest, one study showed a complex relationship between gender, language spoken, and type of program (Condelli, Koch, &

Fletcher, 2000). In this study, 1,573 adults were randomly assigned to treatment programs in New Jersey; mixed results by gender were found. Females in long-term mixed-gender and women-only English-speaking programs had less attrition than males, but no significant differences in attrition were observed between men and women in short-term English-speaking programs and short- and long-term Spanish-speaking programs (Condelli et al., 2000).

Even though population-based studies demonstrate no clear gender differences in treatment retention and completion, some characteristics have been shown to be associated with these outcomes for both men and women, such as greater financial resources, fewer mental health problems, and less severe drug problems (Green et al., 2002; Greenfield, Brooks, et al., 2007; Maglione et al., 2000; Mertens & Weisner, 2000). Studies in women-only samples have found associations between certain characteristics and rates of retention and completion, including better psychological functioning, higher levels of personal stability and social support, lower levels of anger, treatment beliefs, and referral source (Brady & Ashley, 2005; Brown, Kokin, Seraganian, & Shields, 1995; Davis, 1994; Huselid, Self, & Gutierres, 1991; Kelly, Blacksin, & Mason, 2001; Knight et al., 1999; Loneck, Garrett, & Banks, 1997).

Treatment program characteristics may also be associated with retention and completion rates among women. The Alcohol and Drug Services Study (ADSS), conducted between 1996 and 1999 in public and private substance abuse programs, failed to show that receiving treatment at women-only facilities or facilities offering child care services was associated with treatment completion among women when other client and facility characteristics were controlled; however, treatment in these settings was positively correlated with LOS (Brady & Ashley, 2005). The results of this study also indicated that women in nonhospital residential facilities or facilities providing combined mental heath and substance abuse treatment services were more likely to complete planned treatment than women receiving treatment at outpatient nonmethadone facilities. Women receiving combined substance abuse and mental health services were, however, less likely to complete treatment than the women receiving substance abuse treatment alone (odds ratio [OR] = 0.37), which might reflect a greater likelihood of dropout for women with co-occurring disorders (Brady & Ashley, 2005).

A complex relationship between treatment setting, patient characteristics, and treatment retention was found by Roberts and Nishimoto (1996). In this study retention patterns were analyzed across types of services for 141 women in traditional outpatient treatment; 77 women in traditional residential treatment; and 151 women in highly structured, women-focused day treatment. Treatment setting was found to be the most prominent factor in predicting retention (compared with pretreatment and patient characteristics), with greatest retention in women-focused day treatment (45%), followed by traditional residential (26%) and outpatient (21.3%) programs. Even though pretreatment and patient characteristics were not significant predictors overall, an interaction between specific factors and type of settings was found. For example, being married was related to greater retention in outpatient treatment, previous drug treatment was related to greater retention in day treatment, and severity of drug problem and anxiety were related to retention in residential treatment (Roberts & Nishimoto, 1996). Within residential programs, policies allowing children to accompany their mothers in treatment have been associated with better treatment retention (Hughes et al., 1995; Szuster, Rich, Chung, & Bisconer, 1996).

Although the effectiveness of substance abuse treatment for women has been questioned, many studies have found few or no gender differences in treatment outcome across various populations (Acharyya & Zhang, 2003; Alterman, Randall, & McLellan, 2000; Ballesteros, Gonzalez-Pinto, Querejeta, & Arino, 2004; Benishek, Bieschker, Staffelmayr, & Mavis, 1992; Foster, Peters, & Marshall, 2000; Green, Polen, Lynch, Dickinson, & Bennett, 2004; Greenfield et al., 1998; Hser, Huang, Teruya, & Anglin, 2003; Jerrell & Ridgely, 1995; Marsh, Cao,

& D'aunno, 2004; McCance, Carroll, & Rounsaville, 1999; McLellan et al., 1994; Rohse-now, Monti, Martin, Michalec, & Abrams, 2000; Sterling, 2004; Toneatto, Sobell, & Sobell, 1992; Wong, Badger, Sigmon, & Higgins, 2002). Minimal differences in treatment-related improvement between men and women were reported by Acharyya and Zhang (2003) across four treatment modalities (methadone, nonmethadone outpatient, short-term inpatient, and long-term residential). In a prospective naturalistic study of inpatient alcohol treatment, Greenfield found that gender was not a predictor of treatment outcomes (Greenfield et al., 1998), but that there were significant predictors of outcome for both men and women, includ-ing educational attainment (Greenfield et al., 2003), self-efficacy (Greenfield et al., 2000), co-occurring major depression (Greenfield et al., 1998), and a history of sexual abuse (Greenfield et al., 2002). These predictors often vary in prevalence by gender and may, therefore, have greater significance for women's relapse and recovery. A recent meta-analysis of seven studies of brief interventions for hazardous alcohol consumption, delivered in primary care settings, did not find any gender difference in improved treatment outcomes (Ballesteros et al., 2004). A secondary analysis of data from the prospective U.S. National Treatment Improvement Evaluation Study, including 1,123 women and 2,019 men in 50 treatment modalities (Marsh et al., 2004), found that receipt of comprehensive services, including educational, housing, and income support, was related to posttreatment outcomes for both men and women.

In studies that have found gender differences, many have found that women had better outcomes than men, despite differences in populations targeted, types of treatment, problem drug, and treatment settings (Fiorentine et al., 1997; Hser, Evans, & Huang, 2005; Jarvis, 1992; Kosten, Gawin, Kosten, & Rounsaville, 1993; Kranzler, Del Boca, & Rounsaville, 1996; McKay, Lynch, Pettinati, & Shepard, 2003; Project MATCH, 1997; Rivers, Green-baum, & Goldberg, 2001; Sanchez-Craig, Spivak, & Davila, 1991; Satre, Mertens, Arean, & Weisner, 2004; Stephens, Roffman, & Simpson, 1994; Timko, Moos, Finney, & Connell, 2002). For example, a prospective study of 567 women and 506 men with methamphetamine abuse found that women had greater improvement than men on the Addiction Severity Index (ASI) family and medical scores, and similar improvements in all other ASI scores at 3- and 9-month follow-up, despite higher baseline rates of unemployment, child care responsibilities, partners with alcohol or drug use, and psychiatric symptoms (Hser et al., 2005). In the Project MATCH study (1997) results indicated that women may have slightly less severe relapse char-acteristics and be more willing than men to seek help following relapse. However, no interac-tion between gender and treatment modality on treatment outcomes was found.

While female gender, per se, might be associated with similar or better substance abuse treatment outcomes, certain characteristics more frequently seen in women, such as co-occurring psychiatric disorders and history of physical and/or sexual abuse, might be associated with poorer treatment outcomes. Many studies have shown that a co-occurring psychiatric disorder is associated with poorer substance abuse treatment response (Galen, Brower, Gillespie, & Zucker, 2000; Greenfield et al., 1998; Hasin, Endicott, & Keller, 1991; Hesselbrock, 1991; Kranzler et al., 1996; Mueller et al., 1994). The relationship between gender, co-occurring psychiatric disorders, and substance abuse treatment outcomes, how-ever, is complex and may vary depending upon the population studied, the specific sub-stance of abuse, and the co-occurring psychiatric disorders (Greenfield, Brooks, et al., 2007). Studies using all-female samples have shown that women with posttraumatic stress disorder (PTSD) and SUDs had worse outcomes than women without PTSD (Brady et al., 1994; Brown, 2000; Ingersoll, Lu, & Haller, 1995). High rates of co-occurring SUDs and eating disorders among treatment-seeking women with alcohol or drug use disorders (Beary, Lacey, & Merry, 1986; Lacey & Moureli, 1986; Peveler & Fairburn, 1990; Taylor, Peveler, Hib-bert, & Fairburn, 1993) have been reported, with 30–50% of individuals with bulimia and

12–18% with anorexia (National Center on Addiction and Substance Abuse at Columbia University [CASA], 2003), but there are no data on treatment outcomes (Greenfield, Brooks, et al., 2007). Results from mixed-gender samples have shown that co-occurring psychiatric disorders might have different prognostic significance in men and women. A global measure of psychopathology was found to be predictive of more alcohol problems 6 months post-treatment for women, but not for men (Benishek et al., 1992). Another study found that women with co-occurring major depressive disorders had shorter durations of abstinence than women without, whereas the opposite was found for men (Westermeyer, Kopka, & Nugent, 1997). Conversely, in a 1-year follow-up study of 61 men and 57 women with alcohol dependence, following inpatient treatment in Germany, Mann, Hintz, and Jung (2004) showed similar relapse rates for men with or without psychiatric comorbidity, but lower relapse rates among women with, as compared to women without, psychiatric comorbidity. Another study found that men with psychiatric disorders generally, and with major depression or antisocial personality disorders specifically, had worse 1-year substance abuse treatment outcomes, whereas women with co-occurring phobic disorders had better outcomes (Compton, Cotter, Jacobs, Ben-Abdallah, & Spitznagel, 2003).

Reports of histories of physical and/or sexual abuse, with or without PTSD, have been associated with poorer treatment outcomes in some (Comfort, Sockloff, Loverro, & Kaltenbach, 2003; Greenfield et al., 2002; Kang, Magura, Laudet, & Whitney, 1999; Pirard et al., 2005) but not all (Fiorentine, Pilati, & Hillhouse, 1999) studies. Such histories might have different impact on treatment outcomes for men and women. For example, Messina, Wish, and Nemes (2000) showed that a history of physical abuse predicted positive urine drug screens at follow-up for women but not for men. Another study showed that being a victim of domestic violence predicted greater numbers of hours in treatment for men but not for women (Green et al., 2002). Again, those results show a complex relationship between gender, baseline characteristics, and treatment outcomes.

RELATIONSHIP OF GENDER-SPECIFIC VERSUS MIXED-GENDER PROGRAMS WITH TREATMENT OUTCOMES

Based on the available literature, the effect of gender-specific and gender-sensitive programs and services for women on treatment outcomes remains unclear (LaFave & Echols, 1999; Nelson-Zlupko et al., 1995; Schliebner, 1994; Smith & Weisner, 2000; Wilke, 1994). However, only a few randomized trials have examined the relative effectiveness of comparable women-only versus mixed-gender settings (Greenfield, Brooks, et al., 2007; Greenfield, Trucco, McHugh, Lincoln, & Gallop, 2007). In a meta-analysis examining effectiveness of single-gender substance abuse treatment for women, Orwin et al. (2001) concluded that single-gender treatment was effective, and that its strongest impact was on pregnancy outcomes. Psychological well-being, attitudes/beliefs, and HIV risk reduction were also substantially improved by treatment, but psychiatric outcomes improved only modestly. Across studies, treatment resulted in only small improvements in alcohol use, other drug use, and lowered criminal activity (Orwin et al., 2001). However, it is important to note that only a few of the studies compared gender-sensitive or gender-specific treatment to mixed-gender programs, limiting the interpretation of the results (Orwin et al., 2001). Ashley et al. reviewed 38 studies investigating the effect of substance abuse treatment for women on treatment outcomes (Ashley, Marsden, & Brady, 2003). Among those, only seven were randomized, controlled trials. Child care, prenatal care, women-only programs, supplemental services and workshops that addressed women-focused topics, mental health programming, and comprehensive programming were found to have a positive association with treatment completion, LOS, decreased use of substances, reduced mental health symptoms, improved birth outcomes, employment, self-reported health status, and HIV risk reduction (Ashley et al., 2003).

Mixed results have been reported in studies that compared women-only with mixed-gender programs. A study that randomized first-time women patients ($n = 1,573$) to women-only versus mixed-gender treatment programs failed to show a difference between the two types of services when considering treatment refusals and attrition during the first 25 days of treatment (Condelli et al., 2000). In contrast, a study that randomized women with infants and a crack cocaine dependence, whose infants had been exposed prenatally to drugs, to either an intensive, specialized women-only day treatment program, or a traditional mixed-gender outpatient program, found that women in the women-only program had significantly higher retention rates at 4 months (60.2 vs. 46.1%; Strantz & Welch, 1995). In a more recent randomized, controlled trial, outcomes and costs of women-only and mixed-gender day treatment programs were compared (Kaskutas, Zhang, French, & Witbrodt, 2005). One hundred and twenty-two women were randomized to a women-only program with gender-specific programming or one of three standard mixed-gender programs, including two community-based and one hospital-based program. The only significant difference in outcome found was a lower total abstinence during the follow-up period in the women-only program versus the hospital-based program (OR = 0.17). The hospital-based program, however, cost twice as much per week as the women-only program. Limitations were the small sample size and the exclusive focus on day treatment programs (Kaskutas et al., 2005).

In a recent Stage 1 behavioral development trial, Greenfield, Trucco, et al. (2007) developed a manual-based 12-session women's recovery group (WRG) and tested this new treatment in a randomized, controlled trial against a mixed-gender group drug counseling (GDC), an effective manual-based treatment for SUDs. In this study women were randomized to WRG ($n = 16$) or GDC ($n = 7$ women, 10 men). The WRG was equally effective as the mixed-gender GDC in reducing substance use during the 12-week in-treatment phase, but demonstrated significantly greater improvement in reductions in drug and alcohol use over the 6-month posttreatment follow-up phase. In addition, although satisfaction with both groups was high, women were significantly more satisfied with WRG than GDC (Greenfield, Trucco, et al., 2007).

Results from nonrandomized studies have also shown mixed results. Bride (2001) analyzed outcome data for both men and women from an agency that switched from providing mixed-gender to gender-specific groups. The treatment structures used were essentially unchanged after the switch, except that the content of groups was more gender-specific, and the women-specific program was staffed exclusively by women, whereas the other two programs had mixed-gender staff. Results failed to show significant differences in either treatment completion or retention. Another study, this one in Australia, compared outcomes of women attending a women-only residential program with women attending mixed-gender residential and mixed-gender detoxification programs (Copeland et al., 1993). The only major difference between the women-only program and the mixed-gender programs was the women-only environment and the availability of residential child care. There was no difference in degree of change in alcohol- and other drug-associated problems between the women attending the women-only versus mixed-gender programs. However, women attending the women-only programs were significantly more likely to have dependent children, be lesbian, have a history of childhood sexual abuse, and/or have maternal history of substance dependence (Copeland & Hall, 1992). The authors, therefore, suggested that the higher concentration of patients with more complicated histories in the women-only program might have contributed to the lack of difference, and that those patients might have done significantly worse in a mixed-gender program (Copeland et al., 1993).

Comparisons of data from publicly funded residential women-only and mixed-gender drug treatment programs showed that women in women-only programs had significantly longer LOS (87.4 vs. 74.0 days) and significantly higher rates of completion (16.9 vs. 7.6%) than women in mixed-gender programs. In addition, women in women-only programs were significantly more likely to have more complex psychosocial circumstances, including being pregnant, on probation, or homeless, and having longer duration of primary drug use (Grella, 1999). A more recent retrospective study compared treatment outcomes for women with children who were admitted to long-term residential substance abuse programs in Washington State (Claus et al., 2007). A total of 747 women attended seven specialized programs, and a total of 823 women attended nine standard programs. On average, women who attended specialized programs stayed in treatment longer but were somewhat less likely to complete treatment, as compared to women who attended standard programs. Women who attended specialized programs were also more likely to continue care (i.e., enrolling in a step-down treatment modality within 30 days of discharge from long-term residential) than their counterparts who attended standard programs. When treatment completion was taken into account, women who completed specialized programs were far more likely to continue treatment than either women who completed nonspecialized programs or women who did not complete either specialized or standard programs. The author concluded that specialized treatment for women promotes continuing care and that the effect of specialized care was augmented by treatment completion and longer LOS (Claus et al., 2007).

POTENTIAL FACTORS MEDIATING EFFECTIVENESS

Beyond treatment retention and LOS, the current data comparing women-only versus mixed-gender treatment programs are more ambiguous regarding differences in substance abuse treatment outcomes. However, a subgroup of women with SUDs may perceive women-only treatment more positively than mixed-gender treatment, and some women with specialized needs may have better outcomes in those programs. Women-only treatment may be viewed by some women, particularly for women with histories of abuse, as providing a safer atmosphere (Nelson-Zlupko et al., 1996; Swift & Copeland, 1996).

Increasing gender matching between patients and clinicians might be another potentially effective element. However, studies that have investigated the effects of matching patient to clinician gender have reported mixed results. Some studies found no effects of gender matching on outcomes (McKay, Lynch, et al., 2003; Sterling, Gottheil, Weinstein, & Serota, 2001), whereas others found that such matching may be associated with better abstinence outcomes (Fiorentine & Hillhouse, 1999; Sterling, Gottheil, Weinstein, & Serota, 1998; Sterling et al., 2001). The first study by Sterling was conducted with outpatient individual therapy participants and found that women who were paired with female therapists were retained in outpatient treatment for a significantly longer period of time. However, both male and female participants who were paired with a same-sex therapist participated significantly less in Narcotics Anonymous (NA) groups than did those in mixed-gender pairings (Sterling et al., 1998). The authors suggested that the modest positive effect for gender matching in this study may have been partially due to the group treatment modality itself, noting that the impact of gender congruence might be more potent in an individual therapy setting (Sterling et al., 1998). To test this hypothesis, their second study included a similar gender-matching process of patient–clinician in an outpatient individual treatment program for cocaine abuse. They failed to find any positive effect on substance use outcomes, but rather found that both males and females with gender-congruent therapists reported significantly more psychological symptoms at a 9-month follow-up. The authors discounted this finding, however, as being a function of the absolute number of statistical tests that were conducted on their data (Sterling et al., 2001). Fiorentine and Hillhouse (1999) showed that gender congruence was associated with higher levels of perceived therapist empathy for both males and females and that pairing female participants with female therapists was associated with increased abstinence in the 6 months period immediately preceding the 8-month postintake follow-up.

A number of studies has examined services to address psychosocial needs that are more prevalent in women, certain subpopulations, or specialized interventions for a particular subgroup of women, and have demonstrated the effectiveness of women-only programs as they related to the specialized needs of women with substance abuse (Elk et al., 1995; Hien, Cohen, Miele, Litt, & Capstick, 2004; Jansson et al., 1996; Kelly, Halford, & Young, 2000; Linehan et al., 1999; Luthar & Suchman, 2000; Reynolds, Coombs, Lowe, Peterson, & Gayoso, 1995; Volpicelli et al., 2000; Washington, 2001; Welle et al., 1998). For example; mixed-gender programs are less likely to address women's barriers to treatment, such as child care needs and financial concerns (Grella, 1999; Hodgins et al., 1997). For pregnant and parenting women, studies have shown that women-only programs were more likely to have child care services and that those services might be associated with better treatment retention (Brady & Ashley, 2005; Hughes et al., 1995; Szuster et al., 1996). Those programs are also more likely to provide prenatal, postpartum, and well-baby services, as well as psychosocial services for women (Grella, 1999). In a randomized clinical trial (n = 84) comparing standard case management services to a psychosocial enhanced treatment (PET) in an outpatient, gender-specific, group-therapy treatment setting, women in the PET condition reported significantly less cocaine use at 12-month follow-up. In addition, women with more severe psychological symptoms had better retention rates in the PET condition. The authors suggested that the significant outcomes may have been due primarily to the availability of individual therapy, which was the most extensively used PET-only service (Volpicelli et al., 2000).

Several studies have shown greater success using treatments that address problems more common to women with SUDs. Those include services for pregnant women leading to reduction of alcohol use (Reynolds et al., 1995), contingency management to increase abstinence from cocaine in pregnant women (Elk et al., 1995), a comprehensive services model for pregnant women (Jansson et al., 1996), parenting skills for methadone-maintained mothers (Luthar & Suchman, 2000), relapse prevention for women with comorbid PTSD (Hien et al., 2004; Najavits, 2002; Najavits & Ryngala, et al., in press), relapse prevention for women with marital distress and alcohol dependence (Kelly et al., 2000), dialectical behavior therapy for patients with co-occurring borderline personality disorder and drug dependence (Linehan et al., 1999), and prison-based single-gender drug treatment for women offenders (Pelissier et al., 2003), among others (Washington, 2001). Even though more data, in particular from randomized, controlled trials, are needed (Greenfield, Brooks, et al., 2007), the results of currently published studies indicate that specialized interventions might lead to better outcomes for specific subgroups of women. It still remains unclear whether gender-specific services are optimally effective when delivered in the context of non-gender-specific treatment (Nelson-Zlupko et al., 1996) compared with women-only treatment programs.

FUTURE DIRECTIONS

Although gender-specific services have emerged in the last several decades, the relative effectiveness of such services compared with mixed-gender treatment for women, especially for specific subgroups of women, remains unclear. Future studies will be necessary to elucidate the (1) elements of gender-specific treatments that confer benefit for treatment outcome; (2) impact of women's preferences for gender-specific versus mixed-gender treatment on substance abuse outcomes; (3) specific subgroups of women who may benefit from gender-specific treatments; (4) mediators and moderators of outcome of gender-specific treatments; and (5) mechanisms of action of such treatments.

KEY POINTS

- Gender-specific services for SUDs have emerged in response to the growing recognition that women and men differ not only in style, social interaction, and perception of their needs, but also that women with SUDs are characterized by different risk factors, natural history, presenting problems, motivations for treatment, and reason for relapse.
- Mixed-gender programs often fail to address women's specific needs, such as child care. In addition, some women, especially those who have been victimized, report feeling uncomfortable or unsafe in mixed-gender programs.
- Gender-specific treatment may be available as women-only programs or as women-only interventions within mixed-gender programs. The availability of women-only programs is still limited, even though it is recognized that these might better address specific needs such as pregnancy and parenting, co-occurring psychiatric disorders, trauma and victimization, and provide ancillary services such as housing, income support, and social services.
- Studies examining the effect of gender on substance abuse treatment outcomes have shown that gender might not be a predictor of treatment outcome, per se, but that certain characteristics, such as higher rates of psychiatric comorbidities and histories of trauma, might negatively affect treatment outcomes. These characteristics are more prevalent among women than men and may, therefore, have greater impact on treatment outcome in women.
- The effectiveness of gender-specific programs for women on substance abuse treatment outcomes remains unclear based on the available literature. There are emerging data from randomized trials comparing women-only versus mixed-gender programs and treatments and demonstrating some promise for the women-only programs. In particular, the services provided in these women-only programs may have enhanced effectiveness for certain subpopulations, such as pregnant women, women with dependent children, women with histories of trauma, and women with co-occurring psychiatric disorders.

ACKNOWLEDGMENTS

Work on this chapter was supported in part by Grant No. K24 DA019855 from the National Institute on Drug Abuse to Shelly F. Greenfield

REFERENCES

Asterisks denote recommended readings.

Acharyya, S., & Zhang, H. (2003). Assessing sex differences on treatment effectiveness from the Drug Abuse Treatment Outcome Study (DATOS). *American Journal of Drug and Alcohol Abuse*, 29, 415–444.

Alonso, J., Angermeyer, M .C., Bernert, S., Bruffaerts, R., Brugha, T. S., Bryson, H., et al. (2004). 12-month comorbidity patterns and associated factors in Europe: Results from the European

Study of the Epidemiology of Mental Disorders (ESEMeD) project. *Acta Psychiatrica Scandinavica, 109,* 28–37.

Alterman, A. I., Randall, M., & McLellan, A. T. (2000). Comparison of outcomes by gender and for fee-for-service versus managed care: A study of nine community programs. *Journal of Substance Abuse Treatment, 19,* 127–134.

Arfken, C. L., Klein, C., di Menza, S., & Schuster, C. R. (2001). Gender differences in problem severity at assessment and treatment retention. *Journal of Substance Abuse Treatment, 20,* 53–57.

Ashley, O. S., Marsden, M. E., & Brady, T. M. (2003). Effectiveness of substance abuse treatment programming for women: A review. *American Journal of Drug and Alcohol Abuse, 29,* 19–53. (*)

Ballesteros, J., Gonzalez-Pinto, A., Querejeta, I., & Arino, J. (2004). Brief interventions for hazardous drinkers delivered in primary care are equally effective in men and women. *Addiction, 99,* 103–108.

Beary, M. D., Lacey, J. H., & Merry, J. (1986). Alcoholism and eating disorders in women of fertile age. *British Journal of Addiction, 81,* 685–689.

Benishek, L. A., Bieschke, K. J., Staffelmayr, B. E., & Mavis, B. E. (1992). Gender differences in depression and anxiety among alcoholics. *Journal of Substance Abuse, 4,* 235–245.

Brady, K. T., Killeen, T., Saladin, M. E., Dansky, B., & Becker, S. (1994). Comorbid substance abuse and posttraumatic stress disorder: Characteristics of women in treatment. *American Journal on Addictions, 3,* 160–164.

Brady, T., & Ashley, O. (2005). *Women in substance abuse treatment: Results from the Alcohol and Drug Services Study (ADSS).* Substance Abuse and Mental Health Services Administration, Rockville, MD. Available at *www.oas.samhsa.gov/WomenTX/ WomenTX.htm.* (*)

Bride, B. E. (2001). Single-gender treatment of substance abuse: Effect on treatment retention and completion. *Social Work Research, 25,* 223–232.

Brown, P. J. (2000). Outcome in female patients with both substance use and post-traumatic stress disorders. *Alcoholism Treatment Quarterly, 18,* 127–135.

Brown, T. G., Kokin, M., Seraganian, P., & Shields, N. (1995). The role of spouses of substance abusers in treatment: Gender differences. *Journal of Psychoactive Drugs, 27,* 223–229.

Castel, S., Rush, B., Urbanoski, K., & Toneatto, T. (2006). Overlap of clusters of psychiatric symptoms among clients of a comprehensive addiction treatment service. *Psychology of Addictive Behaviors, 20,* 28–35.

Chander, G., & McCaul, M. E. (2003). Co-occurring psychiatric disorders in women with addictions. *Obstetric and Gynecological Clinics of North America, 30,* 469–481.

Claus, R. E., Orwin, R. G., Kissin, W., Krupski, A., Campbell, K., & Stark, K. (2007). Does gender-specific substance abuse treatment for women promote continuity of care? *Journal of Substance Abuse Treatment, 32,* 27–39. (*)

Comfort, M., & Kaltenbach, K. A. (2000). Predictors of treatment outcomes for substance-abusing women: A retrospective study. *Substance Abuse, 21,* 33–45.

Comfort, M., Loverro, J., & Kaltenbach, K. (2000). A search for strategies to engage women in substance abuse treatment. *Social Work in Health Care, 31,* 59–70.

Comfort, M., Sockloff, A., Loverro, J., & Kaltenbach, K. (2003). Multiple predictors of substance-abusing women's treatment and life outcomes. A prospective longitudinal study. *Addictive Behaviors, 28,* 199–224.

Compton, W., Cottler, L. B., Jacobs, J. L., Ben-Abdallah, A., & Spitznagel, E. L. (2003). The role of psychiatric disorders in predicting drug dependence treatment outcomes. *American Journal of Psychiatry, 160,* 890–895.

Condelli, W. S., Koch, M. A., & Fletcher, B. (2000). Treatment refusal/attrition among adults randomly assigned to programs at a drug treatment campus: The New Jersey Substance Abuse Treatment Campus, Seacaucus, NJ. *Journal of Substance Abuse Treatment, 18,* 395–407.

Copeland, J., & Hall, W. (1992). A comparison of women seeking drug and alcohol treatment in a specialist women's and two traditional mixed-sex treatment services. *British Journal of Addiction, 87,* 1293–1302.

Copeland, J., Wayne, H., Didcott, P., & Biggs, V. (1993). A comparison of a specialist women's alcohol and other drug treatment service with two traditional mixed-sex services: Client characteristics and treatment outcome. *Drug and Alcohol Dependence, 32,* 81–92.

Davis, S. (1994). Drug treatment decisions of chemically-dependent women. *International Journal of the Addictions, 29,* 1287–1304.

Dawson, D. A. (1996). Gender differences in the probability of alcohol treatment. *Journal of Substance Abuse Treatment, 8,* 211–225.

Elk, R., Schmitz, J., Spiga, R., Rhoades, H., Andres, R., & Grabowski, J. (1995). Behavioral treatment of cocaine-dependent pregnant women and TB-exposed patients. *Addictive Behaviors, 20,* 533–542.

European Monitoring Center for Drugs and Drug Addiction (EMCDDA). (2006). *Annual report 2006: The state of the drug problem in Europe.* Lisbon: European Monitoring Center for Drugs and Drug Addiction.

Finkelstein, N. (1994). Treatment issues for alcohol- and drug-dependent pregnant and parenting women. *Health and Social Work, 19,* 7–15.

Fiorentine, R., Anglin, M. D., Gil-Rivas, V., & Taylor, E. (1997). Drug treatment: Explaining the gender paradox. *Substance Use and Misuse, 32,* 653–678.

Fiorentine, R., & Hillhouse, M. P. (1999). Drug treatment effectiveness and client–counselor empathy. *Journal of Drug Issues, 29,* 59–74.

Fiorentine, R., Pilati, M. L., & Hillhouse, M. P. (1999). Drug treatment outcomes: Investigating the long-term effects of sexual and physical abuse histories. *Journal of Psychoactive Drugs, 31,* 363–372.

Foster, J. H., Peters, T. J., & Marshall, E. J. (2000). Quality of life measures and outcome in alcohol-dependent men and women. *Alcohol, 22,* 45–52.

Galen, L. W., Brower, K. J., Gillespie, B. W., & Zucker, R. A. (2000). Sociopathy, gender, and treatment outcome among outpatient substance abusers. *Drug and Alcohol Dependence, 61,* 23–33.

Green, C. A., Polen, M. R., Dickinson, D. M., Lynch, F. L., & Bennett, M. D. (2002). Gender differences in predictors of initiation, retention, and completion in an HMO-based substance abuse treatment program. *Journal of Substance Abuse Treatment, 23,* 285–295.

Green, C. A., Polen, M. R., Lynch, F. L., Dickinson, D. M., & Bennett, M. D. (2004). Gender differences in outcomes in an HMO-based substance abuse treatment program. *Journal of Addictive Diseases, 23,* 47–70.

Greenfield, S. F. (2002). Women and alcohol use disorders. In K. H. Pearson, B. Sonwalla, & J. F. Rosenbaum (Eds.), *Women's health and psychiatry* (pp. 67–75). Philadelphia: Lippincott, Williams & Wilkins.

Greenfield, S. F., Brooks, A., Gordon, S., Green, C., Kropp, F., McHugh, R., et al. (2007). Substance abuse treatment entry, retention, and outcome in women: A review of the literature. *Drug and Alcohol Dependence, 86,* 1–21. (Access supplementary material at *hdx.doi.org by entering doi:10.1016/j.drugalcdep.2006. 05.012.*) (*)

Greenfield, S. F., Hufford, M. R., Vagge, L. M., Muenz, L. R., Costello, M. E., & Weiss, R. D. (2000). The relationship of self-efficacy expectancies to relapse among alcohol dependent men and women: A prospective study. *Journal of Studies on Alcohol, 61,* 345–351.

Greenfield, S. F., Kolodziej, M. E., Sugarman, D. E., Muenz, L. R., Vagge, L. M., He, D. Y., et al. (2002). History of abuse and drinking outcomes following inpatient alcohol treatment: A prospective study. *Drug and Alcohol Dependence, 67,* 227–234.

Greenfield, S. F., Sugarman, D. E., Muenz, L. R., Patterson, M. D., He, D. Y., & Weiss, R. D. (2003). The relationship between educational attainment and relapse among alcohol-dependent men and women: A prospective study. *Alcoholism: Clinical and Experimental Research, 27,* 1278–1285.

Greenfield, S. F., Trucco, E., McHugh, R., Lincoln, M., & Gallop, R. (2007). The Women's Recovery Group study: A stage I trial of women-focused group therapy for substance use disorders versus mixed-gender group drug counseling. *Drug and Alcohol Dependence, 90,* 39–47. (*)

Greenfield, S. F., Weiss, R. D., Muenz, L. R., Vagge, L. M., Kelly, J. F., Bello, L. R., et al. (1998). The effect of depression on return to drinking: A prospective study. *Archives of General Psychiatry, 55,* 259–265.

Grella, C. E. (1999). Women in residential drug treatment: Differences by program type and pregnancy. *Journal of Health Care for the Poor and Underserved, 10,* 216–229.

Grella, C. E., & Greenwell, L. (2004). Substance abuse treatment for women: Changes in the settings where women received treatment and types of services provided, 1987–1998. *Journal of Behavioral Health Services and Research, 31,* 367–383.

Grella, C. E., Polinsky, M. L., Hser, Y., & Perry, S. M. (1999). Characteristics of women-only and mixed-gender drug abuse treatment programs. *Journal of Substance Abuse Treatment, 17,* 37–44. (*)

Hansen, H., Alegria, M., Caban, C. A., Pena, M., Lai, S., & Shrout, P. (2004). Drug treatment, health, and social service utilization by substance-abusing women from a community-based sample. *Medical Care, 42*(11), 1117–1124.

Hasin, D. S., Endicott, J., & Keller, M. B. (1991). Alcohol problems in psychiatric patients: 5-year course. *Comprehensive Psychiatry, 32,* 303–318.

Hesselbrock, M. N. (1991). Gender comparison of antisocial personality disorder and depression in alcoholism. *Journal of Substance Abuse, 3,* 205–219.

Hien, D. A., Cohen, L. R., Miele, G. M., Litt, L. C., & Capstick, C. (2004). Promising treatments for women with comorbid PTSD and substance use disorders. *American Journal of Psychiatry, 161,* 1426–1432.

Hodgins, D. C., el-Guebaly, N., & Addington, J. (1997). Treatment of substance abusers: Single- or mixed-gender programs? *Addiction, 92,* 805–812.

Hser, Y., Grella, C., Hubbard, R., Hsieh, S., Fletcher, B., Brown, B., et al. (2001). An evaluation of drug treatments for adolescents in 4 U.S. cities. *Archives of General Psychiatry, 58,* 689–695.

Hser, Y., Huang, D., Teruya, C. M., & Anglin, D. M. (2003). Gender comparisons of drug abuse treatment outcomes and predictors. *Drug and Alcohol Dependence, 72,* 255–264.

Hser, Y. I., Evans, E., & Huang, Y. C. (2005). Treatment outcomes among women and men methamphetamine abusers in California. *Journal of Substance Abuse Treatment, 28,* 77–85.

Hser, Y. I., Huang, D., Teruya, C. M., & Anglin, D. M. (2004). Gender differences in treatment outcomes over a three-year period: A PATH model analysis. *Journal of Drug Issues, 34,* 419–439.

Hughes, P. H., Coletti, S. D., Neri, R. L., Urmann, C. F., Stahl, S., Sicilian, D. M., et al. (1995). Retaining cocaine-abusing women in a therapeutic community: The effect of a child live-in program. *American Journal of Public Health, 85,* 1149–1152.

Huselid, R. F., Self, E. A., & Gutierres, S. E. (1991). Predictors of successful completion of a halfway-house program for chemically-dependent women. *American Journal of Drug and Alcohol Abuse, 17,* 89–101.

Ingersoll, K. S., Lu, I. L., & Haller, D. L. (1995). Predictors of in-treatment relapse in perinatal substance abusers and impact on treatment retention: A prospective study. *Journal of Psychoactive Drugs, 27,* 375–387.

Jansson, L. M., Svikis, D., Lee, J., Paluzzi, P., Rutigliano, P., & Hackerman, F. (1996). Pregnancy and addiction: A comprehensive care model. *Journal of Substance Abuse Treatment, 13,* 321–329.

Jarvis, T. J. (1992). Implications of gender for alcohol treatment research: A quantitative and qualitative review. *British Journal of Addiction, 87,* 1249–1261.

Jerrell, J., & Ridgely, M. (1995). Gender differences in the assessment of specialized treatments for substance abuse among people with severe mental illness. *Journal of Psychoactive Drugs, 27,* 347–355.

Joe, G. W., Simpson, D. D., & Broome, K. M. (1999). Retention and patient engagement models for different treatment modalities in DATOS. *Drug and Alcohol Dependence, 57,* 113–125.

Kang, S., Magura, S., Laudet, A., & Whitney, S. (1999). Adverse effect of child abuse victimization among substance-using women in treatment. *Journal of Interpersonal Violence, 14,* 657–670.

Kaskutas, L. A., Zhang, L., French, M. T., & Witbrodt, J. (2005). Women's programs versus mixed-gender day treatment: Results from a randomized study. *Addiction, 100,* 60–69.

Kauffman, E., Dore, M. M., & Nelson-Zlupko, L. (1995). The role of women's therapy groups in the treatment of chemical dependence. *American Journal of Orthopsychiatry, 65,* 355–363.

Kearney, M. H. (1998). Truthful self-nurturing: A grounded formal theory of women's addiction recovery. *Qualitative Health Research, 8,* 495–512.

Kelly, A. B., Halford, W. K., & Young, R. M. (2000). Maritally distressed women with alcohol problems: The impact of a short-term alcohol-focused intervention on drinking behavior and marital satisfaction. *Addiction, 95*, 1537–1549.

King, A. C., & Canada, S. A. (2004). Client-related predictors of early treatment drop-out in a substance abuse clinic exclusively employing individual therapy. *Journal of Substance Abuse Treatment, 26*, 189–195.

Knight, D. K., Hood, P. E., Logan, S. M., & Chatham, L. R. (1999). Residential treatment for women with dependent children: One agency's approach. *Journal of Psychoactive Drugs, 31*, 339–351.

Kosten, T. A., Gawin, F. H., Kosten, T. R., & Rounsaville, B. J. (1993). Gender differences in cocaine use and treatment response. *Journal of Substance Abuse Treatment, 10*, 63–66.

Kranzler, H. R., Del Boca, F. K., & Rounsaville, B. J. (1996). Comorbid psychiatric diagnosis predicts three-year outcomes in alcoholics: A posttreatment natural history study. *Journal of Studies on Alcohol, 57*, 619–626.

Lacey, J. H., & Moureli, E. (1986). Bulimic alcoholics: Some features of a clinical sub-group. *British Journal of Addiction, 81*, 389–393.

LaFave, L. M., & Echols, L. D. (1999). An argument for choice: An alternative women's treatment program. *Journal of Substance Abuse Treatment, 16*, 345–352.

Lewis, C. (2006). Treating incarcerated women: Gender matters. *Psychiatric Clinics of North America, 29*, 773–789.

Linehan, M. M., Schmidt, H., 3rd, Dimeff, L. A., Craft, J. C., Kanter, J., & Comtois, K. A. (1999). Dialectical behavior therapy for patients with borderline personality disorder and drug-dependence. *American Journal of Addictions, 8*, 279–292.

Loneck, B., Garrett, J., & Banks, S. M (1997). Engaging and retaining women in outpatient alcohol and other drug treatment: The effect of referral intensity. *Health and Social Work, 22*, 38–46.

Luthar, S. S., & Suchman, N. E. (2000). Relational psychotherapy mothers' group: A developmentally informed intervention for at-risk mothers. *Developmental Psychopathology, 12*, 235–253.

Maglione, M., Chao, B., & Anglin, M. D. (2000). Correlates of outpatient drug treatment drop-out among methamphetamine users. *Journal of Psychoactive Drugs, 32*, 221–228.

Mann, K., Hintz, T., & Jung, M. (2004). Does psychiatric comorbidity in alcohol-dependent patients affect treatment outcome? *European Archives of Psychiatry and Clinical Neuroscience, 254*, 172–181.

Marsh, J. C., Cao, D., & D'aunno, T. (2004). Gender differences in the impact of comprehensive services in substance abuse treatment. *Journal of Substance Abuse Treatment, 27*, 289–300. (*)

McCance, E. F., Carroll, K. M., & Rounsaville, B. J. (1999). Gender differences in treatment seeking cocaine abusers: Implications for treatment. *American Journal on Addictions, 8*, 300–311.

McCaul, M. E., Svikis, D. S., & Moore, R. D. (2001). Predictors of outpatient treatment retention: Patient versus substance use characteristics. *Drug and Alcohol Dependence, 62*, 9–17.

McComish, J. F., Greenberg, R., Ager, J., Chruscial, H., & Laken, M. A. (2000). Survival analysis of three treatment modalities in a residential substance abuse program for women and children. *Outcomes Management for Nursing Practice, 4*, 71–77.

McComish, J. F., Greenberg, R., Ager, J., Essenmacher, L., Orgain, L. S., & Bacik, W. J., Jr. (2003). Family-focused substance abuse treatment: A program evaluation. *Journal of Psychoactive Drugs, 35*, 321–331.

McKay, J. R., Gutman, M., McLellan, A. T., Lynch, K. G., & Ketterlinus, R. (2003). Treatment services received in the CASAWORKS for Families program. *Evaluation Review, 27*, 629–655.

McKay, J. R., Lynch, K. G., Pettinati, H. M., & Shepard, D. S. (2003). An examination of potential sex and race effects in a study of continuing care for alcohol- and cocaine-dependent patients. *Alcoholism: Clinical and Experimental Research, 27*, 1321–1323.

McLellan, A. T., Alterman, A. I., Metzger, D. S., Grissom, G. R., Woody, G. E., Luborsky, L., et al. (1994). Similarity of outcome predictors across opiate, cocaine, and alcohol treatments: Role of treatment services. *Journal of Consulting and Clinical Psychology, 62*, 1141–1158.

Mertens, J. R., & Weisner, C. M. (2000). Predictors of substance abuse treatment retention among women and men in an HMO. *Alcoholism: Clinical and Experimental Research, 24*, 1525–1533.

Messina, N., Wish, E., & Nemes, S. (2000). Predictors of treatment outcomes in men and women admitted to a therapeutic community. *American Journal of Drug and Alcohol Abuse, 26*, 207–227.

Mojtabai, R. (2005). Use of specialty substance abuse and mental health services in adults with substance use disorders in the community. *Drug and Alcohol Dependence, 78*, 345–354.

Mueller, T. I., Lavori, T. W., Keller, M. B., Swartz, A., Warshaw, M., Hasin, D., et al. (1994). Prognostic effect of the variable course of alcoholism on the 10-year course of depression. *American Journal of Psychiatry, 151*, 701–706.

Najavits, L. M. (2002). *Seeking safety: A treatment manual for PTSD and substance abuse.* New York: Guilford Press.

Najavits, L. M., Ryngala, D., et al. (in press). Treatment for PTSD and comorbid disorders: A review of the literature. In E. B. Floa, T. M. Keane, M. J. Friedman, & J. Cohen (Eds.), *Effective treatments for PTSD: Practice guidelines from the International Society for Traumatic Stress Studies.* New York: Guilford Press.

National Center on Addiction and Substance Abuse at Columbia University (CASA). (2003). *The formative years: Pathways to substance abuse among girls and young women ages 8–22.* New York: Columbia University.

Nelson-Zlupko, L., Dore, M., Kauffman, E., & Kaltenbach, K. (1996). Women in recovery: Their perceptions of treatment effectiveness. *Journal of Substance Abuse Treatment 13*, 51–59. (*)

Nelson-Zlupko, L., Kauffman, E., & Dore, M. M. (1995). Gender differences in drug addiction and treatment: Implications for social work intervention with substance-abusing women. *Social Work, 40*, 45–54.

O'Hare, T. (1995). Mental health problems and alcohol abuse: Co-occurrence and gender differences. *Health and Social Work, 20*, 207–214.

Orwin, R. G., Francisco, L., & Bernichon, T. (2001). *Effectiveness of women's substance abuse treatment programs: A meta-analysis.* Arlington, VA: Substance Abuse and Mental Health Services Administration. (*)

Peles, E., Schreiber, S., Naumovsky, Y., & Adelson, M. (2007). Depression in methadone maintenance treatment patients: Rate and risk factors. *Journal of Affective Disorders, 99*, 213–220.

Pelissier, B., & Jones, N. (2005). A review of gender differences among substance abusers. *Crime and Delinquency, 51*, 343–372.

Pelissier, B. M., Camp, S. D., Gaes, G. G., Saylor, W. G., & Rhodes, W. (2003). Gender differences in outcomes from prison-based residential treatment. *Journal of Substance Abuse Treatment, 24*, 149–160.

Petry, N. M., & Bickel, W. K. (2000). Gender differences in hostility of opioid-dependent outpatients: Role in early treatment termination. *Drug and Alcohol Dependence, 58*, 27–33.

Peveler, R., & Fairburn, C. (1990). Eating disorders in women who abuse alcohol. *British Journal of Addiction, 85*, 1633–1638.

Pirard, S., Sharon, E., Kang, S. K., Angarita, G. A., & Gastfriend, D. R. (2005). Prevalence of physical and sexual abuse among substance abuse patients and impact on treatment outcomes. *Drug and Alcohol Dependence, 78*, 57–64.

Project MATCH Research Group. (1997). Matching alcoholism treatments to client heterogeneity: Project MATCH posttreatment drinking outcomes. *Journal of Studies on Alcohol, 58*, 7–29.

Reynolds, K. D., Coombs, D. W., Lowe, J. B., Peterson, P. L., & Gayoso, E. (1995). Evaluation of a self-help program to reduce alcohol consumption among pregnant women. *International Journal of the Addictions, 30*, 427–443.

Rivers, S. M., Greenbaum, R. L., & Goldberg, E. (2001). Hospital-based adolescent substance abuse treatment: Comorbidity, outcomes, and gender. *Journal of Nervous and Mental Disease, 189*, 229–237.

Roberts, A. C., & Nishimoto, R. H. (1996). Predicting treatment retention of women dependent on cocaine. *American Journal of Drug and Alcohol Abuse, 22*, 313–333.

Rohsenow, D. J., Monti, P. M., Martin, R. A., Michalec, E., & Abrams, D. B. (2000). Brief coping skills treatment for cocaine abuse: 12-month substance use outcomes. *Journal of Consulting and Clinical Psychology, 68*, 515–520.

Sanchez-Craig, M., Spivak, K., & Davila, R. (1991). Superior outcome of females over males after brief treatment for the reduction of heavy drinking: Replication and report of therapist effects. *British Journal of Addiction, 86*, 867–876.

Satre, D. D., Mertens, J., Arean, P. A., & Weisner, C. (2004). Contrasting outcomes of older versus middle-aged and younger adult chemical dependency patients in a managed care program. *Journal of Studies on Alcohol, 64*, 520–530.

Saunders, B., Baily, S., Phillips, M., & Allsop, S. (1993). Women with alcohol problems: Do they relapse for reasons different to their male counterparts? *Addiction, 88*, 1413–1422.

Sayre, S. L., Schmitz, J. M., Stotts, A. L., Averill, P. M., Rhoades, H. M., & Grabowski, J. J. (2002). Determining predictors of attrition in an outpatient substance abuse program. *American Journal of Drug and Alcohol Abuse, 28*, 55–72.

Schliebner, C. T. (1994). Gender-sensitive therapy: An alternative for women in substance abuse treatment. *Journal of Substance Abuse Treatment, 11*, 511–515.

Schober, R., & Annis, H. M. (1996). Barriers to help-seeking for change in drinking: A gender-focused review of the literature. *Addictive Behaviors, 21*, 81–92.

Simpson, D., Joe, G. W., Broome, K. M., Hiller, M. L., Knight, D. K., & Rowan-Szal, G. A. (1997). Program diversity and treatment retention rates in the drug abuse treatment outcome study (DATOS). *Psychology of Addictive Behaviors, 11*, 279–293.

Smith, W. B., & Weisner, C. (2000). Women and alcohol problems: A critical analysis of the literature and unanswered questions. *Alcoholism: Clinical and Experimental Research, 24*, 1320–1321.

Stark, M. J. (1992). Dropping out of substance abuse treatment: A clinically oriented review. *Clinical Psychology Review, 12*, 93–116.

Stephens, R. S., Roffman, R. A., & Simpson, E. E. (1994). Treating adult marijuana dependence: A test of the relapse prevention model. *Journal of Consulting and Clinical Psychology, 62*, 92–99.

Sterling, R. C. (2004). Gender differences in cue exposure reactivity and 9-month outcomes. *Journal of Substance Abuse and Treatment, 27*, 39–44.

Sterling, R. C., Gottheil, E., Weinstein, S. P., & Serota, R. (1998). Therapist/patient race and sex matching: Treatment retention and 9-month follow-up outcome. *Addiction, 93*, 1043–1050.

Sterling, R. C., Gottheil, E., Weinstein, S. P., & Serota, R. (2001). The effect of therapist/patient race- and sex-matching in individual treatment. *Addiction, 96*, 1015–1022.

Strantz, I. H., & Welch, S. P. (1995). Postpartum women in outpatient drug abuse treatment: Correlates of retention/completion. *Journal of Psychoactive Drugs, 27*, 357–373.

Substance Abuse and Mental Health Services Administration (SAMHSA). (1993). *45 CFR 96: Rules and regulations.* Available at *www.treatment.org/legis/45CFR961.html.*

Substance Abuse and Mental Health Services Administration (SAMHSA). (2004). *Treatment Episode Data Set (TEDS): 1992–2002: National admissions to substance abuse treatment services.* Rockville, MD: Department of Health and Human Services.

Substance Abuse and Mental Health Services Administration (SAMHSA). (2005). *National Survey of Substance Abuse Treatment Services (N-SSATS).* Rockville, MD: Department of Health and Human Services.

Swift, W., & Copeland, J. (1996). Treatment needs and experiences of Australian women with alcohol and other drug problems. *Drug and Alcohol Dependence, 40*, 211–219.

Szuster, R. R., Rich, L. L., Chung, A., & Bisconer, S. W. (1996). Treatment retention in women's residential chemical dependency treatment: The effect of admission with children. *Substance Use and Misuse, 31*, 1001–1013.

Taylor, A. V., Peveler, R. C., Hibbert, G. A., & Fairburn, C. G. (1993). Eating disorders among women receiving treatment for an alcohol problem. *International Journal of Eating Disorders, 14*, 147–151.

Timko, C., Moos, R. H., Finney, J. W., & Connell, E. G. (2002). Gender differences in help-utilization and the 8-year course of alcohol abuse. *Addiction, 97*, 877–889.

Toneatto, A., Sobell, L. C., & Sobell, M. B. (1992). Gender issues in the treatment of abusers of alcohol, nicotine, and other drugs. *Journal of Substance Abuse, 4*, 209–218.

Veach, L. J., Remley, T. P., Jr., Kippers, S. M., & Sorg, J. D. (2000). Retention predictors related to intensive outpatient programs for substance use disorders. *American Journal of Drug and Alcohol Abuse, 26*, 417–428.

Velasquez, M. M., & Stotts, A. L. A. (2003). *Substance abuse and dependence disorders in women.* Thousand Oaks, CA: Sage.

Volpicelli, J., Markman, I., Monterosso, J., Filing, J., & O'Brien, C. (2000). Psychosocially enhanced treatment for cocaine-dependent mothers: Evidence of efficacy. *Journal of Substance Abuse Treatment, 18,* 41–49.

Wallen, J. (1992). A comparison of male and female clients in substance abuse treatment. *Journal of Substance Abuse Treatment, 9,* 243–248.

Washington, O. G. (2001). Using brief therapeutic interventions to create change in self-efficacy and personal control of chemically dependent women. *Archives of Psychiatric Nursing, 15,* 32–40.

Washington Sate Department of Social and Health Services and Department of Health. (1999). *Washington State Mom's Project Perinatal Research and Demonstration Project: The Mom's Project final report.* Olympia, WA: Washington State Department of Social and Health Services.

Weisner, C. (1993). The epidemiology of combined alcohol and drug use within treatment agencies: A comparison by gender. *Journal of Studies on Alcohol, 54,* 268–274.

Weisner, C., & Schmidt, L. (1992). Gender disparities in treatment for alcohol treatment problems. *Journal of the American Medical Association, 268,* 1872–1876.

Welle, D., Falkin, G. P., & Jainchill, N. (1998). Current approaches to drug treatment for women offenders: Project WORTH—Women's Options for Recovery, Treatment, and Health. *Journal of Substance Abuse Treatment, 15,* 151–163.

Westermeyer, J., Kopka, S., & Nugent, S. (1997). Course and severity of substance abuse among patients with comorbid major depression. *American Journal on Addictions, 6,* 284–292.

Wilke, D. (1994). Women and alcoholism: How a male-as-norm bias affects research, assessment, and treatment. *Health and Social Work, 19,* 29–35.

Wong, C. J., Badger, G. J., Sigmon, S. C., & Higgins, S. T. (2002). Examining possible gender differences among cocaine-dependent outpatients. *Experimental and Clinical Psychopharmacology, 10,* 316–323.

CHAPTER 18

Treatment Seeking and Utilization among Women with Substance Use Disorders

Christine E. Grella, PhD

Since the 1970s the field of substance abuse treatment has witnessed enormous changes in the number of treatment providers, forms of treatment financing, and types of treatment modalities available. There has been increasing emphasis on developing, implementing, and disseminating evidence-based treatment for substance use disorders within community-based settings. Moreover, increasingly sophisticated epidemiological surveys have provided a more detailed understanding of the prevalence of substance use within the general population, the characteristics of those who have substance use disorders (SUDs), and the rates at which they receive treatment (Degenhardt, Chiu, Sampson, Kessler, & Anthony, 2007). Further, data collected from national surveys of treatment providers yield a composite picture of the characteristics of individuals participating in treatment and enable comparisons both across time periods and by types of settings in which individuals receive treatment.

These various population surveys and provider surveys, along with clinical research from individual and multisite studies, allow for an in-depth examination of the role of gender in substance abuse treatment participation. The goal of this chapter is to provide a synthesis of research regarding treatment seeking and utilization among women with SUDs, and the implications of this body of research for future research and policy. This chapter examines the influence of gender in the following areas: (1) the prevalence of SUDs and need for treatment in order to provide a context for understanding treatment utilization; (2) the barriers and facilitators of treatment utilization, including the complex and unique impact that being a parent has on treatment participation among women; (3) the pathways into substance abuse treatment through other service delivery systems with which women come into contact; and (4) interventions to increase treatment participation, including coerced treatment and motivational enhancements.

SEX DIFFERENCES IN PREVALENCE OF SUDs AND HELP SEEKING

Data from national prevalence surveys show that a greater proportion of men in the general population have a history of SUDs (both abuse and dependence); however, the sex difference is less pronounced with regard to drug use disorders (Kandel, 2000). For example, in the National Epidemiologic Survey on Alcohol and Related Conditions (NESARC), males are 3.1 times more likely than females to have a lifetime alcohol use disorder, 2.3 times more likely to have alcohol abuse, and 2.6 times more likely to have alcohol dependence (Hasin, Stinson, Ogburn, & Grant, 2007). The differentials are less pronounced with regard to lifetime drug use disorders: males are 2.3 times more likely than females to have a lifetime drug use disorder, 2.2 times more likely to abuse drugs, and 1.9 times more likely to be drug dependent (Compton, Thomas, Stinson, & Grant, 2007). The gap between males and females is smallest with regard to the prevalence of past-year amphetamine use disorders; males are about 1.6 times more likely than females to manifest this disorder. In addition, women are more likely than men to engage in nonmedical use of prescription drugs, particularly narcotic analgesics and tranquilizers; women are twice as likely as men to report past-year abuse of these substances (Simoni-Wastila & Strickler, 2004).

Data from the National Survey on Drug Use and Health, conducted from 2004 to 2006, indicate that an annual average of 6.3 million women (9.4%), ages 18–49, needed treatment for a substance use problem (Office of Applied Studies [OAS]; 2007). Of the women ages 18–49 who met criteria for needing substance use treatment in the past year, 84.2% neither received it nor perceived the need for it. Only 5.5% of women in this age group had a perceived unmet treatment need. The survey further elicited reasons for not receiving substance use treatment among the women with an unmet treatment need: 36.1% stated they were not ready to stop using alcohol or illicit drugs; 34.4% could not cover their treatment costs because of no, or inadequate, health insurance coverage; and 28.9% did not seek substance use treatment because of social stigma.

National survey data have shown that help seeking for substance use problems among the general population is generally low, although it is higher among individuals who have multiple types of substance use problems, as well as co-occurring mental disorders (Wu, Ringwalt, & Williams, 2003). Yet, when controlling for number of disorders and other demographic characteristics, males with at least 1 past-year disorder were approximately 1.7 times more likely than females to report having received substance abuse services. Upon reviewing data from several national surveys, Greenfield and colleagues (2007) concluded that the proportion of women who participate in substance abuse treatment is lower than the population prevalence of SUDs in women relative to men. Hence, although most women with SUDs in the general population do not acknowledge a need for treatment, the rate of unmet treatment need may be greater among women than men.

Despite the high rates of unrecognized need for treatment among women, it is well established that women demonstrate an accelerated progression from initiation of substance use (particularly cannabis, alcohol, and cocaine) to onset of dependence and first admission to treatment, as compared with men (Hernandez-Avilia, Rounsaville, & Kranzler, 2004; Hser, Anglin, & Booth, 1987; Wagner & Anthony, 2007). When women do enter treatment, they typically report a shorter duration of use but more severe disorders (usually measured by symptoms of dependence or by standardized assessments, such as the Addiction Severity Index [ASI]), as compared with men. In particular, women tend to report greater psychological distress and mental health problems, particularly mood and anxiety disorders; more family-related needs, including issues related to parenting, child care, and child custody; more health-related problems; greater exposure to childhood and adult trauma and victimization and associated problems; and more problems related to lack of employment and vocational skills (Brady, Grice, Dustan, & Randall, 1993; Chatham, Hiller, Rowan-Szal, Joe, & Simpson, 1999; Stewart, Gossop, Marsden, Kidd, & Treacy, 2003; Wechsberg, Craddock, & Hubbard, 1998).

SEX DIFFERENCES IN TREATMENT UTILIZATION

Data on treatment admissions in the United States are reported into the Treatment Episodes Data System (TEDS) and provide valuable information on the extent to which women participate in treatment and differences in the characteristics of men and women who enter treatment. These data show that the overall proportion of men to women within the treatment system has remained fairly constant over the past 10 years (1995–2005) at 2:1, with women making up approximately one-third of all treatment admissions (OAS, 2006).

The sources of referral into treatment reveal the differential pathways through which women and men access substance abuse treatment. Nationally, a much higher proportion of men than women are referred into treatment through the criminal justice system (40 vs. 28%), whereas about twice as many women as men access treatment by referral from other community agencies (e.g., welfare, child welfare, health care providers; 15 vs. 6%; OAS, 2006). Other studies have also shown that women are more likely than men to enter treatment via the mental health and child welfare systems, whereas men are more likely to enter treatment through the criminal justice system (Schmidt & Weisner, 1995). Similarly, there are differences between men and women in their sources of payment for treatment, with a greater proportion of men reporting self-pay (26 vs. 18%) and a relatively greater proportion of women being dependent upon public insurance to pay for treatment (26 vs. 12%; OAS, 2006). These differences in source of referral and method of payment suggest that the pathways to treatment for men and women are strongly differentiated based on their economic and employment status, which may serve as either barriers or facilitators of treatment utilization. Moreover, the greater reliance of women upon public insurance to pay for treatment suggests that they are more vulnerable to changes in eligibility for, or reductions in, public insurance coverage for treatment.

In addition to the differential referral pathways into treatment, treatment participation is influenced by the severity of individuals' substance use, their self-perception of the problems and adverse consequences related to their substance use, their access to resources, and the external forces that may support or inhibit treatment entry (Anglin, Hser, & Booth, 1987; Finney & Moos, 1995; Weisner & Schmidt, 1992). Some studies have shown that men and women define their substance use differently, in ways that either hinder or facilitate their treatment entry. In a study of 50 individuals with alcohol dependence in outpatient treatment, half of whom were women, the women frequently failed to identify their drinking as problematic and were adverse to being labeled "alcoholic" (Thom, 1986). They minimized the harmfulness of their drinking and emphasized that their drinking had not impaired their ability to fulfill their roles as wives and mothers. In fact, for many women, drinking with their spouses was integral to their marital relationships, and their spouses contributed to defining their drinking as nonproblematic. In contrast, nearly all of the men in the study who were living with a spouse or partner reported that they had been encouraged or supported by that person to enter treatment (Thom, 1987). Similarly, another study showed that a greater number of negative social consequences related to drinking—such as traffic accidents, arrests, and family-, legal-, and work-related problems—were associated with treatment entry among men but not among women (Weisner, 1993). However, employment and prior treatment history were related to treatment entry for both men and women.

These prior studies were confined to people with alcohol dependence; traditionally, women with alcohol dependence were relatively invisible, compared with men, as they risked being stigmatized as sexually deviant and social outcasts (Blume, 1986). Hence, their problems with alcohol may have remained relatively hidden and therefore triggered no social pressures to enter treatment. Moreover, traditional sex roles and marital relationships may have inhibited treatment participation among women with alcohol dependence. There are similar findings with respect to women with drug use disorders. A study of couples in methadone treatment in the 1980s showed that patterns of drug use and decisions to enter treatment were often made jointly (Anglin, Kao, Harlow, Peters, & Booth, 1987). More recent research has shown that a greater adherence to traditional sex roles among men in methadone treatment is positively related to psychological dominance and "couple drug involvement," which in turn is associated with their perpetration of intimate partner violence (El-Bassel et al., 2004). Men in relationships where both partners used illicit drugs were more than twice as likely as others to perpetrate intimate partner violence and nearly four times as likely to perpetrate "severe" forms of violence (El-Bassel, Gilbert, Wu, Chang, & Fontdevila, 2007). Hence, the threat of intimate partner violence may limit women's ability to enter treatment if drug use is integral to the couple's relationship.

A study conducted with primary drug users demonstrates the contrary influences of marital relationships and social stigma on treatment participation for men and women. Using data from the national Drug Abuse Treatment Outcome Studies, Grella and Joshi (1999) examined the factors associated with having a history of substance abuse treatment among individuals who were sampled from residential, outpatient, hospital inpatient, and methadone maintenance programs. More severe drug use history and greater involvement in criminal behavior were related to prior treatment participation for both men and women. Yet there was a divergence between men and women in the other characteristics that were related to a history of treatment participation. Prior drug treatment among men was associated with higher levels of family opposition to their drug use and more support for their treatment participation. Treatment history among men was also associated with having been referred to treatment by their family, an employer, or the criminal justice system. In contrast, treatment history for women was associated with having been referred by a social worker, having a diagnosis of antisocial personality disorder, having engaged in sex work, or having initiated treatment on their own.

Taken together, this profile suggests that women's treatment participation may be triggered by the greater "deviance" ascribed to their drug use and accompanying behaviors, such as sex work. Hence, women's participation in treatment is inextricably bound up with the greater stigma that is associated with their substance use, vis-à-vis men's. This distinction in social perception and consequences of drug use between men and women becomes even more salient when examining the factors that influence treatment participation among women who are pregnant or mothers of small children.

Given the greater centrality of their role as caregivers for children, the potential effects of treatment participation (or nonparticipation) on their relationships with their children may be a central influence on their decisions regarding whether or not to enter treatment. Several studies have shown that most women entering into substance abuse treatment are mothers of dependent children, and at least half have had contact with child welfare (Conners et al., 2004; Grella, Scott, Foss, Joshi, & Hser, 2003). However, less than half of mothers entering treatment are living with all of their children, and up to one-third have lost their parental rights to at least one child (Knight & Wallace, 2003; Schilling, Mares, & El-Bassel, 2004; Tracy & Martin, 2007). A study utilizing state administrative data showed that among mothers with a history of injection drug use, those who were residing with their children were significantly more likely to enter into methadone maintenance treatment (vs. other forms of treatment) than mothers who did not reside with their children (Lundgren, Schilling, Fitzgerald, Davis, & Amodeo, 2003). Mothers entering into methadone maintenance were also more likely to be employed and stably housed, compared with others, underscoring the importance of access to resources in their ability to care for children as well as participate in treatment.

The influence of children upon parental substance use and mothers' motivation for, and participation in, treatment is complex (Collins, Grella, & Hser, 2003). Children (and pregnancy) may impede treatment participation if women fear it will jeopardize their retaining custody of their children (Haller, Miles, & Dawson, 2003). This factor was evident in a study in which involvement with child welfare was negatively associated with treatment motivation among mothers (Wilke, Kamata, & Cash, 2005). The authors suggested that the negative influence of child-welfare involvement on treatment motivation reflects the practical or emotional issues associated with having to leave children with other caregivers, as well as the fear of losing custody of their children. Similarly, another study found that among mothers who were opiate users, greater parenting responsibility, defined as number of children, was inversely related to number of treatment episodes, although this relationship was moderated by ethnicity and relationship status (McMahon, Winkel, Suchman, & Luthar, 2002). Further, many mothers claim to adopt strategies to limit the effects of their drug use on children, including restricting their use to certain time periods and hiding or disguising their use, thus discounting the harmful effects upon themselves and their children (Baker & Carson, 1999).

Logistical issues and access to resources also facilitate or impede treatment use among women. In a study of women with cocaine dependence and criminal involvement, both in and not in treatment, Saum, Hiller, Leigey, Inciardi, and Surratt (2007) showed that enabling factors, such as being legally employed, having health insurance, having custody of children, and knowing where to go to get treatment appeared to be the most influential predictors of treatment participation (as compared with predisposing and service need factors). In a study of individuals seeking publicly funded treatment in Washington State, women were found to spend longer on a wait list for treatment and to be less likely to eventually enter treatment, compared with men (Downey, Rosengren, & Donovan, 2003). The authors noted that pregnant women, who were given priority for admission to treatment, were excluded from the analyses; hence, women who were not pregnant may have had longer wait times stemming from the remaining limited capacity of inpatient and residential beds for women. They further surmised that women may postpone treatment entry due to lack of child care arrangements, thus prolonging their time on the wait list.

A qualitative study conducted in Australia examined barriers to treatment participation among 32 women who had sustained recovery for more than 1 year without participation in either treatment or self-help groups (Copeland, 1997). The sample identified the following barriers to treatment: social stigma and labeling, lack of awareness of the range of treatment options, concerns about child care, the economic and time costs of residential treatment, concerns about the confrontational approaches that were pervasive in traditional substance abuse treatment, and stereotyped perceptions of treatment services (e.g., the "religious" nature of 12-step groups). Moreover, several studies have shown that women with co-occurring mental disorders and/or who are homeless may be even more reluctant to enter into treatment because of their greater vulnerability, which is often related to histories of trauma and victimization (Padgett, Hawkins, Abrams, & Davis, 2006; Watkins, Shaner, & Sullivan, 1999).

Because of women's multiple vulnerabilities, some have argued that outreach and engagement strategies need to address the complex array of treatment needs that typically accompany substance use among women (Melchior, Huba, Brown, & Slaughter, 1999). Brown, Melchior, Panter, Slaughter, and Huba (2000) posit that women's readiness to make life changes must be assessed across four domains: domestic violence, HIV sexual risk behavior, substance abuse, and mental health. Their resultant help-seeking behaviors reflect a hierarchy of readiness based on the immediacy, or time urgency, of their treatment issues across these domains. Moreover, previous studies have shown that experiences of socioeconomic disadvantage, exposure to community violence, criminal justice system interactions, and access to resources among women vary by ethnicity and influence perceptions of treatment needs and coping behaviors (Amaro et al., 2005, 2007).

PATHWAYS TO SUBSTANCE ABUSE TREATMENT THROUGH OTHER SERVICE DELIVERY SYSTEMS

Since the mid-1980s, major policy initiatives have influenced the pathways into substance abuse treatment for women through other service systems, either through mandated treatment, interventions to screen for substance abuse problems and refer clients to treatment, or cross-system collaborations. These policy changes and interventions are briefly reviewed.

Health Services

The primary health care sector is one of the predominant sources of treatment for individuals with alcohol or drug problems. Findings from the National Comorbidity Survey Replication showed that among individuals with a past-year SUD (either abuse of, or dependence on, alcohol and/or drugs), 26.2% received treatment from the mental health sector (including specialty substance abuse providers), and 18.1% received treatment from the general medical sector, which included treatment from physicians, nurses, and other health care professionals (Wang et al., 2005). Moreover, there was a dramatic increase in treatment for psychiatric disorders (including SUDs) in the general medical sector from 1990 to 2003, and women were more likely than men to be treated in this sector (Kessler et al., 2005).

Patient interactions with health care clinicians provide an important opportunity for screening and referral; hence, there is increased emphasis on developing screening tools and brief interventions for SUDs that can be implemented in primary care settings. In one study individuals screened for SUDs in a hospital emergency department were successfully referred to treatment and other services, including for women's health services such as breast cancer screenings and gynecological exams (Bernstein, Bernstein, & Levenson, 1997). Women who seek emergency medical treatment as a result of intimate partner violence, in which substance abuse is often involved, can be screened and referred to substance abuse treatment, as well as to other needed services (Lipsky, Caetano, Field, & Bazargan, 2005).

An optimal site for screening and referral of women for substance abuse interventions is within reproductive health services, such as obstetrics (Morse, Gehshan, & Hutchins, 1997). One study demonstrated the feasibility of using a brief screener to detect alcohol use among pregnant women in waiting rooms in eight obstetric clinics; 13% scored above the cutoff score indicating at-risk alcohol use (defined as binge drinking or more than one standard drink per week). At-risk use was predicted by smoking and earlier stage of pregnancy, indicating the feasibility of intervening early in pregnancies to reduce potential harm (Flynn, Marcus, Barry, & Blow, 2003).

Criminal Justice System

There has been an influx of women with substance abuse problems into the criminal justice system in the past 20 years, due to changes in sentencing and criminal justice policies that have increased incarceration rates for drug users. Since 1995 the total number of female prisoners in the United States has grown by 53%, as compared to 32% for males (Harrison & Beck, 2005). Much of this increase can be accounted for by changes in sentencing for drug-related crimes, which have disproportionately affected women, particularly women of color (Freudenberg, 2002). As of 2002, 31.5% of female inmates nationally were incarcerated for drug-related crimes, compared with 20.7% of males. Thus, the criminal justice system is increasingly a conduit into substance abuse treatment for both men and women, including in prison-based settings and in community-correctional programs (Grella & Greenwell, 2004).

As with women who enter into community-based treatment, women who enter into the criminal justice system typically have multiple service needs (Alemagno, 2001). These include a greater likelihood of psychiatric disorders, particularly mood and anxiety disorders, compared with male offenders, as well as compared with women in the general population (Jordan, Schlenger, Fairbank, & Caddell, 1996; Pelissier & Jones, 2005; Teplin, Abram, & McClelland, 1996). Female offenders face substantial barriers to obtaining needed services, both in the community and in correctional settings. In one study female offenders were more likely to receive services for mental health needs in prisons than in the community preceding incarceration (Blitz, Wolff, & Paap, 2006). The lack of integrated treatment for female offenders with SUDs and co-occurring mental disorders is especially critical, given that these women are at higher risk for recidivism following their return to the community (Sacks, 2004).

Welfare

Legislation enacted in 1996, generally referred to as "welfare reform," instituted Temporary Assistance for Needy Families (TANF). This state block grant program established federally mandated work requirements and a maximum lifetime 5-year limit to cash aid for clients. Along with these restrictions and requirements, the legislation instituted new expectations for local and state welfare systems, including the option to require screening for substance abuse and referral to treatment services as a condition of participation (Schmidt & McCarty, 2000).

Studies have shown that substance use is more prevalent among welfare recipients, compared with other women with dependent children who do not receive public assistance; however, the self-reported prevalence of illicit drug use is less pervasive than commonly assumed. Using national survey data, Pollack and colleagues showed that 22.3% of female TANF recipients reported illicit drug use, compared to 12.8% of women with dependent children who did not receive TANF (Pollack, Danziger, Jayakody, & Seefeldt, 2002). Among those who need treatment, however, rates of treatment are low. One study showed that fewer than half of TANF participants who were diagnosed with substance dependence at baseline participated in treatment over a 2-year follow-up period (Atkinson, Brown, Montoya, & Bell, 2004). Administrative barriers to the screening, assessment, and referral of drug-dependent recipients to treatment may impede their ability to access and utilize treatment services. Commonly noted barriers are the lack of resources and expertise among caseworkers to screen and assess for SUDs and the limited capacity of treatment systems to provide the comprehensive services needed by these recipients (Metsch & Pollack, 2005).

Although women with SUDs constitute a minority of TANF recipients, they face additional barriers to attaining economic self-sufficiency and are less likely to transition successfully to paid employment than recipients without SUDs (Jayakody, Danziger, & Pollack, 2000; Schmidt, Zabkiewicz, Jacobs, & Wiley, 2007). Given this population's greater impairments and multiple problems, intensive case management services have been developed for these women, which have increased their likelihood of entering and staying in treatment (Morgenstern et al., 2003). Moreover, welfare recipients with SUDs who stay in treatment longer and complete treatment are more likely to be working and not require welfare following treatment discharge, compared with those who do not complete treatment (Metsch, Pereyra, Miles, & McCoy, 2003).

Child Welfare

Greater awareness of the association between parental substance abuse and child abuse and neglect has fostered increased levels of interaction between these two systems in order to encourage coordination of services for child-welfare-involved parents with SUDs. Substance abuse treatment providers and child-welfare agencies are increasingly called upon to collaborate in providing services and making determinations of parental fitness and recommendations for child placement outcomes (Kerwin, 2005). However, historically these two service delivery systems have had differing orientations, goals, and organizational cultures, and these differences have created barriers to increasing coordination of services and case planning (Karoll & Poertner, 2002). Moreover, coordination of services across systems is further impeded when women fear that they may jeopardize custody of their children when they admit to substance abuse problems in child-welfare assessments or if they enter substance abuse treatment (Finkelstein, 1994; Jessup, Humphreys, Brindis, & Lee, 2003).

The development of dependency drug courts (or family drug courts), in which participation in treatment is mandated and supervised by a separate court or judge, has strengthened linkages between child-welfare and substance abuse treatment systems. Several recent evaluations have shown that women referred to substance abuse treatment through dependency drug court enter into treatment sooner and have higher rates of treatment completion, compared with those who are referred from child welfare but are not under court supervision (Boles, Young, Moore, & DiPirro-Beard, 2007; Green, Furrer, Worcel, Burrus, & Finigan, 2007).

Although participation in substance abuse treatment may be made a condition of, or considered as a factor in, the determination of a woman's parental rights, there is little understanding of whether or how participation in substance abuse treatment affects the outcomes of both parents and children within the child-welfare system. A study using state administrative data showed that women who were pregnant or who had custody of minor children were less likely than others to complete substance abuse treatment, although women who had children in foster care were more likely to do so (Scott-Lennox, Rose, Bohlig, & Lennox, 2000). Other studies have shown that mothers who are able to keep their children with them while in residential drug treatment (Hughes et al., 1995), or who retain custody of their infants while in intensive day treatment, have higher rates of treatment retention, particularly among those who are involved with child welfare (Chen et al., 2004) or who are mandated to treatment (Nishimoto & Roberts, 2001).

INTERVENTIONS TO INCREASE TREATMENT PARTICIPATION: COERCION AND MOTIVATIONAL ENHANCEMENTS

The effect of coerced participation in drug abuse treatment has typically been studied by addressing individuals who are involved with the criminal justice system, the majority of whom are men; the extent to which women are coerced into treatment has not been examined to the same extent. Over half of the sample of women participating in the national multisite Women, Co-Occurring Disorders, and Violence Study reported that they had had at least one previous involuntary admission to alcohol, drug abuse, or psychiatric treatment, and 12% reported involuntary admissions to both psychiatric and substance use treatment (Clark et al., 2005). Yet there were no differences between women who had been mandated to treatment and those who had not, either in severity of substance use or psychiatric symptoms. The women who had been mandated to treatment, however, were more likely to have been arrested, suggesting that criminal behavior involvement, rather than clinical severity, is more likely to prompt such a mandate. Similarly, in a statewide treatment outcome study in California, women who were involved with the child-welfare system had lower levels of alcohol use severity and had no differences in psychiatric severity, but who were more likely to have been referred to treatment by the criminal justice system, compared with mothers with no child-welfare involvement (Grella, Hser, & Huang, 2006).

In a longitudinal follow-up study of a cohort that had initially been sampled at the point of treatment referral, external mandate was a much more powerful factor influencing treatment reentry among men over a 6-year follow-up period; there was a 12-fold greater likelihood of moving from *using* to *treatment* for men who were mandated to treatment, compared with women (Grella, Scott, Foss, & Dennis, 2008). Yet the same study showed that self-help participation was more strongly associated with moving from *using* to *recovery* for women. This finding is consistent with the findings from a longitudinal study of individuals who sought help for alcohol problems, showing that women were more likely than men to participate in self-help groups following initial treatment participation, and to have greater reductions in drinking concurrent with their self-help participation over an 8-year follow-up period (Timko, Finney, & Moos, 2005; Timko, Moos, Finney, & Connell, 2002). More recently, these findings have endured over a 16-year follow-up period (Moos, Moos, & Timko, 2006). Thus, whereas men may be influenced more to engage in treatment because of external mandates, women may be more willing to participate in self-help and other activities following treatment exposure.

Increasingly, the willingness of individuals with SUDs to enter and to stay in treatment has become a focus within treatment research. There has been considerable interest in recent years in "unpacking" the construct of treatment motivation and understanding its relationship to eventual treatment engagement and outcomes (Longshore & Teruya, 2006; Wild, Cunningham, & Ryan, 2006). Yet there has been remarkably little examination of sex differences in treatment motivation (Vasilaki, Hosier, & Cox, 2006), particularly in ways that can inform interventions that are designed to increase motivation and enhance treatment engagement and retention (Grella, 2008).

Motivational interventions use therapeutic strategies to increase the individuals' awareness of their substance abuse problems and engage their commitment to behavior change. These interventions can build upon the issues that are central influences on women's treatment participation, such as their identity, self-esteem, health concerns, and relationships with children, other family members, and friends. Moreover, motivational interventions can be tailored to address gender-related differences in differentiation and conception of self and coping styles in ways that increase women's treatment participation (Cook, Epperson, & Gariti, 2005).

In most instances where motivational interventions have been developed specifically for women, they have aimed to promote changes in substance use among pregnant women with SUDs. Pregnancy is viewed as a "window of opportunity" in which women may be particularly receptive to substance abuse interventions that may be embedded with prenatal care (Handmaker & Wilbourne, 2001; Jessup & Brindis, 2005). In one example, a brief motivational intervention was used to address alcohol use among pregnant women in primary health care settings; an empathic, client-centered motivational interview focused on the health of participants' unborn babies (Handmaker, Miller, & Manicke, 1999). Participants who had the highest blood alcohol levels during early pregnancy had greater reductions at a 2-month follow-up if they received the motivational interview, compared with participants who received an informational pamphlet. Similarly, in another experimental study, pregnant women with the highest levels of consumption had significantly greater reductions in alcohol use after a single-session brief intervention, compared with a usual care group; furthermore, the effect was enhanced when the woman's partner participated in the session (Chang et al., 2005). Yet in another study, non-treatment-seeking pregnant women were recruited from prenatal clinics and assigned to two conditions. Both groups received motivational interviewing combined with behavioral incentives, and one group received case management services in addition (Jones, Svikis, Rosado, Tuten, & Kulstad, 2004). Although the addition of case management increased access to needed services, there was no effect of the combined motivational interviewing and behavioral incentives on number of counseling visits or completion (defined as four visits). The authors concluded that the combined intervention may have lacked sufficient intensity to engage these participants in treatment.

FUTURE DIRECTIONS

Building upon this large and growing body of research, future research should continue to track the patterns of treatment and service utilization among women with substance use problems. It will be especially important to understand the factors that facilitate or impede access to treatment for women of differing characteristics, including parental status, and the interventions that increase screening, referral, and treatment entry across different settings. A full understanding of women's treatment utilization requires the integration of epidemiological data on substance use prevalence and need for treatment, health services research on the pathways into treatment and the costs of different service configurations, clinical research on the characteristics of women who enter treatment and their treatment outcomes, and longitudinal studies that track patterns of substance use, treatment utilization, and recovery over time. Such a research base will provide the foundation necessary for fully informed policy initiatives that prioritize substance abuse treatment for women who need it.

KEY POINTS

- The historical legacy of greater stigma associated with alcohol and drug use among women, and the relative invisibility of women's treatment needs, compared with men's (Kandall, 1996), have influenced the pathways into treatment and treatment options available to women.
- As women's alcohol and drug use has neared parity with that of men, particularly among users of stimulants, or, in the case of prescription drug abuse, exceeded that of men, women with substance abuse problems have increasingly entered into treatment, as well as the criminal justice system.
- Heightened public awareness of the potential consequences of maternal substance use on children has focused attention on alcohol and drug use among pregnant and parenting women. The spotlight on mothers, however, has often promoted greater stigma and increased barriers to treatment participation among women who fear incarceration or loss of custody of their children.
- At the same time, policy initiatives focusing on maternal substance abuse have increased fund-

ing and treatment capacity dedicated to pregnant and parenting women (Grella & Greenwell, 2004; Schmidt & Weisner, 1995). An unintended consequence of this policy focus on pregnant and parenting women is that other women, such as older women, may have less access to treatment. However, there has been little investigation into the treatment needs of this population thus far (Hamilton & Grella, 2008).

• Women with SUDs frequently come into contact with other service systems, including mental health, health services, welfare, child welfare, and criminal justice. Various interventions to screen women for SUDs, to refer them to appropriate treatment, and to coordinate delivery of services have been implemented across these systems.

• Future research can build upon this existing body of research on women's treatment utilization by continuing to examine the relationship of treatment need to access and utilization, longitudinal patterns of service use and outcomes, and organizational and system-level factors that improve the delivery of treatment services to women.

REFERENCES

Asterisks denote recommended readings.

Alemagno, S. A. (2001). Women in jail: Is substance abuse treatment enough? *American Journal of Public Health*, *91*(5), 798–800.

Amaro, H., Dai, J., Arevalo, S., Acevedo, A., Matsumoto, A., Nieves, R., et al. (2007). Effects of integrated trauma treatment on outcomes in a racially/ethnically diverse sample of women in urban community-based substance abuse treatment. *Journal of Urban Health*, *84*(4), 508–522.

Amaro, H., Larson, M. J., Gampel, J., Richardson, E., Savage, A., & Wagler, D. (2005). Racial/ethnic differences in social vulnerability among women with co-occurring mental health and substance abuse disorders: Implications for treatment services. *Journal of Community Psychology*, *33*(4), 495–511.

Anglin, M. D., Hser, Y., & Booth, M. W. (1987). Sex differences in addict careers: IV. Treatment. *American Journal of Drug and Alcohol Abuse*, *13*(3), 253–280.

Anglin, M. D., Kao, C. F., Harlow, L. L., Peters, K., & Booth, M. W. (1987). Similarity of behavior within addict couples: Part I. Methodology and narcotics patterns. *International Journal of the Addictions*, *22*(6), 497–524.

Atkinson, J., Brown, V. L., Montoya, I. D., & Bell, D. (2004). Personal adjustment and substance abuse problems in a longitudinal study of TANF recipients and the potential need for treatment. *American Journal of Drug and Alcohol Abuse*, *30*, 643–657.

Baker, P. L., & Carson, A. (1999). "I take care of my kids": Mothering practices of substance-abusing women. *Gender and Society*, *13*(3), 347–363.

Bernstein, E., Bernstein, J., & Levenson, S. (1997). Project ASSERT: An ED-based intervention to increase access to primary care, preventive services, and the substance abuse treatment system. *Annals of Emergency Medicine*, *30*, 181–189.

Blitz, C. L., Wolff, N., & Paap, K. (2006). Availability of behavioral health treatment for women in prison. *Psychiatric Services*, *57*, 356–360.

Blume, S. B. (1986). Women and alcohol. *Journal of the American Medical Association*, *256*, 1467–1469.

Boles, S. M., Young, N. K., Moore, T., & DiPirro-Beard, S. (2007). The Sacramento dependency drug court: Development and outcomes. *Child Maltreatment*, *12*(2), 161–171.

Brady, K. T., Grice, D. E., Dustan, L., & Randall, C. (1993). Gender differences in substance use disorders. *American Journal of Psychiatry*, *150*(11), 1707–1711.

Brown, V. B., Melchior, L. A., Panter, A. T., Slaughter, R., & Huba, G. J. (2000). Women's steps of change and entry into drug abuse treatment: A multidimensional stages of change model. *Journal of Substance Abuse Treatment*, *18*(3), 231–240.

Chang, G., McNamara, T. K., Orav, E. J., Koby, D., Lavigne, A., Ludman, B., et al. (2005). Brief intervention for prenatal alcohol use: A randomized trial. *Obstetrics and Gynecology, 105*(5, Pt. 1), 991–998.

Chatham, L. R., Hiller, M. L., Rowan-Szal, G. A., Joe, G. W., & Simpson, D. D. (1999). Gender differences at admission and follow-up in a sample of methadone maintenance clients. *Substance Use and Misuse, 34*(8), 1137–1165.

Chen, X., Burgdorf, K., Dowell, K., Roberts, T., Porowski, A., & Herrell, J. M. (2004). Factors associated with retention of drug abusing women in long-term residential treatment. *Evaluation and Program Planning, 27*, 205–212.

Clark, C., Becker, M., Giard, J., Mazelis, R., Savage, A., & Vogel, W. (2005). The role of coercion in the treatment of women with co-occurring disorders and histories of abuse. *Journal of Behavioral Health Services and Research, 32*(2), 167–181.

Collins, C., Grella, C. E., & Hser, Y. I. (2003). Effects of gender and level of parental involvement among parents in drug treatment. *American Journal of Drug and Alcohol Abuse, 29*(2), 237–261.

Compton, W. M., Thomas, Y. F., Stinson, F. S., & Grant, B. F. (2007). Prevalence, correlates, disability, and comorbidity of DSM-IV drug abuse and dependence in the United States. *Archives of General Psychiatry, 64*, 566–576.

Conners, N. A., Bradley, R. H., Mansell, L. W., Liu, J. Y., Roberts, T. J., Burgdorf, K., et al. (2004). Children of mothers with serious substance abuse problems: An accumulation of risks. *American Journal of Drug and Alcohol Abuse, 30*, 85–100.

Cook, L. S., Epperson, L., & Gariti, P. (2005). Determining the need for gender-specific chemical dependence treatment: Assessment of treatment variables. *American Journal on Addiction, 14*, 328–338.

Copeland, J. (1997). A qualitative study of barriers to formal treatment among women who self-managed change in addictive behaviours. *Journal of Substance Abuse Treatment, 14*(2), 183–190.

Degenhardt, L., Chiu, W. T., Sampson, N., Kessler, R., & Anthony, J. C. (2007). Epidemiological patterns of extra-medical drug use in the United States: Evidence from the National Comorbidity Study Replication, 2001–2003. *Drug and Alcohol Dependence, 90*(2–3), 210–223.

Downey, L., Rosengren, D. B., & Donovan, D. M. (2003). Gender, waitlists, and outcomes for public-sector drug treatment. *Journal of Substance Abuse Treatment, 25*(1), 19–28.

El-Bassel, N., Gilbert, L., Golder, S., Wu, E., Chang, M., Fontdevila, J., et al. (2004). Deconstructing the relationship between intimate partner violence and sexual HIV risk among drug-involved men and their female partners. *AIDS and Behavior, 8*(4), 429–439.

El-Bassel, N., Gilbert, L., Wu, E., Chang, M., & Fontdevila, J. (2007). Perpetration of intimate partner violence among men in methadone treatment programs in New York City. *American Journal of Public Health, 97*(7), 1230–1232.

Finkelstein, N. (1994). Treatment issues for alcohol- and drug-dependent pregnant and parenting women. *Health and Social Work, 19*(1), 7–15.

Finney, J. W., & Moos, R. H. (1995). Entering treatment for alcohol abuse: A stress and coping model. *Addiction, 90*(9), 1223–1240.

Flynn, H. A., Marcus, S. M., Barry, K. L., & Blow, F. C. (2003). Rates and correlates of alcohol use among pregnant women in obstetrics clinics. *Alcoholism: Clinical and Experimental Research, 27*(1), 81–87.

Freudenberg, N. (2002). Adverse effects of U.S. jail and prison policies on the health and well-being of women of color. *American Journal of Public Health, 92*, 1895–1899.

Green, B. L., Furrer, C., Worcel, S., Burrus, S., & Finigan, M. W. (2007). How effective are family treatment drug courts? Outcomes from a four-site national study. *Child Maltreatment, 12*(1), 43–59.

Greenfield, S. F., Brooks, A. J., Gordon, S. M., Green, C. A., Kropp, F., McHugh, K., et al. (2007). Substance abuse treatment entry, retention, and outcome in women: A review of the literature. *Drug and Alcohol Dependence, 86*(1), 1–21. (*)

Grella, C. E. (2008). From generic to gender-responsive treatment: Changes in social policies, treatment services, and outcomes of substance abuse treatment. *Journal of Psychoactive Drugs, SARC Supplement 5*, 327–343.

Grella, C. E., & Greenwell, L. (2004). Substance abuse treatment for women: Changes in settings where women received treatment and types of services provided, 1987–1998. *Journal of Behavioral Health Services and Research*, 31(4), 367–383.

Grella, C. E., Hser, Y., & Huang, Y. C. (2006). Mothers in substance abuse treatment: Differences in characteristics based on involvement with child welfare. *Child Abuse and Neglect*, 30(1), 55–73.

Grella, C. E., & Joshi, V. (1999). Gender differences in drug treatment careers among clients in the National Drug Abuse Treatment Outcome Study. *American Journal of Drug and Alcohol Abuse*, 25(3), 385–406. (*)

Grella, C. E., Scott, C. K., Foss, M., & Dennis, M. L. (2008). Gender similarities and differences in the treatment, relapse, and recovery cycle. *Evaluation Review*, 32(1), 113–137. (*)

Grella, C. E., Scott, C. K., Foss, M. A., Joshi, V., & Hser, Y. (2003). Gender differences in drug treatment outcomes among participants in the Chicago Target Cities Study. *Evaluation and Program Planning*, 26(3), 297–310.

Haller, D. L., Miles, D. R., & Dawson, K. S. (2003). Factors influencing treatment enrollment by pregnant substance abusers. *American Journal of Drug and Alcohol Abuse*, 29(1), 117–131.

Hamilton, A., & Grella, C. E. (2009). "Honey, drugs don't have no age": Older heroin addicts and gender issues. *Journal of Women and Aging*, 21(1/2).

Handmaker, N. S., Miller, W. R., & Manicke, M. (1999). Findings of a pilot study of motivational interviewing with pregnant drinkers. *Journal of Studies on Alcohol*, 60(2), 285–287.

Handmaker, N. S., & Wilbourne, P. (2001). Motivational interventions in prenatal clinics. *Alcohol Research and Health*, 25(3), 21–29.

Harrison, P. M., & Beck, A. J. (2005). *Prisoners in 2004* (BJS Bulletin, NCJ 210677). Washington, DC: Bureau of Justice Statistics, U.S. Department of Justice. Retrieved October 10, 2006, from *www.ojp.gov/bjs/abstract/p04.htm*.

Hasin, D. S., Stinson, F. S., Ogburn, E., & Grant, B. F. (2007). Prevalence, correlates, disability, and comorbidity of DSM-IV alcohol abuse and dependence in the United States. *Archives of General Psychiatry*, 64(7), 830–842.

Hernandez-Avilia, C. A., Rounsaville, B. J., & Kranzler, H. R. (2004). Opioid-, cannabis-, and alcohol-dependent women show more rapid progression to substance abuse treatment. *Drug and Alcohol Dependence*, 74(2), 265–272.

Hser, Y. I., Anglin, M. D., & Booth, M. W. (1987). Sex differences in addict careers: 3. Addiction. *American Journal of Drug and Alcohol Abuse*, 13(3), 231–251.

Hughes, P. H., Coletti, S. D., Neri, R. L., Urmann, C. F., Stahl, S., Sicilian, D. M., et al. (1995). Retaining cocaine abusing women in a therapeutic community: The effect of a child live-in program. *American Journal of Public Health*, 85, 1149–1152.

Jayakody, R., Danziger, S., & Pollack, H. (2000). Welfare reform, substance use, and mental health. *Journal of Health Politics, Policy and Law*, 25(4), 623–651.

Jessup, M. A., & Brindis, C. D. (2005). Issues in reproductive health and empowerment in perinatal women with substance use disorders. *Journal of Addictions Nursing*, 16, 97–105.

Jessup, M. A., Humphreys, J. C., Brindis, C. D., & Lee, K. A. (2003). Extrinsic barriers to substance abuse treatment among pregnant drug dependent women. *Journal of Drug Issues*, 33(2), 285–304.

Jones, H. E., Svikis, D., Rosado, J., Tuten, M., & Kulstad, J. L. (2004). What if they do not want treatment? Lessons learned from intervention studies of non-treatment seeking, drug-using pregnant women. *American Journal on Addictions*, 13, 342–357.

Jordan, B. K., Schlenger, W. E., Fairbank, J. A., & Caddell, J. M. (1996). Prevalence of psychiatric disorders among incarcerated women: II. Convicted felons entering prison. *Archives of General Psychiatry*, 53, 513–519.

Kandall, S. R. (1996). *Substance and shadow: Women and addiction in the United States*. Cambridge, MA: Harvard University Press.

Kandel, D. B. (2000). Gender differences in the epidemiology of substance dependence in the United States. In E. Frank (Ed.), *Gender and its effects on psychopathology* (pp. 231–252). Washington, DC: American Psychiatric Association.

Karoll, B. R., & Poertner, J. (2002). Judges', caseworkers', and substance abuse counselors' indicators of family reunification with substance-affected parents. *Child Welfare, 81*(2), 249–269.

Kerwin, M. E. (2005). Collaboration between child welfare and substance-abuse fields: Combined treatment programs for mothers. *Journal of Pediatric Psychology, 30*(7), 581–597.

Kessler, R. C., Demler, O., Frank, R. G., Olfson, M., Pincus, H. A., Walters, E. E., et al. (2005). Prevalence and treatment of mental disorders, 1990 to 2003. *New England Journal of Medicine, 352*(24), 2515–2523.

Knight, D. K., & Wallace, G. (2003). Where are the children? An examination of children's living arrangements when mothers enter residential drug treatment. *Journal of Drug Issues, 33*(2), 305–324.

Lipsky, S., Caetano, R., Field, C. A., & Bazargan, S. (2005). The role of alcohol use and depression in intimate partner violence among black and Hispanic patients in an urban emergency department. *American Journal of Drug and Alcohol Abuse, 31*, 225–242.

Longshore, D., & Teruya, C. (2006). Treatment motivation among drug users: A theory based analysis. *Drug and Alcohol Dependence, 81*(2), 179–188.

Lundgren, L. M., Schilling, R. F., Fitzgerald, T., Davis, K., & Amodeo, M. (2003). Parental status of women injection drug users and entry to methadone maintenance. *Substance Use and Misuse, 38*(8), 1109–1131.

McMahon, T. J., Winkel, J. D., Suchman, N. E., & Luthar, S. S. (2002). Drug dependence, parenting responsibilities, and treatment history: Why doesn't mom go for help? *Drug and Alcohol Dependence, 65*(2), 105–114. (*)

Melchior, L. A., Huba, G. J., Brown, V. B., & Slaughter, R. (1999). Evaluation of the effects of outreach to women with multiple vulnerabilities on entry into substance abuse treatment. *Evaluation and Program Planning, 22*(3), 269–277.

Metsch, L. R., Pereyra, M., Miles, C. C., & McCoy, C. B. (2003). Welfare and work outcomes after substance abuse treatment. *Social Service Review, 77*, 237–254.

Metsch, L. R., & Pollack, H. A. (2005). Welfare reform and substance abuse. *Milbank Quarterly, 83*, 65–99.

Moos, R. H., Moos, B. S., & Timko, C. (2006). Gender, treatment, and self-help in remission from alcohol use disorders. *Clinical Medicine and Research, 4*, 163–174.

Morgenstern, J., Nakashian, M., Woolis, D. D., Gibson, F. M., Bloom, N. L., & Kaulback, B. G. (2003). CASAWORKS for families: A new treatment model for substance-abusing parenting women on welfare. *Evaluation Review, 27*(6), 583–596.

Morse, B., Gehshan, S., & Hutchins, E. (1997). *Screening for substance abuse during pregnancy: Improving care, improving health.* Arlington, VA: National Center for Education in Maternal and Child Health.

Nishimoto, R. H., & Roberts, A. C. (2001). Coercion and drug treatment for postpartum women. *American Journal of Drug and Alcohol Abuse, 27*(1), 161–181.

Padgett, D. K., Hawkins, R. L., Abrams, C., & Davis, A. (2006). In their own words: Trauma and substance abuse in the lives of formerly homeless women with serious mental illness. *American Journal of Orthopsychiatry, 76*(4), 461–467.

Pelissier, B., & Jones, N. (2005). A review of gender differences among substance abusers. *Crime and Delinquency, 51*(3), 343–372.

Pollack, H., Danziger, S., Jayakody, R., & Seefeldt, K. (2002). Drug testing welfare recipients: False positives, false negatives, unanticipated opportunities. *Women's Health Issues, 12*(1), 23–31.

Sacks, J. Y. (2004). Women with co-occurring substance use and mental disorders (COD) in the criminal justice system: A research review. *Behavioral Sciences and Law, 22*(4), 449–466.

Saum, C. A., Hiller, M. L., Leigey, M. E., Inciardi, J. A., & Surratt, H. L. (2007). Predictors of substance abuse treatment entry for crime-involved, cocaine-dependent women. *Drug and Alcohol Dependence, 91*(3), 253–259.

Schilling, R., Mares, A., & El-Bassel, N. (2004). Women in detoxification: Loss of guardianship of their children. *Children and Youth Services Review, 26*(5), 463–480.

Schmidt, L., & Weisner, C. (1995). The emergence of problem-drinking women as a special population in need of treatment. In M. Galanter (Ed.), *Recent developments in alcoholism: Alcoholism and women* (pp. 309–334). New York: Plenum Press.

Schmidt, L., Zabkiewicz, D., Jacobs, L., & Wiley, J. (2007). Substance abuse and employment among welfare mothers: From welfare to work and back again? *Substance Use and Misuse, 42*(7), 1069–1087.

Schmidt, L. A., & McCarty, D. (2000). Welfare reform and the changing landscape of substance abuse services for low-income women. *Alcoholism: Clinical and Experimental Research, 24*(8), 1298–1311.

Scott-Lennox, J., Rose, R., Bohlig, A., & Lennox, R. (2000). The impact of women's family status on completion of substance abuse treatment. *Journal of Behavioral Health Services and Research, 27*(4), 366–379.

Simoni-Wastila, L., & Strickler, G. (2004). Risk factors associated with problem use of prescription drugs. *American Journal of Public Health, 94*(2), 266–268.

Stewart, D., Gossop, M., Marsden, J., Kidd, T., & Treacy, S. (2003). Similarities in outcomes for men and women after drug misuse treatment: Results from the National Treatment Outcome Research Study (NTORS). *Drug and Alcohol Review, 22*, 35–41.

Substance Abuse and Mental Health Services Administration. (2006). *Treatment episode data set (TEDS) highlights—2005 national admissions to substance abuse treatment services: 1995–2005.* Rockville, MD: Author. Retrieved November 8, 2007, from *oas.samhsa.gov/teds2k5/ TEDSHi2k5.htm.*

Substance Abuse and Mental Health Services Administration. (2007, October 4). *The NSDUH report: Substance use treatment among women of childbearing age.* Rockville, MD: Author. Retrieved December 11, 2007, from *oas.samhsa.gov/2k7/womenTX/womenTX.cfm.*

Teplin, L. A., Abram, K. M., & McClelland, G. M. (1996). Prevalence of psychiatric disorders among incarcerated women: Pretrial jail detainees. *Archives of General Psychiatry, 53*(6), 505–512.

Thom, B. (1986). Sex differences in help-seeking for alcohol problems: I. The barriers to help-seeking. *British Journal of Addiction, 81*(6), 777–788.

Thom, B. (1987). Sex differences in help-seeking for alcohol problems: II. Entry into treatment. *British Journal of Addiction, 82*(9), 989–997.

Timko, C., Finney, J. W., & Moos, R. H. (2005). The 8-year course of alcohol abuse: Gender differences in social context and coping. *Alcoholism: Clinical and Experimental Research, 29*(4), 612–621.

Timko, C., Moos, R. H., Finney, J. W., & Connell, E. G. (2002). Gender differences in help-utilization and the 8-year course of alcohol abuse. *Addiction, 97*(7), 877–889. (*)

Tracy, E. M., & Martin, T. C. (2007). Children's roles in the social networks of women in substance abuse treatment. *Journal of Substance Abuse Treatment, 32*(1), 81–88.

Vasilaki, E. I., Hosier, S. G., & Cox, W. M. (2006). The efficacy of motivational interviewing as a brief intervention for excessive drinking: A meta-analytic review. *Alcohol and Alcoholism, 41*(3), 328–335.

Wagner, F. A., & Anthony, J. C. (2007). Male–female differences in the risk of progression from first use to dependence upon cannabis, cocaine, and alcohol. *Drug and Alcohol Dependence, 86*(2–3), 191–198.

Wang, P. S., Lane, M., Olfson, M., Pincus, H. A., Wells, K. B., & Kessler, R. C. (2005). Twelve-month use of mental health services in the United States: Results from the National Comorbidity Survey Replication. *Archives of General Psychiatry, 62*(6), 629–640.

Watkins, K. E., Shaner, A., & Sullivan, G. (1999). The role of gender in engaging the dually diagnosed in treatment. *Community Mental Health Journal, 35*, 115–126.

Wechsberg, W. M., Craddock, S. G., & Hubbard, R. L. (1998). How are women who enter substance abuse treatment different than men? A gender comparison from the Drug Abuse Treatment Outcome Study (DATOS). *Drugs and Society, 13*, 97–115.

Weisner, C. (1993). Toward an alcohol treatment entry model: A comparison of problem drinkers in the general population and in treatment. *Alcoholism: Clinical and Experimental Research, 17*(4), 746–752.

Weisner, C., & Schmidt, L. (1992). Gender disparities in treatment for alcohol problems. *Journal of the American Medical Association*, 268(14), 1872–1876.

Wild, C. T., Cunningham, J. A., & Ryan, R. M. (2006). Social pressure, coercion, and client engagement at treatment entry: A self-determination theory perspective. *Addictive Behaviors*, 31, 1858–1872.

Wilke, D. J., Kamata, A., & Cash, S. J. (2005). Modeling treatment motivation in substance-abusing women with children. *Child Abuse and Neglect*, 29, 1313–1323.

Wu, L.-T., Ringwalt, C. L., & Williams, C. E. (2003). Use of substance abuse treatment services by persons with mental health and substance use problems. *Psychiatric Services*, 54(3), 363–369.

CHAPTER 19

Behavioral Couple Therapy

Partner-Involved Treatment for Substance-Abusing Women

William Fals-Stewart, PhD
Wendy K. K. Lam, PhD
Michelle L. Kelley, PhD

Among the various psychosocial interventions presently available to treat alcohol and drug abuse, it could be argued that partner-involved treatments are the most broadly efficacious. There is not only substantial empirical support for the use of couple-based treatments in terms of improvements in primary targeted outcomes, such as substance use and relationship adjustment, but also in other areas that are of clear public health significance, including intimate partner violence (IPV), children's adjustment, and cost–benefit ratio and cost-effectiveness. During the last few decades, programmatic research on the application of partner-involved therapies for substance abuse has been among the most active and fruitful.

Although marital and family therapies for substance abuse have been used with a wide variety of patient populations, the purpose of this chapter is to focus on the application of partner-involved interventions with women who abuse substances and are in intimate relationships. More specifically, we (1) provide a conceptual rationale as to why couple therapy for female patients with substance abuse problems may be particularly appealing, compared to more traditional individual-based approaches; (2) describe theoretical and practical considerations involved when implementing couple therapy with these patients; (3) examine available evidence for the efficacy of couple therapy with female patients who abuse alcohol and drug; and (4) discuss future directions with respect to partner-involved therapies with these patients.

TREATING SUBSTANCE ABUSE AMONG FEMALE PATIENTS WITH SUBSTANCE USE DISORDERS: THE CASE FOR PARTNER-INVOLVED INTERVENTIONS

As highlighted throughout this volume, alcohol and drug use disorders have historically been conceptualized as problems of men. In turn, it has been the study of addictive behavior in men that has shaped our understanding of the etiology, course, and treatment of these disorders (e.g., Jellinek, 1952; Vaillant, 1995). Both researchers and clinicians have posited that, due to significant behavioral, social, and emotional differences between treatment-seeking men and women who abuse substances, the findings from intervention studies that have focused largely or exclusively on men may not generalize to women who suffer with these disorders (e.g., Gerolamo, 2004; Straussner & Zelvin, 1997).

Treatment Response and Outcomes: Women versus Men

Comparisons of men and women entering substance abuse treatment have indicated that women (1) have a briefer transition from substance use to addiction, but tend to enter treatment after a shorter period of regular use (e.g., Grella, Scott, Foss, Joshi, & Hser, 2003; Randall et al., 1999); (2) are younger, poorer, and more likely to have direct responsibility for children (e.g., Brady & Randall, 1999; Oggins, Guydish, & Delucchi, 2001; Stewart, Gossop, & Trakada, 2007); (3) receive less emotional support from their intimate partners and others (Blum, Nielsen, & Riggs, 1998; Kail & Elberth, 2002); (4) are more likely to have partners, friends, and family members who use drugs (e.g., Bendtsen, Dahlström, & Lejman, 2002; Hser, Evans, & Huang, 2005); and (5) have a higher prevalence of psychiatric disorders, such as depression and anxiety (Hernandez-Avila, Rounsaville, & Kranzler, 2004; Kidorf et al., 2004; Sonne, Back, Zuniga, Randall, & Brady, 2003; Webster, Rosen, & McDonald, 2007).

Not surprisingly, several studies have also found differences in substance abuse treatment response and outcomes for male and female patients. For example, one of the few significant predictors of posttreatment outcomes to emerge from Project MATCH (Matching Alcoholism Treatments to Client Heterogeneity), the most comprehensive alcoholism treatment outcome study conducted to date, was sex; women had a significantly higher percentage of days abstinent from alcohol after treatment than men (Project MATCH Research Group, 1998a, 1998b). Similarly, Sanchez-Craig, Leigh, Spivak, and Lei (1989) reported that women with alcohol dependence had greater reductions in heavy and problem drinking after brief outpatient treatment than men. In a study of men and women predominantly in treatment for drug use, women's responses to treatment and self-help participation appeared more consistent in reducing drug use during the follow-up period (Greenfield et al., 2007; Hser, Huang, Teruya, & Anglin, 2004).

Thus, despite what is generally a positive response to intervention, women have been substantially underrepresented in substance abuse treatment programs included in most studies exploring outcomes of different treatments for alcoholism and drug abuse. As a result, the effects of different intervention approaches on women's outcomes are far less understood than they are for men.

The Influence of Partner and Family Relationships of Women with Substance Abuse on Treatment Response and Outcomes

Among the most important characteristics that distinguishes men and women who have substance use disorders (SUDs) is the role of dyadic conflict and relationship stress in problematic substance abuse and relapse. For example, Allan and Cooke (1985) found that, compared to men, women were more likely to drink in response to current life stressors and life events such as marital discord, divorce, and children leaving the home. Consistent with these findings, Annis and Graham (1995) found that women were more likely than men to report heavy drinking in response to negative emotional states and interpersonal conflict with others.

Similarly, relationship issues have been found to affect relapse to substance abuse. Lemke, Brennan, and Schutte (2007) found that family problems and emotional distress were linked to relapse for women with alcohol dependence. Connors, Maisto, and Zywiak (1998) found that women alcohol dependence were significantly more likely than men with alcohol dependence to attribute conflict with their spouse or romantic partner as a primary precipitant for relapse. Although women frequently report using or discontinuing use for the sake of their partner (Sun, 2007), having a partner that abuses alcohol or other psychoactive substances is more strongly related to higher rates of relapse for women than for men (Grella et al., 2003). Clearly, these findings indicate that a woman's recovery attempts appear vulnerable to problems in her relationships and her partner's substance use.

Because family and relationship factors play a critical role in the maintenance and exacerbation of drinking and drug problems, as well as relapses after treatment, interventions specifically designed to address both relationship and substance abuse issues concurrently would seem likely to have particular benefit for women with SUDs. Yet, this viewpoint has not been universally held by alcohol and drug abuse treatment researchers or clinicians. In their influential review of therapies for alcohol dependence, Edwards and Steinglass (1995) reported that studies finding family treatment superior to control treatments in reducing alcohol consumption generally examined more male patients (i.e., an average of 6% of participants in family treatment were women) than those investigations finding no differences in drinking outcomes between family versus control treatments (average of 30% female participants). They argued that, in studies "with a preponderance of male alcoholics, marital or family therapy may be more likely to yield positive results; family therapy for female alcoholics may lose its edge over individual treatment" (p. 502). The authors, however, did not examine whether gender was a moderating variable in the effect size for couple/family therapies versus individual treatments. The contrasting positions set the stage for an empirical evaluation of family-involved therapies for women with SUDs.

Of course, a fundamental issue in any such study is the type of family-involved therapy that should be tested. A family-based treatment approach for alcohol and drug use disorders that may have particular benefit for women is behavioral couple therapy (BCT). During the last 3 decades, various forms of BCT have been associated with positive outcomes for men with alcohol dependence and their families, in terms of reduced drinking and improved relationship adjustment (e.g., McCrady, Hayaki, Epstein, & Hirsch, 2002; O'Farrell, Cutter, Choquette, Floyd, & Bayog, 1992), decreased IPV (e.g., O'Farrell, Murphy, & Stephan, 2004), and reduced emotional and behavioral problems of the couples' children (Kelley & Fals-Stewart, 2002; Kelley & Fals-Stewart, 2007). BCT has also been shown to be effective for reducing drug use and improving dyadic relationships (e.g., Epstein, McCrady, & Morgan, 2007; Fals-Stewart, Kashdan, O'Farrell, & Birchler, 2002; Fals-Stewart, O'Farrell, & Birchler, 2001).

As such, BCT was a natural selection as a family-based treatment to test with women with SUDs. Findings in the BCT trials that have been conducted thus far, which are reviewed later in this chapter, have shown positive effects for BCT with women with SUDs, compared to individual-based treatments and attention controls (Fals-Stewart, Birchler, & Kelley, 2006; Winters, Fals-Stewart, O'Farrell, Birchler, & Kelley, 2002). These findings are extremely encouraging and suggest that BCT may be an important intervention approach with women who seek treatment for alcohol or drug abuse.

BCT FOR SUBSTANCE ABUSE: CONCEPTUAL CONSIDERATIONS AND PRACTICAL APPLICATION

The causal connections between substance use and relationship discord are complex and appear to interact reciprocally. For example, chronic substance use outside the home is correlated with reduced marital satisfaction for spouses (e.g., Dunn, Jacob, Hummon, & Seilhamer, 1987). At the same time, however, stressful marital interactions are related to increased problematic substance use and are related to posttreatment relapse among those who abuse alcohol and drugs (e.g., Fals-Stewart & Birchler, 1994; Maisto, O'Farrell, McKay, Connors, & Pelcovitz, 1988). Thus, the relationship between substance use and marital problems is not unidirectional, with one consistently causing the other, but rather each can serve as a precursor to the other, creating a vicious cycle from which couples that include a partner who abuses drugs or alcohol often have difficulty escaping.

Viewed from a family systems perspective, several familial antecedent conditions and reinforcing consequences of substance use can be identified. Poor communication and problem-solving abilities, arguing, financial stressors, and nagging are common antecedents to substance use. Consequences of substance use can be positively or negatively reinforcing, thus increasing or decreasing the likelihood of future substance use. For instance, certain behaviors by a non-substance-abusing spouse—such as avoiding conflict with the partner with SUDs when he or she is intoxicated, or engaging in caretaking behaviors during or after episodes of drinking or drug taking—can inadvertently reinforce continued substance-using behavior. Partners making disapproving verbal comments about the other's drinking or drug use is perhaps the most commonly observed negative interaction sequela of substance abuse (e.g., Becker & Miller, 1976), and can inadvertently serve to increase the likelihood of future drinking or drug use. Other negative effects of substance use on the family—such as psychological distress of the spouse; increased social, behavioral, academic, and emotional problems among children; and elevated levels of stress in the family system—can lead to, or exacerbate, substance use (Moos, Finney, & Cronkite, 1990).

The strong interrelationship between substance use and family interaction suggests that interventions that address only one aspect of this relationship would be less than optimal. However, traditional interventions for substance abuse, which focus largely on the individual patient with an SUD, often do just that. In contrast, BCT (and, for that matter, family-based treatments for substance abuse in general) have two primary objectives that evolve from a recognition of the interrelationship between substance use and family interaction: (1) eliminate abusive drinking and drug use and harness the support of the family to support the patient's efforts to change and (2) alter dyadic and family interaction patterns to promote a family environment that is more conducive to sobriety. Viewed from a marital or intimate relationship context, a high priority is to change substance-related interaction patterns between partners, such as nagging about past drinking and drug use, and ignoring or otherwise minimizing positive aspects of current sober behavior. Continued discussions about and focus on past or "possible" future drinking or drug use increases the likelihood of relapse (Maisto et al., 1988). Thus, abstinent patients and their partners are encouraged to engage in, and are provided training in, behaviors that are more pleasing to each other.

Taking into account our conceptual understanding of the cyclic interplay between substance use and family distress, the BCT intervention for substance abuse is founded upon two fundamental assumptions. First, family members, specifically spouses or other intimate partners, can reward abstinence. Second, reduction of relationship distress and conflict reduces a very significant set of powerful antecedents to substance use and relapse, thereby leading to improved substance use outcomes.

BCT Treatment Methods

When delivering BCT to a married or cohabiting patient with an SUD, a therapist treats this patient with his or her intimate partner and works to build support for abstinence within the dyadic system. The therapist, with extensive input from the partners, develops, and has the partners enter into, a daily Recovery Contract (which is also referred to as a Sobriety Contract). As part of the contract, partners agree to engage in a daily Sobriety Trust Discussion, in which the partner with an SUD states (if true, of course) his or her success in staying sober and the intention not to drink or use drugs that day (e.g., "I have been sober for the last 24 hours, and it is my intention to stay sober for the next 24 hours"). In turn, the non-substance-abusing partner verbally expresses positive support for the patient's efforts to remain sober (e.g., "Thank you for staying sober and please let me know if there is anything I can do to help you stay sober for the next 24 hours"). For patients with SUDs who are medically cleared and willing, daily ingestion of medications designed to support abstinence (e.g., naltrexone, disulfiram), witnessed and verbally reinforced by the non-substance-abusing partner, is often a component that occurs during the daily Sobriety Trust Discussion. The non-substance-abusing partner records the performance of the Sobriety Trust Discussion (and consumption of medication, if applicable) on a calendar provided by the therapist. As a condition of the Recovery Contract, both partners agree not to discuss past drinking or drug use or fears of future substance use when at home (i.e., between scheduled BCT sessions) during the course of couple treatment. This agreement is put in place to reduce the likelihood of substance-related conflicts occurring outside the safety of the therapy sessions, possibly triggering relapse. Partners are asked to reserve such discussions for the BCT therapy sessions, which can then be monitored and, if needed, mediated by the therapist. Many contracts also include specific provisions for partners' regular attendance at self-help meetings (e.g., Alcoholics Anonymous, Al-Anon), which are also marked on the provided calendar during the course of treatment.

At the start of a typical BCT session, the therapist reviews the calendar to ascertain overall compliance with different components of the contract. The calendar provides an ongoing record of progress that is rewarded verbally by the therapist at each session; it also provides a visual (and temporal) record of problems with adherence that can be addressed each week. When possible, the partners perform behaviors that are aspects of their Recovery Contract (e.g., Sobriety Trust Discussion, consumption of abstinence-supporting medication) in each scheduled BCT session to highlight its importance and to allow the therapist to observe their behaviors and provide corrective feedback as needed.

Through the use of standard couple-based behavioral assignments, BCT also seeks to increase positive feelings, shared activities, and constructive communication—relationship factors that are viewed as conducive to sobriety. In the assignment "Catch Your Partner Doing Something Nice" each partner notices and acknowledges one pleasing behavior performed by the other each day. In the "Caring Day" assignment, each partner plans ahead to surprise the significant other with a day when he or she does some special things to show his or her caring. Planning and engaging in mutually agreed-upon "Shared Rewarding Activities" is important because many families with drug problems have ceased engaging in shared pleasing activities, and such activities have been associated with positive recovery outcomes (Moos et al., 1990). Each activity must involve both partners, either as a couple only or with their children or other adults, and can be performed at or away from home. Teaching "Communication Skills" (e.g., paraphrasing, empathizing, validating) can help the patient with an SUD and his or her partner better address stressors in their relationship and in their lives as they arise, which is also viewed as reducing the risk of relapse.

Relapse prevention planning occurs in the final stages of BCT. At the end of weekly BCT sessions, each couple completes a "Continuing Recovery Plan." This written plan provides an overview of the couple's ongoing post-BCT activities to promote stable sobriety (e.g., continuation of a daily Sobriety Trust Discussion, attending self-help support meetings) and contingency plans if relapses occur (e.g., recontacting the therapist, reengaging in self-help support meetings, contacting a sponsor).

BCT sessions tend to be moderately to highly structured, with the therapist setting a specific agenda for the sessions from the outset of each meeting. A typical BCT session begins with an inquiry about any drinking or use of drugs that has occurred since the last session. Compliance with different aspects of the Recovery Contract that have been negotiated is also reviewed and any difficulties with compliance are discussed and addressed. The session then moves to a detailed review of homework assigned during the previous session and the partners' success in completing the assignments. The therapist then identifies any relationship or other types of problems that may have arisen during the last week that can be addressed in session, with the goal of resolving the problems or designing a plan for resolution. Therapists then introduce new material, such as instruction in, and rehearsal of, skills to be practiced at home during the week. Toward the end of the session, partners are given specific homework assignments to complete during the subsequent week.

During initial sessions, BCT therapists focus on decreasing negative feelings and interactions about past and possible future drinking or drug use, and increasing positive behavioral exchanges between partners. Later sessions engage partners in communication skills training, problem-solving strategies, and negotiating behavior change agreements.

Traditionally, the patient with the SUD and his or her partner are seen together in BCT, typically for 15–20 outpatient couple sessions over 5–6 months, although BCT has been reduced to as few as six sessions (Fals-Stewart, Birchler, & O'Farrell, 2001). BCT can also be delivered as a stand-alone intervention or as an adjunct to standard individual substance abuse counseling. Appropriate candidates for BCT are (1) couples in which partners are married or have cohabited for at least a year; (2) couples in which neither partner has a co-occurring psychiatric condition that may significantly interfere with engaging in BCT (e.g., schizophrenia, psychosis); and (3) dyads in which only one member of the couple has a current problem with alcohol or drug abuse.

BCT for Women and Men: Comparable Outcomes, Different Processes

BCT with men and women who abuse substances have shown comparable effects in terms of substance use reductions, dyadic adjustment, and other outcomes. The BCT intervention is manualized but allows for some modification and changes in emphases, depending on the needs of the patients and the couples. With that stated, it has been our experience that the clinical content of BCT sessions with couples in which a female partner has an SUD focuses substantially more on relationship issues, whereas therapy sessions with couples in which the male partner has the SUD tend to focus more on substance use reduction and elimination. This is not by design, but tends to evolve based on the wants and needs of different couple types entering BCT.

BCT FOR FEMALES WITH SUDs: RESULTS FROM RANDOMIZED CLINICAL TRIALS

Since the 1970s, multiple studies have consistently found that participation in BCT by married or cohabiting patients with SUDs results in significant reductions in substance use, decreased problems related to substance use (e.g., job loss, hospitalization), and improved relationship satisfaction. Recently, investigations exploring other outcomes have found that, compared to traditional individual-based treatments, participation in BCT results in significantly (1) higher reductions in partner violence, (2) greater improvements in the psychosocial functioning of children who live with parents who receive the intervention, and (3) better cost–benefit and cost-effectiveness (for a comprehensive review, see Fals-Stewart, O'Farrell, Birchler, Cordova, & Kelley, 2005).

As noted earlier, these findings are based largely on studies that enrolled men with SUDs and their non-substance-abusing female partners. Recent randomized clinical trials of BCT with female patients with SUDs have demonstrated promising evidence of effectiveness with women (Fals-Stewart et al., 2006; Winters et al., 2002). The following sections describe these studies in detail.

BCT with Female Patients with Alcohol Use Disorder

In a randomized trial that we conducted (Fals-Stewart et al., 2006), participants were heterosexual couples ($n = 138$) in which married or cohabiting women were entering outpatient treatment for an alcohol use disorder. Participating couples were then randomly assigned to one of three equally intensive interventions: (1) a BCT therapy condition, which consisted of individual alcohol counseling plus BCT sessions; (2) an individual-based treatment (IBT) condition, consisting of individual alcohol counseling only; or (3) psychoeducational attention control treatment (PACT) condition, consisting of individual alcohol counseling plus couple-based lectures.

During the first 4 weeks after admission, female patients in each condition participated in an *orientation phase*, during which background and medical information were collected. They also began weekly 12-step facilitation individual counseling sessions with their assigned counselor. During the following 12-week *primary treatment phase*, the female patients randomly assigned to the BCT condition began attending conjoint behavioral couple therapy sessions with their partners one time weekly, in addition to one individual counseling session each week. Female partners assigned to PACT began attending the conjoint psychoeducational lectures with their partners one time weekly, in addition to one individual counseling session weekly. Female partners assigned to the IBT condition attended two individual counseling sessions each week. Thus, during the primary treatment phase, female participants in all conditions were scheduled to receive 24 sessions. For the final 4 weeks, or the *discharge phase*, all female participants were scheduled to meet with their counselor for 12-step individual counseling sessions for one 60-minute session each week. Women in each condition were allowed to attend emergency individual counseling sessions at any time during any treatment phase.

Upon entering the study, at the completion of the discharge phase of treatment, and every 3 months thereafter for 1 year, female patients and their male partners were contacted and interviewed by a research assistant. During each of these assessments, participants were interviewed about the female partner's drinking and the couple's relationship satisfaction and adjustment.

In this randomized study, BCT was significantly more effective in terms of improving outcomes along different dimensions of drinking behavior and relationship adjustment than the other treatment conditions. More specifically, compared to female patients who received IBT or PACT, those who participated in BCT with their non-substance-abusing partners reported significantly fewer days of drinking and higher levels of dyadic adjustment during a 12-month posttreatment follow-up period. Additionally, the positive effects of BCT on drinking and dyadic adjustment were more enduring during the posttreatment period than the positive effects of IBT or PACT, as evidenced by the slower rate of return to drinking and slower reductions in relationship satisfaction during follow-up.

Although drinking behavior and relationship satisfaction were the primary targets of the BCT intervention, the comparatively positive results for BCT were observed in other significant areas of psychosocial adjustment. In particular, women who participated in BCT reported fewer total negative consequences as a result of drinking during the year after treatment, particularly in terms of interpersonal, intrapersonal, and social responsibility consequences, than women who participated in IBT or PACT. Couples participating in BCT versus those participating in IBT or PACT reported fewer days of partner violence incidents, both in terms of male-to-female and female-to-male physical aggression. Because IPV is a significant and prevalent problem among alcoholic dyads, in general, identification and use of interventions that serve to reduce it in this population, as well as substance use, may be particularly important.

BCT with Female Patients with Drug Use Disorder

In a similarly designed study, Winters et al. (2002) conducted a randomized trial with married or cohabitating female patients with SUDs ($n = 60$) who were entering an outpatient treatment program. Participating couples were randomly assigned to one of two equally intensive treatment conditions: one treatment package consisted of IBT only, based on cognitive-behavioral therapy (CBT) for substance abuse; the other condition was BCT, consisting of individual- and CBT-based therapy plus BCT. Measures of drug use and dyadic functioning were collected pretreatment, during treatment, posttreatment, and at quarterly intervals thereafter for 1 year.

The couples in the BCT condition reported significantly greater marital satisfaction during treatment and through the 3-month posttreatment follow-up than the couples in which the female partner received IBT. The female patients in the BCT condition also reported lower frequency of substance use during treatment and throughout the 1-year posttreatment, when compared to the female patients in the IBT group.

In both our studies (Fals-Stewart et al., 2006; Winters et al., 2002), participants who received BCT had better within-treatment and posttreatment outcomes across several areas of substance use behavior and couple functioning. However, in the Winters et al. investigation of women in treatment primarily for drug abuse, differences in substance use and dyadic adjustment between the two treatments (i.e., BCT and IBT) diminished over the course of the 12-month follow-up period; in contrast, group differences in these domains of functioning increased during posttreatment follow-up for female patients with alcohol use disorder (Fals-Stewart et al., 2006). It is not clear why the effects of BCT were more robust with the female patients with the alcohol disorder, given the highly manualized treatment. However, differences in the sociodemographic and relationship characteristics of participants across the two studies suggest some plausible explanations. Females with SUDs from the Winters et al. study reported more formidable, multifaceted psychosocial problems (i.e., lower socioeconomic status, multiple current substance use diagnoses) and lower dyadic adjustment at baseline than the women entering alcohol treatment in the Fals-Stewart et al. study. These women appeared to spend more session time diffusing partner conflict and addressing substance-abuse-related crises than the female patients with alcohol problems, who appeared to use more session time on couple-based skills to enhance relationships and support for sobriety (Fals-Stewart et al., 2006).

BCT with "Double-Trouble" Couples

It is important to highlight that published studies of BCT have recruited couples in which only one partner met criteria for a current SUD. Couples in which both partners use drugs (i.e., double-trouble couples) have been far more difficult to treat, primarily because, in contrast to couples with one non-substance-abusing partner, there appears to be little support from within the dyadic system for sobriety. In fact, for dual-using couples, the more time partners reported spending together using substances, the stronger and more negative the association between length of time abstinent and dyadic adjustment; the inverse of this relationship is found for couples with only one partner with an SUD (Fals-Stewart, Birchler, & O'Farrell, 1999). Recently, a pilot study (Birchler & Fals-Stewart, 2007) examined the comparative efficacy of (1) a hybrid treatment of BCT plus contingency management (BCT + CM), (2) a standard BCT package without CM, (3) and treatment as usual (TAU). In this small-scale randomized clinical trial, participants were women with SUDs entering treatment for substance abuse (n = 60) who were married to, or in a stable relationship with, a male partner who met *DSM-IV* criteria for a current SUD. Couples were randomly assigned to one of the three conditions noted earlier. BCT + CM consisted of 32 sessions conducted over a 12-week period. Twelve sessions consisted of couple therapy, and the remaining sessions were 12-step facilitation sessions for the female partner only. Partners received vouchers contingent upon session attendance and providing clean urine and breath samples three times weekly. Standard BCT consisted of 12 BCT and 20 individual counseling sessions; vouchers were not provided in this condition. The TAU condition consisted of 32 individual counseling sessions for the female patients only; no CM procedures were used in this condition. Couples who received BCT + CM provided fewer positive urine samples during treatment, had a higher percentage of days abstinent during treatment and the year after treatment, and had higher levels of dyadic adjustment after treatment completion than couples in the other conditions. Although this was only a pilot study, the findings indicate that BCT + CM is a promising hybrid treatment for these very challenging couples in which both partners abuse substances.

FUTURE DIRECTIONS

Much work remains to examine whether BCT effects significant and meaningful changes for women with SUDs through a research program of empirically based, randomized clinical trials that is comparable to that which has been established for men with SUDs. Gaps in BCT research exist for both males and females with SUDs. However, given the unique gender-specific contextual issues faced by many women who attempt sobriety, the effectiveness of BCT and other family-based treatments must be explored independently for women. In particular, investigations in the following areas seem most critical to address the issues facing women with SUDs and their intimate partners: (1) moving beyond whether BCT works to an examination of *how* it works; (2) exploration of whether adaptations of BCT might offer even stronger treatment options for unique women's contexts (e.g., women who abuse drugs vs. alcohol, women who are a partner in a double-trouble couple, and lesbian couples); (3) addition of other intervention components to standard BCT specifically targeted to enhance important secondary outcomes, particularly enhancements of parenting and child functioning, decreases in IPV and HIV risk behaviors, and addressing issues specific to women with same-sex partners; and (4) dissemination of BCT to community-based programs to address treatment access and availability issues facing women with SUDs.

The "How" of BCT: Mechanisms of Action

Although the results of multiple randomized clinical trials indicate that BCT works, no studies, to date, have empirically established *how* it works. More precisely, the mechanisms of action that produce the observed outcomes have not been tested empirically. As described earlier, the general theoretical rationale for the effects of BCT on substance abuse has been that certain dyadic interactions serve as inadvertent reinforcement for continued substance use or relapse and that relationship distress in general is a trigger for substance use. In turn, the BCT intervention package that has evolved from this rationale involves (1) teaching and promoting methods to reinforce sobriety within the dyad (e.g., engaging in the Recovery Contract), (2) improving communication skills to address problems and conflict appropriately when it arises, and (3) encouraging participation in relationship enhancement exercises (e.g., Shared Rewarding Activities) to increase dyadic adjustment.

However, it is not clear if participation in any or all of these aspects of the BCT intervention results in the improvements observed. For example, although most BCT studies have found that participation in BCT results in improvements in relationship adjustment and reductions in substance use, none has conducted a formal test of mediation to determine if changes in relationship adjustment (i.e., either during treatment or after treatment completion) partially or fully mediate the relationship between type of treatment received (e.g., BCT, individual counseling, an attention control) and substance use outcomes. Indeed, it is important to highlight that most studies have generally failed to find strong relationships between theoretical mechanisms of action of different interventions and subsequent outcomes, both in general psychotherapy (e.g., Orlinski, Grawe, & Parks, 1994; Stiles & Shapiro, 1994), and in substance abuse treatment (e.g., Longabaugh & Wirtz, 2001). The apparently heightened sociodemographic and relationship complexities of females with SUDs seeking therapy may threaten the sustainability of effects and their recovery attempts. Thus, it is particularly important for future studies of women with SUDs to test formally the theoretical mechanisms thought to underlie the observed BCT effects.

BCT for Different Types of Couples and Partners

Although BCT has been the subject of multiple clinical trials in the last three decades, the vast majority of these studies has focused on heterosexual couples in which only one partner was an identified patient with an SUD. Moreover, the studies for alcohol and drug dependence have evolved on separate tracks. In nearly all cases, studies include either patients who report that their primary substance of abuse is alcohol *or* those who report that their primary drug of abuse is something other than alcohol. To increase the ecological validity of BCT research, participant inclusion must be broadened to capture the wide array of couples that typically enter clinical practice.

For example, the majority of BCT approaches have excluded patients whose partners met criteria for current alcohol or SUD. This exclusion criterion has particular salience for females with SUDs, whose non-substance-abusing male partners are most likely to leave the relationship before the couple enters treatment (Fals-Stewart et al., 1999). Thus, these couples may not be adequately represented in treatment-based investigations. Instead, studies have repeatedly found that the majority or significant minority of married or cohabiting females with alcohol or substance-abusing problems entering treatment are involved with partners who also abuse drugs (e.g., Fals-Stewart et al., 1999, 2006; Laudet, Magura, Furst, Kumar, & Whitney, 1999). The pilot study conducted by Gorman, Klostermann, Fals-Stewart, Birchler, and O'Farrell (2004) examining BCT with CM for dual-using couples, offers great promise for future efforts to reach these couples. A larger randomized trial is needed to determine the effectiveness of this BCT + CM therapy for these dual-using couples. Such an approach would serve not only the needs of many female patients initially entering treatment, but would also have the effect of reaching patients' intimate male partners who might not otherwise seek help for alcohol or drug use problems.

A criticism of BCT is that there has been a nearly exclusive application to heterosexual couples. It is widely recognized that partners in gay and lesbian couples have unique individual and relationship needs, and that findings from research with heterosexual couples may not generalize to same-sex couples (e.g., Mohr & Fassinger, 2006). A recent small-scale randomized clinical trial comparing BCT versus individual-based treatment for substance dependence with gay and lesbian couples found that BCT was more effective in reducing substance use frequency and relationship satisfaction than individual-based treatment (Fals-Stewart, O'Farrell, & Birchler, 2007). Although these findings are promising, they are far from definitive and highlight the need for further research on the use of BCT with these couples.

Lastly, it is also not clear if the demarcation between alcohol dependence and drug dependence of female patients, which is standard in BCT studies, continues to be necessary or useful. Although the distinctions between these patient populations may very well have been more defined 30 years ago, when BCT research began in earnest, the boundaries between these patient groups have become increasingly blurred over time. In most instances, female patients now entering treatment for an SUD meet criteria for multiple SUDs. It is plausible that the sociocultural differences between women with drug- versus alcohol dependence continue to be important and clinically relevant and, as such, warrant separation of these groups. It is a question that deserves greater empirical scrutiny.

Additions to Standard BCT Targeted to Enhance Secondary Outcomes

Although participation in BCT appears to have a positive impact on important secondary outcomes, the next phase of research needs to examine if these effects can be enhanced if the BCT intervention were modified to specifically target these outcome domains (in addition to substance use and relationship satisfaction). Some preliminary research is now underway with males with SUDs and their female partners to examine the effect of adding such circumscribed interventions to the standard BCT intervention package to determine if such outcomes can be further improved. Parallel investigations for women with SUDs and their male partners will be especially important to address the psychosocial contexts that are highly relevant to them.

For example, we completed a study exploring the impact of adding parent skills training to BCT to ascertain the effect on school-age children living with participating parents (Fals-Stewart, Fincham, Vendetti, & Kelley, 2003). In this study 72 couples who were raising a school-age child and in which the male partners abused drugs were randomly assigned to one of four conditions: (1) a 24-session manualized BCT condition, consisting of 12-sessions of BCT plus 12 sessions of 12-step group drug counseling (Daley, Mercer, & Carpenter, 1998); (2) a 24-session manualized Parent Skills plus BCT (PSBCT) condition, consisting of 6 sessions of BCT, 6 sessions of parent skills training, and 12 sessions of 12-step group drug counseling; (3) a manualized 24-session parent skills (PS) training condition, consisting of 12 sessions of parent skills training and 12 sessions of group drug counseling; or (4) a manualized 24-session group drug counseling condition for the male partner only. Parents and children were assessed at baseline, posttreatment, and quarterly thereafter for 12 months. Substance use frequency, dyadic adjustment, and children's emotional and behavioral adjustment were measured at each assessment point. Although participants who received BCT and PSBCT had equivalent substance use frequency and relationship outcomes during the posttreatment follow-up period, with participants having superior outcomes in these areas to those who received PS or group counseling, children whose parents received PSBCT had higher levels of psychosocial functioning (i.e., reductions in internalizing and externalizing symptoms) during and after treatment completion than children whose parents were assigned to BCT, PS, or group counseling.

These findings suggest that the positive effects of standard BCT on children's emotional and behavioral adjustment can be enhanced with the addition of parent skills training. These findings have particular relevance for women with SUDs, who often maintain primary caregiving responsibilities for custodial children. In addition, the results of the study have implications for similarly designed investigations intended to explore the effects of adding other components to standard BCT to enhance secondary outcomes of interest. Pilot studies are also underway to determine if components added to BCT intended to reduce HIV risk behaviors, IPV, and issues facing lesbians with SUDs will also enhance the effects of standard BCT on these secondary outcomes.

Dissemination to Community-Based Settings

Although it has strong research support for its efficacy, BCT is not yet widely used in community-based alcoholism and drug abuse treatment settings. A national survey was conducted of 398 randomly selected U.S. substance abuse treatment programs that treated adults to determine the proportion of settings that use different family- and couple-based therapies (Fals-Stewart & Birchler, 2001). Based on responses from program administrators, 27% of the facilities provided some type of couple-based service mostly confined to assessment, that included couples. Less than 5% of the agencies used behaviorally oriented couple therapy, and none used BCT specifically.

In this survey program administrators were also queried about significant barriers to adoption of BCT; two primary concerns were raised. BCT was viewed as too costly to deliver, requiring too many sessions in its standard form. In addition, most BCT studies used master's-level therapists as treatment providers, but most community-based treatment programs employ counselors with less formal education or clinical training. Thus, the concern was that counselors who typically work in substance abuse treatment programs, most of whom have undergraduate degrees or less and have little formal clinical training, could not deliver BCT as effectively as master's-level therapists.

Two recently completed studies addressed each of these concerns regarding the use of BCT with men who abused substances. First, we evaluated the effectiveness of a briefer version of BCT. Brief BCT (six couple sessions and six individual sessions) and standard BCT were significantly more effective than IBT or PACT in terms of male partners' percentage of days abstinent and other outcome indicators during the year after treatment (Fals-Stewart, O'Farrell, & Birchler, 2001). Furthermore, brief BCT and standard BCT produced equivalent posttreatment outcomes. A second parallel study with male patients who were drug dependent produced similar findings as with the male patients who were alcohol dependent (Fals-Stewart, Klostermann, Yates, O'Farrell, & Birchler, 2005).

We also examined the differential effect of BCT based on counselors' educational background, comparing outcomes of couples randomly assigned to be treated by either bachelor's- or master's-level counselors in delivering BCT (Fals-Stewart & Birchler, 2002). Results for 48 men with alcohol dependence and their female partners showed that, in comparison to master's-level counselors, bachelor's-level counselors were equivalent in terms of adherence ratings to a BCT treatment manual, but were rated lower in terms of quality of treatment

delivery. However, couples who received BCT from the bachelor's- and master's-level counselors reported equivalent (1) levels of satisfaction with treatment, (2) relationship happiness
during treatment, (3) levels of relationship adjustment, and (4) percentage of days abstinent
(for patients with alcohol dependence) at posttreatment, 3-, 6-, 9-, and 12-month follow-
up.

The findings of these investigations suggest that the primary identified barriers to BCT
implementation in community-based settings (i.e., concerns about counselors with limited
educational backgrounds and that BCT required too many sessions) either were not found
when tested (i.e., no differential effectiveness of BCT based on counselors' educational background) or could be effectively overcome (i.e., use of an abbreviated version of BCT). Taken
together, the results of these studies suggest that BCT could potentially be delivered effectively
in the context of community-based substance abuse treatment programs, with one caveat:
These studies targeted male patients; comparable investigations are needed for women with
SUDs.

KEY POINTS

- Among female patients diagnosed with SUDs, dyadic and familial factors play a particularly
  salient role in etiology and maintenance of drinking and drug use behavior, as well as in relapse
  among patients who achieve stable periods of abstinence.
- Addressing these relationship and family factors may be a critical aspect of effective treatment
  efforts with married or cohabiting female patients diagnosed with SUDs.
- Three decades of research indicate that BCT is more effective, in terms of substance use,
  relationship quality, and family adjustment, than individual-based treatments for married or
  cohabiting males with SUDs and their non-substance-abusing female partners.
- Consistent with the findings of BCT with male patients, the results of two randomized clinical
  trials with married or cohabiting female patients with SUDs and their non-substance-abusing male partners revealed that BCT was more efficacious than individual-based treatments
  across multiple domains of functioning.
- More trials are needed to examine not only whether or not BCT is effective for married or
  cohabiting females with SUDs, but also to explore how it works (i.e., its mechanisms of action)
  and how it might be modified to meet the unique needs of different couple types (lesbian
  couples, dual-substance-using partners) .

REFERENCES

Asterisks denote recommended readings.

Allan, C. A., & Cooke, D. J. (1985). Stressful life events and alcohol misuse in women: A critical
  review. *Journal of Studies on Alcohol, 46,* 147–152.
Annis, H. M., & Graham, J. M. (1995). Profile types on the Inventory of Drinking Situations: Implications for relapse prevention counseling. *Psychology of Addictive Behaviors, 9,* 176–182.
Becker, J. V., & Miller, P. M. (1976). Verbal and nonverbal marital interaction patterns of alcoholics
  and nonalcoholics. *Journal of Studies on Alcohol, 37,* 1616–1624.
Bendtsen, P., Dahlström, M., & Lejman, B. P. (2002). Sociodemographic gender differences in patients
  attending a community-based alcohol treatment center. *Addictive Behaviors, 27,* 21–33.
Birchler, G. R., & Fals-Stewart, W. (2007, June). *Learning sobriety together.* Workshop presented at the
  Smart Marriages Conference, Denver, CO.

Blum, L. N., Nielsen, N. H., & Riggs, J. A. (1998). Alcoholism and alcohol abuse among women: Report of the Council on Scientific Affairs. *Journal of Women's Health, 7,* 861–871.

Brady, K. T., & Randall, C. L. (1999). Gender differences in substance use disorders. *Psychiatric Clinics of North America, 22,* 241–252.

Connors, G. J., Maisto, S. A., & Zywiak, W. H. (1998). Male and female alcoholics' attributions regarding the onset and termination of relapses and the maintenance of abstinence. *Journal of Substance Abuse, 10,* 27–42.

Daley, D., Mercer, D., & Carpenter, G. (1998). *Group drug counseling manual.* Holmes Beach, FL: Learning Publications.

Dunn, N. J., Jacob, T., Hummon, N., & Seilhamer, R. A. (1987). Marital stability in alcoholic-spouse relationships as a function of drinking pattern and location. *Journal of Abnormal Psychology, 96,* 99–107.

Edwards, M. E., & Steinglass, P. (1995). Family therapy treatment outcomes for alcoholism. *Journal of Marital and Family Therapy, 21,* 475–490.

Epstein, E. E., McCrady, B. S., & Morgan, T. J. (2007). Couples treatment for drug-dependent males: Preliminary efficacy of a stand alone outpatient model. *Addictive Disorders and Their Treatment, 6,* 21–37.

Fals-Stewart, W., & Birchler, G. R. (1994). *Marital functioning among substance-abusing patients in outpatient treatment.* Poster presented at the Annual Meeting of the Association for Advancement of Behavior Therapy, San Diego, CA.

Fals-Stewart, W., & Birchler, G. R. (2001). A national survey of the use of couples therapy in substance abuse treatment. *Journal of Substance Abuse Treatment, 20,* 277–283.

Fals-Stewart, W., & Birchler, G. R. (2002). Behavioral couples therapy for alcoholic men and their intimate partners: The comparative effectiveness of master's- and bachelor's-level counselors. *Behavior Therapy, 33,* 123–147.

Fals-Stewart, W., Birchler, G. R., & Kelley, M. L. (2006). Learning Sobriety Together: A randomized clinical trial examining behavioral couples therapy with alcoholic female patients. *Journal of Consulting and Clinical Psychology, 74,* 579–591. (*)

Fals-Stewart, W., Birchler, G. R., & O'Farrell, T. J. (1999). Drug-abusing patients and their intimate partners: Dyadic adjustment, relationship stability, and substance use. *Journal of Abnormal Psychology, 108,* 11–23. (*)

Fals-Stewart, W., Birchler, G. R., & O'Farrell, T. J. (2001, July). Use of abbreviated couples therapy in substance abuse treatment. In J. V. Cordova (Chair), *Approaches to brief couples therapy: Application and efficacy.* Symposium conducted at the World Congress of Behavioral and Cognitive Therapies, Vancouver, BC.

Fals-Stewart, W., Fincham, F., Vendetti, K., & Kelley, M. L. (2003, August). *The effect of adding parent skills training to behavioral couples therapy.* Poster presented at the 110th annual convention of the American Psychological Association, Toronto, ON.

Fals-Stewart, W., Kashdan, T. B., O'Farrell, T. J., & Birchler, G. R. (2002). Behavioral couples therapy for drug-abusing patients: Effects on partner violence. *Journal of Substance Abuse Treatment, 22,* 87–96.

Fals-Stewart, W., Klostermann, K., Yates, B. T., O'Farrell, T. J., & Birchler, G. R. (2005). Brief relationship therapy for alcoholism: A randomized clinical trial examining clinical efficacy and cost-effectiveness. *Psychology of Addictive Behaviors, 19,* 363–371.

Fals-Stewart, W., O'Farrell, T. J., & Birchler, G. R. (2001, June). Both brief and extended behavioral couples therapy produce better outcomes than individual treatment for alcoholic patients. In T. J. O'Farrell (Chair), *Behavioral couples therapy for alcohol and drug problems: Recent advances.* Symposium conducted at the 24th annual scientific meeting of the Research Society on Alcoholism, Montreal, QU.

Fals-Stewart, W., O'Farrell, T. J., & Birchler, G. R. (2007, November). Behavioral couples therapy for gay and lesbian couples. In T. J. O'Farrell (Chair), *Behavioral couples therapy for addictive disorders: New applications.* Symposium conducted at the annual meeting of the Association for the Advancement of Behavioral and Cognitive Therapies, Philadelphia, PA.

Fals-Stewart, W., O'Farrell, T. J., Birchler, G. R., Cordova, J., & Kelley, M. L. (2005). Behavioral couples therapy for alcoholism and drug abuse: Where we've been, Where we are, and where we're going. *Journal of Cognitive Psychotherapy, 30,* 1479–1495. (*)

Gerolamo, A. M. (2004). State of the science: Women and the nonpharmacological treatment of substance abuse. *Journal of the American Psychiatric Nurses Association, 10,* 181–189.

Gorman, C., Klostermann, K., Fals-Stewart, W., Birchler, G. R., & O'Farrell, T. J. (2004). *Treatment for dual drug-abusing couples: The effectiveness of contingency management plus couples therapy.* Poster presented at the 38th Annual Meeting of the Association for the Advancement of Behavior Therapy, New Orleans.

Greenfield, S. F., Brooks, A. J., Gordon, S. M., Green, C. A., Kropp, F., McHugh, K., et al., (2007). Substance abuse treatment entry, retention, and outcome in women: A review of the literature. *Drug and Alcohol Dependence, 86,* 1–21.

Grella, C. E., Scott, C. K., Foss, M. A., Joshi, V., & Hser, Y. I. (2003). Gender differences in drug treatment outcomes among participants in the Chicago Target Cities Study. *Evaluation and Program Planning, 26,* 297–310.

Hernandez-Avila, C. A., Rounsaville, B. J., & Kranzler, H. R. (2004). Opioid-, cannabis- and alcohol-dependent women show more rapid progression to substance abuse treatment. *Drug and Alcohol Dependence, 74,* 265–272.

Hser, Y., Evans, E., & Huang, Y. (2005). Treatment outcomes among women and men methamphetamine abusers in California. *Journal of Substance Abuse Treatment, 28,* 77–85.

Hser, Y., Huang, D., Teruya, C., & Anglin, M. D. (2004). Diversity of drug abuse treatment utilization patterns and outcomes. *Evaluation and Program Planning, 27,* 309–319.

Jellinek, E. M. (1952). Phases of alcohol addiction. *Quarterly Journal of Studies on Alcohol, 13,* 673–684.

Kail, B. L., & Elberth, M. (2002). Moving the Latina substance abuser toward treatment: The role of gender and culture. *Journal of Ethnicity in Substance Abuse, 1,* 3–16.

Kelley, M. L., & Fals-Stewart, W. (2002). Couples versus individual-based therapy for alcoholism and drug abuse: Effects on children's psychosocial adjustment. *Journal of Consulting and Clinical Psychology, 70,* 417–427. (*)

Kelley, M. L., & Fals-Stewart, W. (2007). Treating paternal alcoholism with Learning Sobriety Together: Effects on adolescents versus preadolescents. *Journal of Family Psychology, 21,* 435–444. (*)

Kidorf, M., Disney, E. R., King, V. L., Neufeld, K., Beilenson, P. L., & Bronner, R. K. (2004). Prevalence of psychiatric and substance use disorders in opioid abusers in a community syringe exchange program. *Drug and Alcohol Dependence, 74,* 115–122.

Laudet, A., Magura, S., Furst, R. T., Kumar, N., & Whitney, S. (1999). Male partners of substance-abusing women in treatment: An exploratory study. *American Journal of Drug and Alcohol Abuse, 25,* 607–627.

Lemke, S., Brennan, P. L., & Schutte, K. K. (2007). Upward pressures on drinking: Exposure and reactivity in adulthood. *Journal of Studies on Alcohol and Drugs, 68,* 437–445.

Longabaugh, R., & Wirtz, P. W. (Eds.). (2001). *Project MATCH hypothesis: Results and causal chain analyses. Project MATCH Monograph Series,* Vol. 8 (NIH Publication No. 01-4238). Washington, DC: U.S. Department of Health and Human Services.

Longabaugh, R., Wirtz, P. W., Beattie, M., Noel, N., & Stout, R. (1995). Matching treatment focus to patient social investment and support: 18-month follow-up results. *Journal of Consulting and Clinical Psychology, 63,* 296–307.

Maisto, S. A., O'Farrell, T. J., McKay, J., Connors, G. J., & Pelcovitz, M. A. (1988). Alcoholics' attributions of factors affecting their relapse to drinking and reasons for terminating relapse events. *Addictive Behaviors, 13,* 79–82.

McCrady, B. S., Hayaki, J., Epstein, E. E., & Hirsch, L. S. (2002). Testing hypothesized predictors of change in conjoint behavioral alcoholism treatment for men. *Alcoholism: Clinical and Experimental Research, 26,* 463–470.

Mohr, J. J., & Fassinger, R. E. (2006). Sexual orientation identity and romantic relationship quality in same-sex couples. *Personality and Social Psychology Bulletin, 8,* 1085–1099.

Moos, R. H., Finney, J. W., & Cronkite, R. C. (1990). *Alcoholism treatment, context, process, and outcome.* New York: Oxford University Press.

O'Farrell, T. J., Cutter, H. S. G., Choquette, K. A., Floyd, F. J., & Bayog, R. D. (1992). Behavioral marital therapy for male alcoholics: Marital and drinking adjustment during two years after treatment. *Behavior Therapy, 23,* 529–549.

O'Farrell, T. J., Murphy, C. M., & Stephan, S. H. (2004). Partner violence before and after couples-based alcoholism treatment for male alcoholic patients: The role of treatment involvement and abstinence. *Journal of Consulting and Clinical Psychology, 72,* 202–217.

Oggins, J., Guydish, J., & Delucchi, K. (2001). Gender differences in income after substance abuse treatment. *Journal of Substance Abuse Treatment, 20,* 215–224.

Orlinski, D. E., Grawe, K., & Parks, B. K. (1994). Process and outcome in psychotherapy—Noch einmal. In A. E. Bergin & S. L. Garfield (Eds.), *Handbook of psychotherapy and behavior change* (pp. 270–283). New York: Wiley.

Project MATCH Research Group. (1998a). Matching alcoholism treatments to client heterogeneity: Treatment main effects and matching effects on drinking during treatment. *Journal of Studies on Alcohol, 59,* 631–639.

Project MATCH Research Group. (1998b). Matching alcoholism treatment to client heterogeneity: Project MATCH three-year drinking outcomes. *Alcoholism: Clinical and Experimental Research, 22,* 1300–1311.

Randall, C. L., Roberts, J. S., DelBoca, F. K., Carroll, K. M., Connors, G. J., & Matson, M. E. (1999). Telescoping of landmark events associated with drinking: A gender comparison. *Journal of Studies on Alcohol, 60,* 252–260.

Sanchez-Craig, M., Leigh, G., Spivak, K., & Lei, H. (1989). Superior outcomes of females over males after a brief treatment for reduction of heavy drinking. *British Journal of Addiction, 84,* 395–404.

Sonne, S. C., Back, S. E., Zuniga, C. D., Randall, C. L., & Brady, K. T. (2003). Gender differences in individuals with comorbid alcohol dependence and post-traumatic stress disorder. *American Journal on Addictions, 12,* 412–423.

Stewart, D., Gossop, M., & Trakada, K. (2007). Drug dependent parents: Childcare responsibilities, involvement with treatment services, and treatment outcomes. *Addictive Behaviors, 32,* 1657–1668.

Stiles, W. B., & Shapiro, D. A. (1994). Disabuse of the drug metaphor: Psychotherapy process–outcome correlation. *Journal of Consulting and Clinical Psychology, 62,* 942–948.

Straussner, S. L. A., & Zelvin, E. (Eds.). (1997). *Gender and addiction: Men and women in treatment.* Northvale, NJ: Jason Aronson.

Sun, A. (2007). Relapse among substance-abusing women: Components and processes. *Substance Use and Misuse, 42,* 1–21.

Vaillant, G. E. (1995). *The natural history of alcoholism revisited.* Cambridge, MA: Harvard University Press.

Webster, J. M., Rosen, P. J., & McDonald, H. S. (2007). Mental health as a mediator of gender differences in employment barriers among drug abusers. *American Journal of Drug and Alcohol Abuse, 33,* 259–265.

Winters, J., Fals-Stewart, W., O'Farrell, T. J., Birchler, G. R., & Kelley, M. L. (2002). Behavioral couples therapy for female substance-abusing patients: Effects on substance use and relationship adjustment. *Journal of Consulting and Clinical Psychology, 70,* 344–355. (*)

PART V

SPECIFIC SUBSTANCES

CHAPTER 20

Women, Girls, and Alcohol

Sherry H. Stewart, PhD
Dubravka Gavric, BA
Pamela Collins, BA

Traditionally, alcohol use disorders were thought to be a problem largely affecting men. Thus, women were underrepresented in theory and research on the nature, development, and maintenance of this disorder (Amaro, Blake, Schwartz, & Flinchbaugh, 2001). Women and girls were also underserved in treatment centers and in prevention programming. Fortunately, it is increasingly recognized that alcohol touches the lives of most girls and women in our society, whether because they are drinkers themselves or they have been affected by a family member or partner's drinking (Poole & Dell, 2005). Moreover, it is now better understood that a substantial portion of girls and women are at risk for, or already experience, alcohol abuse and dependence, and that females show different drinking patterns, as well as risk and maintenance factors, for alcohol use disorders. There is now considerable evidence that women with alcohol problems have unique alcohol treatment and prevention needs relative to their male counterparts.

This chapter begins with a review of the evidence for the *convergence hypothesis*— the notion that the gender gap in various indices of alcohol use/misuse is closing. We cite data suggesting that women develop problem drinking at a later age than men, on average, but progress to alcohol dependence more quickly. We discuss mechanisms that have been advanced to explain this "telescoping effect" among women and review evidence on sex differences in drinking motives and implications for prevention and treatment. Common forms of comorbid psychological disorders faced by women with alcohol use disorders (i.e., eating disorders, borderline personality, depression, anxiety, and post-traumatic stress) are discussed along with implications for improving treatment efficacy for women. Finally, sex differences in treatment seeking for alcohol problems are discussed, and potential barriers for women in accessing treatment for alcohol problems are identified. We review the literature to determine whether women-specific and gender-sensitive programming has been successful in addressing women clients' traditional underrepresentation in alcohol treatment and in improving their treatment outcome.

THE CONVERGENCE HYPOTHESIS

Although alcohol is the most common substance used by women (e.g., Adlaf, Begin, & Sawka, 2005), studies that have examined alcohol use and abuse across societies and cultures consistently confirm that men exceed women in both absolute drinking levels and rates of alcohol misuse (Wilsnack, Vogeltanz, Wilsnack, & Harris, 2000). However, with the changing roles of women in Western society beginning around the 1970s, research reports began to suggest that women's drinking levels and drinking problems were increasing and more closely approximating those seen among men (Kalant, 1980). This notion of women's consumption patterns "catching up" with those of men in more recent years is referred to as the "convergence hypothesis" (Greenfield & Room, 1997).

Let us first examine why there might be sex differences in drinking levels before we turn to a critical examination of the evidence for the convergence hypothesis. The two major theoretical perspectives that help explain sex differences in drinking behavior emphasize either biological or sociocultural explanatory factors. The biological perspective holds that, at similar doses of alcohol, women reach higher peak blood alcohol levels than do men for a number of reasons (Haas & Peters, 2000). In comparison to men, women on average have a lower body weight, have a smaller proportion of water volume in their bodies, and have lower levels of alcohol-metabolizing enzymes (Ammon, Schafer, Hofmann, & Klotz, 1996). Thus, their resultant higher blood alcohol levels per unit of alcohol consumed could lead women to drink less to obtain the same effects as men (Marshall, Kingstone, Boss, & Morgan, 1983). Because of these biological differences, some recommend that epidemiological surveys need to first adjust alcohol quantity or volume measures for sex differences in body fluid and body weight before examining overall sex differences in consumption levels (e.g., Mercer & Khavari, 1990).

The sociocultural explanation contends that gender-specific social roles cause women and men to drink differently. For example, traditional beliefs dictate that drinking affects women's social responsibilities and behavior more adversely than men's. In effect, intoxication in a woman was thought to signal a failure of control over her family relationships and social/public behavior (Child, Barry, & Bacon, 1965). From a sociocultural perspective, the traditional stigmatization of heavy drinking among women was thought to exert a protective influence, in effect keeping women's consumption lower, on average, than that of men, since women would fear being judged negatively for excessive drinking. Together, these various biological and sociocultural factors may help explain why men drink more heavily, on average, than women and are at greater risk for alcohol use disorders.

But despite these well-established sex differences in drinking levels and rates of alcohol problems, there is considerable research evidence supporting the convergence hypothesis. For example, Keyes, Grant, and Hasin (2008) examined a sample of 42,693 adults in the 2001–2002 National Epidemiologic Survey on Alcohol and Related Conditions (NESARC). Outcomes included largest number of drinks consumed in the participant's lifetime; frequent binge drinking (defined as drinking 5+ drinks once per week or more during the period of heaviest drinking); and alcohol abuse and dependence diagnoses according to the fourth edition, text revised, of the *Diagnostic and Statistical Manual of Mental Disorders* (American Psychiatric Association, 2000). Outcomes were examined as a function of birth cohort and sex. The authors conducted analyses to examine whether birth cohorts (i.e., born 1913–1932, 1933–1949, 1950–1967, or 1968–1984) affected the magnitude of sex differences in the lifetime prevalence of these four outcomes. An interaction between birth cohort and sex was significant for all four alcohol outcomes, with sex differences in the prevalence of all four drinking measures decreasing in the cohorts born more recently. Keyes and colleagues suggest several explanations for their findings. First, there may be a true cohort effect whereby drinking behaviors (and the potential risks for alcohol use disorders) are indeed converging between men and women born after the 1960s. Mechanisms for such a true cohort effect might include women's increased socialization to traditional male roles, exposure to print advertising increasing the social acceptability and decreasing the negative perceptions associated with drinking in women (Poole & Dell, 2005), increases in women working outside the home (since work stress is often related to drinking), and decreases in women having children (increasing women's exposure to drinking contexts outside of the home). Alternatively, since norms have changed in our society regarding the need for women to adhere to certain "moral" codes of behavior (e.g., the traditional norm that "proper" women abstain from heavy drinking), these changing norms may have resulted in women feeling more comfortable in accurately self-reporting their drinking without concern of being stigmatized. In other words, due to a general relaxation of sex roles and reduced stigmatization in more recent years, evidence for convergence may be based on a decrease in underreporting among women, rather than on an actual increase in women's drinking (Babcock, 1996). Regardless of why the gender gap in alcohol use disorders is narrowing, findings such as these suggest that women in younger cohorts are in particular need of targeted prevention and intervention efforts.

The findings of Keyes et al. (2008) are very consistent with those of another recent population survey by Grucza, Bucholz, Rice, and Bierut (2008). These researchers employed data from two large, national epidemiological surveys conducted in the United States. They used repeated cross-sectional analysis to compare lifetime drinking and lifetime prevalence of alcohol dependence across birth cohorts that were temporally adjacent and surveyed at the same age. This method enabled estimates of cross-cohort differences while controlling for effects due to age. The results showed few significant cross-cohort differences among groups of men compared at similar ages. In marked contrast, women born between 1954 and 1963 were at significantly increased risk for lifetime drinking, and those who drank were at significantly increased risk for lifetime alcohol dependence, compared with the immediately preceding birth cohort born between 1944 and 1953. Moreover, the 1944–1953 cohort of women was also at significantly increased risk for lifetime drinking compared with their predecessors (i.e., women in the birth cohort both from 1934 to 1943). The authors concluded that there have been substantial increases in drinking and alcohol dependence among women but not men in our culture over the past several decades (Grucza et al., 2008), providing further evidence for the convergence hypothesis.

In fact, evidence for the convergence hypothesis is emerging internationally (e.g., Kraus, Bloomfield, Augustin, & Reese, 2000; Roche & Deehan, 2002). For example, using data from a population survey conducted in New Zealand, McPherson, Casswell, and Pledger (2004) examined the results of a large study (4,000–5,000+ participants ages 14–65) conducted in 1995 and 2000 to compare women's and men's alcohol consumption patterns and problems. Both surveys employed quantity and frequency measures to determine alcohol consumption. This study found significant gender convergence (defined as women's alcohol consumption moving toward that of the men) on all quantity measures and also for frequency of consumption, but with greater convergence observed in the younger age groups. The authors offered several possible social explanations for this convergence, including increases in rates of women living alone, cohabiting, working in nontraditional roles, and not having children. The authors contended that policy issues also contribute to this convergence. For example, they argue that policy shifts involving more readily accessible alcohol (e.g., in cafes and supermarkets) create conditions where more younger women are drinking publicly and consuming larger quantities of alcohol.

In summary, studies from around the world provide quite consistent evidence of gender convergence and suggest that this convergence appears particularly pronounced among younger women (i.e., women born since the advent of the women's movement). In fact, in recent years, several alarming trends in female adolescent alcohol use have emerged. Recent findings indicate an increased rate of alcohol involvement among adolescent girls, with a decline in the age of girls' first use, higher rates of alcohol use initiation, and an increased involvement of adolescent girls in alcohol-related crime (e.g., Grant & Dawson, 1997). Such findings suggest the need for further attention to monitoring trends in females' drinking behavior and to developing targeted prevention programming for younger women.

TELESCOPING EFFECTS

The fact that alcohol use and misuse is on the rise among young women today is particularly concerning, given that girls and women appear more vulnerable to the effects of alcohol than boys and men. One such consistent gender difference in the alcohol research field is the finding that women tend to have shorter drinking histories before seeking treatment, yet the severity of their problems upon treatment entry rivals that of men. This phenomenon has been termed "telescoping" and has found support in a multitude of research studies (Piazza, Vrbka, & Yeager, 1989). For example, several studies have found that although women report the beginning of regular drinking patterns at a significantly later age than men, their entry into addiction treatment actually occurs earlier than for their male counterparts (e.g., Johnson, Richter, Kleber, McLellan, & Carise, 2005). In addition, research has shown that at the time of entry into a treatment program, women present with more severe symptoms than males, despite their shorter drinking history (e.g., Hernandez-Avila, Rounsaville, & Kranzler, 2004).

There are several possible explanations for the faster progression of alcohol-related problems found in women. One possibility focuses on biological differences between the sexes, discussed earlier in this chapter in the convergence hypothesis section (Ammon et al., 1996). These biological differences are thought to make females more vulnerable to the effects of alcohol. Taken together, differences in body weight, proportion of body water, and alcohol metabolism result in higher blood–alcohol concentrations in women versus men, which make women more susceptible to the negative effects of alcohol, especially under conditions of prolonged use (Brady & Randall, 1999). Perhaps due to this increased sensitivity, females with alcohol dependence consistently report more medical problems than males with alcohol dependence, despite having been drinking for shorter periods of time. Examples of such medical conditions include diseases of the liver (e.g., fatty liver), malnutrition, gastrointestinal hemorrhage, obesity, anemia, ulcers, hypertension, cardiovascular diseases, and brain atrophy (e.g., Frezza et al., 1990; Mann et al., 2005). In addition, compared to men, women with alcohol dependence are significantly more likely to exhibit a number of comorbid psychiatric conditions, as we cover in later sections of this chapter (e.g., Bjork, Dougherty, & Moeller, 1999). A higher prevalence rate of such medical and psychiatric conditions may make women more likely to seek treatment earlier relative to the onset of their heavy drinking.

A second possible explanation for the telescoping effect found in women involves sociocultural factors. In general, heavy drinking is viewed much more negatively when it occurs in women as opposed to men. Such stigmatization has several implications. On the one hand, it may serve as a protective factor that prevents women from engaging in heavy drinking and thus protects them against the development of alcohol-related problems. On the other hand, it may cause women to conceal their drinking behavior and prevent them from receiving treatment until their alcohol-related problems have become quite severe (Blankfield, 1990). A sociocultural theory of the telescoping effect has received support from numerous studies, which have found that sex differences in alcohol problem severity at treatment intake disappear in younger cohorts, among which societal sanctions against heavy drinking by women are lessened. For example, one study examined the telescoping of alcohol-related events and found significant sex differences, but only in the older age groups (Randall et al., 1999). In this study, significant sex differences present in the older cohorts either diminished or disappeared altogether when examining only the youngest participants. Randall and her colleagues suggested that the diminished results in the younger participants may reflect a change in societal norms, such that males and females are both entering treatment earlier than in previous generations. Another study, by Johnson et al. (2005), found similar results. Women reported initiating regular alcohol use at a later age than men, but began drinking to reach intoxication at an earlier stage of their drinking career than men—findings that suggest that women are progressing more rapidly from initial alcohol use to hazardous drinking. However, these findings were true for only the older cohort (30+ years); no significant sex differences in the rate of this progression were found in the younger cohorts. These findings suggest a sociocultural basis for telescoping.

A final explanation provided for telescoping effects cites women's higher utilization of health care services, in general (Randall et al., 1999). Based on this explanation, women's increased willingness to seek professional help would make them more likely then men to enter addiction treatment soon after they realize they have a problem with alcohol, potentially explaining women's earlier treatment-seeking behavior relative to the onset of their heavy drinking. However, this explanation does not help us understand the higher severity of alcohol-related problems women present with upon treatment entry. A study conducted by Dawson (1996) may provide an explanation. This study found that although men were more likely than women to receive treatment for alcohol-related problems, this difference disappeared in the most severely affected patients. Thus, although women are far less likely to receive treatment for alcohol-related problems, those who do enter addiction treatment are more likely exhibit severe symptoms. This finding, combined with women's increased use of general health care services, suggests that women with mild-to-moderate alcohol-related problems may seek help from sources other than formal addiction services (e.g., family physicians, psychologists, psychiatrists), and thus be underrepresented in research studies where participants for alcohol-related research are drawn from those who utilize addiction services. We come back to such issues of women's accessing and utilization of alcohol treatment in the last section of this chapter.

Based on the research discussed here, it is clear that there are significant sex differences in alcohol use patterns. Much research suggests that women begin drinking later than men, but that there is a faster progression from drinking onset to alcohol-related problems among women than men with alcohol dependence, although this telescoping effect may be decreasing in the younger age ranges. Although there is ample evidence suggesting the existence of the telescoping effect, the exact mechanisms and causes of it are still not clear, and further research is necessary.

MOTIVES FOR DRINKING AMONG WOMEN

In this section we examine whether girls and women might drink for different reasons than boys and men. As mentioned earlier, research suggests different drinking patterns among

men and women, with men generally demonstrating higher rates of alcohol use, more negative consequences of alcohol use, and increased rates of alcohol use disorder (e.g., O'Malley
& Johnston, 2002). Some emerging research evidence also suggests that reasons for drinking,
or "drinking motives," might also vary by sex and that different motives may be associated
with alcohol use for men versus women. Women appear more likely to drink to reduce negative affect and/or to deal with emotional pain (i.e., for "coping" motives). In contrast, men
are more likely to drink to enhance pleasurable emotional states and in reaction to social
pressure (i.e., for "enhancement" and "conformity" motives; e.g., Annis & Graham, 1995;
Schall, Weede, & Maltzman, 1991). Cooper (1994) found that although the relations of
various drinking motives to patterns of use were largely invariant across gender, conformity
motives were more strongly correlated with greater drinking for men than for women.

Harrell and Karim (2008) examined sex differences in the relations of drinking motives
to various indices of alcohol use and misuse in a college student sample of 266 females and
140 males with a mean age of 19 years. As hypothesized, the authors found that among
males, drinking to "feel high" (i.e., enhancement drinking) was significantly correlated with
problems related to alcohol use and with frequency of alcohol use and frequency of binge
drinking. With the females, alcohol-related problems were associated with self-reported
depressive symptoms. The authors concluded that the motivation to drink to "feel high" is
the way that boys and men are socialized in our culture when it comes to alcohol, and thus
enhancement motives are more often related to greater drinking behavior and more alcohol
problems among young men than women. They concluded that for young women, negative
affective spheres are the more relevant motivation for drinking.

Such findings could have positive implications in terms of tailoring gender-specific prevention and treatment efforts. With regard to preventing or treating heavy drinking and
problem use, young women may benefit from training in negative emotion regulation strategies, whereas young men may benefit most from learning to manage peer pressure and from
finding alternate sources of arousal enhancement.

ALCOHOL USE DISORDERS
AND MENTAL HEALTH COMORBIDITY IN WOMEN

As we discussed earlier in the telescoping section, women appear more vulnerable to the
effects of alcohol in terms of being more prone to the development of adverse medical conditions as a consequence of their drinking. Women with alcohol use disorders also appear more
likely to display a variety of comorbid mental health conditions, relative to men with alcohol
use disorders. In this section we discuss several of the more common forms of comorbid mental health disorders faced by many women with alcohol problems; namely, eating disorders,
borderline personality disorder, depression, and anxiety disorders, including posttraumatic
stress disorder (PTSD).

Eating Disorder Comorbidity

Many research studies have found that the co-occurrence of alcohol use problems and disordered eating is common in women. Although the exact rate of comorbidity varies across
studies, a comprehensive review by Holderness, Brooks-Gunn, and Warren (1994) found
that as many as 49% of women with eating disorders are also diagnosed with alcohol abuse/
dependence, and as many 89% report alcohol use that does not meet the criteria for abuse/
dependence. Furthermore, this finding has been supported in clinical as well as nonclinical

samples (e.g., Bulik, Sullivan, McKee, Wehzin, & Kaye, 1994; Dansky, Brewerton, & Kilpatrick, 2000). In addition, just as high rates of alcohol use problems have been found in women with eating disorders, the converse is also true. That is, women who have problems with alcohol use demonstrate a higher prevalence of eating disorders (e.g., Stewart, Brown, Devoulyte, Theakston, & Larsen, 2006). Although increased rates of alcohol problems are found in all types of eating disorders, the finding is most robust among those women with bulimia nervosa and those with the binge–purge subtype of anorexia nervosa, as opposed to those with restricting anorexia nervosa (e.g., Dunn, Larimer, & Neighbors, 2001).

Alcohol abuse and binge eating share several important features that may explain their high rates of co-occurrence. For example, individuals with either disorder have a tendency to lose control, engage in excessive behavior, and experience feelings of depression, anger, guilt, powerlessness, or self-loathing in response to a binge drinking or eating episode. Given these similarities, researches have postulated several theories, all of which propose that alcohol use disorders and eating disorders may have the same underlying cause. One such theory proposes that women suffering from either an alcohol use or eating disorder may engage in "symptom substitution." For example, one study found that a patient who was abusing alcohol began exhibiting symptoms of bulimia while trying to abstain from alcohol use, and that these bulimic symptoms disappeared once the patient returned to previous heavy drinking patterns (Cepik, Arikan, Boratav, & Isik, 1995). Similarly, Cowan and Devine (2008) found that patients recovering from alcohol use disorders demonstrated high rates of disordered eating, such as binge eating, substituting food for alcohol use, and using food to diminish alcohol cravings. These findings were especially prominent during the early alcoholism recovery phase. Although there is some evidence for the symptom substitution hypothesis, this theory fails to explain the underlying mechanisms and motivations common to both alcohol use and eating disorders (Stewart & Brown, 2007). In addition, if symptom substitution were the primary reason for the high comorbidity of these disorders, one would expect to find increased alcohol use in patients recovering from eating disorders, and this has not been reported in the literature (Mitchell, Pyle, Eckert, & Hatsukami, 1990).

A second possible explanation for the high coexistence of alcohol use and eating disorders proposes that both disorders provide a coping mechanism for dealing with stressful life events (Anderson, Simmons, Martens, Ferrierr, & Sheehy, 2006). A body of research demonstrates that the motivation for women's alcohol use comes from their desire to regulate negative emotional states, and that this motivation is related to an increase in alcohol use problems (e.g., Birch, Stewart, & Brown, 2007). Similarly, disordered eating may also provide a way for women to cope with stress and negative emotions—a notion that has found support in the literature (e.g., Sherwood, Crowther, & Ben-Porath, 2000). Both alcohol misuse and binge eating may provide relief from stressful life events and may serve as a mechanism by which to manage unpleasant states (Stewart, Brown, et al., 2006). For example, both alcohol use and binge eating have been related to depression, and both may serve as a mechanism to alleviate sad mood (Stice, Burton, & Shaw, 2004).

A third explanation that has been provided to account for the high comorbidity of alcohol use and eating disorders comes from the finding that individuals suffering from both disorders tend to display elevated levels of impulsivity and difficulties with behavioral regulation (e.g., Marczinski, Combs, & Fillmore, 2007). Impulsivity is defined as a tendency to react in a rapid and unplanned manner to both internal and external stimuli, and to do so without consideration for the possible longer-term negative consequences of such actions (Moeller et al., 2001). Recent research has examined the effects of alcohol on impulsivity, and findings suggest that alcohol interferes with an individual's ability to inhibit inappropriate reactions (Fillmore, 2003). In addition, one study found that in comparison to a control group, people who engaged in binge drinking showed significantly higher impairments in behavioral control while under the influence of alcohol (Marczinski et al., 2007). These finding suggest that even moderate doses of alcohol may decrease behavioral inhibition and thereby increase the probability of impulsive behavior such as binge eating. As mentioned earlier in this section, the majority of comorbid alcohol problems in women with eating disorders occurs in women suffering from bulimia nervosa as opposed to anorexia nervosa (restricting subtype). It is possible that the impairments in behavioral inhibition found in women with bulimia makes them more susceptible to binge eating, whereas the rigid self-regulating behavior of women with the restrictive subtype of anorexia makes them better able to control their impulsiveness. Such impulse control may also provide an explanation for the lower rates of alcohol use disorders found in women with restrictive anorexia.

Family history provides a fourth possible explanation for the high comorbidity of alcohol use and eating disorders. Research has demonstrated that a high proportion of women who suffer from eating disorders has alcoholism in the family history (e.g., Lilenfeld et al., 1997). In a literature review, Holderness et al. (1994) found that among women with bulimia, family alcoholism rates were as high as 82% in some studies. In comparison, among individuals with anorexia, the prevalence of familial alcoholism was around 20%. Families in which alcohol misuse is prevalent are likely to be characterized by environments that are unstable, chaotic, negative, lacking in cohesion, and unpredictable, and in which family members are unable to provide necessary emotional support for the children (e.g., Coniglio, 1993). Such environments are unlikely to meet children's needs; thus, these children may later seek alternate sources for meeting their emotional needs, such as via heavy drinking and binge eating (Stewart & Brown, 2007).

Borderline Personality Disorder Comorbidity

There is ample research evidence documenting high cooccurrence rates of alcohol use disorders and borderline personality disorder (e.g., Trull, Sher, Minks-Brown, Durbin, & Burr, 2000)—one of the more common personality disorders among women (Durand, Barlow, & Stewart, 2008). In a literature review, Trull et al. (2000) found that as many as 49% of participants with borderline personality disorder also exhibited symptoms of alcohol use or dependence, and that 14% of individuals with alcohol use disorders also exhibited borderline personality symptoms. Research has shown that borderline personality disorder is among the most common Axis II disorders in alcohol-abusing populations. For example, one study found that 18% of individuals entering alcoholism treatment also had a comorbid diagnosis of bipolar disorder (Verheul et al., 2000). The high rates of comorbidity between these two disorders are troubling, in that there is evidence to suggest an increase in severity and adverse consequences when the two disorders occur in the same individual (e.g., Links, Heslegrave, Mitton, van Reekum, & Patrick, 1995). For example, Griggs and Tyrer (1981) showed that individuals suffering from both alcohol use and borderline personality disorders have worse treatment outcomes in group therapy. Miller, Abrams, Dulit, and Fyer (1993) reported that, in comparison to women who were diagnosed with borderline personality disorder alone, women with comorbid borderline personality disorder and alcohol abuse had higher rates of unemployment and prostitution and lower levels of education.

Several theories have been proposed to explain the high co-occurrence of alcohol use and borderline personality disorders in women. One such theory proposes that women with these disorders share certain personality characteristics, such as impulsivity, which may make the development of both disorders more likely. In fact, one of the diagnostic criteria for borderline disorder is impulsivity or a failure to plan for the future (DSM-IV-TR; American

Psychiatric Association, 2000). Likewise, individuals diagnosed with alcohol use disorders generally exhibit higher rates of impulsive behavior than are found in the general population (e.g., Fillmore, 2003). These findings can be interpreted in a number of ways. On the one hand, it is possible that impulsivity is a shared characteristic in individuals who are affected by both disorders. On the other hand, it is possible that women with borderline personality disorder have an inherent tendency toward impulsive behavior, and that this makes them increasingly likely to misuse alcohol in situations where less impulsive individuals would discontinue drinking (Trull et al., 2000).

Family history has also been implicated as a possible explanation for the comorbidity of alcohol use and borderline personality disorders (e.g., Paris, 2000). This body of research suggests that the comorbidity of alcohol use and borderline personality can be attributed to genetic factors. However, there is also evidence to suggest that individuals with both disorders have significantly more troubling childhoods. For example, one study found that patients with borderline personality disorder experienced significantly higher rates of family violence and sexual abuse in childhood (Bandelow et al., 2005). These findings suggest that an interaction between genetics and environment may predispose individuals to suffer from both disorders.

Another explanation that attempts to explain the high co-occurrence rates of alcohol use and borderline personality disorders in women focuses on affective regulation, or the ability to regulate one's internal mood sates. One of the key diagnostic features of borderline personality disorder is affective instability (American Psychological Association, 2000), and a recent line of research has demonstrated that patients with borderline personality exhibit higher rates of affective instability, compared to healthy controls (e.g., Russell, Moskowitz, Zuroff, Sookman, & Paris, 2007). As was mentioned previously, the use of alcohol as a coping mechanism for dealing with negative affect is common among women with alcohol use problems (Birch et al., 2007). Thus, it is possible that the higher levels of emotional dysregulation in patients with borderline personality lead them to use alcohol as a way of coping with their ever-fluctuating emotional states.

Depression Comorbidity

Alcohol use disorders and depression are highly comorbid conditions. The odds ratio (OR) for someone with an alcohol use disorder to experience depression at some point in his or her lifetime is 4.8 (Grant et al., 2004). There are sex differences in the rate of comorbid depression among individuals with alcoholic dependence. Even after accounting for the higher prevalence of depression among women, women with alcohol use disorders are significantly more likely to experience a comorbid depression than men with alcohol use disorders. In other words, women with alcohol dependence have a higher OR for comorbid depression (relative to gender-specific base rates) than men with alcohol dependence (i.e., OR of 4.05 and 2.95 for women versus men with alcohol use disorders, respectively; Kessler et al., 1997).

Another area in which interesting sex differences occur among those with alcohol use disorders is with respect to the distinction between independent comorbid depression and alcohol-induced co-morbid depression. DSM-IV-TR (American Psychiatric Association, 2000) places importance on, and provides a clear distinction between, depression that is "independent" versus "alcohol-induced." To be considered an independent depression, the individual must have either a history of depression prior to the onset of the alcohol use disorder or must have experienced depression during a substantially lengthy period of alcohol abstinence (DSM-IV-TR; American Psychiatric Association, 2000). In contrast, alcohol-induced depression is considered a secondary consequence of heavy alcohol use and is expected to remit within 4–6 weeks of abstinence (Schuckit et al., 1997). Among those with co-occurring alcoholism and depression, women are more likely to have an independent depression (66%), whereas men are more likely to have an alcohol-induced depression (78%) (e.g., Zilberman, Tavares, Blume, & el-Guebaly, 2003).

The higher rates of independent depression among women with alcohol use disorders may have important clinical implications for at least two reasons. First, independent depression may be linked with greater severity of alcohol problems and with more difficulties during the alcoholism treatment process. For example, some studies have linked independent depression with more frequent alcohol abuse relapses and with more suicide attempts than alcohol-induced depression (e.g., Ramsey, Kahler, Read, Stuart, & Brown, 2004). And recent findings from our research group show that for women with alcohol problems, compared to men with alcohol problems, independent depression is associated with a more complex clinical presentation (e.g., more comorbid anxiety disorders) as well as more severe substance use problems (Sabourin & Stewart, in press). Second, by definition, independent depression is not expected to remit with alcohol abstinence (DSM-IV-TR; American Psychiatric Association, 2000). Thus, women with co-occurring depression are more likely than men with co-occurring depression to require treatment services that specifically address their depression either concurrently or sequentially with their alcoholism treatment (e.g., Brown, Evans, Miller, Burgess, & Mueller, 1997). An integrated treatment approach that considers the interrelations between women's experiences of depression and their alcohol misuse is likely to be of most benefit, given the involvement of these women in a vicious cycle of self-medication for depression with alcohol misuse whereby each disorder appears to mutually maintain the other (Brown & Stewart, 2008).

Anxiety Disorder and PTSD Comorbidity

Whereas alcohol use disorders are more common in men, anxiety disorders are more common in women (e.g., Lewis, Bucholz, Spitznagel, & Shayka, 1996). However, when we compare ORs calculated using sex-specific base rates, some interesting patterns emerge in terms of sex differences in the comorbidity of alcohol use disorders with anxiety disorders (Kushner, Krueger, Frye, & Peterson, 2008). When examining comorbidity across specific anxiety disorder categories with alcohol abuse and alcohol dependence in the National Co-Morbidity Survey (Kessler et al., 1997), no positive associations were found for men between alcohol abuse and any of the specific anxiety disorders examined (i.e., generalized anxiety disorder [GAD], panic disorder with or without agoraphobia, social phobia, simple phobia, and PTSD). In fact, PTSD and GAD both have negative associations with alcohol abuse in men! For example, men with PTSD are only half as likely as men without PTSD to have a comorbid alcohol abuse diagnosis. In contrast, several of these ORs were positive for women, and across all anxiety disorders, the odds ratio was 1.8. In other words, women with any anxiety disorder were about twice as likely as women without anxiety disorders to be diagnosed with a comorbid alcohol abuse diagnosis; the corresponding OR for men was 1.0 across all anxiety disorders, indicating no association between anxiety disorders overall and alcohol abuse for men. A similar gender difference is present in the ORs for the comorbidity of anxiety disorders with alcohol dependence, in that the OR is stronger in women than in men (of 3.1 vs. 2.2, respectively; Kessler et al., 1997; see review in Kushner et al., 2008). Considering all anxiety and alcohol use disorders together, women with any anxiety disorder are approximately one-third more likely to have a comorbid alcohol use disorder, as compared to their male counterparts (overall ORs of 2.5 and 1.6, respectively). Thus, although there is comorbidity between anxiety disorders and alcohol use disorders in both genders, this form of comorbidity is favored in women.

It is not currently clear why this sex difference favoring comorbid anxiety disorders in women with alcohol dependence exists. One possibility, suggested by Kushner et al. (2008), is that women and men may be prone to different subtypes of alcohol use disorder. For example, Cloninger (1987) distinguishes between individuals with Type I alcohol dependence, who drink to escape from or to cope with anxiety, and Type II individuals who drink for other reasons. According to Cloninger's theory, both types are prone to different forms of mental health comorbidity, with Type I specifically prone to "neurotic" psychopathology (i.e., anxiety disorders). Consistent with Cloninger's (1987) original theory, there is some evidence that more women than men fall into the Type I category (e.g., Sannibale & Hall, 1998), which might help explain why women with alcohol dependence have a greater propensity toward comorbid anxiety disorders.

Although both men and women with PTSD are at increased risk for alcohol dependence (ORs of 3.2 and 3.6, respectively; Kessler et al., 1997), women with alcohol dependence report qualitatively different traumatic life experiences than do men with alcohol dependence (e.g., Back et al., 2000). For example, a review by Stewart, Grant, Ouimette, and Brown (2006) reveals that women are more likely than men to report histories of rape/sexual assault, childhood sexual abuse, and domestic violence. On the other hand, men are more likely to report histories of traumatic accidents, having been stabbed or shot at, and having experienced sudden serious injuries. And even though comorbid PTSD is a problem for many individuals with alcohol dependence (Stewart, Grant, et al., 2006), gender nonetheless appears important in the comorbidity of PTSD and alcohol use disorders in clinical samples. For example, in a study by Clark et al. (1997), even though there were no overall sex differences in PTSD comorbidity rates in their sample of adolescents with alcohol dependence, PTSD and alcohol abuse were more strongly associated among the adolescent girls than among the adolescent boys. Moreover, order-of-onset data suggest that PTSD precedes the development of alcohol use disorders more often in comorbid females than in comorbid males (Deykin & Buka, 1997). Both of the above findings are consistent with a self-medication explanation of comorbid PTSD and alcohol use disorders in women (Stewart, Grant, et al., 2006). The above findings also suggest that comorbid women may be particularly likely to benefit from an integrated treatment approach where both problems are addressed simultaneously in a treatment program that directly recognizes the interconnectedness of the trauma, PTSD, and alcohol abuse (Riggs & Foa, 2008; Stewart & Conrod, 2008).

WOMEN-SPECIFIC ALCOHOL TREATMENT SERVICES

Concerns have been raised about the effects of gender on the alcoholism treatment process and the fact that women face more barriers to treatment than men (e.g., Greenfield, Brooks, et al., 2007; Hodgins, el-Guebaly, & Addington, 1997). We still have a ways to go to fully understand how sex differences affect treatment process and outcome, and how to design treatment programs to best meet the unique needs of women with alcohol problems (Smith & Weisner, 2000). Hodgins et al. (1997) have provided a review of the literature from the 1970s to the 1990s as it pertains to gender and treatment of substance use disorders, including alcohol disorders. They conclude that because of the differential history and course of their alcohol use disorders, and differences in rates and types of victimization and comorbid disorders, women and men may benefit from different treatment approaches. They suggest that single-gender groups are preferable due to the tendency of male domination in number and style at alcohol treatment programs. Histories of victimization by men, sexual orientation issues, and sex-role conflict are other factors that may make same-gender groups optimal for treatment-seeking alcoholic women.

Three main stages need to be considered in determining whether an alcoholism treatment program has the potential to be successful (Green, Polen, Dickinson, Lynch, & Bennett, 2002): (1) treatment access—that is, the potential client must be able to contact the treatment facility to access service; (2) treatment initiation—the client must actually begin to attend the treatment sessions following initial access; and (3) treatment completion—the client must stay in treatment long enough to complete the program (including any treatment aftercare). There may be sex differences at some or all of these stages. Research suggests that treatment seeking is affected by gender in that women are less likely than men to receive alcohol treatment (Dawson, 1996) or seek treatment for alcohol abuse problems (Brennan, Moos, & Kim, 1993). There are many possible reasons for these sex differences. Some reasons that have been identified include child care responsibilities, poverty, greater stigma for women with alcohol use disorders, lack of transportation to alcohol treatment facilities, or inadequate health care coverage, to name but a few. In a literature review on gender bias and other issues in the utilization, effectiveness, and scope of treatment services for alcohol problems in women, Walitzer and Connors (1997) suggest that treatment professionals may be less likely to offer their services to women than to men, because they regard women's drinking problems as less severe or because they assume that treatment will help women less than men. They also suggest that women who abuse alcohol tend to seek help from general mental health services instead of alcohol treatment programs because they feel uncomfortable in these programs, which have been designed largely for, and which mostly serve, men.

Once treatment is initiated, women appear to have less social support, fewer family resources (Timko, Finney, & Moos, 2005), and more family responsibilities than do men; women report higher levels of stress (Timko et al., 2005), are less likely to be married or to have spouses who refer them to treatment, are more likely to identify problems other than drinking as their primary problem, are more likely to have been abused, have higher rates of comorbid mental health problems (e.g., anxiety and depression), have greater dysfunction in their families of origin, and are more likely to feel stigmatized, than men initiating treatment (Green et al., 2002; Greenfield, Brooks, et al., 2007). As mentioned earlier in this chapter in the section on telescoping, women who present for treatment of an alcohol use disorder have more severe alcohol abuse problems than their male counterparts presenting for treatment (e.g., Foster, Peters, & Marshall, 2000; Timko, Moos, Finney, & Connell, 2002). Moreover, on average, women entering alcoholism treatment have been shown to be younger, less educated, to have lower incomes, and to be less likely to be employed than men entering treatment (e.g., Green et al., 2002; Greenfield, Brooks, et al., 2007; Timko et al., 2002). With respect to treatment retention, women are more likely to drop out of treatment, and they attend fewer therapy sessions, on average, than do men. It has been shown that women who are married, unemployed, or who have higher incomes are more likely to stay in treatment than other women. Furthermore, African American women are less likely than European American women to stay in treatment for alcoholism (Mammo & Weinbaum, 1993).

In response to these gender barriers to accessing, initiating, and remaining in alcohol treatment among women, over the last 20 years a variety of women-specific alcohol treatments and programs have been developed and evaluated. For example, in a classic controlled study, Dahlgren and Willander (1989) randomly assigned women with early alcohol problems to treatment in either a regular ward/alcoholism treatment center or a women-only outpatient or residential setting, and conducted follow-up on these women over a 2-year period. Results showed a more successful rehabilitation outcome in the "experimental" group with the women-only treatment format; the women needed less hospital care for alcoholism, displayed lower mortality, had fewer relapses to heavy drinking, evidenced greater work capacity, and evidenced greater positive social adjustment than women assigned to the regular (non-gender-specific) treatment center. Participants in the women-only treatment group also reported better social drinking outcomes than those assigned to the regular (non-gender-specific) program. Improvements relative to baseline were also noted for the women assigned to the regular (non-gender-specific) program but to a lesser extent than in the women specific group. The authors argued that not only do their results suggest superior outcomes for women-specific programs, but that specialized female units/programs may be able to attract women to come for help earlier. They reason that treatment at a specialized department with only female clients should be a less intimidating alternative for women with alcohol problems than treatment at a traditional mixed-gender institution/program.

Since the time of early studies such as that of Dahlgren and Willander (1989), many investigations have been conducted on the subject of alcohol treatment programming for women. A recent example is a randomized controlled trial conducted by Greenfield, Trucco, McHugh, Lincoln, and Gallop (2007), in which a new manual-based women-only treatment was compared to an effective manual-based mixed-gender treatment control group. Women with substance use disorders (mainly alcohol dependence) were randomized to one of the two 12-week group treatments. No significant differences in substance use outcomes were found between treatment groups at treatment completion. However, during the 6-month follow-up, members of the women-only treatment group demonstrated a pattern of continued reductions in substance use, whereas women in the mixed-gender control treatment group showed a worsening of outcomes. In addition, women with alcohol dependence in the women-only group showed significantly greater reductions in average drinks per drinking day than women with alcohol dependence in the mixed-gender group at the 6-month follow-up. Moreover, satisfaction with treatment ratings were significantly higher among women assigned to the women-only treatment than among women assigned to the mixed-gender control group. The researchers concluded that women-focused single-gender group treatments may enhance longer-term clinical outcomes (e.g., reductions in drinking quantity) among women with substance use disorders (SUDs).

In a comprehensive review of the literature, Ashley, Marsden, and Brady (2003) evaluated the effectiveness of substance abuse treatment programming for women, including women-specific treatments for alcohol problems. They examined 38 published, peer-reviewed studies from 1980 to 2000 that investigated whether substance abuse treatment services improved outcomes in women. The review explored six specific program components of women's treatment programs: (1) child care, (2) prenatal care, (3) women-only admission, (4) supplemental services that address women-focused issues, (5) mental health programming, and (6) comprehensive programming. Findings consistently showed improved treatment outcomes based on the six measures. Certain components, such as access to child care, prenatal care, and mental health programming, helped to reduce barriers to treatment entry and retention for women. These women-centered services provide emotional and tangible support to allow women to concentrate on their recovery and help them feel less stigmatized. Women-centered treatment programs also offer a more attractive alternative to women suffering from past abuse, lesbian women, and sex workers.

A recent literature review by Greenfield, Brooks, et al. (2007) revealed that whereas women are less likely to enter treatment than their male counterparts, once in treatment, gender was not a significant predictor of treatment retention, completion, or outcome. Greenfield, Brooks, et al. (2007) reviewed 280 relevant articles gleaned from Medline and PsycInfo from the years 1975 to 2005. They drew the following conclusions: (1) Women with alcohol use disorders are less likely than their male counterparts to enter treatment over their lifetime; (2) to help women access alcoholism treatment, it should address their needs, such as child care, perinatal care, and family services; and (3) factors such as lower levels of psychiatric symptoms, higher socioeconomic status, and social support have been associated with better retention of women in substance abuse treatment. The authors concluded that their review does not substantiate previous beliefs that women with alcohol dependence suffer worse treatment outcomes than their male counterparts. They assert that gender should no longer be the focus in predicting alcoholism treatment outcome. Instead, certain target characteristics that vary by gender, such as socioeconomic status, co-occurring psychiatric disorders, history of victimization, therapist–client gender matching, and relapse patterns all should be seen as modifiable gender-related predictors of treatment outcomes. They also concluded that their literature review does support the notion that certain subgroups of women (e.g., women with trauma histories, women with alcohol dependence and co-occurring PTSD or borderline personality disorder) do benefit from gender-specific treatment programming with regard to treatment entry, retention, and outcomes.

KEY POINTS

- On average, men drink more heavily than women and are at greater risk, overall, for the development of alcohol use disorders.
- Women are nonetheless at substantial risk for a number of reasons, including gender convergence and their greater vulnerability to the adverse effects of alcohol. For example, women progress from drinking to heavy drinking and dependence more quickly than do men—a phenomenon known as "telescoping."
- Men and women with problematic heavy drinking differ in the reasons for drinking. Generally speaking, alcohol problems are more related to attempts to cope with depression among women, whereas male drinking is more motivated by peer pressure and by desires to enhance positive moods.
- Women with alcohol problems evidence different forms of comorbid mental health problems than their male counterparts. For example, independent depression is more common in females than males with alcohol dependence, and PTSD tends to precede alcohol problems more often in comorbid women. These patterns of comorbidity are consistent with a pattern of self-medication of negative emotional states among women with alcohol use disorders.
- Given their different trauma histories, unique mental health comorbidities, and their generally more severe presentation at treatment outset, many have suggested that women with alcohol use problems require separate alcohol treatment programs and services that are single-gendered in order to draw them into treatment and better engage them in the treatment process.
- Evidence is accumulating that such gender-specific alcohol treatment services are achieving their goals of better treatment engagement and retention of women with alcohol problems. This is likely because these services better meet female patients' unique needs and provide them with an environment in which they feel safer to discuss such personal issues as trauma histories and emotional difficulties that are so often closely tied to their alcohol misuse.

REFERENCES

Asterisks denote recommended readings.

Adlaf, E. M., Begin, P., & Sawka, E. (2005). *Canadian Addiction Survey (CAS): A national survey of Canadians' use of alcohol and other drugs. Prevalence of use and related harms: Detailed report.* Ottawa, Canada: Canadian Centre on Substance Abuse.

Amaro, H., Blake, S., Schwartz, P., & Flinchbaugh, L. (2001). Developing theory-based substance abuse prevention programs for young adolescent girls. *Journal of Early Adolescence, 21,* 256–293.

American Psychiatric Association. (2000). *Diagnostic and statistical manual of mental disorders* (4th ed., text rev.). Washington, DC: Author.

Ammon, E., Schafer, C., Hofmann, U., & Klotz, U. (1996). Disposition and first-pass metabolism of ethanol in humans: Is it gastric or hepatic and does it depend on gender? *Clinical Pharmacology and Therapeutics, 59,* 503–513.

Anderson, D. A., Simmons, A. M., Martens, M. P., Ferrier, A. G., & Sheehy, M. J. (2006). The relationship between disordered eating behaviour and drinking motives in college-age women. *Eating Behaviors, 7,* 419–422.

Annis, H., & Graham, J. (1995). Profile types on the Inventory of Drinking Situations: Implications for relapse prevention counseling. *Psychology of Addictive Behaviors, 9,* 176–182.

Ashley, O. S., Marsden, M. E., & Brady, T. M. (2003). Effectiveness of substance abuse treatment programming for women: A review. *American Journal of Drug and Alcohol Abuse, 29,* 19–53.

Babcock, M. (1996). Does feminism drive women to drink? Conflicting themes. *International Journal on Drug Policy, 7,* 158–165.

Back, S., Dansky, B. S., Coffey, S. F., Saladin, M. E., Sonne, S., & Brady, K. T. (2000). Cocaine dependence with and without post-traumatic stress disorder: A comparison of substance abuse, trauma history, and psychiatric co-morbidity. *American Journal on Addictions, 9,* 51–62. (*)

Bandelow, B., Krause, J., Wedekind, D., Broocks, A., Hajak, G., & Rüther, E. (2005). Early traumatic life events, parental attitudes, family history, and birth risk factors in patients with borderline personality disorder and healthy controls. *Psychiatry Research, 134,* 169–179.

Birch, C. D., Stewart, S. H., & Brown, C. G. (2007). Exploring differential patterns of situational risk for binge eating and heavy drinking. *Addictive Behaviors, 32,* 433–448.

Bjork, J. M., Dougherty, D. M., & Moeller, F. G. (1999). Symptomatology of depression and anxiety in female "social drinkers." *American Journal of Drug and Alcohol Abuse, 25,* 173–182.

Blankfield, A. (1990). Female alcoholics: The expression of alcoholism in relation to gender and age. *Acta Psychiatrica Scandinavica, 81,* 448–452.

Brady, K. T., & Randall, C. L. (1999). Gender differences in substance use disorders. *Psychiatric Clinics of North America, 22,* 241–252. (*)

Brennan, P. L., Moos, R. H., & Kim, J. Y. (1993). Gender differences in the individual characteristics and life contexts of late-middle-aged and older problem drinkers. *Addiction, 88,* 781–790.

Brown, C. G., & Stewart, S. H. (2008). Exploring women's use of alcohol as self-medication for depression among women receiving community-based treatment for alcohol problems. *Journal of Prevention and Intervention in the Community, 35,* 33–47.

Brown, R. A., Evans, D. M., Miller, I. W., Burgess, E. S., & Mueller, T. I. (1997). Cognitive-behavioral treatment for depression in alcoholism. *Journal of Consulting and Clinical Psychology, 65,* 715–726.

Bulik, C. M., Sullivan, P. M., McKee, M., Wehzin, T. E., & Kaye, W. H. (1994). Characteristics of bulimic women with and without alcohol abuse. *American Journal of Drug and Alcohol Abuse, 20,* 273–283.

Cepik, A., Arikan, Z., Boratav, C., & Isik, E. (1995). Bulimia in a male alcoholic: A symptom substitution in alcoholism. *International Journal of Eating Disorders, 17,* 201–204.

Child, I. L., Barry, H., & Bacon, M. K. (1965). Sex differences. *Quarterly Journal of Studies on Alcohol*(Suppl. 3), 49–61.

Clark, D. B., Pollock, N., Bukstein, O. G., Mezzich, A. C., Bromberger, J. T., & Donovan, J. E. (1997).

Gender and co-morbid psychopathology in adolescents with alcohol dependence. *Journal of the American Academy of Child and Adolescent Psychiatry, 36*, 1195–1203.

Cloninger, R. C. (1987). Neurogenetic adaptive mechanisms in alcoholism. *Science, 236*, 410–416.

Coniglio, C. (1993). Making connections: Family alcoholism and the development of eating problems. In C. Brown & K. Jasper (Eds.), *Consuming passions: Feminist approaches to weight preoccupation and eating disorders* (pp. 235–250). Toronto: Second Story Press.

Cooper, M. (1994). Motivations for alcohol use among adolescents: Development and validation of a four-factor model. *Psychological Assessment, 6*, 117–128.

Cowan, J., & Devine, C. (2008). Food, eating, and weight concerns of men in recovery from substance addiction. *Appetite, 50*, 33–42.

Dahlgren, L., & Willander, A. (1989). Are special treatment facilities for female alcoholics needed? A controlled 2-year follow-up study from a specialized female unit (EWA) versus a mixed male/female treatment facility. *Alcoholism: Clinical and Experimental Research, 13*, 499–504.

Dansky, B. S., Brewerton, T. D., & Kilpatrick, D. G. (2000). Comorbidity of bulimia nervosa and alcohol use disorders: Results from the National Women's Study. *International Journal of Eating Disorders, 27*, 180–190.

Dawson, D. A. (1996). Gender differences in the probability of alcohol treatment. *Journal of Substance Abuse, 8*, 211–225.

Deykin, E. Y., & Buka, S. L. (1997). Prevalence and risk factors for posttraumatic stress disorder among chemically dependent adolescents. *American Journal of Psychiatry, 154*, 752–757.

Dunn, E. C., Larimer, M. A., & Neighbors, C. (2001). Alcohol and drug-related negative consequences in college students with bulimia nervosa and binge eating disorder. *International Journal of Eating Disorders, 32*, 171–178.

Durand, M., Barlow, D. H., & Stewart, S. H. (2008). *Abnormal psychology: Essentials.* Toronto: Thomson-Nelson.

Fillmore, M. T. (2003). Drug abuse as a problem of impaired control: Current approaches and findings. *Behavioral and Cognitive Neuroscience Reviews, 2*, 179–197.

Foster, J. H., Peters, T. J., & Marshall, E. J. (2000). Quality of life measures and outcome in alcohol-dependent men and women. *Alcohol, 22*, 45–52.

Frezza, M., Di Padova, C., Pozzato, G., Terpin, M., Baraona, E., & Lieber, C. S. (1990). High blood alcohol levels in women: The role of decreased gastric alcohol dehydrogenase activity and first-pass metabolism. *New England Journal of Medicine, 322*, 95–99.

Grant, B. F., & Dawson, D. A. (1997). Age at onset of alcohol use and its association with DSM-IV alcohol abuse and dependence: Results from the National Longitudinal Alcohol Epidemiological Survey. *Journal of Substance Abuse, 9*, 103–110.

Grant, B. F., Stinson, F. S., Dawson, D. A., Chou, S. P., Dufour, M. C., Compton, W., et al. (2004). Prevalence and co-occurrence of substance use disorders and independent mood and anxiety disorders. *Archives of General Psychiatry, 61*, 807–816.

Green, C. A., Polen, M. R., Dickinson, D. M., Lynch, F. L., & Bennett, M. D. (2002). Gender differences in predictors of initiation, retention, and completion in an HMO-based substance abuse treatment program. *Journal of Substance Abuse Treatment, 23*, 285–295.

Greenfield, S. F., Brooks, A. J., Gordon, S. M., Green, C. A., Kropp, F., McHugh, R. K., et al. (2007). Substance abuse treatment entry, retention, and outcome in women: A review of the literature. *Drug and Alcohol Dependence, 86*, 1–21. (*)

Greenfield, S. F., Trucco, E. M., McHugh, R. K., Lincoln, M. F., & Gallop, R. (2007). The Women's Recovery Group Study: A Stage I trial of women-focused group therapy for substance use disorders versus mixed-gender group drug counselling. *Drug and Alcohol Dependence, 90*, 39–47.

Greenfield, T. K., & Room, R. (1997). Situational norms for drinking and drunkenness: Trends in the U.S. adult population, 1979–1990. *Addiction, 92*, 33–47.

Griggs, M. A., & Tyrer, P. J. (1981). Personality disorders in panic patients: Response to termination of antipanic medication. *Journal of Personality Disorders, 2*, 303–315.

Grucza, R. A., Bucholz, K. K., Rice, J. P., & Bierut, L. J. (2008). Secular trends in the lifetime prevalence of alcohol dependence in the United States: A re-evaluation. *Alcoholism: Clinical and Experimental Research, 32*, 763–770.

Haas, A. L., & Peters, R. H. (2000). Development of substance abuse problems among drug-involved offenders: Evidence for the telescoping effect. *Journal of Substance Abuse, 12*, 241–253.

Harrell, Z. A. T., & Karim, N. M. (2008). Is gender relevant only for problem alcohol behaviors? An examination of correlates of alcohol use among college students. *Addictive Behaviors, 33*, 359–365.

Hernandez-Avila, C. A., Rounsaville, B. J., & Kranzler, H. R. (2004). Opioid-, cannabis-, and alcohol-dependent women show more rapid progression to substance abuse treatment. *Drug and Alcohol Dependence, 74*, 265–272.

Hodgins, D. C., el-Guebaly, N., & Addington, J. (1997). Treatment of substance abusers: Single or mixed gender programs? *Addictions, 92*, 802–812. (*)

Holderness, C. C., Brooks-Gunn, J., & Warren, M. P. (1994). Co-morbidity of eating disorders and substance abuse: Review of the literature. *International Journal of Eating Disorders, 16*, 1–34.

Johnson, P. B., Richter, L., Kleber, H. D., McLellan, A. T., & Carise, D. (2005). Telescoping of drinking-related behaviors: Gender, racial/ethnic, and age comparisons. *Substance Use and Misuse, 40*, 1139–1151.

Kalant, O. J. (1980). *Alcohol and drug problems in women: Research advances in alcohol and drug problems.* New York: Plenum Press.

Kessler, R. C., Crum, R. M., Warner, L. A., Nelson, C. B., Schulenberg, J., & Anthony, J. C. (1997). Lifetime co-occurrence of DSM-III-R alcohol abuse and dependence with other psychiatric disorders in the National Comorbidity Survey. *Archives of General Psychiatry, 54*, 313–321.

Keyes, K. M., Grant, B. F., & Hasin, D. S. (2008). Evidence for a closing gender gap in alcohol use, abuse, and dependence in the United States population. *Drug and Alcohol Dependence, 93*, 21–29. (*)

Kraus, L., Bloomfield, K., Augustin, R., & Reese, A. (2000). Prevalence of alcohol use and the association between onset of use and alcohol-related problems in a general population sample in Germany. *Addiction, 95*, 1389–1401.

Kushner, M. G., Krueger, R., Frye, B., & Peterson, J. (2008). Epidemiological perspectives on co-occurring anxiety disorders and substance use disorder. In S. H. Stewart & P. J. Conrod (Eds.), *Anxiety and substance use disorders: The vicious cycle of comorbidity* (pp. 3–17). New York: Springer.

Lewis, C. E., Bucholz, K. K., Spitznagel E., & Shayka, J. J. (1996). Effects of gender and co-morbidity on problem drinking in a community sample. *Alcoholism: Clinical and Experimental Research, 20*, 466–476.

Lilenfeld, L. R., Kaye, W. H., Greeno, C. G., Merikangas, K. R., Plotnicov, K., Pollice, C., et al. (1997). Psychiatric disorders in women with bulimia nervosa and their first-degree relatives: Effects of co-morbid substance dependence. *International Journal of Eating Disorders, 22*, 253–264.

Links, P. S., Heslegrave, R. J., Mitton, J. E., van Reekum, R., & Patrick, J. (1995). Borderline personality disorder and substance abuse: Consequences of co-morbidity. *Canadian Journal of Psychiatry, 40*, 9–14.

Mammo, A., & Weinbaum, D. F. (1993). Some factors that influence dropping out from outpatient alcoholism treatment facilities. *Journal of Studies on Alcohol, 54*, 92–101.

Mann, K., Ackermann, K., Croissant, B., Mundle, G., Nakovics, H., & Diehl, A. (2005). Neuroimaging of gender differences in alcohol dependence: Are women more vulnerable? *Alcoholism: Clinical and Experimental Research, 29*, 896–901.

Marczinski, C. A., Combs, S. W., & Fillmore, M. T. (2007). Increased sensitivity to the diminishing effects of alcohol in binge drinkers. *Psychology of Addictive Behaviors, 21*, 346–354.

Marshall, A. W., Kingstone, D., Boss, M., & Morgan, M. Y. (1983). Ethanol elimination in males and females: Relationship to the menstrual cycle and body composition. *Hepatology, 3*, 701–706.

McPherson, M., Casswell, S., & Pledger, M. (2004). Gender convergence in alcohol consumption and related problems: Issues and outcomes from comparisons of New Zealand survey data. *Addiction, 99*, 738–748.

Mercer, P. W., & Khavari, K. A. (1990). Are women drinking more like men? An empirical examination of the convergence hypothesis. *Alcoholism: Clinical and Experimental Research, 14*, 461–466.

Miller, F. T., Abrams, T., Dulit, R., & Fyer, M. (1993). Substance use in borderline personality disorder. *American Journal of Alcohol and Drug Abuse, 19*, 491–497.

Mitchell, J. E., Pyle, R. L., Eckert, E. D., & Hatsukami, D. (1990). The influence of prior alcohol and drug abuse problems on bulimia nervosa treatment outcome. *Addictive Behaviors*, *15*, 169–173.

Moeller, F. G., Barratt, E. S., Fischer, C. J., Dougherty, D. M., Schmitz, J. M., & Swann, A. C. (2001). Psychiatric aspects of impulsivity. *American Journal of Psychiatry*, *158*, 1783–1793.

O'Malley, P., & Johnston, L. (2002). Epidemiology of alcohol and other drug use among American college students. *Journal of Studies on Alcohol*, *14*, 23–49.

Paris, J. (2000). Childhood precursors of borderline personality. *Psychiatric Clinics of North America*, *23*, 77–88.

Piazza, N. J., Vrbka, J. L., & Yeager, R. D. (1989). Telescoping of alcoholism in women alcoholics. *International Journal of the Addictions*, *24*, 19–28.

Poole, N., & Dell, C. A. (2005). *Girls, women, and substance use*. Ottawa, ON: Canadian Centre on Substance Abuse.

Ramsey, S. E., Kahler, C. W., Read, J. P., Stuart, G. L., & Brown, R. A. (2004). Discriminating between substance-induced and independent depressive episodes in alcohol dependent patients. *Journal of Studies on Alcohol*, *65*, 672–676.

Randall, C. L., Roberts, J. S., Del Boca, F. K., Carroll, K. M., Connors, G. J., & Mattson, M. E. (1999). Telescoping of landmark events associated with drinking: A gender comparison. *Journal of Studies on Alcohol*, *60*, 252–260.

Riggs, D. S., & Foa, E. B. (2008). Treatment for co-morbid post-traumatic stress disorder and substance use disorders. In S. H. Stewart & P. J. Conrod (Eds.), *Anxiety and substance use disorders: The vicious cycle of co-morbidity* (pp. 119–137). New York: Springer.

Roche, A. M., & Deehan, A. (2002). Women's alcohol consumption: Emerging patterns, problems, and public health implications. *Drug and Alcohol Review*, *21*, 169–178.

Russell, J. J., Moskowitz, D. S., Zuroff, D. C., Sookman, D., & Paris, J. (2007). Stability and variability of affective experience and interpersonal behaviour in borderline personality disorder. *Journal of Abnormal Psychology*, *116*, 578–588.

Sabourin, B. C., & Stewart, S. H. (in press). Patterns of depression–substance use disorder comorbidity in women seeking addictions treatment. In J. Gallivan & S. Cooper (Eds.), *Determinants of women's health: A holistic approach to women's psychological and physical well-being. A book of selected papers from the 2008 Section of Women and Psychology (SWAP) Institute*. Sydney, Nova Scotia: Cape Breton University Press.

Sannibale, C., & Hall, W. (1998). An evaluation of Cloninger's typology of alcohol abuse. *Addiction*, *93*, 1241–1249.

Schall, M., Weede, T., & Maltzman, I. (1991). Predictors of alcohol consumption by university students. *Journal of Alcohol and Drug Education*, *37*, 72–80

Schuckit, M. A., Tipp, J. E., Bergman, M., Reigh, W., Hesselbrock, V. M., & Smith, T. L. (1997). Comparison of induced and independent major depressive disorders in 2,945 alcoholics. *American Journal of Psychiatry*, *154*, 948–956.

Sherwood, N. E., Crowther, J. H., & Ben-Porath, Y. S. (2000). The perceived function of eating for bulimic, subclinical bulimic, non-eating disordered women. *Behavior Therapy*, *31*, 777–793.

Smith, W. B., & Weisner, C. (2000). Women and alcohol problems: A critical analysis of the literature and unanswered questions. *Alcoholism: Clinical and Experimental Research*, *24*, 1320–1321.

Stewart, S. H., & Brown, C. G. (2007). The relationship between disordered eating and substance use problems among women: A critical review. In L. Greaves, N. Poole, & J. Greenbaum (Eds.), *Highs and lows: Canadian perspectives on women and substance use* (pp. 157–163). Toronto: Centre for Addiction and Mental Health.

Stewart, S. H., Brown, C. G., Devoulyte, K., Theakston, J., & Larsen, S. E. (2006). Why do women with alcohol problems binge eat? Exploring connections between binge eating and heavy drinking in women receiving treatment for alcohol problems. *Journal of Health Psychology*, *11*, 409–425. (*)

Stewart, S. H., & Conrod, P. J. (2008). Anxiety disorder and substance use disorder co-morbidity: Common themes and future directions. In S. H. Stewart & P. J. Conrod (Eds.), *Anxiety and substance use disorders: The vicious cycle of co-morbidity* (pp. 239–257). New York: Springer.

Stewart, S. H., Grant, V. V., Ouimette, P., & Brown, P. J. (2006). Are gender differences in posttraumatic stress disorder rates attenuated in substance use disorder patients? *Canadian Psychology, 47*, 110–124. (*)

Stice, E., Burton, E. M., & Shaw, H. (2004). Prospective relations between bulimic pathology, depression, and substance abuse: Unpacking co-morbidity in adolescent girls. *Journal of Consulting and Clinical Psychology, 72*, 62–71.

Timko, C., Finney, J. W., & Moos, R. H. (2005). The 8-year course of alcohol abuse: Gender differences in social context and coping. *Alcoholism: Clinical and Experimental Research, 29*, 612–621.

Timko, C., Moos, R. H., Finney, J. W., & Connell, E. G. (2002). Gender differences in help-utilization and the 8-year course of alcohol abuse. *Addiction, 97*, 877–889.

Trull, T. J., Sher, K. J., Minks-Brown, C., Durbin, J., & Burr, R. (2000). Borderline personality disorder and substance use disorders: A review and integration. *Clinical Psychology Review, 20*, 235–253. (*)

Verheul, R., Kranzler, H. R., Poling, J., Tennen, H., Ball, S., & Rounsaville, B. J. (2000). Co-occurrence of Axis I and Axis II disorders in substance abusers. *Acta Psychiatrica Scandinavica, 101*, 110–118.

Walitizer, K. S., & Connors, G. J. (1997). Gender and treatment of alcohol-related problems. In R. W. Wilsnack & S. C. Wilsnack (Eds.), *Gender and alcohol: Individual and social perspectives* (pp. 445–461). New Brunswick, NJ: Rutgers Center of Alcohol Studies.

Wilsnack, R. W., Vogeltanz, N. D., Wilsnack, S. C., & Harris, T. R. (2000). Gender differences in alcohol consumption and adverse drinking consequences: Cross-cultural patterns. *Addiction, 95*, 251–265. (*)

Zilberman, M. L., Tavares, H., Blume, S. B., & el-Guebaly, N. (2003). Substance use disorders: Sex differences and psychiatric comorbidities. *Canadian Journal of Psychiatry, 48*, 5–13.

CHAPTER 21

Treatment of Nicotine Dependence in Women

Kenneth A. Perkins, PhD

Tobacco smoking kills about 5 million people annually worldwide (Ezzati & Lopez, 2003), or about one person every 6 seconds, and smoking may be particularly pernicious for women. Recent research on the health consequences of cigarette smoking indicates that smoking produces greater risks in the primary smoking-related illnesses among women than men. Not only did lung cancer overtake breast cancer as the leading cancer killer of women in the 1980s, the risk of lung cancer due to smoking may be greater in women than men, particularly after controlling for age and amount of smoking exposure (International Early Lung Cancer Action Program Investigators, 2006). Similarly, the relative risk of myocardial infarction (MI, or heart attack) due to smoking is about twofold greater in women than men (Prescott, Hippe, Schnohr, Ole Hein, & Vestbo, 1998). The deterioration in lung function due to smoking may be more rapid in women versus men (Dransfield, Davis, Gerald, & Bailey, 2006), explaining women's greater risk of chronic obstructive pulmonary disease (COPD). Thus, evidence suggests that the risks for the three main causes of premature morbidity and mortality from smoking are higher in women than men.

Furthermore, smoking carries health risks in women that are not seen in men, such as risks to fetal development in pregnant women who smoke, including greater infant mortality from sudden infant death syndrome (SIDS) and other causes, and greater infant morbidity due to low birthweight and impaired infant lung function (DiFranza, Aligne, & Weitzman, 2004). Maternal smoking, possibly more than paternal smoking, is also associated with greater risk of the offspring suffering from adverse effects of secondhand smoke exposure and of becoming adults who smoke (Buka, Shenassa, & Niaura, 2003). Smoking also increases the risk of other health problems in women that are not relevant to men. Smoking hastens the onset of menopause and is associated with increased menstrual bleeding and duration of dysmenorrhea (Hornsby, Wilcox, & Weinberg, 1998). Women who smoke have a more difficult time becoming pregnant, even with *in vitro* fertilization, and are at increased risk of spontaneous abortion. Beyond these risks specific to women, smoking also has other consequences that are experienced by both men and women but may be more salient to women. For example, smoking increases facial wrinkling by decreasing the elasticity of the skin and connective tissue, and smoking decreases bone density (Ernster et al., 1995).

Compounding the greater health risks of smoking in women is evidence that women tend to have more difficulty than men quitting smoking and remaining abstinent. Although not invariably found, this sex difference appears to be generally true overall, regardless of whether individuals try to quit as part of a formal program or on their own (Fortmann & Killen, 1994). For example, nationwide surveys of smoking behavior in representative samples of several hundred thousand Americans are conducted on a regular basis by the Centers for Disease Control and Prevention (2006). From these results, it is often possible to determine how many respondents ever smoked and how many among those who ever smoked have quit, also called "former smokers." Population-based data from 2002, presented in Rodu and Cole (2007), show that, among women age 35 or over (i.e., those old enough to have had extensive opportunity to quit), 31.5 million have ever smoked and 17.4 million are former smokers, making a "quit ratio" (the ratio of former smokers to ever smokers) of 55.2%. Among men age 35 or over, 38.0 million have ever smoked and 22.5 million are former smokers, for a quit ratio of 59.2%. Although seemingly a small sex difference in quit ratio, it nevertheless translates nationally (United States) into more than one million fewer women who have quit smoking than would be expected if there was no difference at all in the rates of successful smoking cessation among men and women. Other research examining results of formal clinical trials also suggests that women are less successful than men in quitting smoking (e.g., Perkins, 2001; Piper et al., 2007; Scharf & Shiffman, 2004; Wetter et al., 1999). This differential rate of quitting may help explain why the rate of smoking has decreased less sharply over the past 50 years among all adult women, from about 30 to 18%, than among adult men, from about 55 to 24%, as of 2005 (Giovino, 2007).

Because they have greater difficulty quitting, women could be viewed as a very large subpopulation of smokers requiring greater attention and effort by health care providers to improve their cessation rates. Further, because women suffer from greater risk of smoking-related illness, one could argue that an increase in quit rates among women could generate a greater reduction in the overall adverse impact of smoking on public health than the same increase in quit rates among men. This chapter discusses research examining the greater difficulty of quitting in women, along with possible reasons for this difficulty and approaches to improving smoking cessation treatment in women. An overview of factors that contribute to nicotine dependence is presented first, with an emphasis on ways in which these factors may differ between men and women. The second section of the chapter is devoted to sex differences in response to the Federal Drug Administration (FDA)-approved cessation medications, particularly nicotine patch as well as other medications. The last section discusses obstacles to quitting more often faced by women than men and outlines possible counseling treatment approaches to overcoming these obstacles.

SEX DIFFERENCES IN NICOTINE AND NON-NICOTINE INFLUENCES ON DEPENDENCE

Tobacco dependence is acquired and maintained through both pharmacological and nonpharmacological factors, as with any drug dependence. Effective treatment for smoking cessation requires adequately addressing both sets of factors (Perkins, Conklin, & Levine, 2008). The primary pharmacological factor is *nicotine*, the main psychoactive ingredient of tobacco. The nonpharmacological factors are extensive but consist mostly of the environmental stimuli that commonly accompany nicotine intake via smoking. The most obvious of these stimuli are "cues" that are *proximal* to (i.e., temporally contiguous with and integral to) the act of smoking, such as the sight, smell, and taste of a lit cigarette. These proximal cues are rather similar for most smokers since lit cigarettes mostly look and smell alike (Conklin, 2006). Far more variable and underappreciated in clinical research are the wide range of stimuli that are *distal* to, or set the stage for, the act of smoking. Those distal stimuli are mostly environments or people that often accompany smoking and can come to be conditioned to smoking, such that they may elicit urges to smoke even in the absence of any proximal cues. For this reason, distal cues may precipitate relapse when abstinent individuals come into contact with them. Examples of these distal cues include favorite smoking locations or contexts, such as an easy chair in one's home, friends with whom one smokes, or activities often done while smoking, such as drinking alcohol (Conklin, 2006). These distal influences may be very important for individuals who are trying to remain abstinent, as avoiding familiar environments and smoking friends is likely much more difficult than avoiding proximal cues of lit cigarettes.

Differences in Nicotine Response

Little research has examined sex differences in the contribution of pharmacological and non-pharmacological factors to tobacco dependence. However, based on our research and that of others, we find that the smoking behavior of women seems to be influenced less by nicotine and more by non-nicotine factors, compared to the smoking behavior of men (Perkins, 1996, 2008; Perkins, Donny, & Caggiula, 1999). Note that this sex difference appears to be specific to smoking reinforcement and effects promoting reinforcement (e.g., "reward"), and not a broad sex difference in all responses to nicotine and non-nicotine factors. Because the sex differences in the relative contribution of these factors to smoking behavior act in opposite directions, and because smoking inextricably contains both nicotine and non-nicotine factors, it is often difficult to see any significant sex differences merely from observations of typical smoking behavior. Identifying these differences requires isolating the influences of nicotine and non-nicotine factors by manipulating one of the factors and holding the other factors constant. Such manipulations are difficult to do in clinical studies but can be accomplished in controlled laboratory research on acute smoking behavior. Examples of this research are presented below.

Regarding sex differences in the influence of nicotine, two general potential explanations involve a difference in either the pharmacokinetics or the pharmacodynamics of nicotine. Pharmacokinetic differences, such as faster or slower uptake or metabolism of the drug, would result in differences in blood nicotine concentration, which would obviously affect the observed response. Although recent findings suggest that women may metabolize nicotine about 10% more quickly than men (Benowitz, Lessov-Schlaggar, Swan, & Jacob, 2006), this is not likely an important reason for the difference in smoking behavior responses due to nicotine. Such a difference would produce lower blood levels of nicotine in women versus men, and so women would exhibit smaller responses to *all* effects of nicotine, such as physiological, mood, and behavioral responses, and not just responses specific to smoking behavior. This type of across-the-board sex difference in nicotine effects is contrary to the vast literature on acute nicotine effects in humans (Benowitz & Hatsukami, 1998; Perkins et al., 1999).

Thus, the source of the difference in nicotine's influence on smoking seems to be pharmacodynamic—that is, to differences in sensitivity to certain pharmacological actions of the drug. In other words, the varying influence of nicotine on smoking behavior of men and women appears to be due to differences in tissue sensitivity, to how they respond to a given level of nicotine in the body (or more specifically, in the brain areas relevant to nicotine reinforcement). Evidence for sex differences in pharmacodynamic influences of nicotine on smoking behavior comes from several lines of research. First, laboratory studies manipulating nicotine content in cigarettes show that women are less sensitive than men to this manipulation on ratings of reward (e.g., "liking") and in a measure of reinforcement, how much they will work to obtain puffs on the cigarettes (Perkins, Jacobs, Sanders, & Caggiula, 2002; Perkins et al., 2006). Second, women often self-administer less nicotine than do men when it is available in novel forms, such as via nasal spray, even after correcting for differences in body weight. An example of such research is shown in Figure 21.1. In this study (Perkins et al., 1996), men and women attempting to quit smoking were randomized to either a nicotine or placebo experimental nasal spray to use, ad lib, during the first week of quitting. Men self-administered nicotine spray twice as much as the placebo, demonstrating that nicotine per se was reinforcing, but women self-administered nicotine spray no more often than placebo. Third, when pretreated with nicotine spray and then allowed to smoke ad lib, men "compensated" for the nicotine pretreatment by reducing their ad lib smoking, but women did so to a lesser degree (Perkins, Grobe, Stiller, Fonte, & Goettler, 1992). This observation suggests that men may regulate their nicotine intake around a certain level to a stricter extent than women. Such regulation of nicotine intake is thought to be a critical feature of dependence (U.S. Department of Health and Human Services, 1988).

Differences in Non-Nicotine Responses

In contrast to the sex difference in the effects of nicotine, some research indicates that the smoking behavior of women may be more responsive to non-nicotine factors, compared to the smoking behavior of men. Most of this limited body of research focuses on the influence

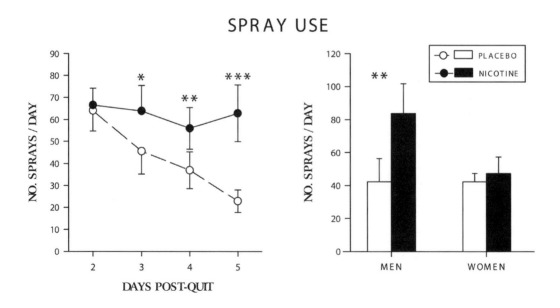

FIGURE 21.1. *Left*: Mean ± *SEM* number of sprays self-administered across each of 4 days of spray access by participants randomized to an experimental nicotine (2.5 μg/kg/spray) or placebo nasal spray who maintained continuous abstinence during the quit week. *Right*: Mean ± *SEM* number of sprays self-administered daily by continuously abstinent men versus women randomized to nicotine versus placebo spray. *$p < .05$; **$p < .01$; ***$p < .001$ for differences between groups. From Perkins et al. (1996, Figs, 1 and 2). Copyright 1996 by the American Psychological Association. Reprinted by permission.

of *proximal* smoking cues (e.g., sight and smell of lit cigarette), but the potential breadth of these sex differences across smoking-related environmental stimuli may be very wide. Regarding sex differences in responses to proximal smoking cues, we have found that blocking the ability of the smoker to taste/smell cigarette smoke while smoking decreases reward ratings and ad lib smoking behavior more in women than in men (Perkins, Gerlach, et al., 2001). However, blocking the ability to see the lit cigarette or the smoke did not differentially affect men and women. An earlier study found that the presence (vs. absence) of a lit cigarette in an ashtray increased responding on a task to earn opportunities to smoke to a greater extent in women than in men (Perkins, Epstein, Grobe, & Fonte, 1994). It is interesting to note that comparable sex differences have been found in rodent research on nicotine self-administration: Nicotine-associated cues (light or tone) increased responding to obtain nicotine in female rats more than in male rats (Chaudhri et al., 2005). Such cross-species consistency suggests a rather basic difference due to biological sex in the effects of proximal cues for nicotine or smoking.

Another way to view these proximal smoking cues is as nonverbal information on the availability of smoking or nicotine. In other words, seeing a lit cigarette signals that nicotine is readily available to the smoker. Complementing such nonverbal information is verbal information on the availability of smoking or nicotine, which can be manipulated by oral or written instructions to a person, such as indicating that a cigarette does or does not contain nicotine (Perkins, Sayette, Conklin, & Caggiula, 2003). Other verbal and nonverbal information about the enticing effects of smoking is routinely provided to people who smoke in the form of cigarette packaging and advertisements. Such information can increase a person's expectancies for nicotine intake, which in turn may elicit increases in craving or urges to smoke. We have found that women are generally more responsive than men to such verbal information. In fact, in these short-term studies, verbal information about nicotine dose may alter reward ratings and ad lib smoking in women to a greater degree than the actual presence or absence of nicotine in the cigarette (Perkins, Doyle, Ciccocioppo, et al., 2006; Perkins, Jacobs, Ciccocioppo, et al., 2004).

Indirect support for the notion that women are more responsive to smoking-related stimuli also comes from tobacco industry documents that summarize industry research on smoking preferences in men and women. The content of these documents is reported by Carpenter, Wayne, and Connolly (2005, 2007). For example, Brown & Williamson (B&W) Company documents state that "young women, much more so than men, would be likely to smoke a flavored cigarette" and "female taste-related preference included: 'satisfying flavor, real smoking enjoyment, mild taste'" (Carpenter et al., 2005, p. 840). British–American Tobacco (BAT) documents indicated that "the research shows that the role of smoking for males concerns satisfaction, while for females it concerns sensory pleasure" (Carpenter et al., 2005, p. 840), and "the role of smoking relates to emotions and sensory pleasure for women, and habit and reward for men" (Carpenter et al., 2007, p. 140). Aside from affecting the development of brands and, therefore, the sensory effects of smoking those brands, these perceived sex differences guided print advertising of cigarette brands aimed at men or women. Thus, they formed some of the verbal information about the cigarettes presented to men and women who smoke and were exposed to those ads, in addition to nonverbal information represented by proximal smoking cues.

Contrasting with this research on sex differences in the influence of proximal cues is the virtual absence of research on *distal* cues for smoking in *any* smoking-related study, and not just in studies comparing men and women (Conklin, 2006; Conklin, Robin, Perkins, Salkeld, & McClernon, 2008). As noted, distal cues are essentially the context of smoking, such as the environments or people around whom one typically smokes. Whereas some distal cues may be very common among those who smoke, such as a bar or bus stop, others may be specific to particular individuals, such as their favorite chair, their car, or their closest friend who smokes (Conklin, 2006). Such influences may be harder to avoid after quitting than the influence of proximal cues, since abstinent individuals cannot easily avoid their friends, their car, or locations in their home where they used to smoke. Thus, coming into contact with these distal stimuli can set in motion an increased urge to smoke, which may lead to relapse, even in the absence of proximal smoking stimuli (Conklin et al., 2008). Men and women may differ in the intensity of their responses (i.e., craving, smoking) to such distal cues, which could help explain sex differences in relapse risk, but no research, to date, has systematically examined this possibility. If identified, treatment research could focus on developing methods to extinguish responses to distal cues (Conklin, 2006).

In summary, women tend to have greater difficulty quitting smoking, compared with men, and this difficulty helps perpetuate the stubbornly high rates of smoking-related morbidity and mortality in women. The acute factors promoting smoking may differ in relative importance between men and women, as nicotine may be less influential and non-nicotine factors such as smoking cues (proximal, perhaps distal) more influential in women than in men. These differences are relevant to smoking cessation treatment in women, which is addressed in the remainder of this chapter.

SEX DIFFERENCES IN CESSATION MEDICATION RESPONSE

The sex differences in the influence of nicotine and non-nicotine factors on smoking behavior, noted above, have implications for smoking cessation treatment in women versus men. For example, if the smoking behavior of women is less responsive to nicotine than is the smoking behavior of men, then treatments relying on nicotine replacement therapy (NRT) may be less successful in women versus men. This appears to be the case, at least for treatment with the nicotine patch (Perkins, 2001; Perkins & Scott, 2008). In addition, one would expect that medications not containing nicotine may show little sex difference in efficacy, and that, too, appears to be the case (e.g., Scharf & Shiffman, 2004), although few such analyses have included long-term follow-up data. Conversely, if the smoking behavior of women is more responsive than that of men to non-nicotine factors, then treatments that address such factors (e.g., coping with proximal cues) may be more successful in women versus men. Very little research has examined this latter question, although there is reason to think this may be the case, as is discussed in a later section on counseling approaches with women who smoke. This section of the chapter evaluates sex differences in the clinical efficacy of the FDA-approved medications for smoking cessation.

Sex Differences in Treatment Effects of Nicotine Replacement

Clinical outcome in smoking cessation trials is usually dichotomous, as subjects are either abstinent or not abstinent (i.e., relapsed) at follow-up. Consequently, very large sample sizes (e.g., several hundred) are needed just to have adequate statistical power to determine the main effects of a medication versus placebo. Adding the between-subjects factor of sex to detect an interaction of sex by medication would require several thousand subjects to have adequate power (Perkins & Scott, 2005). Because almost all clinical trials are not designed, and thus not powered, to detect sex differences in outcome, even a twofold or greater difference in the effects of medication in men versus women usually turns out to be nonsignificant (e.g., Shiffman, Sweeney, & Dresler, 2005; Wetter et al., 1999). Thus, an adequate test of the possibility of sex differences in clinical response to treatment requires meta-analysis, or collapsing results across many similar studies.

Several such meta-analyses have been conducted to examine sex differences in NRT response. In a meta-analysis of placebo-controlled trials involving four of the NRT formulations (gum, patch, inhaler, and spray), the 1-year cessation rates due to nicotine versus placebo were lower in women compared to men (Cepeda-Benito, Reynoso, & Erath, 2004). However, this sex difference in medication efficacy may very well be sensitive to NRT formulation. For example, in one open-label trial (i.e., not involving a placebo condition), women responded more poorly than men to NRT gum, patch, and spray, but women responded better than men to the inhaler (West et al., 2001).

Because the transdermal patch is the formulation most commonly used, with some 25% of all individuals with nicotine dependence having tried it (Bansal, Cummings, Hyland, & Giovino, 2004), sex differences in response to an NRT patch may have the most significance for public health. We recently followed up a meta-analysis of 11 placebo-controlled patch trials that concluded that men and women did not differ significantly in patch response (Munafo, Bradburn, Bowes, & David, 2004), adding three additional trials not included in the earlier analysis (Perkins & Scott, 2008). These 14 trials constituted the only placebo-controlled nicotine patch trials for which data on cessation outcome at 6-month follow-up were available to us separately for men and women. Even then, most of the results by sex had to be requested by Munafo et al. from the trial investigators because only 1 of the 11 studies in the Munafo et al. (2004) analysis actually reported outcome by sex in the publication. (Munafo et al. [2004] rightly criticized the clinical literature in smoking cessation for ignoring the reporting of outcome results by sex, because this prevents identification of potential sex differences.) In our updating of the Munafo et al. (2004) meta-analysis, we found that the increase in abstinence due to nicotine versus placebo patch was only half as large in women as in men, as shown in Figure 21.2. The odds ratios (ORs) for abstaining due to nicotine patch were highly significant for both men (OR = 2.20) and women (OR = 1.61), but nevertheless differed significantly (interaction OR of 1.40, 95% confidence interval = 1.02–1.93, p = .04). However, contrary to many reports (e.g., Piper et al., 2007; Scharf & Shiffman, 2004; Wetter et al., 1999), we did not find a significantly lower quit rate in women than men treated with placebo patch (i.e., no lower overall quit rate in women vs. men), as also shown in Figure 21.2. Thus, not every examination of quit rates via all cessation methods necessarily shows significantly poorer quit rates in women versus men, although many do, and we are aware of none that has ever shown the reverse—better quit rates in women versus men.

Whether a similar sex difference in efficacy would be seen for the other NRT formulations is not known but warrants testing (Cepeda-Benito et al., 2004; West et al., 2001). Results of many, but certainly not all, trials of nicotine versus placebo gum suggest a similarly poorer outcome in women versus men (see Perkins, 2001). Other research suggests that nicotine gum may be less effective in relieving nicotine withdrawal in women versus men (Hatsukami, McBride, Pirie, Hellerstedt, & Lando, 1991). Less efficacy in alleviating withdrawal perhaps indicates a sex difference in the negative reinforcing effects of nicotine rather than, or in addition to, a difference in positive reinforcing effects.

From a practical standpoint, however, NRT, including patch, should remain a key medication for women trying to quit smoking; the nicotine patch is safe, easy to use, easy to obtain (e.g., it does not require a prescription), and inexpensive relative to other medications. The NRT patch also helps women quit smoking, just not as much as it appears to help men, on average (Figure 21.2). Furthermore, some women may be very sensitive to nicotine's effects on smoking behavior and respond very well to an NRT patch, whereas some men may be more sensitive to the non-nicotine effects on smoking behavior and not respond very well

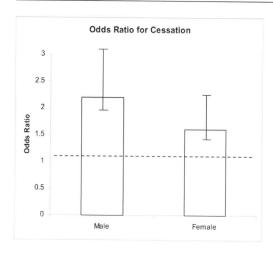
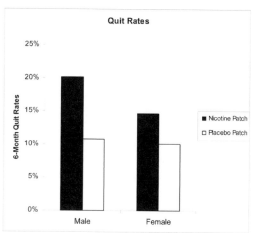

FIGURE 21.2. Odds ratios (OR, *left*) and absolute quit rates (*right*) for men and women from a meta-analysis of 14 clinical trials (*n* = 6,250) comparing 6-month cessation outcome due to nicotine versus placebo patch. ORs are the odds of abstinence among those randomized to nicotine versus placebo patch by the follow-up period. OR of 1.0 indicates no effect of nicotine over placebo. Also shown are the 95% confidence intervals (CI) for each OR. Data from Perkins and Scott (2008).

to an NRT patch. Thus, from the standpoint of an individual woman who smokes, the patch may be an effective option. However, given the literature showing generally poorer outcome with nicotine patch in women versus men (Perkins & Scott, 2008), women and their health care providers need to be aware that women may be more likely than men to require additional treatment options in order to quit successfully. These options include non-nicotine medications and counseling, either separate from or in addition to NRT. Each of these is discussed next.

Sex Differences in Treatment Effects of Non-Nicotine Medications

Less research attention has been focused on sex differences in the efficacy of cessation medications other than NRT. However, where they have been examined, no comparable sex difference has been observed in the efficacy of these other medications. The first non-NRT medication approved by the FDA for smoking cessation was bupropion (Zyban). In a meta-analysis of 12 placebo-controlled bupropion trials (Scharf & Shiffman, 2004), bupropion was equally effective in men and women, with ORs for abstinence of 2.53 and 2.47, respectively, at the end of the treatment period (typically 7–10 weeks; compare with the difference between men and women in ORs for NRT patch in Figure 21.2). This meta-analysis also found significantly lower overall cessation rates in women versus men, regardless of treatment (OR = 0.77). Thus, in these trials, women had more difficulty quitting in general, as found by others, but they were no less likely to be helped by bupropion. However, the lack of examination of abstinence over longer follow-up periods beyond the end of treatment is potentially important because some evidence with NRT indicates that the sex difference in efficacy is greater with longer duration of follow-up (Cepeda-Benito et al., 2004).

To date, the only other FDA-approved cessation medication is varenicline (Chantix), which is a drug specifically designed by its manufacturer, Pfizer, to act as a partial agonist of certain nicotine receptors in the brain (alpha$_4$beta$_2$ subtype) believed to be critical to smoking reinforcement. Relatively few controlled trials have been published with varenicline, but, as with bupropion, this medication appears to be equally efficacious in men and women. In the largest varenicline trial, with over 1,000 participants (Gonzales et al., 2006), the ORs for abstinence due to medication at the end of 12 weeks of treatment were similar between men (OR = 3.75) and women (OR = 3.63). However, although outcome results for 1-year follow-up were reported in this varenicline trial, there was no mention as to whether or not sex differences in outcome at 1 year were analyzed. Thus, as with the meta-analysis of bupropion trials (Scharf & Shiffman, 2004), omission of analyses of sex differences at longer duration of follow-up prevents a more comprehensive evaluation of whether men and women differ in long-term clinical response to varenicline.

Most other medications tested in clinical trials but not yet approved by the FDA for smoking cessation, including mecamylamine, clonidine, and naltrexone, may be equally or more efficacious in women than in men, at least during active treatment (Perkins, 2001). Therefore, although sex differences in long-term follow-up of non-nicotine medication effects on cessation have not been adequately examined, the apparent lack of poorer outcome in women versus men when treated with these medications indicate that the sex difference in response to NRT is specific to nicotine. If confirmed, this research would suggest that non-nicotine medications, or treatments not relying on any medications (see below), may warrant greater consideration in the treatment of women wanting to quit smoking, in the absence of contraindications for their use.

In summary, the NRT patch (and perhaps other NRT formulations) appears to be less effective in women than in men, on average, whereas non-nicotine medications are equally effective in women and men. These results are consistent with the basic research, described previously, indicating that smoking in women is less influenced by nicotine than is the smoking of men. Yet, comprehensive meta-analyses of sex differences in medication effects have examined only the NRT patch and bupropion, and systematic evaluation of sex differences in the long-term clinical outcome results with other medications and treatments is needed before firm conclusions can be reached.

COUNSELING APPROACHES TO IMPROVE CESSATION IN WOMEN

The discussion of sex differences in medication response is important because of the current emphases on medication use in clinical settings and on medication development in the search for improved interventions for cessation. However, in many respects, the sex difference in medication response is a very small part of why men and women may differ in ability to quit smoking. Many other obstacles to quitting may be more salient or common in women and thus may better explain their greater difficulty in quitting. Addressing these obstacles may require enhancing some elements of standard counseling that are more relevant for women, or providing adjunct interventions tailored to particular women who smoke, based on their needs.

Enhancing Standard Counseling in Women

Increase Medication Efficacy

Counseling is essential even when medications are recommended to people wanting to quit. Key components of counseling should include increasing patients' motivation to quit, educating them about what they can and cannot expect from medications, and teaching them ways to cope with smoking cues, as well as following up on problems and progress after the quit day (Perkins et al., 2008). Not only may women gain at least as much as men from such counseling, but some evidence suggests that counseling can enhance the effects of medication more in women than men. In the meta-analysis of NRT formulations discussed previously, Cepeda-Benito et al. (2004) found that NRT had no effect at 6-month follow-up in women given little or no counseling but was effective in women given high-intensity counseling. By contrast, they found that NRT was effective in men regardless of counseling intensity. Because minimal counseling is far more common in the real world than intense counseling, the poorer response of women than men to NRT may be overcome by routinely providing intense counseling to women who want to quit smoking. Yet, in our meta-analysis of NRT patch trials (Perkins & Scott, 2008), we did not find that higher-intensity counseling enhanced the response of women to the nicotine patch.

Compounding this issue of the influence of counseling on NRT response is the fact that physicians and other health care providers are only *half as likely to recommend* cessation medications for women who smoke compared to men who smoke (Steinberg, Akincigil, Delnevo, Crystal, & Carson, 2006). Thus, a starting point for improving cessation counseling in women may be ensuring that practitioners are trained to provide women with equal access to the tools available to help them quit smoking, including medications.

Increase Coping with Cues

In standard cognitive-behavioral cessation counseling, individuals preparing to quit are given strategies to cope with smoking cues that may elicit urges to smoke and thereby jeopardize their efforts to remain abstinent (Perkins et al., 2008). For example, they are told to avoid places where smoking is likely to occur (e.g., bars), and if that is not possible, to engage in cognitive and behavioral efforts to divert their attention from the cues (e.g., keep busy with a task, conduct an activity incompatible with smoking). Because women appear to be more responsive to such cues (Perkins, 2008; Perkins, Gerlach, et al., 2001), they may benefit more from such counseling advice, although this notion has not been formally tested. However, at least one study showed that women were more likely than men to relapse following an early lapse (i.e., any brief smoking exposure), suggesting that avoiding early lapse is particularly important for women (Borelli, Papandonatos, Spring, Hitsman, & Niaura, 2004). Consequently, counseling to improve women's ability to cope with smoking urges without lapsing soon after the quit day could greatly increase their long-term success in abstaining.

Increase Social Support

People who smoke tend to have more success with quitting if they receive support from friends or family through the early phases of quitting. This influence may be even more important in women, as some women may feel less supported by spouses when trying to quit, compared to men (e.g., Neff & Karney, 2005). Providing extra assistance on getting support from friends or others may increase the abstinence success of women.

Overcoming Particular Obstacles to Quitting

Reduce Concerns about Cessation-Induced Weight Gain

Half of all women who smoke, or about 10 million in the United States, express concern about gaining weight after they quit smoking. This proportion is at least twice the prevalence of weight gain concern among men who smoke (Pirie, Murray, & Luepker, 1991). Moreover, women tend to gain a bit more weight than men after quitting, about 8–10 pounds on average (Williamson et al., 1991). Young women are over three times more likely than men to cite weight gain as a cause of smoking relapse (Swan, Ward, Carmelli, & Jack, 1993). Individuals who are concerned about cessation-induced weight gain are less intent on quitting (Weekley, Klesges, & Relyea, 1992), may experience greater withdrawal severity upon quitting (Pinto, Borrelli, King, et al., 1999), are more likely to drop out of cessation treatment (Mizes et al., 1998), and are more likely to relapse (Meyers et al., 1997), compared to those who are not concerned about weight gain.

Regarding treatment options, the most common assumption has been to recommend concurrent dieting while quitting smoking so that the resulting weight gain can be prevented (Hall, Tunstall, Vila, & Duffy, 1992). However, dieting while trying to quit smoking has not been shown to enhance quit success *or* attenuate long-term weight gain (see Perkins, 1994). We have proposed an alternative approach: the use of cognitive-behavioral therapy (CBT) to directly reduce weight gain *concerns* rather than prevent the weight gain itself (Perkins, Levine, Marcus, & Shiffman, 1997). We tested this idea in women expressing concern about cessation-induced weight gain. All participants were given routine cessation counseling plus one of three adjuncts: CBT for weight concerns, behavioral dieting, or nonspecific social support that did not address weight (i.e., "standard" counseling; Perkins, Marcus, et al., 2001). Total contact time between patients and counselors was equal across these three treatment conditions; no medication was provided. We found that such a CBT treatment more than doubled 1-year smoking cessation rates beyond standard cessation counseling, whereas a behavioral dieting program did not significantly improve cessation (see Figure 21.3). Continuous abstinence in women receiving the CBT was nearly 30% at 6 months and over 20% at 1 year—comparable to or better than medication trials (e.g., see Figure 21.2).

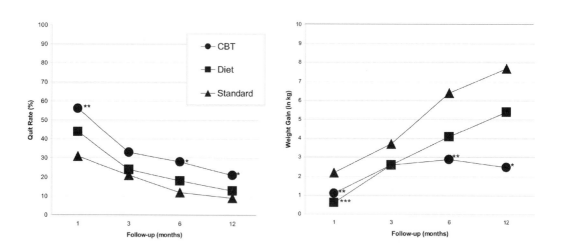

FIGURE 21.3. *Left*: Continuous smoking abstinence across the 1-year follow-up period in weight-concerned women who smoke given cessation counseling plus one of three adjunct components— cognitive-behavioral therapy to reduce weight concerns (CBT), behavioral weight control (DIET), or nonspecific social support that did not address weight (STANDARD). *Right*: Weight gain across the 1-year follow-up period in abstinent participants of each treatment group. *$p < .05$; **$p < .01$; ***$p < .001$ for the difference from the STANDARD (reference) group. Adapted from Perkins, Marcus, Levine, et al. (2001). Copyright 2001 by the American Psychological Association. Adapted by permission.

As described in detail elsewhere (Perkins et al., 1997, 2007; Perkins, Marcus, et al., 2001), this CBT involves challenging participants' assumptions about weight and shape and their thinking about the relationship of smoking with food, encouraging *moderate* snacking, and emphasizing the far greater health improvement due to quitting smoking versus avoiding modest weight gain. This counseling requires relatively long and frequent contacts and so may not be practical in brief one-on-one counseling. Cessation medications may also differentially affect weight gain; for example, bupropion and perhaps nicotine gum attenuate the amount of cessation-induced weight gain during the period of medication use but not long term (Doherty, Militello, Kinnunen, & Garvey, 1996; Hurt et al., 1997). Thus, because weight gain occurs eventually in those using bupropion or nicotine gum, counseling to increase acceptance of modest weight gain also applies to interventions that involve medications, and not just cessation counseling used alone.

Address Comorbid Depression

Women are twice as likely as men to suffer from the clinical disorder of depression. Because current depression, if not a history of depression, can interfere with a quit attempt (Hall et al., 1996), the greater prevalence of depression in women could partly account for their greater difficulty quitting. Monitoring a depressed patient's clinical state and compliance with prescribed antidepressant medications as part of counseling for smoking cessation would help promote increased abstinence.

Aside from the disorder of depression, the symptom of negative affect (e.g., sad mood, anxiety) is a critical facet of tobacco withdrawal in most affected individuals that is strongly predictive of smoking relapse (Kenford et al., 2002). Women may be more likely to view smoking as a way to manage their mood (Brandon & Baker, 1991), and negative mood after quitting may predict relapse more strongly in women than men (Borland, 1990). To combat this possible reason for greater relapse risk in women, adjunct mood management counseling may help alleviate depressive symptoms that emerge after quitting (Hall et al., 1996). Moreover, choice of cessation medication may influence the severity of such symptoms; bupropion, for example, is also an antidepressant that may help alleviate negative affect more than other cessation medications. Recall that bupropion has been shown to be equally effective for smoking cessation in women and men (Scharf & Shiffman, 2004).

Treat Smoking in Pregnant Women

Pregnant women who smoke present some unusual challenges to health care providers. First, the impact of their smoking on the fetus is a major public health issue, as noted in the introduction. Second, because of concerns over the possible effects of medications on fetal development, cessation often is supported solely by counseling alone, which may make quitting more difficult. (However, NRT is believed to be generally safe and worth considering for use by pregnant women who cannot quit smoking without medication; Benowitz & Dempsey, 2004.) Third, despite having less access to cessation medications, pregnant women who smoke actually have a very high likelihood of quitting successfully, until they give birth—after which about 65% resume smoking within the following 6 months (McBride & Pirie, 1990). Thus, very often, the challenge to providers is as likely to be the prevention of relapse after extended abstinence as it is to be initiating abstinence in recalcitrant pregnant women who smoke.

Counseling in this context may first require a more sensitive approach to assessing smoking status, due to the social stigma of continuing to smoke while pregnant. Over 20% of pregnant women claiming to be abstinent may in fact still be smoking (England et al., 2007). Giving pregnant women several response options (e.g., they have cut down but not quit) may be more successful in identifying women currently smoking than asking yes–no questions about current or recent smoking. Biochemical validation of smoking status by expired-air carbon monoxide or saliva cotinine is needed to identify pregnant women who smoke, as well as verify abstinence after the quit day in all supposedly abstinent women, especially during follow-up after the women give birth.

The same standard counseling steps appropriate for others who smoke can be used with pregnant women, although the intensity may need to be greater, since women unable to quit after learning they are pregnant may be particularly nicotine dependent. Important here may be increasing social support for cessation from the woman's partner (if willing) or from others. Novel nonmedication approaches to encouraging cessation may also be warranted, such as offering economic incentives to quitting (confirmed biochemically). Incentives can be vouchers exchangeable for baby supplies or other useful goods. This approach (contingency management) has been used frequently to reduce illicit drug use and has been shown to be very successful in fostering abstinence in pregnant women (Donatelle et al., 2004). Moreover, frequent contact by electronic means, such as via telephone counseling, may be cost-effective and more practical during follow-up than repeated in-person contacts in this population (Parker et al., 2007).

Attenuate Withdrawal Severity in Premenopausal Women

A woman's menstrual cycle phase may influence the intensity of withdrawal-related symptoms after quitting. Although the research findings are not necessarily consistent, women who quit during the luteal phase of their cycle (last 2 weeks of a 28-day cycle) may have more withdrawal, craving, and depressed mood than women who quit during the follicular phase (first 2 weeks of 28-day cycle; Perkins et al., 2000). Therefore, encouraging a woman to choose a quit date in the beginning of her menstrual cycle (i.e., during the follicular phase), especially if she is concerned about nicotine withdrawal, may help foster abstinence, although replication of this finding is necessary.

In summary, counseling that addresses the non-nicotine factors that contribute to smoking may be more effective in women than in men, but this notion has not been systematically tested. Other factors may also impede smoking cessation in women more than in men, such as the greater prevalence of depression or influence of negative mood during withdrawal, concerns about cessation-induced weight gain, menstrual cycle influences in worsening withdrawal, greater need for social support, and special problems posed by smoking during pregnancy. Counseling can effectively address these obstacles to improve smoking cessation rates in women.

FUTURE DIRECTIONS

Despite greater attention to sex differences in smoking and cessation treatment in recent research, many facets of nicotine dependence and smoking behavior remain underexplored. First, too little research has examined possible mechanisms to explain these sex differences, including those in the relative influence of nicotine and non-nicotine factors on smoking behavior. Research on the effects of other drugs, such as cocaine, suggests the presence of sex differences similar to those with smoking, as women may be less responsive to pharmacological and more responsive to nonpharmacological factors, compared with men (e.g., Lukas,

Sholar, Fortin, Wines, & Mendelson, 1996; Robbins, Ehrman, Childress, & O'Brien, 1999). However, this research is limited and not programmatic. Hormonal differences between men and women may help explain these sex differences, although smoking *behavior* has not been shown to vary reliably as a function of menstrual cycle phase, when hormone levels in women change sharply, despite the possible influence of cycle phase on withdrawal severity (Perkins et al., 2000), noted previously.

Second, the laboratory and clinical research discussed here indicates the presence of sex differences in the factors maintaining smoking behavior in dependent adults, but little research has determined whether these differences may play a role in the onset of smoking in teens. Some surveys suggest that the factors promoting smoking onset may differ between boys and girls, such as the relative influence of peers or family who smoke (e.g., Leatherdale, Manske, & Kroeker, 2006). Other studies suggest that girls may be more responsive to certain imagery used in cigarette advertising (Shadel, Niaura, & Abrams, 2004). However, the absence of laboratory studies of smoking behavior in teens prevents discovery of possible sex differences in the influence of nicotine and non-nicotine factors on acute smoking reinforcement and reward during early smoking experiences. If girls are influenced more by non-nicotine factors, prevention efforts could focus on ways to counter these factors during smoking experimentation.

A third area of future research would be to determine the breadth of the non-nicotine factors that differentially influence smoking reinforcement and reward in women and men. As outlined, proximal smoking cues (e.g., a lit cigarette) and verbal information about nicotine dose appear to influence smoking behavior more in women than in men. Distal cues (i.e., smoking contexts) may similarly influence smoking behavior more in women than in men. Thus, environments that set the stage for smoking may be more likely to precipitate smoking in women than in men, even in the absence of overt proximal cues for smoking (Conklin, 2006). Relatedly, perhaps social influences on smoking are greater in women than in men, as suggested by the possibly greater therapeutic influence of social support for cessation in women. The presence of friends or others smoking may increase smoking reinforcement and reward more in women than in men, but no controlled studies examining this notion have been published. Men and women may also differ in reinforcement from the motor effects of smoking (e.g., handling a cigarette, inhaling smoke). Although this idea has not formally been tested, an unpublished 1998 survey by the American Lung Association found that women smokers who failed to quit were more likely than men to say they relapsed because they "missed having something to do with their hands" and "missed the comfort of something to hold."

Finally, greater attention should be paid to improving nonmedication treatments for smoking cessation, primarily behavioral counseling, which have largely been ignored in recent decades with the shift in emphasis to medications (Piasecki & Baker, 2001). Many of the obstacles to quitting faced by women require counseling to teach them strategies to cope or otherwise overcome the obstacles. Enhancements in counseling would improve cessation rates in all who smoke, given that many of these obstacles are faced by men as well as women, if often to a lesser degree.

KEY POINTS

• Women tend to have greater difficulty in quitting smoking, compared to men, and this difficulty compounds the higher risks of smoking-related morbidity and mortality suffered by women, compared to men.

- The acute factors promoting smoking may differ in relative importance between men and women. Nicotine may be less influential, whereas non-nicotine factors, such as smoking cues, may be more influential in women than in men.
- These differences have implications for improving smoking cessation treatment, as NRT patch and perhaps other formulations appear to be less effective in women than in men, and non-nicotine medications are equally effective in women and men.
- Another implication of these differences is that counseling to address the non-nicotine factors in smoking should be more effective in women than in men, but this notion has not been systematically tested.
- Other factors may also impede smoking cessation in women more than in men, such as the greater prevalence of depression or greater influence of negative mood during withdrawal, concerns about cessation-induced weight gain, menstrual cycle influences in worsening withdrawal, greater need for social support, and special problems posed by smoking during pregnancy. Counseling can effectively address these obstacles to improve smoking cessation rates in women.
- Future research is needed to identify the specific mechanisms responsible for these sex differences, determine whether they may influence the onset of smoking and not just smoking persistence, examine what other non-nicotine factors may be more influential in women than men, and develop better counseling to address the obstacles to smoking cessation in women as well as all who smoke.

ACKNOWLEDGMENTS

Preparation of this chapter was supported by Grant Nos. DA16483, DA19478, and P50 DA/CA84718 from the National Institute on Drug Abuse (NIDA). Some of my research described here was supported by Grant No. DA12655 from NIDA.

REFERENCES

Asterisks denote recommended readings.

Bansal, M. A., Cummings, K. M., Hyland, A., & Giovino, G. A. (2004). Stop-smoking medications: Who uses them, who misuses them, and who is misinformed about them? *Nicotine and Tobacco Research*, 6(Suppl.), S303–S310.

Benowitz, N. L., & Dempsey, D. A. (2004). Pharmacotherapy for smoking cessation during pregnancy. *Nicotine and Tobacco Research*, 6(Suppl.), S189–S202.

Benowitz, N. L., & Hatsukami, D. K. (1998). Gender differences in the pharmacology of nicotine addiction. *Addiction Biology*, 3, 383–404.

Benowitz, N. L., Lessov-Schlaggar, C. N., Swan, G. E., & Jacob, P. (2006). Female sex and oral contraceptive use accelerate nicotine metabolism. *Clinical Pharmacology and Therapeutics*, 79, 480–488.

Borland, R. (1990). Slip-ups and relapse in attempts to quit smoking. *Addictive Behaviors*, 15, 235–245.

Borrelli, B., Papandonatos, G., Spring, B., Hitsman, B., & Niaura, R. (2004). Experimenter-defined quit rates for smoking cessation: Adherence improves outcomes for women but not for men. *Addiction*, 99, 378–385.

Brandon, T. H., & Baker, T. B. (1991). The Smoking Consequences Questionnaire: The subjective expected utility of smoking in college students. *Psychological Assessment*, 3, 484–491.

Buka, S. L., Shenassa, E. D., & Niaura, R. (2003). Elevated risk of tobacco dependence among offspring of mothers who smoked during pregnancy: A 30-year prospective study. *American Journal of Psychiatry, 160,* 1978–1984.

Carpenter, C. M., Wayne, G. F., & Connolly, G. N. (2005). Designing cigarettes for women: New findings from the tobacco industry documents. *Addiction, 100,* 837–851.

Carpenter, C. M., Wayne, G. F., & Connolly, G. N. (2007). The role of sensory perception in the development and targeting of tobacco products. *Addiction, 102,* 136–147.

Centers for Disease Control and Prevention. (2006). Cigarette smoking among adults—United States, 2005. *Morbidity and Mortality Weekly Report, 55,* 1145–1148.

Cepeda-Benito, A., Reynoso, J. T., & Erath, S. (2004). Meta-analysis of the efficacy of nicotine replacement therapy for smoking cessation: Differences between men and women. *Journal of Consulting and Clinical Psychology, 72,* 712–722. (*)

Chaudhri, N., Caggiula, A. R., Donny, E. C., Booth, S., Gharib, M. A., Craven, L. A., et al. (2005). Sex differences in the contribution of nicotine and nonpharmacological stimuli to nicotine self-administration in rats. *Psychopharmacology, 180,* 258–266.

Conklin, C. A. (2006). Environments as cues to smoke: Implication for human extinction-based research and treatment. *Experimental and Clinical Psychopharmacology, 14,* 12–19.

Conklin, C. A., Robin, N., Perkins, K. A., Salkeld, R., & McClernon, F. J. (2008). Proximal versus distal cues to smoke: The effects of environments on smokers' cue reactivity. *Experimental and Clinical Psychopharmacology, 16,* 207–214.

DiFranza, J. R., Aligne, C. A., & Weitzman, M. (2004). Prenatal and postnatal environmental tobacco smoke exposure and children's health. *Pediatrics, 113*(Suppl.), 1007–1015.

Doherty, K., Militello, F. S., Kinnunen, T., & Garvey, A. J. (1996). Nicotine gum dose and weight gain after smoking cessation. *Journal of Consulting and Clinical Psychology, 64,* 799–807.

Donatelle, R. J., Hudson, D., Dobie, S., Goodall, A., Hunsberger, M., & Oswald, K. (2004). Incentives in smoking cessation: Status of the field and implications for research and practice with pregnant smokers. *Nicotine and Tobacco Research, 6*(Suppl. 2), S163–S179. (*)

Dransfield, M. T., Davis, J. J., Gerald, L. B., & Bailey, W. C. (2005). Racial and gender differences in susceptibility to tobacco smoke among patients with chronic obstructive pulmonary disease. *Respiratory Medicine, 100,* 1110–1116.

England, L. J., Grauman, A., Qian, C., Wilkins, D. G., Schisterman, E. F., Yu, K. F., et al. (2007). Misclassification of maternal smoking status and effects on an epidemiologic study of pregnancy outcomes. *Nicotine and Tobacco Research, 9,* 1005–1013.

Ernster, V. L., Grady, D., Miike, R., Black, D., Selby, J., & Kerlikowske, K. (1995). Facial wrinkling in men and women, by smoking status. *American Journal of Public Health, 85,* 78–82.

Ezzati, M., & Lopez, A. D. (2003). Estimates of global mortality attributable to smoking in 2000. *Lancet, 362,* 847–852.

Fortmann, S. P., & Killen, J. D. (1994). Who shall quit? Comparison of volunteer and population-based recruitment in two minimal-contact smoking cessation studies. *American Journal of Epidemiology, 140,* 39–51.

Giovino, G. A. (2007). The tobacco epidemic in the United States. *American Journal of Preventive Medicine, 33*(Suppl. 6), S318–S326.

Gonzales, D., Rennard, S. I., Nides, M., Oncken, C., Azoulay, S., Billing, C. B., et al. (2006). Varenicline, an a4b2 nicotinic acetylcholine receptor partial agonist, vs. sustained-release bupropion and placebo for smoking cessation. *Journal of the American Medical Association, 296,* 47–55.

Hall, S. M., Munoz, R. F., Reus, V. I., Carol, D., Humfleet, G. L., & Hartz, D. T. (1996). Mood management and nicotine gum in smoking treatment: A therapeutic contact and placebo controlled study. *Journal of Consulting and Clinical Psychology, 64,* 1003–1009.

Hall, S. M., Tunstall, C. D., Vila, K. L., & Duffy, J. (1992). Weight gain prevention and smoking cessation: Cautionary findings. *American Journal of Public Health, 82,* 799–803.

Hatsukami, D., McBride, C., Pirie, P., Hellerstedt, W., & Lando, H. (1991). Effects of nicotine gum on prevalence and severity of withdrawal in female cigarette smokers. *Journal of Substance Abuse, 3,* 427–440.

Hornsby, P. P., Wilcox, A. J., & Weinberg, C. R. (1998). Cigarette smoking and disturbance of menstrual function. *Epidemiology, 9,* 193–198.

Hurt, R. D., Sachs, D. P., Glover, E. D., Offord, K. P., Johnston, J. A., Khayrallah, M. A., et al. (1997). A comparison of sustained-release bupropion and placebo for smoking cessation. *New England Journal of Medicine, 337,* 1195–1202.

International Early Lung Cancer Action Program Investigators. (2006). Women's susceptibility to tobacco carcinogens and survival after diagnosis of lung cancer. *Journal of the American Medical Association, 296,* 180–184. (*)

Kenford, S. L., Smith, S. S., Wetter, D. W., Jorenby, D. E., Fiore, M. C., & Baker, T. B. (2002) Predicting relapse back to smoking: Contrasting affective and physical models of dependence. *Journal of Consulting and Clinical Psychology, 70,* 216–227.

Leatherdale, S. T., Manske, S., & Kroeker, C. (2006). Sex differences in how older students influence younger student smoking behaviour. *Addictive Behaviors, 31,* 1308–1318.

Lukas, S. E., Sholar, M. B., Fortin, M., Wines, J., & Mendelson, J. H. (1996). Sex differences in plasma cocaine levels and subjective effects after acute cocaine administration in human volunteers. *Psychopharmacology, 125,* 346–354.

McBride, C. M., & Pirie, P. L. (1990). Postpartum smoking relapse. *Addictive Behaviors, 15,* 165–168.

Meyers, A. W., Klesges, R. C., Winders, S. E., Ward, K. D., Peterson, B. A., & Eck, L. H. (1997). Are weight concerns predictive of smoking cessation? A prospective analysis. *Journal of Consulting and Clinical Psychology, 66,* 448–452.

Mizes, J. S., Sloan, D. M., Segraves, K., Spring, B., Pingitore, R., & Kristeller, J. (1998). The influence of weight related variables on smoking cessation. *Behavior Therapy, 29,* 371–385.

Munafo, M., Bradburn, M., Bowes, L., & David, S. (2004). Are there sex differences in transdermal nicotine replacement therapy patch efficacy? A meta-analysis. *Nicotine and Tobacco Research, 6,* 769–776.

Neff, L. A., & Karney, B. R. (2005). Gender differences in social support: A question of skill or responsiveness? *Journal of Personality and Social Psychology, 88,* 79–90.

Parker, D. R., Windsor, R. A., Roberts, M. B., Hecht, J., Hardy, N. V., Strolla, L. O., et al. (2007). Feasibility, cost, and cost-effectiveness of a telephone-based motivational intervention for underserved pregnant smokers. *Nicotine and Tobacco Research, 9,* 1043–1051.

Perkins, K. A. (1994). Issues in the prevention of weight gain after smoking cessation. *Annals of Behavioral Medicine, 16,* 46–52.

Perkins, K. A. (1996). Sex differences in nicotine vs. non-nicotine reinforcement as determinants of tobacco smoking. *Experimental and Clinical Psychopharmacology, 4,* 166–177.

Perkins, K. A. (2001). Smoking cessation in women: Special considerations. *CNS Drugs, 15,* 391–411.

Perkins, K. A. (2008). Sex differences in nicotine reinforcement and reward: Influences on the persistence of tobacco smoking. In R. Bevins & A. R. Caggiula (Eds.), *The motivational impact of nicotine and its role in tobacco use* (pp. 143–169). New York: Springer-Verlag.

Perkins, K. A., Conklin, C. A., & Levine, M. D. (2008). *Cognitive-behavioral treatment of smoking cessation.* New York: Routledge. (*)

Perkins, K. A., Donny, E., & Caggiula, A. R. (1999). Sex differences in nicotine effects and self-administration: Review of human and animal evidence. *Nicotine and Tobacco Research, 1,* 301–315. (*)

Perkins, K. A., Doyle, T., Ciccocioppo, M., Conklin, C., Sayette, M., & Caggiula, A. R. (2006). Sex differences in the influence of nicotine and dose instructions on subjective and reinforcing effects of smoking. *Psychopharmacology, 184,* 600–607.

Perkins, K. A., Epstein, L. H., Grobe, J. E., & Fonte, C. (1994). Tobacco abstinence, smoking cues, and the reinforcing value of smoking. *Pharmacology, Biochemistry, and Behavior, 47,* 107–112.

Perkins, K. A., Gerlach, D., Vender, J., Grobe, J. E., Meeker, J., & Hutchison, S. (2001). Sex differences in the subjective and reinforcing effects of visual and olfactory cigarette smoke stimuli. *Nicotine and Tobacco Research, 3,* 141–150. (*)

Perkins, K. A., Grobe, J. E., D'Amico, D., Fonte, C., Wilson, A., & Stiller, R. L. (1996). Low-dose nicotine nasal spray use and effects during initial smoking cessation. *Experimental and Clinical Psychopharmacology, 4,* 157–165.

Perkins, K. A., Grobe, J. E., Stiller, R. L., Fonte, C., & Goettler, J. E. (1992). Nasal spray nicotine replacement suppresses cigarette smoking desire and behavior. *Clinical Pharmacology and Therapeutics*, *52*, 627–634.

Perkins, K. A., Jacobs, L., Ciccocioppo, M., Conklin, C. A., Sayette, M., & Caggiula, A. (2004). The influence of instructions and nicotine dose on the subjective and reinforcing effects of smoking. *Experimental and Clinical Psychopharmacology*, *12*, 91–101.

Perkins, K. A., Jacobs, L., Sanders, M., & Caggiula, A. R. (2002). Sex differences in the subjective and reinforcing effects of cigarette nicotine dose. *Psychopharmacology*, *163*, 194–201. (*)

Perkins, K. A., Levine, M., Marcus, M., Shiffman, S., D'Amico, D., Miller, A., et al. (2000). Tobacco withdrawal in women and menstrual cycle phase. *Journal of Consulting and Clinical Psychology*, *68*, 176–180.

Perkins, K. A., Levine, M. D., Marcus, M. D., & Shiffman, S. (1997). Addressing women's concerns about weight gain due to smoking cessation. *Journal of Substance Abuse Treatment*, *14*, 173–182.

Perkins, K. A., Marcus, M. D., Levine, M. D., D'Amico, D., Miller, A., Broge, M., et al. (2001). Cognitive-behavioral therapy to reduce weight concerns improves smoking cessation outcome in weight concerned women. *Journal of Consulting and Clinical Psychology*, *69*, 604–613. (*)

Perkins, K. A., Sayette, M., Conklin, C. A., & Caggiula, A. R. (2003). Placebo effects of tobacco smoking and other nicotine intake. *Nicotine and Tobacco Research*, *5*, 695–709.

Perkins, K. A., & Scott, J. (2005). Comment on Shiffman and colleagues, "Nicotine patch and lozenge are effective in women." *Nicotine and Tobacco Research*, *7*, 915–916.

Perkins, K. A., & Scott, J. (2008). Sex differences in long-term smoking cessation rates due to nicotine patch. *Nicotine and Tobacco Research*, *10*, 1245–1251. (*)

Piasecki, T. M., & Baker, T. B. (2001). Any further progress in smoking cessation treatment? *Nicotine and Tobacco Research*, *3*, 311–323.

Pinto, B. M., Borrelli, B., King, T. K., Bock, B. C., Clark, M. M., Roberts, M., et al. (1999). Weight control smoking among sedentary women. *Addictive Behaviors*, *24*, 75–86.

Piper, M. E., Federman, E. B., McCarthy, D. E., Bolt, D. M., Smith, S. S., Fiore, M. C., et al. (2007). Efficacy of bupropion alone and in combination with nicotine gum. *Nicotine and Tobacco Research*, *9*, 947–954.

Pirie, P. L., Murrary, D. M., & Luepker, R. V. (1991). Gender differences in cigarette smoking and quitting in a cohort of young adults. *American Journal of Public Health*, *81*, 324–327.

Prescott, E., Hippe, M., Schnohr, P., Ole Hein, H., & Vestbo, J. (1998). Smoking and risk of myocardial infarction in women and men: Longitudinal population study. *British Medical Journal*, *316*, 1043–1047.

Robbins, S. J., Ehrman, R. N., Childress, A. R., & O'Brien, C. P. (1999). Comparing levels of cocaine cue reactivity in male and female outpatients. *Drug and Alcohol Dependence*, *53*, 223–230.

Rodu, B., & Cole, P. (2007). Declining mortality from smoking in the United States. *Nicotine and Tobacco Research*, *9*, 781–784.

Scharf, D., & Shiffman, S. (2004). Are there gender differences in smoking cessation, with and without bupropion? Pooled and meta-analyses of clinical trials of bupropion SR. *Addiction*, *99*, 1462–1469. (*)

Shadel, W. G., Niaura, R., & Abrams, D. B. (2004). Adolescents' responses to the gender valence of cigarette advertising imagery: The role of affect and the self-concept. *Addictive Behaviors*, *29*, 1735–1744.

Shiffman, S., Sweeney, C. T., & Dresler, C. M. (2005). Nicotine patch and lozenge are effective for women. *Nicotine and Tobacco Research*, *7*, 119–127.

Steinberg, M. B., Akincigil, A., Delnevo, C. D., Crystal, S., & Carson, J. L. (2006). Gender and age disparities for smoking cessation treatment. *American Journal of Preventive Medicine*, *30*, 405–412.

Swan, G. E., Ward, M. M., Carmelli, D., & Jack, L. M. (1993). Differential rates of relapse in subgroups of male and female smokers. *Journal of Clinical Epidemiology*, *46*, 1041–1053.

U.S. Department of Health and Human Services. (1988). *The health consequences of smoking: Nicotine addiction. A report of the U.S. Surgeon General*. Washington, DC: U.S. Public Health Service.

Weekley, C. K., Klesges, R. C., & Relyea, G. (1992). Smoking as a weight-control strategy and its relationship to smoking status. *Addictive Behaviors, 17,* 259–271.

West, R., Hajek, P., Nilsson, F., Foulds, J., May, S., & Meadows, A. (2001). Individual differences in preferences for and responses to four nicotine replacement products. *Psychopharmacology, 153,* 225–230.

Wetter, D., Kenford, S. L., Smith, S. S., Fiore, M. C., Jorenby, D. E., & Baker, T. B. (1999). Gender differences in smoking cessation. *Journal of Consulting and Clinical Psychology, 67,* 555–562.

Williamson, D. F., Madans, J., Anda, R. F., Kleinman, J. C., Giovino, G. A., & Byers, T. (1991). Smoking cessation and severity of weight gain in a national cohort. *New England Journal of Medicine, 324,* 739–745.

CHAPTER 22

Gender and Prescription Opioid Addiction

Sudie E. Back, PhD
Rebecca Payne, MD

Prescription opioid abuse and dependence are a significant problem for both men and women. In this chapter we briefly review the scope of the problem and discuss potential reasons for the recent upsurge. In the remaining sections, we review gender differences in rates of opioid abuse and dependence, sources and reasons for using prescription opioids, likelihood of being prescribed an opioid medication, comorbidity, routes of administration, and treatment. Finally, because of the important role that chronic pain plays in prescription opioid use, gender differences in pain and factors that affect pain are reviewed

This is a relatively new area of study, and the findings regarding gender differences are limited. The goal of this chapter, however, is to synthesize the research on gender and prescription opioids, to date, and offer suggestions for future investigations to expand and improve upon the current state of knowledge.

EPIDEMIOLOGY

Prescription opioid use, abuse, and dependence are on the rise (Blanco et al., 2007; Cicero, Inciardi, & Munoz, 2005; Rawson, Maxwell, & Rutkowski, 2007). According to the Substance Abuse and Mental Health Services Administration's (SAMHSA) 2006 National Survey on Drug Use and Health (NSDUH; $n = 67,802$), 20.4 million Americans ages 12 and older reported using illicit drugs in the past month, with 5.2 million having used prescription opioids nonmedically (SAMHSA, 2007a). Between 1992 and 2003, rates of prescription opioid abuse increased 141% (National Center on Addiction and Substance Abuse at Columbia University [CASA], 2005). This increased rate of abuse was twice as high as increased rates of marijuana, five times as high as cocaine, and 60 times as high as heroin (CASA, 2005). Table 22.1 lists commonly abused prescription opioids. Oxycodone and hydrocodone are the most commonly abused and the most frequently reported to emergency departments (EDs) and poison control centers (Back et al., in press; Cicero et al., 2005, 2007; Hughes, Bogdan, & Dart, 2007; Inciardi et al., 2006; Rosenblum et al., 2007; SAMHSA, 2007b; Zacny et al., 2003).

TABLE 22.1. Commonly Abused Prescription Opioids

Generic name	Trade name
Oxycodone[a]	OxyContin, Percocet, Percodan, Roxicodone, Tylox
Hydrocodone[a]	Vicodin, Lortab, Hycodan
Methadone	Dolophine
Morphine	Duramorph, Roxanol, MS Contin, Oramorph
Hydromorphone	Dilaudid
Fentanyl	Duragesic, Sublimaze, Actiq
Buprenorphine	Subutex, Suboxone, Buprenex
Codeine	Empirin; Tylenol 1, 2, 3
Meperidine	Demerol
Propoxyphene	Darvon

[a]The most commonly abused prescription opioids.

ED visits, another indication of abuse, have increased substantially over the past few years. In 2005 almost 600,000 people were treated in EDs across the country for nonmedical use of prescription drugs, with 23% more women than men being admitted for this reason (SAMHSA, 2007b). From 2004 to 2005, ED visits related to opioids rose 24% from 158,284 to 196,225 (SAMHSA, 2007b). ED visits related specifically to narcotic analgesics rose 21%, with the most commonly reported narcotics being hydrocodone (51,225), oxycodone (42,810), methadone (41,216), morphine (15,183), and fentanyl (9,160) (SAMHSA, 2007b).

Similarly, rates of DSM-IV prescription opioid abuse and dependence have increased (Zacny et al., 2003). Using data from two large national surveys, the 1991–1992 National Longitudinal Alcohol Epidemiologic Survey (n = 42,862; Grant et al., 1992) and the 2001–2002 National Epidemiologic Survey on Alcohol and Related Conditions (NESARC, n = 43,093; Grant et al., 2003), Blanco and colleagues (2007) compared the prevalence of nonmedical prescription drug use disorders. The findings revealed a statistically significant increase in rates of nonmedical prescription opioid abuse or dependence: They had tripled (0.1–0.3%) over the 10-year span (Blanco et al., 2007).

Hypothesized reasons for the striking increase in use and abuse include the fact that, in comparison to other drugs such as heroin or cocaine, (1) prescription opioids can be relatively easily obtained in a variety of settings (e.g., EDs, primary care physicians, pain clinics, the Internet), (2) they may be more socially accepted by peers, (3) they are less likely than other street drugs to be adulterated, and (4) their purchase and possession are less closely monitored (Blanco et al., 2007; Cicero et al., 2005; Compton & Volkow, 2006; Ling, Wesson, & Smith, 2003). Significant increases in the production and distribution of prescription opioids over the past decade are also likely related to the increase in use and abuse. For example, from 1997 to 2001, the supply of oxycodone increased 348%, and from 1992 to 2002 prescriptions for oxycodone increased 380% (CASA, 2005).

One of the most unique features of prescription opioids, in contrast to other commonly abused substances, is that they are endorsed and prescribed by physicians. They serve as a primary treatment for medical conditions and are a legitimate means of improving functioning for many patients. Because of this, some individuals may have a false sense of safety regarding prescription opioids, and misconceptions regarding the risk of harm from using them nonmedically (Compton & Volkow, 2006). Physicians have received criticism for the undertreatment of pain syndromes (Gajraj & Hervias-Sanz, 1998), which might also contribute to the rise in prescribed opioids. Given the increase in opioid prescriptions to treat pain, one might hypothesize that increased nonmedical prescription opioid use reflects progression of available medical treatments for pain. However, this is unlikely given that the highest prevalence of nonmedical prescription opioid use is found among the youngest age groups, and disorders of chronic pain tend to be found in middle- to older-age people (Blanco, 2007).

Gender and Epidemiology

For most substances of abuse, men consistently demonstrate higher rates of use, abuse, and dependence as compared to women (Grant et al., 2004; Kessler et al., 2005; SAMHSA, 2007a; Stinson et al., 2005). In contrast, the data regarding prescription opioids are equivocal. Using data from the 1991 National Household Survey on Drug Abuse (NHSDA), which sampled over 32,000 individuals 12 years and older, Simoni-Wastila, Ritter, and Strickler (2004) found that women were more likely than men to use prescription drugs nonmedically. In fact, the odds of nonmedical use of narcotic analgesics were 41% higher for women than men (Simoni-Wastila et al., 2004). In another large epidemiological survey, the 1987 National Medical Expenditure Survey, Simoni-Wastila (2000) also found that significantly more women than men used narcotic analgesics.

In contrast, more recent findings suggest that women and men are equally likely to use prescription opioids nonmedically (Zacny et al., 2003) or that men evidence higher rates of use (Tetrault et al., 2008). For example, no gender differences in use were found in the 2001–2002 NESARC (Blanco et al., 2007). The 2006 NSDUH also reported similar rates of past-month use for men and women (SAMHSA, 2007a). In addition, the 2006 NSDUH reported that rates of nonmedical use from 2005 to 2006 increased for males but not females (SAMHSA, 2007a).

Among college populations, the findings are also equivocal. McCabe at al. (2005b) reported that men had significantly higher rates of both lifetime (17.4% men vs. 15.7% women) and past-year (10.1% men vs. 8.7% women) prescription pain medication use. In addition, men were significantly more likely than women to report being asked to divert their medications. Interestingly, McCabe found that attending a more competitive college was a risk factor for prescription opioid use for men but not women (McCabe, Teter, Boyd, Knight, & Wechsler, 2005). Another more recent study conducted by McCabe, Cranford, Boyd, and Teter (2007) failed to find appreciable gender differences in lifetime or past-year rates of nonmedical prescription opioid use.

Among treatment-seeking samples, some studies suggest that men are more likely than women to abuse prescription opioids (Chabal, Erjavec, Jacobson, Mariano, & Chaney, 1997; Cicero et al., 2005). Data from the Researched Abuse, Diversion, and Addiction-Related Surveillance (RADAR) system, which compiles data from law enforcement, poison control centers, methadone maintenance treatment clinics, and other "key informants" across the country, indicates that about 65% of OxyContin (oxycodone) abusers are men (Cicero et al., 2005). Similarly, Carise and colleagues (2007) conducted a large-scale national study (*n* = 27,816) of 157 addiction treatment programs in the United States and found that the majority of patients who abused OxyContin were men (69%). In contrast to these findings, Rosenblum et al. (2007) investigated past month prescription opioid abuse among patients at 72 methadone maintenance treatment programs across 33 states (*n* = 5,663) and found that women were more likely than men to report past-month abuse (70.2% women vs. 65.3% men).

With regard to studies mentioned above, differences in settings and sources of data collection (e.g., poison control centers, methadone maintenance clinics, law enforcement agencies) and the type of prescription opioids assessed may help explain the discrepancies. Furthermore, the inconsistencies found across the literature may be due, in part, to the varying definitions used to assess the problem of prescription opioids. For example, the terms *use, misuse, nonmedical use, aberrant behaviors, abuse, dependence,* and *pseudoaddiction* are often used and can generate confusion (Ling et al., 2003; Lusher, Elander, Bevan, Telfer, & Burton, 2006; SAMHSA, 2006; Zacny et al., 2003). Table 22.2 includes examples of the various terms and definitions commonly seen in the literature. Although it is beyond the scope of this chapter to address the advantages and disadvantages of these various terms, we include them to help readers understand potential sources of variability in the extant literature, and to highlight the need for greater consensus among investigators with regard to these terms and their definitions.

Age and Gender

Teenagers and young adults are at particularly high risk of abusing prescription opioids (Blanco et al., 2007; Colliver, Kroutil, Dai, & Gfroerer, 2006; Hughes et al., 2007; Johnston, O'Malley, Bachman, & Schulenberg, 2006; Rosenblum et al., 2007; SAMHSA, 2007a; Zacny et al., 2003). Data from the 2006 Monitoring the Future study found that 9% of 12th-grade students reported using narcotic pain relievers (Johnson et al., 2006). Several large studies of college students, some with over 14,000 participants, indicate an 11–18% lifetime

TABLE 22.2. Common Terms and Definitions Used to Investigate and Characterize the Spectrum of Prescription Opioid Use

Nonmedical use: Use of a prescription opioid that was not prescribed to a person or was taken simply for the experience or feeling it caused.

Misuse: Incorrect use of an opioid medication (e.g., taking more than was prescribed, taking it more often than was prescribed, using it for a purpose other than that for which it was prescribed).

Abuse: A maladaptive pattern of use leading to clinically significant impairment or distress, as evidenced by one or more DSM-IV diagnostic criteria in the past 12 months (e.g., recurrent failure to fulfill major obligations at work, school, or home; recurrent use in situations in which it is physically hazardous; continued use despite having recurrent social or interpersonal problems caused or exacerbated by the use).

Dependence: Often used synonymously with *addiction*. A maladaptive pattern of use that indicates a loss of control and clinically significant impairment or distress, as evidenced by three or more DSM-IV diagnostic criteria in the past 12 months (e.g., tolerance, withdrawal symptoms, persistent desire or unsuccessful efforts to cut down or quit, taking more of the substance than was planned). Note that a patient can be "addicted" to, or dependent on, a substance, per DSM-IV criteria, without having physiological dependence.

Physiological dependence: Tolerance for a medication, emergence of withdrawal symptoms upon cessation of the medication, or continued use of the medication to prevent withdrawal symptoms. Note that a patient may have physiological dependence without being "addicted" or meeting DSM-IV criteria for dependence.

Pseudoaddiction: Drug-seeking and other behaviors that are phenotypically consistent with psychological dependence but actually result from insufficient pain treatment or pain relief. Once the pain is adequately treated, the drug-seeking and other related behaviors typically cease.

Aberrant behaviors: Behaviors related to using a medication in a way other than it was prescribed; for example, unauthorized dose escalations, borrowing medications from family or friends, running out of medications and needing early refills, obtaining medications from more than one doctor, and using an alternative route of administration (e.g., crushing and snorting).

Note. The items listed in this table are examples of terms frequently used in the literature. This table is not meant to serve as an exhaustive or definitive list.

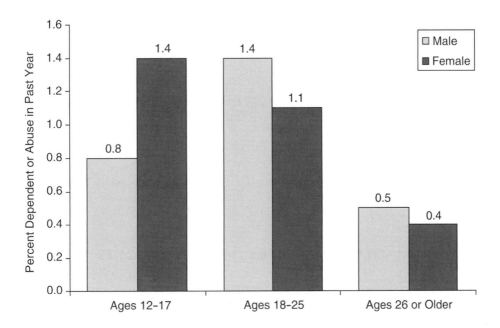

FIGURE 22.1. Substance dependence or abuse for nonmedical use of pain relievers in the past year, by age group and gender: Annual averages based on 2002–2004. Data from Colliver, Kroutil, Dai, and Gfroerer (2006).

prevalence rate and 4–10% past-year rate of nonmedical prescription opioid use (McCabe, Teter, Boyd, Knight, et al., 2005).

Interestingly, there appears to be an interaction between age and gender with regard to heightened times of vulnerability. As illustrated in Figure 22.1, among youths 12–17 years of age, females have been shown to have higher rates of prescription opioid abuse and dependence, but among youths ages 18–25, males have been shown to have higher rates (Colliver et al., 2006).

GENDER DIFFERENCES IN PRESCRIPTIONS FOR OPIOIDS

Some studies suggest that women are more likely than men to be prescribed an abusable medication (McCabe, Teter, & Boyd, 2005; Simoni-Wastila, 2000; Simoni-Wastila et al., 2004; Sullivan, Edlund, Steffick, & Unutzer, 2005). A large-scale study including over 38,000 individuals in the United States found that women were 48% more likely than men to use an abusable prescription drug, particularly narcotic analgesics (Simoni-Wastila, 2000). This finding has also been shown among young adult populations, with women being more likely than men to be prescribed a prescription pain medication in the past year (27.2% women vs. 20.7% men; McCabe, Teter, & Boyd, 2005). While the reasons for this remain unclear, the higher rates of prescriptions among women could be related to increased rates of pain conditions or a greater propensity among women to seek treatment and report symptoms (Simoni-Wastila, 2000). Regardless of the reasons for this gender disparity, women have increased access to prescription opioids, which may increase their risk of misuse, abuse, or dependence.

REASONS FOR USING PRESCRIPTION OPIOIDS

In response to press reports describing OxyContin addiction occurring within an appropriate course of medical treatment among "drug naïve" individuals, Carise and colleagues (2007) examined OxyContin use in 157 addiction programs across the United States. Of patients who endorsed using OxyContin (n = 1,425), the majority (78%) reported that it had not been prescribed to them for a medical reason, and 86% reported using it to "get high or get a buzz."

McCabe, Cranford, Boyd, and Teter (2007) surveyed 4,580 college students at a large Midwestern public institution and found that the most common reason for nonmedical prescription opioid use was to relieve pain (63.0%) and to get "high" (31.9%). Men were significantly more likely than women to report using prescription opioids to get "high" (39.4% men vs. 24.4% women) or for "experimentation" (35.3% men vs. 18.4% women).

SOURCES OF PRESCRIPTION OPIOIDS

The majority of individuals who misuse prescription opioids appear to obtain them from friends or relatives (cf. Carise et al., 2007; SAMHSA, 2007b). Among young adults, men are significantly more likely than women to obtain prescription opioids from peers or a drug dealer (McCabe, Teter, Boyd, et al., 2005; McCabe, Teter, Boyd, Knight, et al., 2005). Although not statistically significant, more women than men report obtaining prescription opioids from their partner (10% women vs. 6% men; McCabe, Teter, Boyd, Knight, et al., 2005).

Young women are also more likely than young men to obtain prescription drugs from their parents or other family members (up to 36% women vs. up to 20% men; McCabe, Teter, Boyd, Knight, et al., 2005; McCabe, Teter, & Boyd, 2005; McCabe, Cranford, et al., 2007). Usually, parents have previously obtained the medication for a legitimate medical reason, and they subsequently give their unused medication to their daughters when they report pain (e.g., having a severe headache). While not given to "get high," parents must be cautioned against this practice. It is unlikely that parents provide the proper caution around potential drug interactions and dangers associated with prescription opioid use (McCabe, Teter, & Boyd, 2005). In addition, research has shown that the earlier exposure to prescription opioids, the more likely a person is to misuse them later on in life (Colliver et al., 2006). One study found that college students who had taken prescription opioids during elementary school were two times more likely than their counterparts to engage in past-year illicit use (McCabe, Teter, & Boyd, 2005). Another more recent study by McCabe, West, Morales, Cranford, and Boyd (2007) showed that for every year nonmedical prescription drug use was delayed, the risk of developing future prescription drug abuse was reduced by 5%.

ROUTES OF ADMINISTRATION

To date, no appreciable gender differences in routes of administration have been reported. Most individuals ingest prescription opioids orally (Carise et al., 2007; McCabe, Cranford, et al., 2007, 2007), although a recent study found that a minority (16% of men, 11% of women) reported crushing and snorting them (McCabe, Cranford, et al., 2007). Among 121 chronic pain outpatients, 9% of men and 2% of women reported using alternative routes of administration (Back et al., in press).

COMORBIDITY

Both men and women who abuse prescription opioids evidence high rates of other substance use and substance use disorders (SUDs; Carise et al., 2007; CASA, 2005; Kreek, 2000; McCabe & Teter, 2007; Simoni-Wastila et al., 2004). Individuals who have used prescription opioids nonmedically, in comparison to individuals who have not, are four times more likely to binge drink, eight times more likely to use marijuana, and 13 times more likely to use cocaine (McCabe, Teter, & Boyd, 2005). For young adults, the risk of abusing additional substances is particularly high if the source of their prescription opioids is peers, if they are motivated to use for reasons other than pain relief, or if they use non-oral routes of administration (McCabe, Teter, & Boyd, 2005; McCabe, Cranford, et al., 2007; McCabe & Teter, 2007).

Rates of comorbid psychiatric conditions are also high among individuals who use and abuse prescription opioids (Kreek, 2000). Data from a nationally representative sample of the general population (n = 9,279) found that individuals who use prescription opioids have significantly higher rates of mental health disorders, such as major depressive disorder, dysthmia, panic disorder, and generalized anxiety disorder (Sullivan et al., 2005). Anecdotal evidence also posits high rates of physical and sexual abuse histories among women with opioid dependence who present to primary care clinics (O'Conner, 2007).

Among treatment-seeking patients with opioid dependence, Jones, Johnson, Bigelow, and Strain (2004) used the Addiction Severity Index (ASI) and the Structured Interview for DSM-IV (SCID) to assess substance use, other psychiatric conditions, and psychosocial characteristics. Compared to men, women had significantly higher rates of medical, economic, and occupational problems, and major depressive disorder. In addition, men were more likely than women to have an Axis II disorder, antisocial personality disorder, and more frequent alcohol, cannabis, and/or cocaine use (Jones et al., 2004). It is unclear, however, what type of opioids patients were using in this study. Thus, the generalizabitlity to patients with prescription opioid dependence is unknown. In a similar study, Hernandez-Avila, Rounsaville, and Kranzler (2004) used the ASI and SCID to assess treatment-seeking patients with opioid dependence. Again, the form of opioid dependence was not specified, so the findings may not generalize well to patients with prescription opioid dependence. With that caveat in mind, evidence of "telescoping" (i.e., shorter time from onset of substance use to the development of problems) among women with opioid dependence was found, as evidenced by significantly fewer years of pretreatment use among women as compared to men (Hernandez-Avila et al., 2004). Furthermore, women reported more psychiatric, medical, and occupational impairment than men (Hernandez-Avila et al., 2004).

Among general hospital patients (n = 952), one study investigated rates of prescription drug dependence and comorbid psychiatric disorders, and found that women were more likely than men to be dependent on prescription drugs (53% vs. 37%), and that the majority (66.7%) of patients dependent on prescription drugs had at least one comorbid Axis I condition (Fach, Bischof, Schmidt, & Rumpf, 2007). The most common comorbid disorders were anxiety (e.g., specific phobia, panic disorder with agoraphobia), other SUDs (e.g., alcohol), and affective disorders (e.g., major depressive disorder, dysthmia, bipolar disorder). Consistent with the general population, women evidenced significantly higher rates of affective disorders, and men evidenced significantly higher rates of other SUDs (Fach et al., 2007). Unfortunately, the findings were not broken down by type of prescription drug, so rates of comorbidity among patients with prescription opioid dependence in this study is unknown.

CHRONIC PAIN

The study of prescription opioid use disorders and chronic pain are intimately linked, as opioid medications are one of the most common means of treating pain. Chronic pain, often defined as pain that persists for 3–6 months, is a common medical condition. One study estimated the point prevalence of chronic pain among adults in the United States to be 15% (range = 2–40%; Verhaak, Kerssens, Dekker, Sori, & Bensing, 1998). International data also demonstrate high rates of chronic pain, ranging from 16 to 50% in community samples (Blyth et al., 2001; Elliott et al., 1999; Eriksen, Jensen, Sjogren, Ekholm, & Rasmussen, 2003).

Gender and Chronic Pain

In comparison to men, women typically report more frequent and more intense pain, report pain in a greater number of locations throughout the body, have longer-lasting pain, and experience more interference with daily activities as a result of pain (Barsky, Peekna, & Borus, 2001; Blyth et al., 2001; Holdcroft & Berkley, 2006; Kepler et al., 1991; Torrance, Smith, Bennett, & Lee, 2006; Unruh, 1996; Verhaak et al., 1998). In the 2000 Danish National Health and Morbidity Survey (n = 10,066), women had 1.2–1.6 higher odds of reporting chronic pain than men (Eriksen et al., 2003).

Women also have higher rates of chronic pain conditions than men. For example, musculoskeletal pain, one of the most common forms of chronic pain that typically affects the hip, neck, back, and shoulder areas, is significantly more common among women than men (Jacobs, Hammerman-Rozenberg, Cohen, & Stressman, 2006; Unruh, 1996; Wijnhoven, de Vet, & Picavet, 2006). Osteoarthritis, rheumatoid arthritis, and fibromyalgia are also more prevalent in women than men (Felson, 1988; LeResche, 2000; Verbrugge, Lepkowski, & Konkol, 1991; Verbrugge, 1995).

Irritable bowel syndrome (IBS) is another chronic pain condition with a higher prevalence in women than men (Kim et al., 2006). In fact, approximately two-thirds of patients with IBS are women (Drossman, Whitehead, & Camilleri, 1997). Some chronic pain conditions, including IBS, appear to be particularly influenced by hormonal factors (Houghton, Lear, Jackson, & Whorwell, 2002; Whitehead et al., 1990). Temporomandibular joint (TMJ) pain and migraine headaches are more prevalent in women and appear to follow a bell-shaped curve over the course of the lifespan, with higher occurrences during women's reproductive years (LeResche, 2000). In general, recurrent pain in women has been found to correlate with estrogen plasma levels (Aloisi & Bonifazi, 2006). Postmenopausal women on estrogen replacement therapy experience an increased incidence of TMJ (Dao & LeResche, 2000).

The Role of Hormones in Chronic Pain

Pain is a highly complex phenomenon. A number of factors likely contribute to the experience of pain (e.g., genetics, sociocultural factors, cellular differences; Berkley, 1998). As mentioned earlier, hormonal differences may play an important role in the experience of pain and could help explain the substantial gender disparities observed in this area. In the following section, we briefly review the menstrual cycle phase before discussing how hormonal dynamics may influence gender differences in pain. Please refer to Chapter 3 in this volume for a more detailed review of the menstrual cycle.

The Menstrual Cycle

Hormone levels fluctuate across the life cycle. Briefly, the three phases of the menstrual cycle are the follicular phase, ovulation, and luteal phase. The first day of menstrual flow is, by convention, considered day 1 of the cycle. During the follicular phase (days 1–14), follicle-stimulating hormone (FSH) and luteinizing hormone (LH) receptors are up-regulated, and FSH and LH bind to these receptors and stimulate the synthesis of estradiol. Levels of estradiol continue to rise throughout the follicular phase; levels of progesterone are low during the follicular phase. Following ovulation, estradiol levels decrease.

The luteal phase (days 15–28) is characterized by increasing levels of progesterone, which functions to further prepare the endometrium for implantation of the corpus luteum, should fertilization occur. If fertilization does not occur, the corpus luteum regresses and no longer produces estradiol and progesterone, thereby causing an abrupt decrease in hormone plasma levels. The loss of progesterone results in the inability to sustain a prepared endometrium and the menstrual flow is initiated, marking the end of the luteal phase.

Hormonal Changes and Pain

Clinical studies suggest that pain sensitivity may change across the menstrual cycle (Aloisi & Bonifazi, 2006; Hellstrom & Anderberg, 2003; Korszun et al., 2000). This variability is important because such changes in pain sensitivity could represent heightened times of vulnerability to prescription opioid misuse or abuse among women. In addition, a greater understanding of how hormonal changes over the menstrual cycle affect pain perception could provide possible avenues for treatment interventions for pain.

Recurrent pain in women has been found to correlate with estrogen plasma levels (Aloisi & Bonifazi, 2006); however, this relationship has not been consistently demonstrated. For example, increased levels of pain, depression, and subjective stress have been reported during the luteal phase, when both estrogen and progesterone levels are high (Korszun et al., 2000). Hellstrom and Anderberg (2003), however, noted that self-reported pain was higher during the menstrual and premenstrual phases of the cycle, when estrogen levels are lower.

As stated earlier, pain is a complex phenomenon, and investigations of experimentally induced pain provide inconclusive results regarding gender differences (Berkley, 1997; Fillingim & Maixner, 1995). It may be that pain threshold differences across the menstrual cycle are dependent upon the type of experimental pain induced (Aloisi, 2003). For example, some studies report the highest pain threshold for electrical stimulation during the luteal phase, whereas others report the highest pain thresholds for thermal or mechanical stimuli during the follicular phase (Aloisi, 2003). Methodological discrepancies (e.g., definition of menstrual cycle phases, pain stimulus used, number of cycles assesses) and other study limitations (e.g., small sample sizes) preclude more definitive statements regarding changes in pain across the menstrual cycle at this time (Sherman & LeResche, 2006).

SPECIAL POPULATIONS: ELDERLY WOMEN

In recent years the aging population has received more attention as people are living longer and health care costs continue to rise. Women comprise the majority of older patients in the health care system, which may be attributable to better survival rates of women than men at all ages (Newman & Brach, 2001). It is estimated that one-third of women age 70 or older have difficulty performing activities of daily living (Kramarow, Lentzner, Rooks, Weeks, & Saydah, 1999). Musculoskeletal pain is a common cause of such disability (Leveille, Fried, & Guranik, 2002). Furthermore, women have worse outcomes on health-related quality of life measures than men (Emery et al., 2004; Hopman et al., 2000; Michelson, Bolund, Nilsson, & Brandburg, 2000), which may be attributable to the higher prevalence of chronic conditions and disabilities in elderly women (Centers for Disease Control, 2007).

Almost half (43%) of adults age 65 and older are estimated to enter a nursing home before death (Kemper & Murtaugh, 1991). With the increasing use of nursing homes and the recognition of the detrimental effects of pain on quality of life, pain control among older adults has received increasing attention. Pain is apt to be underdiagnosed in older adults (Gloth, 2001). Treating pain in this population poses clinical dilemmas for physicians related to the changing pharmacokinetics, pharmacodynamics, organ function (specifically liver and kidneys), volume of distribution, and body composition that accompany the aging process (Wilder-Smith, 2005). To date, very little research on chronic opioid use in older adults exists (Wilder-Smith, 2005), and what has been studied primarily focused on patients with cancer.

In nononcological investigations, opioid use has been shown to result in higher initial plasma levels in older adults, secondary to reduced volume of distribution, with no further effects from aging (Lemmens, Burm, Hennis, Gladines, & Bovill, 1990; Matteo, Schwartz, Ornstein, Young, & Chang, 1990; Sear, Hand, & Moore, 1989; Singleton, Rosen, & Fisher, 1988). No differences attributable to the pharmacokinetics in older adults were found with a single dose of dihydrocodeine. However, with repeated dosing, a 25% age-related increase in plasma concentrations was found, with a greater effect in women. This finding was likely attributable to decreased plasma clearance (Davies, Castleden, McBurney, & Jagger, 1989) and may place elderly women at a higher risk for adverse events (i.e., respiratory depression, hypotension, altered sensorium) with chronic opiate use. Similarly, in a small study using transdermal fentanyl patches, plasma concentrations doubled in older adults (67–87 years old), compared to younger counterparts (19–27), over 60 hours (2.0 vs. 0.9 ng/mL) (Holdsworth et al., 1994). In this study the young group ($n = 6$) was all male and the majority of the older group ($n = 10$) was female. With the increasing age of the population and prevalence of chronic pain conditions, the use and abuse of prescription opiates among elderly women and men deserves further research.

TREATMENT

Like most patients with SUDs, the majority of individuals with prescription opioid use disorders do not receive treatment. Data from the 2001–2002 NESARC (Grant, Moore, Shepard, & Kaplan, 2003) found that 24.2% of individuals with prescription drug abuse or dependence received treatment (Blanco et al., 2007). This was an increase from a decade ago, however, when only 15.8% reportedly received treatment (Blanco et al., 2007).

There are several treatment challenges unique to patients with prescription opioid use disorders. First, patients may be reluctant to disclose problems with prescription opiate use to the same physician who prescribes their medications. They may fear, for example, that doing so would negatively impact their future medical treatment. Patients who previously used prescriptions opioids to treat a pain condition may also be reluctant to seek substance use treatment for fear that it will result in the return of their pain symptoms (Blanco et al., 2007). Moreover, individuals with prescription opioid use disorders may perceive themselves as fundamentally different from patients seeking treatment for other drugs of abuse, such as alcohol, marijuana, or stimulants. Prescription opioid patients may be deterred from seeking treatment by the stigma associated with alcohol and drug abuse, particularly if they became addicted through "accidental" misuse during the process of treating a pain condition. Patients who "accidentally" become dependent on prescription opioids are unlikely to present to specialty addiction clinics for help (Rawson et al., 2007).

Although a number of pharmacological agents, particularly buprenorphine, has proven effective in the treatment of opioid use disorders (Fudala et al., 2003; Ling et al., 2005; Ling & Wesson, 2003; Stine, Greenwald, & Kosten, 2003), few studies have included gender analyses. In a randomized, 16-week clinical trial examining the safety and side effect profiles of buprenorphine and methadone among patients with intravenous opioid dependence (n = 164, 71% male), Lofwall (2005) reported that the side effect profiles were similar for both medications, with minimal gender differences. Those differences that were found (e.g., levels of serum glutamic oxalacetic and pyruvic transaminase) were deemed of little clinical significance (Lofwall, 2005).

At this time, no gender-specific treatments for prescription opioid abuse or dependence have been tested. One pilot study recently tested a manual-based, 12-session group treatment for women with opioid dependence (n = 8) enrolled in a methadone maintenance treatment program (Najavits, Rosier, Nolan, & Freeman, 2007). The findings were promising and revealed significant improvements in drug use and low rates of attrition among women. Testing manual-based treatments such as this one, which was adapted to prescription opioid use disorders, would be a useful next step.

FUTURE DIRECTIONS

As is evident from the research reviewed in this chapter, there is much room for advancement in the study of gender and prescription opioid dependence. In particular, research on early identification, treatment, and risk factors for men and women is critical. Guidelines for early detection, including the development of effective screening tools, are needed to help identify men and women with problematic or "aberrant" behaviors that confer an increased risk for future abuse or dependence. Research to enhance understanding about which aberrant behaviors or signs of misuse are the most predictive of future abuse or dependence would be helpful. In addition, it would be important to determine whether those behaviors most predictive of future problems differ for men and women.

Similarly, research on gender-specific risk factors is needed. Investigations of the risk of use or relapse across the menstrual cycle (MC) phase among women with prescription opioid abuse, with and without chronic pain conditions, would be of interest. If women's pain sensitivity changes during the MC phase, then it is reasonable to hypothesize that this increased sensitivity could lead to increased risk of prescription opioid misuse or abuse. A better understanding of how estrogen and other gonadal hormonal fluctuations influence risk of use or relapse among women may help lead to improved treatment interventions.

Very little research, to date, has examined gender differences in response to pharmacological or psychosocial treatments. Investigators are encouraged to power sample sizes adequately so that gender analyses can be conducted (e.g., differences in rates and reasons for attrition, factors predictive of positive treatment response, MC phase effects on relapse, response to aftercare).

Increased knowledge regarding whether different opioid medications carry different abuse liabilities for men as compared to women would help inform treatment decisions. With this knowledge, physicians would be able to more carefully select the ideal treatment for men and women in need of prescription opioid medication. This would also help balance the need to provide effective medical treatment while minimizing the risk of addiction.

Clearly, treatments for pain that have decreased abuse liability are needed. Opioid analgesics with low-abuse profiles and more effective nonopioid medications would be helpful for both men and women with chronic pain conditions (Compton & Volkow, 2006). Novel approaches to treating pain among adolescents and young adults, in particular, are also needed. Early exposure to prescription opioids has been associated with increased risk of abuse later in life (McCabe et al., 2005b, 2007c), so efforts to minimize that risk are important.

Lastly, the field of prescription opioid research would benefit from greater consensus with regard to the meaning of the terms that are widely used in the medical and scientific community, for example: *misuse, abuse,* or *aberrant behaviors* (Zacny et al., 2003). Such a consensus would afford greater consistency across studies, enhance interpretability of findings, and improve ability to replicate findings in future studies. Ultimately, greater consensus in the terms and definitions used will help increase the likelihood and speed at which meaningful discoveries will be identified.

KEY POINTS

- Prescription opioid use, abuse, and dependence are on the rise; the findings regarding gender differences are equivocal.
- Teenagers and young adults are at particularly high risk. Among youths ages 12–17, females have higher rates of prescription opioid abuse and dependence, but among youths ages 18–25, males have higher rates.
- Women are more likely than men to be prescribed prescription opioids.
- Women are more likely than men to present at EDs for reasons related to nonmedical prescription drug use.
- Young women are more likely then men to obtain prescription opioids from their parents or other relatives. Young men are more likely than women to obtain prescription opioids from peers or drug dealers.
- No appreciable gender differences in routes of administration have been found; the majority of individuals ingest prescription opioids orally.
- Rates of comorbid SUDs and other psychiatric conditions are high among individuals with opioid abuse or dependence. Similar to the general population, data suggest that women have higher rates of comorbid affective disorders, whereas men have higher rates of concurrent SUDs and antisocial personality disorders. Women also have greater impairment in medical, economic, and occupational functioning.
- Chronic pain conditions are more prevalent in women as compared to men, which may increase women's exposure to prescription opioids.
- Some evidence suggests that prescription opiates display different pharmacokinetic and pharmacodynamic properties in elderly patients, which may place them at a higher risk of adverse events with dosages that are typically well tolerated in younger populations.
- To date, no studies of gender-specific treatments for prescription opioids have been conducted.

ACKNOWLEDGMENTS

Work on this chapter was supported in part by Grant No. K23 DA021228 from the National Institute on Drug Abuse to Sudie E. Back.

REFERENCES

Asterisks denote recommended readings.

Aloisi, A. M. (2003). Gonadal hormones and sex differences in pain reactivity. *Clinical Journal of Pain*, *19*(3), 168–174.

Aloisi, A. M., & Bonifazi, M. (2006). Sex hormones, central nervous system, and pain. *Hormones and Behavior*, *50*(1), 1–7.

Back, S. E., Payne, R., Waldrop, A. E., Smith, A., Reeves, S., & Brady, K. T. (in press). Prescription opioid aberrant behaviors: A pilot study of gender differences. *Clinical Journal of Pain*.

Barsky, A. J., Peekna, H. M., & Borus, J. F. (2001). Somatic symptom reporting in females and males. *Journal of General Internal Medicine*, *16*(4), 266–275.

Berkley, K. J. (1997). Sex differences in pain. *Behavioral and Brain Science*, *20*(3), 371–380.

Berkley, K. J. (1998). *Sexual differences and pain: A constructive issue for the millennium*. Abstract for the 1998 NIH Gender and Pain conference. Retrieved December 18, 2007, from *painconsortium. nih.gov/genderandpain/abstracts/KBerkley.htm*.

Blanco, C., Alderson, D., Ogburn, E., Grant, B. F., Nunes, E. V., Hatzenbuehler, M. L., et al. (2007). Changes in the prevalence of non-medical prescription drug use and drug use disorders in the United States: 1991–1992 and 2001–2002. *Drug and Alcohol Dependence*, *90*(2–3), 252–260.

Blyth, F. M., March, L. M., Brnabic, A. J. M., Jorm, L. R., Williamson, M., & Cousins, M. J. (2001). Chronic pain in Australia: A prevalence study. *Pain*, *89*(2–3), 127–134.

Carise, D., Dugosh, K. L., McLellan, A. T., Camilleri, A., Woody, G. E., & Lynch, K. G. (2007). Prescription Oxycontin abuse among patients entering addiction treatment. *American Journal of Psychiatry*, *164*(11), 1750–1756. (*)

Centers for Disease Control. (2007). *Health related quality of life*. Retrieved December 21, 2007, from *www.cdc.gov/hrqol/*.

Chabal, C., Erjavec, M. K., Jacobson, L., Mariano, A., & Chaney, E. (1997). Prescription opiate abuse in chronic pain patients: Clinical criteria, incidence, and predictors. *Clinical Journal of Pain*, *13*(2), 150–155.

Cicero, T. J., Dart, R. C., Inciardi, J. A., Woody, G. E., Schnoll, S., & Munoz, A. (2007). The development of a comprehensive risk-management program for prescription opioid analgesics: Researched abuse, diversion, and addiction-related surveillance (RADARS). *Pain Medicine*, *8*(2), 157–170.

Cicero, T. J., Inciardi, J. A., & Munoz, A. (2005). Trends in abuse of Oxycontin and other opioid analgesics in the United States: 2002–2004. *Journal of Pain*, *6*(10), 662–672.

Colliver, J. D., Kroutil, L. A., Dai, L., & Gfroerer, J. C. (2006). *Misuse of prescription drugs: Data from the 2002, 2003, and 2004 National Surveys on Drug Use and Health* (DHHS Publication No. SMA 06-4192, Analytic Series A-28). Rockville, MD: Substance Abuse and Mental Health Services Administration, Office of Applied Studies.

Compton, W. M., & Volkow, N. D. (2006). Major increases in opioid analgesic abuse in the United States: concerns and strategies. *Drug and Alcohol Dependence*, *81*(2), 103–107. (*)

Dao, T. T., & LeResche, L. (2000). Gender differences in pain. *Journal of Orofacial Pain*, *14*(3), 169–184.

Davies, K. N., Castleden, C. M., McBurney, A., & Jagger, C. (1989). The effect of ageing on the pharmacokinetics of dihydrocodeine. *European Journal of Clinical Pharmacology*, *37*(4), 375–379.

Drossman, D. A., Whitehead, W. E., & Camilleri, M. (1997). Irritable bowel syndrome: A technical review for practice guideline development. *Gastroenterology*, *112*(6), 2120–2137.

Elliott, A. M., Smith, B. H., Penny, K. I., Smith, B. H., Penny, K. I., Smith, W. C., et al. (1999). The epidemiology of chronic pain in the community. *Lancet, 354*(9186), 1248–1254.

Emery, C. F., Frid, D. J., Engebretson, T. O., Alonzo, A. A., Fish, A., Ferketich, A. K., et al. (2004). Gender differences in quality of life among cardiac patients. *Psychosomatic Medicine, 66*(2), 190–197.

Eriksen, J., Jensen, M. K., Sjogren, P., Ekholm, O., & Rasmussen, N. K. (2003). Epidemiology of chronic non-malignant pain in Denmark. *Pain, 106*(3), 221–228.

Fach, M., Bischof, G., Schmidt, C., & Rumpf, H. J. (2007). Prevalence of dependence on prescription drugs and associated mental disorders in a representative sample of general hospital patients. *General Hospital Psychiatry, 29*(3), 257–263.

Felson, D. T. (1988). Epidemiology of hip and knee osteoarthritis. *Epidemiology Review, 10,* 1–28.

Fillingim, R. B., & Maixner, W. (1995). Gender differences in response to noxious stimuli. *Pain Forum, 4*(4), 209–221.

Fudala, P. J., Bridge, T. P., Herbert, S., Williford, W. O., Chiang, C. N., Jones, K., et al. (2003). Office-based treatment of opiate addiction with a sublingual-tablet formulation of buprenorphine and naloxone. *New England Journal of Medicine, 349*(10), 949–958.

Gajraj, N. M., & Hervias-Sanz, M. (1998). Opiate abuse or undertreatment? *Clinical Journal of Pain, 14*(1), 90–91.

Gloth, F. M., 3rd. (2001). Pain management in older adults: Prevention and treatment. *Journal of the American Geriatric Society, 49*(2), 188–199.

Grant, B. F., Dawson, D. A., Stinson, F. S., Chou, S. P., Dufour, M. C., & Pickering, R. P. (2004). The 12-month prevalence and trends in DSM-IV alcohol abuse and dependence: United States, 1991–1992 and 2001–2002. *Drug and Alcohol Dependence, 74*(3), 223–234.

Grant, B. F., Harford, T. C., Dawson, D. A., Chou, S. P., Dufour, M., & Pickering, R. P. (1992). Prevalence of DSM-IV alcohol abuse and dependence: United States, 1992. *Alcohol Health and Research World, 18,* 243–248.

Grant, B. F., Moore, T. C., Shepard, J., & Kaplan, K. (2003). *Source and accuracy statement for Wave 1 of the 2001–2002 National Epidemiologic Survey on Alcohol and Related Conditions.* Bethesda, MD: National Institute on Alcohol Abuse and Alcoholism. Retrieved January 3, 2008, from *niaaa. census.gov/pdfs/source_and_accuracy_statement.pdf.*

Hellstrom, B., & Anderberg, U. M. (2003). Pain perception across the menstrual cycle phases in women with chronic pain. *Perceptual Motor Skills, 96*(1), 201–211.

Hernandez-Avila, C. A., Rounsaville, B. J., & Kranzler, H. R. (2004). Opioid-, cannabis-, and alcohol-dependent women show more rapid progression to substance abuse treatment. *Drug and Alcohol Dependence, 74*(3), 265–272.

Holdcroft, A., & Berkley, K. J. (2006). Sex and gender differences in pain and its relief. In S. B. McMahan & M. Koltzenburg (Eds.), *Wall and Melzack's textbook of pain* (pp. 1181–1197). Philadelphia: Elsevier/Churchill Livingstone.

Holdsworth, M. T., Forman, W. B., Killilea, T. A., Nystrom, K. M., Paul, R., Brand, S. C., et al. (1994). Transdermal fentanyl disposition in elderly subjects. *Gerontology, 40*(1), 32–37.

Hopman, W. M., Towheed, T., Anastassiades, T., Tenenhouse, A., Poliquin, S., Berger, C., et al. (2000). Canadian normative data for the SF-36 health survey. Canadian Multicentre Osteoporosis Study Research Group. *Canadian Medical Association Journal, 163*(3), 265–271.

Houghton, L. A., Lea, R., Jackson, N., & Whorwell, P. J. (2002). The menstrual cycle affects rectal sensitivity in patients with irritable bowel syndrome but not healthy volunteers. *Gut, 50*(4), 471–474.

Hughes, A. A., Bogdan, G. M., & Dart, R. C. (2007). Active surveillance of abused and misused prescription opioids using poison center data: A pilot study and descriptive comparison. *Clinical Toxicology (Phila), 45*(2), 144–151.

Inciardi, J. A., Cicero, T. J., Munoz, A., Adams, E. H., Geller, A., Senay, E. C., et al. (2006). The diversion of Ultram, Ultracet, and generic tramadol HCL. *Journal of Addictive Diseases, 25*(2), 53–58.

Jacobs, J. M., Hammerman-Rozenberg, R., Cohen, A., & Stressman, J. (2006). Chronic back pain among the elderly: Prevalence, associations, and predictors. *Spine, 31*(7), E203–E207.

Johnston, L. D., O'Malley, P. M., Bachman, J. G., & Schulenberg, J. E. (2006, December 21). National press release, *"Teen drug use continues down in 2006, particularly among older teens; but use of prescription-type drugs remains high."* Retrieved January 3, 2008, from *www.monitoringthefuture.org/pressreleases/06drugpr.pdf.*

Jones, H. E., Johnson, R. E., Bigelow, G., & Strain, E. C. (2004). Differences at treatment entry between opioid-dependent and cocaine-dependent males and females. *Addictive Disorders and Their Treatment, 3*(3), 110–121.

Kemper, P., & Murtaugh, C. M. (1991). Lifetime use of nursing home care. *New England Journal of Medicine, 324*(9), 595–600.

Kepler, K. L., Standifer, K. M., Paul, D., Kest, B., Pasternak, G. W., & Bodnar, R. J. (1991). Gender effects and central opioid analgesia. *Pain, 45*(1), 87–84.

Kessler, R. C., Berglund, P., Demler, O., Jin, R., Merikangas, K. R., & Walters, E. E. (2005). Lifetime prevalence and age-of-onset distributions of DSM-IV disorders in the National Comorbidity Survey Replication. *Archives of General Psychiatry, 62*(6), 593–602.

Kim, S. H., Rhee, P., Park, J., Lee, J. H., Kim, Y., Kim, J. J., et al. (2006). Gender-related differences in visceral perception in health and irritable bowel syndrome. *Journal of Gastroenterology and Hepatology, 21*(2), 468–473.

Korszun, A., Young, E. A., Engleberg, N. C., Masterson, L., Dawson, E. C., Spindler, K., et al. (2000). Follicular phase hypothalamic–pituitary–gonadal axis function in women with fibromyalgia and chronic fatigue syndrome. *Journal of Rheumatology, 27*(6), 1526–1530.

Kramarow, E., Lentzner, H., Rooks, R., Weeks, J., & Saydah, S. (1999). *Health and aging chartbook: Health, United States.* Hyattsville, MD: National Center for Health Statistics.

Kreek, M. J. (2000). Gender differences in the effects of opiates and cocaine: Treatment implications. In E. Frank (Ed.), *Gender and its effects on psychopathology* (pp. 281–299). Washington, DC: American Psychiatric Association.

Lemmens, H. J., Burm, A. G., Hennis, P. J., Gladines, M. P., & Bovill, J. G. (1990). Influence of age on the pharmacokinetics of alfentanil: Gender dependence. *Clinical Pharmacokinetics, 19*(5), 416–422.

LeResche, L. (2000). Epidemiologic perspectives on sex differences in pain. In R. B. Fillingim (Ed.), *Sex, gender and pain: Progress in pain research and management* (pp. 233–249). Seattle, WA: IASP Press.

Leveille, S. G., Fried, L., & Gurainik, J. M. (2002). Disabling symptoms: What do older women report? *Journal of General Internal Medicine, 17*(10), 766–773.

Ling, W., Amass, L., Shoptaw, S., Annon, J. J., Hillhouse, M., Babcock, D., et al. (2005). A multicenter randomized trial of buprenorphine–naloxone versus clonidine for opioid detoxification: Findings from the National Institute on Drug Abuse Clinical Trials Network. *Addiction, 100*(8), 1090–1100.

Ling, W., & Wesson, D. R. (2003). Clinical efficacy of buprenorphine: Comparisons to methadone and placebo. *Drug and Alcohol Dependence, 70*(2 Suppl.), S49–S57.

Ling, W., Wesson, D. R., & Smith, D. E. (2003). *Abuse of prescription opioids.* In A. W. Graham, T. K. Schultz, M. F. Mayo-Smith, R. K. Ries, & B. B. Wilford (Eds.), *Principles of addiction medicine* (pp. 1483–1492). Chevy Chase, MD: American Society of Addiction Medicine.

Lofwall, M. R. (2005). Comparative safety and side effect profiles of buprenorphine and methadone in the outpatient treatment of opioid dependence. *Addictive Disorders and Their Treatment, 4*(2), 49–64.

Lusher, J., Elander, J., Bevan, D., Telfer, P., & Burton, B. (2006). Analgesic addiction and pseudoaddiction in painful chronic illness. *Clinical Journal of Pain, 22*(3), 316–324.

Matteo, R. S., Schwartz, A. E., Ornstein, E., Young, W. L., & Chang, W. J. (1990). Pharmacokinetics of sufentanil in the elderly surgical patient. *Canadian Journal of Anaesthesiology, 37*(8), 852–856.

McCabe, S. E., Cranford, J. A., Boyd, C. J., & Teter, C. J. (2007). Motives, diversion, and routes of administration associated with nonmedical use of prescription opioids. *Addictives Behaviors, 32*(3), 562–575.

McCabe, S. E., & Teter, C. J. (2007). Drug use related problems among nonmedical users of prescription stimulants: A web-based survey of college students from a Midwestern university. *Drug and Alcohol Dependence, 91*(1), 69–76. (*)

McCabe, S. E., Teter, C. J., & Boyd, C. J. (2005). Illicit use of prescription pain medication among college students. *Drug and Alcohol Dependence, 77*(1), 37–47.

McCabe, S. E., Teter, C. J., Boyd, C. J., Knight, J. R., & Wechsler, H. (2005). Nonmedical use of prescription opioids among U.S. college students: Prevalence and correlates from a national survey. *Addictive Behaviors, 30*(4), 789–805.

McCabe, S. E., West, B. T., Morales, M., Cranford, J. A., & Boyd, C. J. (2007). Does early onset of non-medical use of prescription drugs predict subsequent prescription drug abuse and dependence? Results from a national study. *Addiction, 102*(12), 1920–1930.

Michelson, H., Bolund, C., Nilsson, B., & Brandburg, Y. (2000). Health-related quality of life measured by the EORTC QLQ-C30 reference values from a large sample of Swedish population. *Acta Oncologica, 39*(4), 477–484.

Najavits, L. M., Rosier, M., Nolan, A. L., & Freeman, M. C. (2007). A new gender-based model for women's recovery from substance abuse: Results of a pilot outcome study. *American Journal of Drug and Alcohol Abuse, 33*(1), 5–11.

National Center on Addiction and Substance Abuse at Columbia University (CASA). (2005, July). *Under the counter: The diversion and abuse of controlled prescription drugs in the U.S.* Retrieved January 4, 2008, from *www.casacolumbia.org/supportcasa/item.asp?cID=12&PID=138.*

Newman, A. B., & Brach, J. S. (2001). Gender gap in longevity and disability in older persons. *Epidemiology Review, 23*(2), 343–350.

O'Conner, P. G. (2007). Improving substance abuse treatment for women: A golden opportunity. *Substance Abuse, 28*(2), 1–2.

Rawson, R. A., Maxwell, J., & Rutkowski, B. (2007). Oxycontin abuse: Who are the users? *American Journal of Psychiatry, 164*(11), 1634–1636.

Rosenblum, A., Parrino, M., Schnoll, S. H., Fong, C., Maxwell, C., Cleland, C. M., et al. (2007). Prescription opioid abuse among enrollees into methadone maintenance treatment. *Drug and Alcohol Dependence, 90*(1), 64–71.

Sear, J. W., Hand, C. W., & Moore, R. A. (1989). Studies on morphine disposition: Plasma concentrations of morphine and its metabolites in anesthetized middle-aged and elderly surgical patients. *Journal of Clinical Anesthesiology, 1*(3), 164–169.

Sherman, J. J., & LeResche, L. (2006). Does experimental pain response vary across the menstrual cycle? A methodological review. *American Journal of Physiology: Regulatory, Integrative, and Comparative Physiology, 291*(2), R245–R256.

Simoni-Wastila, L. (2000). The use of abusable prescription drugs: The role of gender. *Journal of Women's Health and Gender Based Medicine, 9*(3), 289–297.

Simoni-Wastila, L., Ritter, G., & Strickler, G. (2004). Gender and other factors associated with the nonmedical use of abusable prescription drugs. *Substance Use and Misuse, 39*(1), 1–23. (*)

Singleton, M. A., Rosen, J. I., & Fisher, D. M. (1988). Pharmacokinetics of fentanyl in the elderly. *British Journal of Anaesthesiology, 60*(6), 619–620.

Stine, S. M., Greenwald, M. K., & Kosten, T. R. (2003). Pharmacologic interventions for opioid addiction. In A. W. Graham, T. K. Schultz, M. F. Mayo-Smith, R. K. Ries, & B. B. Wilford (Eds.), *Principles of addiction medicine* (pp. 735–750), Chevy Chase, MD: American Society of Addiction Medicine.

Stinson, F. S., Grant, B. F., Dawson, D. A., Ruan, W. J., Huang, B., & Saha, T. (2005). Comorbidity between DSM-IV alcohol and specific drug use disorders in the United States: Results from the National Epidemiologic Survey on Alcohol and Related Conditions. *Drug and Alcohol Dependence, 80*(1), 105–116.

Substance Abuse and Mental Health Services Administration (SAMHSA). (2006). *Prescription medications: Misuse, abuse, dependence, and addiction* (DHHS Publication No. SMA 06-4175). Rockville, MD: U.S. Department of Health and Human Services.

Substance Abuse and Mental Health Services Administration (SAMHSA). (2007a). *Results from the 2006 National Survey on Drug Use and Health: National Findings* (DHHS Publication No. SMA 07-4293). Rockville, MD: U.S. Department of Health and Human Services.

Substance Abuse and Mental Health Services Administration. (2007b). *Drug Abuse Warning Network,*

2005: National estimates of drug-related emergency department visits (DHHS Publication No. SMA 07-4256). Rockville, MD: U.S. Department of Health and Human Services.

Sullivan, M. D., Edlund, M. J., Steffick, D., & Unutzer, J. (2005). Regular use of prescribed opioids: Association with common psychiatric disorders. *Pain, 119*(1–3), 95–103.

Tetrault, J. M., Desai, R. A., Becker, W. C., Fiellin, D. A., Concato, J., & Sulliva, L. E. (2008). Gender and non-medical use of prescription opioids: Results from a National US survey. *Addiction, 103*, 258–268.

Torrance, N., Smith, B. H., Bennett, M. I., & Lee, A. J. (2006). The epidemiology of chronic pain of predominately neuropathic origin: Results from a general population survey. *Journal of Pain, 7*(4), 281–289.

Unruh, A. M. (1996). Gender variations in clinical pain experience. *Pain, 65*(2–3), 123–167.

Verbrugge, L. M. (1995). Women, men, and osteoarthritis. *Arthritis Care and Research, 8*(4), 212–220.

Verbrugge, L. M., Lepkowski, J. M., & Konkol, L. L. (1991). Levels of disability among U.S. adults with arthritis. *Journal of Gerontology, 46*(2), S71–S83.

Verhaak, P. F. M., Kerssens, J. J., Dekker, J., Sorbi, M. J., & Bensing, J. M. (1998). Prevalence of chronic benign pain disorder among adults: a review of the literature. *Pain, 77*(3), 231–239.

Whitehead, W. E., Cheskin, L. J., Heller, B. R., Robinson, J. C., Crowell, M. D., Benjamin, C., et al. (1990). Evidence for exacerbation of irritable bowel syndrome during menses. *Gastroenterology, 98*(6), 1485–1489.

Wijnhoven, H. A., de Vet, H. C., & Picavet, H. S. (2006). Prevalence of musculoskeletal disorders is systematically higher in women than in men. *Clinical Journal of Pain, 22*(8), 717–724.

Wilder-Smith, O. H. G. (2005). Opioid use in the elderly. *European Journal of Pain, 9*(2), 137–140.

Zacny, J., Bigelow, G., Compton, P., Foley, K., Iguchi, M., & Sannerud, C. (2003). College on Problems of Drug Dependence taskforce on prescription opioid non-medical use and abuse: Position statement. *Drug and Alcohol Dependence, 69*(3), 215–232. (*)

CHAPTER 23

Women and Marijuana Dependence

Issues and Opportunities

Aimee L. McRae-Clark, PharmD, BCPP
Kimber L. Price, PhD, MSCR

Marijuana is the most commonly abused illicit drug in the United States; however, marijuana use disorders have been relatively understudied, to date. In particular, little research has focused on sex-specific interventions or treatments for marijuana-related problems. This chapter reviews the prevalence of marijuana use disorders and discusses sex-related patterns in initiation and continued marijuana use. Current treatment options for marijuana use disorders are also presented and opportunities for increasing research in marijuana-dependence issues related to women are highlighted.

PREVALENCE OF MARIJUANA USE DISORDERS

The 2004 National Survey on Drug Use and Health (NSDUH) indicates that more than 96.6 million (40.2%) of Americans 12 years of age or older have tried marijuana at least once in their lifetime, and almost 25.4 million (10.6%) have used marijuana in the past year (Substance Abuse and Mental Health Services Administration [SAMHSA], 2005). It is estimated that approximately 10% of individuals who ever use marijuana become daily users, and lifetime prevalence rates of marijuana dependence have been estimated at 4% of the population (Anthony & Helzer, 1991; Anthony, Warner, & Kessler, 1994; Johnston, O'Malley, & Bachman, 1995).

A comparison of past-year marijuana use, abuse, and dependence prevalence rates between 1991 and 1992 and 2001 and 2002 found that although prevalence of use remained stable at approximately 4% of the population, the prevalence of DSM-IV abuse or dependence increased significantly from 1.2 to 1.5% (Compton, Grant, Colliver, Glantz, & Stinson, 2004). Of note, increased rates of use were observed among 18- to 29-year-old African American and Hispanic women, and increased rates of abuse or dependence were observed for women overall. Among past-year marijuana users, overall rates of past-year abuse or dependence increased from 30.2% in 1991–1992 to 35.6% in 2001–2002. Increases were noted in rates of marijuana use disorders for both male (33.9–38.9%) and female (22.7–

29.2%) past-year users. Rates of current marijuana use and dependence among males overall were approximated at 2.2% in the 2001–2002 National Epidemiologic Survey on Alcohol and Related Conditions (NESARC), compared to 0.8% in females (Compton et al., 2004).

INITIATION AND PROGRESSION OF MARIJUANA USE

In general, the estimated age at first marijuana use has been younger in males than in females; however, this gap appears to be closing. During the late 1960s, the mean age at first marijuana use for males ranged from 18 to 19 years, and in the late 1990s ranged from 16 to 17 years. For females, the mean age at first marijuana use was, on average, 20 years in the 1960s, and in the 1990s, it had decreased to around 17 years. In 1999 the average age of new male marijuana users was 16.4 years, and the average age of new female marijuana users was 17.6 years, based on data from the National Household Survey on Drug Abuse (Gfroerer, Wu, & Penne, 2002).

It has been suggested that sex differences in prevalence of drug use might be influenced by differences in opportunities to use substances, rather than differences in the likelihood of dependence or abuse once drug use has occurred (Van Etten, Neumark, & Anthony, 1999). An analysis of epidemiological data collected in the National Household Surveys on Drug Abuse from 1979 to 1994 found that although males were more likely than females to have initial opportunities to use marijuana, there were few male–female differences in progression to drug use once an opportunity to use had occurred (Van Etten & Anthony, 1999).

Sex differences in progression from first use to dependence on cannabis have also been examined (Wagner & Anthony, 2007). Among male marijuana users, the estimated risk of dependence was 1% in the first year after initial use, reached 4% per year 2 years later, and then declined. The risk of becoming dependent for females remained stable at approximately 1% for up to 5 years after marijuana use initiation. These data suggest significant male–female differences in the risk of becoming marijuana dependent during the years immediately following initiation of marijuana use.

Although not conclusively demonstrated, there is emerging evidence suggesting that women may have a faster progression to marijuana dependence than men and may experience more deleterious effects as a result of their drug use. An evaluation of sex effects on progression to treatment entry found that women experienced fewer years of regular use of marijuana before entering treatment (Hernandez-Avila, Rounsaville, & Kranzler, 2004). This finding is congruent with similar "telescoped courses" reported in women using alcohol and other drugs of abuse (Longshore, Hsieh, & Anglin, 1993; Piazza, Vrbka, & Yeager, 1989; Randall et al., 1999; White, Brady, & Sonne, 1996).

PATTERNS OF USE

Males are almost three times more likely to report daily marijuana use compared with females (2.0 vs. 0.7%) according to the National Survey of Drug Use and Health's Report: Daily Marijuana Users (Substance Abuse and Mental Health Services Administration [SAMHSA], 2004). An analysis of the concordant use of marijuana and alcohol in women revealed that nondependent marijuana users consume marijuana earlier in the day than alcohol and use both substances most heavily on weekends (Lex, Griffin, Mello, & Mendelson, 1986). In contrast to findings for stimulant drugs, there does not appear to be a strong effect of menstrual-cycle phase in response to marijuana (for review, see Terner & de Wit, 2006).

For example, the affects of acute marijuana smoking on pulse rate and mood did not differ across the follicular, luteal, and ovulatory phases of the menstrual cycle in women, and did not differ between women and men (Lex, Mendelson, Bavli, Harvey, & Mello, 1984). An analysis of self-reported marijuana use diaries over three consecutive menstrual cycles revealed the amount of marijuana used did not differ across menstrual-cycle phase of women in the absence of severe premenstrual dysphoria (Griffin, Mendelson, Mello, & Lex, 1986). In addition, marijuana use by women on a clinical research ward did not consistently vary by menstrual-cycle phase (Mello & Mendelson, 1985); however, women who did increase marijuana use during the premenstrual phase also reported higher levels of premenstrual dysphoria as compared to women whose marijuana use decreased or remained unchanged. Analysis of the Premenstrual Assessment Form (PAS) showed that the dysphoric symptoms (depression, anxiety, mood lability, anger, irritability, and impaired social functioning), rather than the physical symptoms associated with premenstrual tension were more closely related to increased marijuana use during this menstrual-cycle phase. These studies suggest that any changes in marijuana use across the menstrual phase may only be detectable in a subset of women who suffer premenstrual dysphoric disorder (PMDD) or severe premenstrual syndrome (PMS). While further evidence is needed to support this, it is congruent with evidence suggesting varied usage during the premenstrual phase of alcohol and benzodiazepines in women who suffer from these disorders (Terner & de Wit, 2006).

ADVERSE EFFECTS AND MEDICAL CONSEQUENCES

Marijuana can be ingested orally, but most commonly it is administered by inhalation. After marijuana is smoked, up to 59% of the principal psychoactive component, tetrahydrocannabinol (THC), is absorbed. Intoxication develops within minutes after smoking marijuana, and subjective effects generally last for 3–4 hours. Marijuana intoxication initially can cause a period of anxiety, which is followed by feelings of well-being, decreased alertness, and mild euphoria. Perceptions of time and spatial awareness may also be distorted (Galanter & Kleber, 2004). A community survey of adverse effects associated with marijuana use found that anxiety, panic attacks, and development of psychotic symptoms were commonly reported (Thomas, 1996). Of note, significantly more females (32%) than males (13%) reported experiencing panic attacks following marijuana use.

Acute and chronic effects of marijuana use on neuropsychological functioning have been evaluated (for review, see Verdejo-Garcia, Lopez-Torrecillas, Gimenez, & Perez-Garcia, 2004). Laboratory experiments where controlled doses of marijuana were administered revealed acute effects of marijuana on attention processes (Solowij, Mitchie, & Fox, 1995), free recall, and other memory functions (Heishman, Arasteh, & Stitzer, 1996). To examine residual effects of marijuana use, several studies have examined neuropsychological functioning in groups with varying levels of marijuana use after some period of abstinence. For example, after 1 day of abstinence from marijuana, participants with a history of heavy marijuana use showed deficits in memory of word lists and mental flexibility when compared with infrequent marijuana smokers (Pope & Yurgelun-Todd, 1996). A follow-up study reported that those with heavy marijuana use exhibited cognitive deficits at least 7 days following use; however, by day 28 of abstinence, there were no significant differences on test performance among groups of current heavy users, former users, and a control group (Pope, Gruber, Hudson, Huestis, & Yurgelun-Todd, 2001). In addition, a meta-analysis of residual neurocognitive effects of marijuana use found only a subtle yet significant effect of long-term heavy marijuana use on selective memory impairment (Grant, Gonzalez, Carey, Natarajan,

& Wolfson, 2003). These studies indicate that the neuropsychological impairments associated with marijuana use may be more reflective of residual rather than long-term effects.

Of interest, there may be a differential gender effect on some aspects of neuropsychological functioning in those who use marijuana. A comparison of heavy and light marijuana smokers found no overall differences on tests of attention (Pope, Jacobs, Mialet, Yurgelun-Todd, & Gruber, 1997). However, when analyzed separately, women who smoked heavily performed worse on a test of visual–spatial memory than did those who smoked lightly. No differences in performance were observed for men who smoked heavily versus lightly. Although speculative, the authors suggest that women may be more vulnerable to adverse effects of marijuana in certain areas of cortical functioning.

CONSEQUENCES OF MARIJUANA USE ON REPRODUCTION AND PREGNANCY

Marijuana use may have deleterious effects on female reproductive hormones and possibly on reproductive function. Animal studies have shown suppressions of ovarian function and amenorrhea with marijuana use. In a clinical population, Mendelson and colleagues (Mendelson et al., 1986) reported suppression of plasma luteinizing hormone and prolactin levels after marijuana administration during the luteal phase of the menstrual cycle. However, a study of women with chronic marijuana use found no changes in either luteinizing hormone or prolactin (Block, Farinpour, & Schlechte, 1991). This discrepancy suggests that marijuana may exert acute effects on reproductive hormones, and that hormone levels may return to normal after a brief period of abstinence (Greenfield & O'Leary, 1999).

Of great concern, marijuana is one of the substances most frequently used by pregnant women (Huizink & Mulder, 2006). Self-reported use of marijuana during pregnancy has been estimated in the National Pregnancy and Health Survey (1996) at 2.9%. Marijuana use during pregnancy has been correlated with nonoptimal birth outcomes including low birth weight (Hatch & Bracken, 1986; Zuckerman et al., 1989) and decreased length of gestation (Fried, Watkinson, & Willan, 1984; Fried & Willan, 1990).

Two large longitudinal cohorts (the Ottawa Prenatal Prospective Study and the Maternal Health Practices and Child Development Study) have been used to prospectively follow the impact of marijuana exposure *in utero* on behavioral and cognitive outcomes in offspring (Fried, 2002; Richardson & Day, 1998). Findings from both studies show that there may be an association between prenatal exposure to marijuana and nervous system functioning, manifested by increased tremors and altered sleep patterns (Huizink & Mulder, 2006). At ages 6 and 10, more hyperactive, impulsive, and delinquent behaviors were noted in children who were exposed prenatally to marijuana (Fried, Watkinson, & Gray, 1992; Goldschmidt, Day, & Richardson, 2000; Leech, Richardson, Goldschmidt, & Day, 1999). Decreased cognitive functioning has also been reported (Fried & Watkinson, 1990). These findings persisted after controlling for confounding factors such as income, maternal age and education, and gestation, among others. In this report, the authors do note that postnatal lifestyle factors may affect cognitive performance, though the effects of marijuana use during pregnancy also may contribute. Reduced academic performance in children who were exposed prenatally to marijuana at 10 years of age has also been reported (Goldschmidt, Richardson, Cornelius, & Day, 2004).

Also of interest is the impact of prenatal marijuana exposure on subsequent substance use. Adolescents born to mothers who reported use of marijuana during pregnancy have been shown to be at increased risk for initiation of both cigarette and marijuana smoking, compared to offspring of mothers who did not report marijuana use while pregnant (Porath

& Fried, 2005). This relationship appeared to be dose-responsive, and the association was stronger in male than in females adolescents.

PSYCHIATRIC COMORBIDITY ASSOCIATED WITH MARIJUANA USE DISORDERS

Data from the National Co-Morbidity Survey (NCS) found that 90% of individuals with marijuana dependence had a lifetime psychiatric disorder compared with 55% of individuals without marijuana dependence (Agosti, Nunes, & Levin, 2002). Marijuana dependence was strongly associated with alcohol dependence, antisocial personality disorder, and conduct disorder. Early conduct problems have been strongly associated with early marijuana use initiation, and one report found this association to be significantly stronger in girls than in boys (Pederson, Mastekaasa, & Wichstrom, 2001).

Individuals with a lifetime diagnosis of marijuana dependence who reported recent use were twice as likely to have a mood or anxiety disorder as were individuals without lifetime marijuana dependence (Agosti et al., 2002). An increased risk of depression in those who use marijuana has been previously reported (Bovasso, 2001; Troisi, Pasani, Saracco, & Spalleta, 1998); however, sex differences in this comorbidity have not been well explored.

An examination of marijuana use among individuals who smoke daily tobacco reported that both presence and frequency of marijuana use predicted anxiety symptoms (Bonn-Miller, Vujanovic, Feldner, Bernstein, & Zvolensky, 2005). Anxiety has also been related to continued marijuana use, as users of marijuana report that its use relieved unpleasant feeling states, such as anxiety (Gruber, Pope, & Oliva, 1997). Following the September 11, 2001, terrorist attacks, an increase in use of marijuana as well as alcohol and cigarettes was reported, and an association between development of posttraumatic stress disorder (PTSD) and increased marijuana use was found (Vlahov et al., 2002). An examination of posttraumatic stress symptom severity and motivations for marijuana use found a significant relationship between symptom severity and coping-oriented marijuana use motives (Bonn-Miller, Vujanovic, Feldner, Bernstein, & Zvolensky, 2007); sex differences were not explored in this sample.

Social anxiety disorder (SAD) is also associated with elevated rates of marijuana dependence. The NCS found a lifetime prevalence rate of marijuana dependence of 29.0% in individuals with SAD (Agosti et al., 2002), and the National Epidemiologic Survey on Alcohol and Related Conditions (NESARC) reported a prevalence rate of marijuana use disorders of 17.8% in respondents with social phobia (Conway, Compton, Stinson, & Grant, 2006). Recent research has suggested that sex differences may exist in this relationship between problematic marijuana use and SAD (Buckner, Mallott, Schmidt, & Taylor, 2006). In a non-referred sample, SAD symptoms were positively associated with marijuana use disorders in women. A similar correlation was not observed in males; however, it should be noted that a small number of males endorsed symptoms of SAD in this study, which may have prevented detection of such a relationship. Further, analyses conducted on data collected in the NESARC did not find any significant sex differences (Conway et al., 2006).

CURRENT TREATMENT OPTIONS FOR MARIJUANA USE DISORDERS

Until recently, relatively little research has focused on the treatment of marijuana abuse or dependence (Gold, Frost-Pineda, & Jacobs, 2004; McRae, Budney, & Brady, 2003; Nordstrom & Levin, 2007). The establishment of a valid and reliable marijuana withdrawal syndrome has been documented in controlled laboratory and clinical studies (Budney, Hughes, Moore, & Novy, 2001; Budney, Novy, & Hughes, 1999; Copersino et al., 2006; Kouri & Pope, 2000) as well as reports of significant psychosocial and psychiatric impairment, and multiple signs of dependence in marijuana users (Budney, Radonovich, Higgins, & Wong, 1998; McRae, Hedden, Malcolm, Carter, & Brady, 2007) have increased research interest in this area. However, no studies, to date, have evaluated sex differences in response to treatment.

Some recent research has focused on the potential use of medications to treat the symptoms associated with marijuana withdrawal. Common symptoms associated with marijuana withdrawal include irritability, anxiety, restlessness, appetite changes, and sleep disturbances (Budney et al., 1999; Budney et al., 2001). Pharmacotherapy for marijuana withdrawal presumes that such symptoms may contribute to difficulty in maintaining abstinence, and therefore minimizing withdrawal symptoms could be useful in treating marijuana dependence. Controlled laboratory studies have been conducted to evaluate the utility of several medications for moderating the symptoms of marijuana withdrawal, producing mixed results. Bupropion and divalproex did not show adequate potential as treatment medications (Haney et al., 2001; Haney et al., 2004). More positive results were found with nefazodone, but its utility may be limited due to potential adverse effects such as hepatotoxicity (Haney, Hart, Ward, & Foltin, 2003). To date, oral THC has shown the most promise in this area (Haney et al., 2004). Administration of oral THC, at a dose of 10 mg five times daily, decreased marijuana craving and withdrawal symptoms such as anxiety, trouble sleeping, and chills. In this investigation, the dose of oral THC used was not associated with any intoxication effects. These results were recently replicated in an outpatient study of the effects of oral THC on withdrawal symptoms (Budney, Vandery, Hughes, Moore, & Bahrenburg, 2007). Further studies are needed to evaluate the use of medications to treat marijuana withdrawal, and to determine if reducing withdrawal symptoms will prevent relapse in an abstinent individual.

To date, there has been only one published randomized, placebo-controlled trial examining a pharmacotherapeutic intervention for marijuana dependence (Levin et al., 2004). Thirteen subjects received a 2-week placebo lead-in and then were randomized to receive divalproex sodium or placebo for 6 weeks, in conjunction with cognitive-behavioral relapse prevention therapy. At the end of 6 weeks, subjects were crossed over to receive the alternate treatment condition. Both treatment groups reported a reduction in self-reported marijuana use, marijuana craving, and irritability over the course of the trial, with no significant group main effects. Also, little sustained abstinence was reported, and the rate of positive urine drug screens was high in both groups.

Cognitive-behavioral, motivational enhancement, and contingency management therapies have all been demonstrated to be efficacious for reducing marijuana use in the limited number of studies conducted, to date (Budney, Higgins, Radonovich, & Novy, 2000; Copeland, Swift, Roffman, & Stephens, 2001; Marijuana Treatment Project Research Group, 2004; Stephens, Roffman, & Curtin, 2000; Stephens, Roffman, & Simpson, 1994). Most interventions tested have been adapted from those used with other substance dependence disorders. Several studies have failed to demonstrate differences in outcome between brief interventions and more intensive cognitive-behavioral therapy (CBT) interventions; however, the largest controlled trial, the Marijuana Treatment Project, found an extended CBT intervention to be more effective than brief motivational therapy. Contingency management treatments are also likely to be effective and may enhance outcomes when combined with other approaches such as more traditional psychotherapies (Budney et al., 2000).

The populations studied in the majority of trials have been predominantly male, likely reflective of the increased prevalence of marijuana use dependence among men. The lack of enrollment of women in clinical trials has largely prevented analyses to determine if there are sex-related responses to treatment.

FUTURE DIRECTIONS

As research continues to focus on the effects of, and treatment development for, marijuana use disorders, attention should be given to sex-related outcomes. Because females may be more susceptible to development of marijuana dependence or more likely to experience adverse effects from both acute and chronic use, sex-specific treatments may be advantageous. Addressing comorbidities, such as SAD and PTSD, which commonly co-occur in women with marijuana dependence, may also improve treatment outcomes.

KEY POINTS

- Little research has focused on sex differences in marijuana use disorders.
- Preliminary evidence suggests more deleterious effects and possible accelerated course of marijuana dependence for women, compared to men; however, more research is needed.
- Use of marijuana during pregnancy has been associated with negative fetal and postnatal outcomes.
- Psychiatric comorbidity commonly occurs in individuals with marijuana dependence, and some sex differences have been reported.
- Few interventions, in general, have been shown to be helpful in treatment of marijuana dependence, and no sex-specific research studies have yet been conducted.

REFERENCES

Asterisks denote recommended readings.

Agosti, V., Nunes, E., & Levin, F. (2002). Rates of psychiatric comorbidity among U.S. residents with lifetime cannabis dependence. *American Journal of Drug and Alcohol Abuse, 28,* 643–652.
Anthony, J. C., & Helzer, J. E. (1991). Syndromes of drug abuse and dependence. In L. N. Robins & D. A. Regier (Eds.), *Psychiatric disorders in America* (pp. 116–154). New York: Free Press.
Anthony, J. C., Warner, L. A., & Kessler, R. C. (1994). Comparative epidemiology of dependence on tobacco, alcohol, controlled substances, and inhalants: Basic findings from the National Comorbidity Survey. *Experimental and Clinical Psychopharmacology, 2,* 244–268.
Block, R. I., Farinpour, R., & Schlechte, J. A. (1991). Effects of chronic marijuana use on testosterone, luteinizing hormone, follicle stimulating hormone, prolactin, and cortisol in men and women. *Drug and Alcohol Dependence, 28,* 121–128.
Bonn-Miller, M. O., Vujanovic, A. A., Feldner, M. T., Bernstein, A., & Zvolensky, M. J. (2007). Post-traumatic stress symptom severity predicts marijuana use coping motives among traumatic event-exposed marijuana users. *Journal of Traumatic Stress, 20,* 577–586.
Bonn-Miller, M. O., Zvolensky, M. J., Leen-Feldner, E. W., Feldner, M. T., & Yartz, A. R. (2005). Marijuana use among daily tobacco smokers: Relationship to anxiety-related factors. *Journal of Psychopathology and Behavioral Assessment, 27,* 279–289.
Bovasso, G. B. (2001). Cannabis abuse as a risk factor for depression. *American Journal of Psychiatry, 158,* 2033–2037.

Buckner, J. D., Mallott, M. A., Schmidt, N. B., & Taylor, J. (2006). Peer influence and gender differences in problematic cannabis use among individuals with social anxiety. *Anxiety Disorders*, *20*, 1087–1102.

Budney, A. J., Higgins, S. T., Radonovich, P. L., & Novy, P. L. (2000). Adding voucher-based incentives to coping skills and motivational enhancement improves outcomes during treatment for marijuana dependence. *Journal of Consulting and Clinical Psychology*, *68*, 1051–1061.

Budney, A. J., Hughes, J. R., Moore, B. A., & Novy, P. L. (2001). Marijuana abstinence effects in marijuana smokers maintained in their home environment. *Archives of General Psychiatry*, *58*, 917–924.

Budney, A. J., Novy, P. L., & Hughes, J. R. (1999). Marijuana withdrawal among adults seeking treatment for marijuana dependence. *Addiction*, *94*, 1311–1321.

Budney, A. J., Radonovich, K. J., Higgins, S. T., & Wong, C. J. (1998). Adults seeking treatment for marijuana dependence: A comparison with cocaine-dependent treatment seekers. *Experimental and Clinical Psychopharmacology*, *6*, 419–426.

Budney, A. J., Vandery, R. G., Hughes, J. R., Moore, B. A., & Bahrenburg, B. (2007). Oral delta-9-tetrahydrocannabinnol suppresses cannabis withdrawal symptoms. *Drug and Alcohol Dependence*, *86*, 22–29.

Compton, W. M., Grant, B. F., Colliver, J. D., Glantz, M. D., & Stinson, F. S. (2004). Prevalence of marijuana use disorders in the United States, 1991–1992 and 2001–2002. *Journal of the American Medical Association*, *291*, 2114–2121. (*)

Conway, K. P., Compton, W., Stinson, F. S., & Grant, B. F. (2006). Lifetime comorbidity of DSM-IV mood and anxiety disorders and specific drug use disorders: Results from the National Epidemiologic Survey on Alcohol and Related Conditions. *Journal of Clinical Psychiatry*, *67*, 247–257.

Copeland, J., Swift, W., Roffman, R., & Stephens, R. (2001). A randomized controlled trial of brief cognitive-behavioral interventions for cannabis use disorder. *Journal of Substance Abuse Treatment*, *21*, 55–64.

Copersino, M. L., Boyd, S. J., Tashkin, D. P., Huestis, M. A., Heisman, S. J., Dermand, J. C., et al. (2006). Cannabis withdrawal among non-treatment-seeking adult cannabis users. *American Journal on Addictions*, *15*, 8–14.

Fried, P. A. (2002). Conceptual issues in behavioral teratology and their application in determining long-term sequelae of prenatal marihuana exposure. *Journal of Child Psychology and Psychiatry*, *43*, 81–102.

Fried, P. A., & Watkinson, B. (1990). 36- and 48-month neurobehavioral follow-up of children prenatally exposed to marijuana, cigarettes, and alcohol. *Journal of Developmental and Behavioral Pediatrics*, *11*, 49–58.

Fried, P. A., Watkinson, B., & Gray, R. (1992). A follow-up study of attentional behavior in 6-year old children exposed prenatally to marihuana, cigarettes, and alcohol. *Neurotoxicology and Teratology*, *14*, 299–311.

Fried, P. A., Watkinson, B., & Willan, A. (1984). Marijuana use during pregnancy and decreased length of gestation. *American Journal of Obstetrics and Gynecology*, *150*, 23–27.

Galanter, M., & Kleber, H. D. (Eds.). (2004). *Textbook of substance abuse treatment*. Washington, DC: American Psychiatric Association.

Gfroerer, J. C., Wu, L. T., & Penne, M. A. (2002). *Initiation of marijuana use: Trends, patterns, and implications* (Analytic Series: A-17, DHHS Publication No. SMA 02-3711). Rockville, MD: Substance Abuse and Mental Health Administration, Office of Applied Studies.

Gold, M. S., Frost-Pineda, K., & Jacobs, W. S. (2004). Cannabis. In M. Galanter & H. D. Kleber (Eds.), *Textbook of substance abuse treatment* (pp. 167–188). Washington, DC: American Psychiatric Association.

Goldschmidt, L., Day, N. L., & Richardson, G. L. (2000). Effects of prenatal marijuana exposure on child behavior problems at age 10. *Neurotoxicology and Teratology*, *22*, 325–336.

Goldschmidt, L., Richardson, G. A., Cornelius, M. D., & Day, N. L. (2004). Prenatal marijuana and alcohol exposure and academic achievement at age 10. *Neurotoxicology and Teratology*, *26*, 521–532.

Grant, I., Gonzalez, R., Carey, C. L., Natarajan, L., & Wolfson, T. (2003). Non-acute (residual) neurocognitive effects of cannabis use: A meta-analytic study. *Journal of the International Neurospsychological Society*, 9, 679–689.

Greenfield, S. F., & O'Leary, G. (1999). Sex differences in marijuana use in the United States. *Harvard Review of Psychiatry*, 6, 297–303.

Griffin, M. L., Mendelson, J. H., Mello, N. K., & Lex, B. W. (1986). Marijuana use across the menstrual cycle. *Drug and Alcohol Dependence*, 18, 213–224.

Gruber, A. J., Pope, H. G., & Oliva, P. (1997). Very long-term users of marijuana in the United States. *Substance Use and Misuse*, 32, 249–264.

Haney, M., Hart, C. L., Vosburg, S. K., Nasser, J., Bennett, A., Zubaran, C., et al. (2004). Marijuana withdrawal in humans: Effects of oral THC or divalproex. *Neuropsychopharmacology*, 29, 158–170.

Haney, M., Hart, C. L., Ward, A. S., & Foltin, R. W. (2003). Nefazodone decreases anxiety during marijuana withdrawal in humans. *Psychopharmacology (Berl)*, 165, 157–165.

Haney, M., Ward, A. S., Comer, S. D., Hart, C. L., Foltin, R. W., & Fishman, M. W. (2001). Bupropion SR worsens mood during marijuana withdrawal in humans. *Psychopharmacology (Berl)*, 155, 171–179.

Hatch, E. E., & Bracken, M. B. (1986). Effect of marijuana use in pregnancy on fetal growth. *American Journal of Epidemiology*, 124, 986–993.

Heishman, S. J., Arasteh, K., & Stitzer, M. L. (1996). Comparative effects of alcohol and marijuana on mood, memory and performance. *Pharmacology, Biochemistry, and Behavior*, 58, 93–101.

Hernandez-Avila, C. A., Rounsaville, B. J., & Kranzler, H. R. (2004). Opioid-, cannabis-, and alcohol-dependent women show more rapid progression to substance abuse treatment. *Drug and Alcohol Dependence*, 74, 265–272.

Huizink, A. C., & Mulder, E. J. H. (2006). Maternal smoking, drinking, or cannabis use during pregnancy and neurobehavioral and cognitive functioning in human offspring. *Neuroscience and Biobehavioral Reviews*, 30, 24–41. (*)

Johnston, L. D., O'Malley, P. M., & Bachman, J. G. (1995). *National survey results on drug use from the monitoring the future study, 1975–1994, Vol. 1*. U.S. Washington, DC: Department of Health and Human Services.

Kouri, E. M., & Pope, H. G. (2000). Abstinence symptoms during withdrawal from chronic marijuana use. *Experimental and Clinical Psychopharmacology*, 8, 483–492.

Leech, S. L., Richardson, G. A., Goldschmidt, L., & Day, N. L. (1999). Prenatal substance exposure: Effects on attention and impulsivity of 6-year-olds. *Neurotoxicology and Teratology*, 21, 109–118.

Levin, F. R., McDowell, D., Evans, S., Nunes, E., Akerele, E., Donovan, S., et al. (2004). Pharmacotherapy for marijuana dependence: A double-blind, placebo-controlled pilot study of divalproex sodium. *American Journal on Addictions*, 13, 21–32.

Lex, B. W., Griffin, M. L., Mello, N. K., & Mendelson, J. H. (1986). Concordant alcohol and marihuana use in women. *Alcohol*, 3, 193–200.

Lex, B. W., Mendelson, J. H., Bavli, S., Harvey, K., & Mello, N. K. (1984). Effects of acute marijuana smoking on pulse rate and mood states in women. *Psychopharmacology*, 84, 178–187.

Longshore, D., Hsieh, S., & Anglin, M. D. (1993). Ethnic and gender differences in drug users' perceived need for treatment. *International Journal of the Addictions*, 28, 539–558.

Marijuana Treatment Project Research Group. (2004). Brief treatments for cannabis dependence: Findings from a randomized multisite trial. *Journal of Consulting and Clinical Psychology*, 72, 455–466.

McRae, A. L., Budney, A. J., & Brady, K. T. (2003). Treatment of marijuana dependence: A review of the literature. *Journal of Substance Abuse Treatment*, 24, 369–376.

McRae, A. L., Hedden, S. L., Malcolm, R. J., Carter, R. E., & Brady, K. T. (2007). Characteristics of cocaine- and marijuana-dependent subjects presenting for medication treatment trials. *Addictive Behaviors*, 32, 1433–1440.

Mello, N. K., & Mendelson, J. H. (1985). Operant acquisition of marijuana in women. *Journal of Pharmacology and Experimental Therapeutics*, 235, 162–171.

Mendelson, J. H., Mello, N. K., Ellingboe, J., Skupny, A. S. T., Lex, B. W., & Griffin, M. (1986). Marijuana smoking suppresses luteinizing hormone in women. *Journal of Pharmacology and Experimental Therapeutics, 237,* 862–866.

National Pregnancy and Health Survey. (1996). *Drug use among women delivering live births: 1992, 1996* (National Institute of Health Publication No. 96-3819). Rockville, MD: U.S. Department of Health and Human Services, National Institute on Drug Abuse.

Nordstrom, B. R., & Levin, F. R. (2007). Treatment of cannabis use disorders: A review of the literature. *American Journal of Addictions, 16,* 331–342. (*)

Pederson, W., Mastekaasa, A., & Wichstrom, L. (2001). Conduct problems and early cannabis initiation: A longitudinal study of gender differences. *Addiction, 96,* 415–431.

Piazza, N. J., Vrbka, J. L., & Yeager, R. D. (1989). Telescoping of alcoholism in women alcoholics. *International Journal of the Addictions, 24,* 19–28.

Pope, H. G., Gruber, A. J., Hudson, J. I., Huestis, M. A., & Yurgelun-Todd, D. (2001). Neuropsychological performance in long-term cannabis users. *Archives of General Psychiatry, 58,* 909–915.

Pope, H. G., Jacobs, A., Mialet, J.-P., Yurgelun-Todd, D., & Gruber, S. (1997). Evidence for a sex-specific residual effect of cannabis on visuospatial memory. *Psychotherapy and Psychosomatics, 66,* 179–184. (*)

Pope, H. G., & Yurgelun-Todd, D. (1996). The residual effects of heavy marijuana use in college students. *Journal of the American Medical Association, 275,* 521–527.

Porath, A. J., & Fried, P. A. (2005). Effects of prenatal cigarette and marijuana exposure on drug use among offspring. *Neurotoxicology and Teratology, 27,* 267–277.

Randall, C. L., Roberts, J. S., Del Boca, F. K., Carroll, K. M., Connors, G. J., & Mattson, M. E. (1999). Telescoping of landmark events associated with drinking: A gender comparison. *Journal of Studies on Alcohol, 60,* 252–260.

Richardson, G. A., & Day, N. L. (1998). Epidemiologic studies of the effects of prenatal cocaine exposure on child development and behavior. In W. Sliker, Jr. & L. W. Chang (Eds.), *Handbook of developmental neurotoxicology* (pp. 487–496). San Diego, CA: Academic Press.

Solowij, N., Mitchie, P. T., & Fox, A. M. (1995). Differential impairments of selective attention due to frequency and duration of cannabis use. *Biological Psychiatry, 37,* 731–739.

Stephens, R. S., Roffman, R. A., & Curtin, L. (2000). Comparison of extended versus brief treatments for marijuana use. *Journal of Consulting and Clinical Psychology, 68,* 898–908.

Stephens, R. S., Roffman, R. A., & Simpson, E. E. (1994). Treating adult marijuana dependence: A test of the relapse prevention model. *Journal of Consulting and Clinical Psychology, 62,* 92–99.

Substance Abuse and Mental Health Services Administration (2004). *The NSDUH Report: Daily Marijuana Users* (Based on the 2003 *National Survey on Drug Use and Health: National Findings* (Office of Applied Studies, NSDUH Series H-25, DHHS Publication No. SMA 04-3964). Rockville, MD: U.S. Department of Health and Human Services.

Substance Abuse and Mental Health Services Administration (2005). *Results from the 2004 National Survey on Drug Use and Health: National Findings* (Office of Applied Studies, NSDUH Series H-28, DHHS Publication No. SMA 05-4062). Rockville, MD: U.S. Department of Health and Human Services.

Terner, J. M., & de Wit, H. (2006). Menstrual cycle phase and responses to drugs of abuse in humans. *Drug and Alcohol Dependence, 84,* 1–13.

Thomas H. (1996). A community survey of adverse effects of cannabis use. *Drug and Alcohol Dependence, 42,* 201–207.

Troisi, A., Pasani, A., Saracco, M., & Spalletta, G. (1998). Psychiatric symptoms in male cannabis users not using other illicit drugs. *Addiction, 4,* 487–492.

Van Etten, M. L., & Anthony, J. C. (1999). Comparative epidemiology of initial drug opportunities and transitions to first use: Marijuana, cocaine, hallucinogens, and heroin. *Drug and Alcohol Dependence, 54,* 117–125.

Van Etten, M. L., Neumark, Y. D., & Anthony, J. C. (1999). Male–female differences in the earliest stages of drug involvement. *Addiction, 94,* 1413–1419.

Verdejo-Garcia, A., Lopez-Torrecillas, F., Gimenez, C. O., & Perez-Garcia, M. (2004). Clinical implications and methodological challenges in the study of neuropsychological correlates of cannabis, stimulant, and opioid abuse. *Neuropsychology Review*, *14*, 1–35.

Vlahov, D., Galea, S., Resnick, H., Ahern, J., Boscarino, J. A., Bucuvalas, M., et al. (2002). Increased use of cigarettes, alcohol, and marijuana among Manhattan, New York, residents after the September 11th terrorist attacks. *American Journal of Epidemiology*, *155*, 988–996.

Wagner, F. A., & Anthony, J. C. (2007). Male–female differences in the risk of progression from first use to dependence upon cannabis, cocaine, and alcohol. *Drug and Alcohol Dependence*, *86*, 191–198. (*)

White, K. A., Brady, K. T., & Sonne, S. (1996). Gender differences in patterns of cocaine use. *American Journal on Addiction*, *5*, 259–261.

Zuckerman, B., Frank, D. A., Hingson, R., Amaro, H., Levenson, S. M., Kayne, H., et al. (1989). Effects of maternal marijuana and cocaine use on fetal growth. *New England Journal of Medicine*, *320*, 762–768.

CHAPTER 24

Sex Differences in Vulnerability to Stimulant Abuse

A *Translational Perspective*

Wendy J. Lynch, PhD
Marc N. Potenza, MD, PhD
Kelly P. Cosgrove, PhD
Carolyn M. Mazure, PhD

Women have historically had lower rates of drug abuse and dependence compared to men, which has led to the impression that they are less vulnerable to drug abuse than men. However, accumulating evidence suggests that women are not less vulnerable to drug abuse than men, and, with regard to certain aspects of drug abuse, may be more vulnerable than men. Examination of this issue is particularly important in light of recent epidemiological data showing that the longstanding trend for greater drug use and abuse among males as compared to females is getting smaller among adult populations and is no longer apparent in younger populations. Adult females are now equally likely as adult males to use and abuse methamphetamine and other stimulant drugs. Female adolescents are now equally or more likely as male adolescents to smoke cigarettes and use and abuse illicit drugs, including cocaine and amphetamines (Substance Abuse and Mental Health Services Administration, 2007). In this chapter, we address questions of sex differences in vulnerability to drug abuse, focusing on several key components of stimulant abuse, including *initiation of use, the progression to addiction, relapse to use*, and *treatment*. In order to examine more fully the biological basis of sex differences in stimulant abuse, we have included a discussion of both clinical and preclinical findings. Such an integration of preclinical/animal studies and clinical research may be critical for addressing questions regarding sex differences in biological vulnerability to stimulant abuse that can then be translated into more effective, sex-appropriate treatment and prevention strategies. In this chapter, the term "sex" refers to a biological difference between males and females (Committee on Understanding the Biology of Sex and Gender Differences, 2001).

DO WOMEN AND MEN DIFFER
IN THE INITIATION OF DRUG USE?

The belief that men have a greater biological vulnerability to drug abuse than women stems from the fact that prevalence rates of drug use and abuse/dependence, including the use and abuse of cocaine and cigarettes, among adults have historically been higher in men than women (see Table 24.1; Adults [18+]). This belief, however, is not supported by current rates of methamphetamine and other stimulant drug use among adult males and females, current rates of drug use among adolescent males and females (see Table 24.1; Adolescents [12–17]), or by recent results from preclinical studies. For example, results from studies comparing male and female rodents on rates of acquisition of stimulant self-administration have revealed either a lack of a sex difference, or more commonly, the opposite effect, with females acquiring the self-administration of cocaine, methamphetamine, and nicotine more readily than males (for reviews, see Becker & Hu, 2008; Carroll, Lynch, Roth, Morgan, & Cosgrove, 2004; Lynch, Roth, & Carroll, 2002; Lynch, 2006). A review of the literature indicates that female rats will also work harder than males to obtain deliveries of cocaine, methamphetamine, and nicotine, suggesting that these drugs may be more reinforcing in females, compared to males (Becker & Hu, 2008; Carroll et al., 2004; Lynch, 2006; Lynch et al., 2002). Together, these results suggest that females are at least equally, if not more, vulnerable to the reinforcing effects of stimulants.

While there is evidence to support sex differences in a number of biological factors that may contribute to biological vulnerability to stimulant abuse, results from preclinical studies indicate that ovarian hormones may be particularly important during initiation of drug use. For example, blocking estrogen, either by the administration of the anti-estrogen tamoxifen in intact females or by surgically removing the ovaries, abolishes sex differences in rates of acquisition of cocaine self-administration in rats, and this effect is reversed by estrogen replacement (Becker & Hu, 2008; Carroll et al., 2004; Lynch, 2006; Lynch et al., 2002). Additionally, progesterone, when coadministered with estradiol, attenuates the estradiol-induced enhancement of cocaine self-administration during the acquisition phase (Jackson, Robinson, & Becker, 2006) and decreases preference for a cocaine-associated environment

TABLE 24.1. Gender Differences in the Prevalence of Illicit Drug, Cocaine, Stimulant, and Cigarette Use and Abuse/Dependence in Adults and Adolescents

	Adults (18+)		Adolescents (12–17)	
	Males	Females	Males	Females
Current use				
Illicit drugs	4.6	2.9*	4.5	5.2*
Cocaine	1.4	0.7*	0.4	0.4
Stimulants[a]	0.5	0.4	0.6	0.7
Cigarettes	29.9	23.7*	10.1	11.1*
Abuse/dependence				
Illicit drugs	1.9	1.0*	1.5	2.4*
Cocaine	1.0	0.5*	0.2	0.4*
Stimulants	0.1	0.1	0.2	0.5*
Cigarettes	12.9	10.3*	3.1	3.0

[a]Includes methamphetamine and the nonmedical use of other amphetamines.
*$p < .05$.

in female rodents (Quinones-Jenab et al., 2001). Notably, laboratory studies in humans also reveal that the subjective response to various drugs of abuse, including stimulants, differs with menstrual cycle phase (Terner & de Wit, 2006), that estrogen enhances responsiveness to stimulants in women (Justice & de Wit, 2000), and that progesterone attenuates the subjective effects of cocaine in women (Sofuoglu, Mitchell, & Kosten, 2004). These results suggest that ovarian hormones influence the reinforcing effects of stimulants in females.

However, even if hormonal influences, or other biological factors, lead to a vulnerability to drug abuse in women that is comparable or greater than that in men, in order to account for differences between men and women in prevalence rates, women must be protected by other, nonbiological factors. A number of social factors have been identified that differentiate women from men, such as drug use opportunity, which is lower for women than men, and child care responsibilities, which are greater for women than men (Copeland, 1997). A factor that appears to be of major importance is the societal response to drug use in women. Drug use in women is more stigmatized (e.g., social disapproval) than in men. This protective factor, however, may be lessening, in that societal views are changing such that drug use in women is becoming less stigmatized and, consequently, more likely (Nicolaides, 1996). We do know that rates of drug use, particularly stimulant use among women have increased in recent years and that, among adolescents, rates of use and abuse/dependence of illicit drugs, including cocaine, methamphetamine, and other stimulants, are comparable or even greater in females compared to males. These results, combined with the preclinical data, suggest that females are at least equally as vulnerable as males to stimulant abuse and highlight the need for prevention efforts that specifically target adolescent females and young women, particularly since some of the societal factors that have traditionally served to protect women appear to be lessening.

DOES THE PROGRESSION TO ADDICTION DIFFER BETWEEN MEN AND WOMEN?

The progression (or time course) to addiction appears accelerated in women, a phenomenon termed "telescoping" (Brady & Randall, 1999). That is, once initiating substance use, women develop the medical, behavioral, psychological, and social problems characteristic of substance abuse and progress more rapidly through the landmark stages of dependence (e.g., regular drinking or loss of control; Brady & Randall, 1999). This phenomenon has been described extensively in the alcohol literature, and results have shown that, compared to men, women meet criteria for alcohol dependence after fewer years of alcohol use and despite less alcohol consumption (Diehl et al., 2007; Piazza, Vrbka, & Yeager, 1989). A similar phenomenon has been noted for dependence on stimulants drugs including cocaine, nicotine, caffeine, d-amphetamine, and methamphetamine (Griffin & Weiss, 1989; Westermeyer & Boedicker, 2000), as well as other addictive disorders such as gambling (Tavares et al., 2003).

Little information is available on the biological basis for sex differences in the time course to addiction. Part of the reason for this knowledge gap is that "addiction" paradigms have only just been developed in laboratory animals over the past few years. Although there are no complete animal models of addiction, animal models do exist for key elements of addiction, including escalation of intake over time, a transition from controlled to uncontrolled use, and increased intake or motivation for the drug following chronic exposure. Extended drug availability appears to be critical for producing these characteristics (Koob & Kreek, 2007; Roberts, Morgan, & Liu, 2007). A handful of studies have compared males and females under extended drug-access conditions (i.e., 5-hour to 24-hour daily drug availability), and the results from these studies have demonstrated that compared to male rats, female rats self-administer more cocaine, show a more diurnally dysregulated pattern of use, show a greater escalation in their intake of cocaine over time, and a greater increase in motivation for the drug following an abstinence period (Lynch & Taylor, 2004; Roth & Carroll, 2004).

These preliminary findings with cocaine corroborate the clinical data of an escalated course to addiction in women and suggest that such sex differences may be due to biological factors. This biological vulnerability may result from a number of factors, including hormonal, neurochemical, and pharmacokinectics factors, with evidence to support a role for each. For example, estrogen promotes escalation of cocaine self-administration, whereas progesterone inhibits escalation of cocaine self-administration in female rats under extended-access conditions (Larson, Anker, Gliddon, Fons, & Carroll, 2007). Dopamine transporter density and dopamine release and uptake rates are greater in women and female rats compared to men and male rats in brain regions that have been implicated in drug abuse (Mozley, Gur, Mozley, & Gur, 2001; Walker, Rooney, Wightman, & Kuhn, 2000). Results from laboratory animals have demonstrated important interactions of estrogen and dopamine in such regions, which appear to underlie the heightened response in females to drugs of abuse, particularly stimulants (Becker, 1999). This enhanced dopaminergic transmission may cause women to become addicted after less drug exposure. Although the pharmacokinetic profile of cocaine itself has been mixed, with some studies showing sex and/or hormonal effects (e.g., Lukas et al., 1996; Mendelson et al., 1999) and others reporting no sex or hormonal effects (e.g., Bowman et al., 1999; Evans & Foltin, 2004, 2006; Festa et al., 2004), cocaine metabolites do appear to differ by sex and hormonal status (Evans & Foltin, 2004; Festa et al., 2004).

Nonbiological mechanisms may also contribute to differences between men and women in the progression to addiction. For example, it has been suggested that the telescoping effect may reflect a difference in seeking medical treatment or a difference in self-reports of disease progression. We do know that, compared to men, women visit health care providers more frequently in their lifetime and use the medical system to a greater extent (Badley, 2001); thus they may be more likely to seek treatment for an addictive disorder, and they may seek it sooner in the course of the disorder. If, however, the prediction that women are at an increased biological risk during the transition from regular use to addiction is true, then the implication is that the window of opportunity for drug intervention is shorter in women than men.

DO MEN AND WOMEN DIFFER IN VULNERABILITY TO RELAPSE?

Studies investigating sex differences in rates of relapse are sparse, and the results differ between drugs. One area that has received considerable attention for sex differences is for relapse to cigarette smoking. Although the data are somewhat controversial, the majority of these studies have indicated that women tend to be more likely than men to relapse to cigarette smoking during an unaided cessation attempt (Perkins, 2001). Women and men may also differ with regard to the cues that trigger craving and subsequent relapse. Various types of stimuli are known to precipitate relapse in individuals with drug and alcohol dependence, including internal cues such, as reexposure to small "priming" doses of the drug, and external cues, such as specific locations and people associated with the drug. It has been suggested that the external-drug-associated cues may be more likely to elicit craving in women, whereas internal drug cues may be more likely to elicit craving in men. This finding may be particularly true for cigarette dependence, with research showing that craving is increased in females who smoke but not males following exposure to cues associated with smoking (Field & Duka, 2004). This interpretation is consistent with findings showing that olfactory and taste cues are an important determinant of smoking satisfaction in females, but not males who smoke, and with clinical and preclinical findings that females are less sensitive than males to the discriminatory stimulus effects of nicotine (Perkins et al., 2001). Similar results have been observed for stimulants, although perhaps less robustly. For example, among individuals with cocaine dependence, women have been reported to be equally likely (Fox et al., 2006) or more likely than men to report cocaine craving in response to cocaine-associated cues (Elman, Karlsgodt, & Gastfriend, 2001).

Though the contribution of biological factors to drug relapse has been widely investigated, using the rat reinstatement model of relapse, only a handful of studies has examined sex differences using reinstatement models, and these studies have focused on cocaine. Consistent with clinical data on craving during a cocaine abstinence period, females exhibit more drug-seeking behavior than do males during a cocaine-free period (i.e., they respond at higher levels during extinction; Fuchs, Evans, Mehta, Case, & See, 2005; Lynch & Carroll, 2000). Moreover, cocaine-seeking behavior during abstinence remains elevated for a longer period of time in females, compared to males (Kerstetter, Aguilar, Parrish, & Kippin, 2008). However, unlike the human situation, following exposure to *cocaine-associated cues*, females responded at equal or lower levels than males (Fuchs et al., 2005), whereas, following exposure to *priming injections of cocaine*, females responded at higher levels than did males (Lynch & Carroll, 2000).

These preliminary preclinical studies with cocaine suggest that there is a biological basis involved in vulnerability to drug use relapse that is deferentially influenced in males and females by internal and external cues, although the exact nature of this relationship is unclear. Such biological differences may result in differences in functional and neurochemical changes in the brains of individuals with drug dependence. For example, compared to healthy controls, men with cocaine dependence showed decreased perfusion in the anterior cingulate and frontal cortex, areas implicated in decision making and response inhibition. Compared to healthy controls, women with cocaine dependence showed increased perfusion in the posterior cingulate, an area implicated in cue-induced relapse (Tucker, Browndyke, Gottschalk, Cofrancesco, & Kosten, 2004). Following cocaine-associated cues, women with cocaine dependence showed less activation in the amygdala, insula, orbitofrontal, and ventral cingulate cortices and greater activation of the central sulcus and widely distributed frontal cortical areas, compared to men with cocaine dependence (Kilts, Gross, Ely, & Drexler, 2004). Additionally, it has been reported that women who abuse cocaine have fewer perfusion abnormalities in the cortex than men and that women who use crack cocaine have less neuronal damage in the frontal cortex than men, suggesting that the toxic effects of cocaine on the brain may be less severe in women than men (Chang, Ernst, Strickland, & Mehringer, 1999). Consistently, the neurotoxicity associated with chronic methamphetamine use may be more severe in males versus females, and estrogen may underlie this difference (Dluzen & McDermott, 2002). These findings indicate sex differences in the effects of stimulants in the brain and suggest that the underlying processes that lead to drug craving may differ between men and women and that there may be sex differences in the neural correlates of craving under drug-cued situations. Results from preclinical studies showing that estrogen enhances dopamine release and alters stimulant-induced dopamine release in the striatum suggest that hormones may underlie sex differences in the neurochemical effects of chronic drug exposure and contribute to sex differences in relapse to drug use.

Together, these preliminary clinical and preclinical data suggest that women and men may require different relapse prevention programs. The hypothesis that women are more sensitive to the environmental cues associated with smoking, whereas men are more sensitive to the nicotine cues, is of particular interest because it implies that treatments that reduced the cues associated with cigarette smoking (e.g., extinction training) would be more effective at treating drug abuse in women, compared to men, whereas treatments that reduced the primary reinforcing effects (e.g., nicotinic/dopaminergic manipulations) may be more effective in men. However, sex differences during the relapse phase is an understudied and complicated area of research that is believed to be influenced by a complex interplay of psychological, social, and biological factors. Further research is necessary to understand the exact nature of sex differences during relapse to stimulant use.

DO MEN AND WOMEN DIFFER IN TREATMENT OUTCOME FOR DRUG ABUSE?

Behavioral Therapies

The majority of drug abuse treatment programs have used a cognitive-behavioral therapeutic approach, and numerous studies have compared men and women following such treatment. The results from these studies have shown that despite observations that women have more comorbid problems, greater psychological distress, and more medical problems (Brady & Randall, 1999; Cohen, Greenberg, Uri, Halpin, & Zweben, 2007; DiNitto, Webb, & Rubin, 2002; Stevens, Estrada, Murphy, McKnight, & Tims, 2004; Walitzer & Dearing, 2006; Zweben et al., 2004), they generally do as well as (e.g., Alterman, Randall, & McLellan, 2000; Westhuis, Gwaltney, & Hayashi, 2001; Wong, Badger, Sigmon, & Higgins, 2002) if not better than (e.g., Hser, Evans, & Huang, 2005; Hser, Huang, Teruya, & Douglas Anglin, 2003; Weiss, Martinez-Raga, Griffin, Greenfield, & Hufford, 1997) men in treatment. A notable exception is nicotine dependence, for which women often have worse outcomes than men (Perkins, 2001).

Although it would not be possible to model cognitive-behavioral therapy in laboratory animals, several investigators have examined the effects of environmental manipulations on drug use, and two of these studies have compared the effects in males and females (Bardo, Klebaur, Valone, & Deaton, 2001; Cosgrove & Carroll, 2003). Consistent with the clinical data, the results from these preclinical studies have shown that alternative nondrug reinforcers and other forms of environmental enrichment (i.e., inclusion of novel objects and social partners) produce a similar or even greater suppression of cocaine (Cosgrove & Carroll, 2003) and amphetamine (Bardo et al., 2001) self-administration in females compared to males. The biological basis for this effect is not yet understood.

Pharmacotherapies

Reports of sex-difference analyses in clinical trials and laboratory studies with potential pharmacotherapies have been infrequent, perhaps in part due to small numbers of female participants. An area that does have information regarding sex differences in pharmacotherapeutic effects is smoking research. Nicotine replacement therapy (NRT), the most widely used form of cessation treatment, has been speculated to be a less effective treatment method in women than men, based on findings that nicotine plays a lesser role in regulating smoking and cessation in women (Perkins, 2001). Indeed, data from numerous studies have revealed lower quit rates in women receiving NRT, compared to men (for review see Cepeda-Benito, Reynoso, & Erath, 2004), supporting the hypothesis that NRT is less effective for women. However, Shiffman, Sweeney, and Dresler (2005) suggested that a sex difference in treatment outcome may not reflect a difference in response to NRT but, rather, may reflect a sex difference in nicotine dependence. This interpretation is supported by their finding of parallel differences between men and women in the placebo and in the treatment groups and by findings showing that women have lower quit rates even without NRT or any other treatment (Shiffman et al., 2005). NRT does appear to have longer-lasting efficacy, compared to placebo, in males than in females (Cepeda-Benito et al., 2004), and some studies have shown that sex differences are stronger in the NRT group as compared to the placebo group (Wetter et al., 1999). If men and women do differ in their biological response to NRT, then one would expect to see parallel findings in animal models of relapse; that is, the NRT would decrease nicotine-seeking behavior to a lesser extent in female animals compared to male animals. Although this possibility has not yet been investigated in animal studies, the preclinical data do show that there are sex differences in response to nicotine alone versus nicotine paired with visual stimuli, with the most robust differences observed under the nicotine plus visual stimuli conditions (Chaudhri et al., 2005).

Sex differences have also been reported for the effects of bupropion on smoking cessation, with men benefiting more than women from bupropion treatment (Swan et al., 2003). However, results from a recent meta-analysis suggest that the sex difference observed in bupropion trials may be attributable to lower quit rates in women, compared to men, whether treated with bupropion or placebo (Scharf & Shiffman, 2004). Bupropion does, however, appear to negate the general disadvantage women have in quitting smoking among certain populations of females who smoke (i.e., those who smoke lightly; Collins et al., 2004). Results from animal studies have shown that bupropion is effective at reducing different components related to nicotine dependence, including reinforcement and withdrawal severity; however, its effects have not yet been compared between males and females.

Although there are no approved treatments for cocaine abuse, preliminary preclinical results have revealed sex differences in the effects of the GABA-ergic drug baclofen on cocaine self-administration, with a more pronounced effect in females compared to males (Campbell, Morgan, & Carroll, 2002). In contrast, naltrexone was reported to be more effective at reducing cocaine use in men, as compared to women, in a population of patients with co-occurring cocaine and alcohol dependence (Pettinati et al., 2007). Similarly findings have recently been reported for the efficacy of bupropion in decreasing methamphetamine use, with men showing greater reductions compared to women, in a population having low-to-moderate use at baseline (Elkashef et al., 2008).

Although sex difference in the effects of potential pharmacotherapies have been infrequent, the results from the few studies that have been conducted have often revealed sex differences indicating that different biological mechanisms underlie addictive states in men and women. The implication of these results is that optimal pharmacotherapies for treating drug abuse may differ between women and men. These results also highlight the need to conduct future clinical trials with large enough samples to address sex and hormone-specific questions (Wetherington, 2007).

FUTURE DIRECTIONS

Despite historically lower rates of drug use and abuse/dependence among women, the available literature on sex differences indicates that women are not less vulnerable to drug abuse than men. In fact, in some cases, women may be more vulnerable, particularly with regard to the progression to addiction, which appears to be accelerated in women (see Figure 24.1). The convergence of the clinical and preclinical data with regard to sex differences indicates

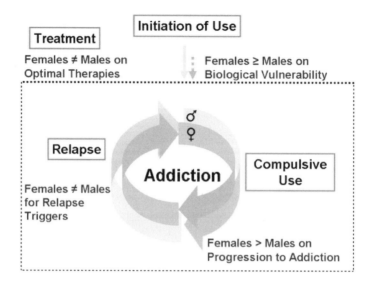

FIGURE 24.1. Sex differences during the different phases of the addiction process. Females appear to have an increased biological vulnerability to stimulant abuse than do males and have a faster progression through landmark phases associated with stimulant abuse than do males. Sex differences have also been noted during the relapse phase, with evidence to suggest that the cues used to trigger craving and drug-seeking behaviors differ between males and females. The optimal therapeutic strategies for treating stimulant abuse may differ between men and women.

that the biological vulnerability to drug abuse in men and women may be driven by neurochemical differences and hormonal influences. Historically, the number of women using and abusing drugs has been constrained by societal factors. The narrowing of differences between males and females in rates of initiation of drug use is concerning, given biological data suggesting that females appear in some ways more vulnerable to stimulant abuse than males. In order to target prevention and treatment efforts in vulnerable populations (e.g., adolescents) most effectively, sex-specific strategies should be considered. However, it is not yet clear whether differences in initiation of use represent a lasting trend that will correspond to changes in the rates of abuse among adult women and men. Thus, further research is necessary to investigate cohort differences and to evaluate sex differences in social/environmental constraints and their influence on, and interaction with, biological factors. Modeling social/environmental influences in biological experiments with animals represents a powerful approach to advancing our understanding of addictive processes in females and males. These investigations, in conjunction with human studies, should further inform a sex-specific model regarding differences in drug abuse, and such a model should significantly advance prevention and treatment strategies for drug abuse.

KEY POINTS

- During drug initiation, women appear to be at least equally, if not more, vulnerable to the reinforcing effects of stimulants as compared to men. In females, estrogen appears to enhance the reinforcing effects of stimulants, an effect that appears to be due to interactions of estrogen and dopamine.

- The progression to addiction appears to be accelerated in women. The concordance of the clinical and preclinical findings suggests that this effect is due to biological differences between males and females, with some evidence to support a role of estrogen in mediating the enhanced vulnerability in females.
- Biological vulnerability to relapse to stimulant use appears to be deferentially influenced between men and women by internal and external cues. These differences may reflect differences in the neurobiology mediating these types of reinstatement.
- The optimal behavioral and pharmacological treatment for treating stimulant abuse may differ between men and women.

ACKNOWLEDGMENTS

This work was supported by grants from the National Institutes of Health Offices of Research on Women's Health and the National Institute on Drug Abuse (Nos. DA018978, DA11717, DA016556, DA114038, DA01667, and DA08227). We would like to acknowledge the Research and Development Program at the University of Virginia, the Yale Interdisciplinary Women's Health Research Scholar Program on Women and Drug Abuse (Carolyn Mazure, Principal Investigator), the Specialized Centers of Research on Women's Health (Rajita Sinha, Principal Investigator), and the Women and Addictive Disorders Core of Women's Health Research at Yale.

REFERENCES

Asterisks denote recommended readings.

Alterman, A. I., Randall, M., & McLellan, A. T. (2000). Comparison of outcomes by gender and for fee-for-service versus managed care: A study of nine community programs. *Journal of Substance Abuse Treatment*, 19(2), 127–134.

Badley, E. M. (2001). Gender differences in access and use of health care services. *Journal of Rheumatology*, 28(10), 2145–2146.

Bardo, M. T., Klebaur, J. E., Valone, J. M., & Deaton, C. (2001). Environmental enrichment decreases intravenous self-administration of amphetamine in female and male rats. *Psychopharmacology*, 155(3), 278–284.

Becker, J. B. (1999). Gender differences in dopaminergic function in striatum and nucleus accumbens. *Pharmacology, Biochemistry, and Behavior*, 64(4), 803–812. (*)

Becker, J. B., & Hu, M. (2008). Sex differences in drug abuse. *Frontiers in Neuroendocrinology*, 29(1), 36–47.

Bowman, B. P., Vaughan, S. R., Walker, Q. D., Davis, S. L., Little, P. J., Scheffler, N. M., et al. (1999). Effects of sex and gonadectomy on cocaine metabolism in the rat. *Journal of Pharmacology and Experimental Therapeutics*, 290(3), 1316–1323.

Brady, K. T., & Randall, C. L. (1999). Gender differences in substance use disorders. *Psychiatric Clinics of North America*, 22(2), 241–252. (*)

Campbell, U. C., Morgan, A. D., & Carroll, M. E. (2002). Sex differences in the effects of baclofen on the acquisition of intravenous cocaine self-administration in rats. *Drug and Alcohol Dependence*, 66(1), 61–69.

Carroll, M. E., Lynch, W. J., Roth, M. E., Morgan, A. D., & Cosgrove, K. P. (2004). Sex and estrogen influence drug abuse. *Trends in Pharmacological Sciences*, 25(5), 273–279.

Cepeda-Benito, A., Reynoso, J. T., & Erath, S. (2004). Meta-analysis of the efficacy of nicotine replacement therapy for smoking cessation: Differences between men and women. *Journal of Consulting and Clinical Psychology*, 72(4), 712–722.

Chang, L., Ernst, T., Strickland, T., & Mehringer, C. M. (1999). Gender effects on persistent cerebral metabolite changes in the frontal lobes of abstinent cocaine users. *American Journal of Psychiatry*, *156*(5), 716–722.

Chaudhri, N., Caggiula, A. R., Donny, E. C., Booth, S., Gharib, M. A., Craven, L. A., et al. (2005). Sex differences in the contribution of nicotine and nonpharmacological stimuli to nicotine self-administration in rats. *Psychopharmacology*, *180*(2), 258–266.

Cohen, J. B., Greenberg, R., Uri, J., Halpin, M., & Zweben, J. E. (2007). Women with methamphetamine dependence: Research on etiology and treatment. *Journal of Psychoactive Drugs*, *4*, 347–351. (*)

Collins, B. N., Wileyto, E. P., Patterson, F., Rukstalis, M., Audrain-McGovern, J., Kaufmann, V., et al. (2004). Gender differences in smoking cessation in a placebo-controlled trial of bupropion with behavioral counseling. *Nicotine and Tobacco Research*, *6*(1), 27–37.

Committee on Understanding the Biology of Sex and Gender Differences. (2001). *Exploring the biological contributions to human health: Does sex matter?* Edited by T. M. Wizemann & M. L. Pardue. Washington, DC: Institute of Medicine National Academy Press.

Cosgrove, K. P., & Carroll, M. E. (2003). Effects of a non-drug reinforcer, saccharin, on oral self-administration of phencyclidine in male and female rhesus monkeys. *Psychopharmacology*, *170*(1), 9–16.

Diehl, A., Croissant, B., Batra, A., Mundle, G., Nakovics, H., & Mann, K. (2007). Alcoholism in women: Is it different in onset and outcome compared to men? *European Archives of Psychiatry and Clinical Neuroscience*, *257*(6), 344–351.

DiNitto, D. M., Webb, D. K., & Rubin, A. (2002). Gender differences in dually-diagnosed clients receiving chemical dependency treatment. *Journal of Psychoactive Drugs*, *34*(1), 105–117.

Dluzen, D. E., & McDermott, J. L. (2002). Estrogen, anti-estrogen, and gender: Differences in methamphetamine neurotoxicity. *Annals of the New York Academy of Sciences*, *965*, 136–156.

Elkashef, A. M., Rawson, R. A., Anderson, A. L., Li, S. H., Holmes, T., Smith, E. V., et al. (2008). Bupropion for the treatment of methamphetamine dependence. *Neuropsychopharmacology*, *33*(5), 1162–1170.

Elman, I., Karlsgodt, K. H., & Gastfriend, D. R. (2001). Gender differences in cocaine craving among non-treatment-seeking individuals with cocaine dependence. *American Journal of Drug and Alcohol Abuse*, *27*(2), 193–202.

Evans, S. M., & Foltin, R. W. (2004). Pharmacokinetics of intravenous cocaine across the menstrual cycle in rhesus monkeys. *Neuropsychopharmacology*, *29*(10), 1889–1900.

Evans, S. M., & Foltin, R. W. (2006). Pharmacokinetics of repeated doses of intravenous cocaine across the menstrual cycle in rhesus monkeys. *Pharmacology, Biochemistry, and Behavior*, *83*(1), 56–66.

Festa, E. D., Russo, S. J., Gazi, F. M., Niyomchai, T., Kemen, L. M., Lin, S. N., et al. (2004). Sex differences in cocaine-induced behavioral responses, pharmacokinetics, and monoamine levels. *Neuropharmacology*, *46*(5), 672–687.

Field, M., & Duka, T. (2004). Cue reactivity in smokers: The effects of perceived cigarette availability and gender. *Pharmacology, Biochemistry, and Behavior*, *78*(3), 647–652.

Fox, H. C., Garcia, M., Jr., Kemp, K., Milivojevic, V., Kreek, M. J., & Sinha, R. (2006). Gender differences in cardiovascular and corticoadrenal response to stress and drug cues in cocaine dependent individuals. *Psychopharmacology*, *185*(3), 348–357.

Fuchs, R. A., Evans, K. A., Mehta, R. H., Case, J. M., & See, R. E. (2005). Influence of sex and estrous cyclicity on conditioned cue-induced reinstatement of cocaine-seeking behavior in rats. *Psychopharmacology*, *179*(3), 662–672.

Griffin, M. L., Weiss, R. D., Mirin, S. M., & Lange, U. (1989). A comparison of male and female cocaine abusers. *Archives of General Psychiatry*, *46*(2), 122–126.

Hser, Y. I., Evans, E., & Huang, Y. C. (2005). Treatment outcomes among women and men methamphetamine abusers in California. *Journal of Substance Abuse Treatment*, *28*(1), 77–85.

Hser, Y. I., Huang, D., Teruya, C., & Douglas Anglin, M. (2003). Gender comparisons of drug abuse treatment outcomes and predictors. *Drug and Alcohol Dependence*, *72*(3), 255–264. (*)

Jackson, L. R., Robinson, T. E., & Becker, J. B. (2006). Sex differences and hormonal influences on acquisition of cocaine self-administration in rats. *Neuropsychopharmacology*, *31*(1), 129–138.

Justice, A. J., & de Wit, H. (2000). Acute effects of estradiol pretreatment on the response to *d*-amphetamine in women. *Neuroendocrinology*, 71(1), 51–59.

Kerstetter, K. A., Aguilar, V. R., Parrish, A. B., & Kippin, T. E. (2008). Protracted time-dependent increases in cocaine-seeking behavior during cocaine withdrawal in female relative to male rats. *Psychopharmacology*, 198(1), 63–75.

Kilts, C. D., Gross, R. E., Ely, T. D., & Drexler, K. P. (2004). The neural correlates of cue-induced craving in cocaine-dependent women. *American Journal of Psychiatry*, 161(2), 233–241. (*)

Koob, G., & Kreek, M. J. (2007). Stress, dysregulation of drug reward pathways, and the transition to drug dependence. *American Journal of Psychiatry*, 164(8), 1149–1159.

Larson, E. B., Anker, J. J., Gliddon, L. A., Fons, K. S., & Carroll, M. E. (2007). Effects of estrogen and progesterone on the escalation of cocaine self-administration in female rats during extended access. *Experimental and Clinical Psychopharmacology*, 15(5), 461–471.

Lukas, S. E., Sholar, M., Lundahl, L. H., Lamas, X., Kouri, E., Wines, J. D., et al. (1996). Sex differences in plasma cocaine levels and subjective effects after acute cocaine administration in human volunteers. *Psychopharmacology*, 125(4), 346–354.

Lynch, W. J. (2006). Sex differences in vulnerability to drug self-administration. *Experimental and Clinical Psychopharmacology*, 14(1), 34–41.

Lynch, W. J., & Carroll, M. E. (2000). Reinstatement of cocaine self-administration in rats: Sex differences. *Psychopharmacology*, 148(2), 196–200.

Lynch, W. J., Roth, M. E., & Carroll, M. E. (2002). Biological basis of sex differences in drug abuse: Preclinical and clinical studies. *Psychopharmacology*, 164, 121–137.

Lynch, W. J., & Taylor, J. R. (2004). Sex differences in the behavioral effects of 24-h/day access to cocaine under a discrete trial procedure. *Neuropsychopharmacology*, 29(5), 943–951.

Mendelson, J. H., Mello, N. K., Sholar, M. B., Siegel, A. J., Kaufman, M. J., Levin, J. M., et al. (1999). Cocaine pharmacokinetics in men and in women during the follicular and luteal phases of the menstrual cycle. *Neuropsychopharmacology*, 21(2), 294–303.

Mozley, L. H., Gur, R. C., Mozley, P. D., & Gur, R. E. (2001). Striatal dopamine transporters and cognitive functioning in healthy men and women. *American Journal of Psychiatry*, 158(9), 1492–1499.

Perkins, K. A. (2001). Smoking cessation in women: Special considerations. *CNS Drugs*, 15(5), 391–411. (*)

Perkins, K. A., Gerlach, D., Vender, J., Grobe, J., Meeker, J., & Hutchison, S. (2001). Sex differences in the subjective and reinforcing effects of visual and olfactory cigarette smoke stimuli. *Nicotine and Tobacco Research*, 3(2), 141–150.

Piazza, N. J., Vrbka, J. L., & Yeager, R. D. (1989). Telescoping of alcoholism in women alcoholics. *International Journal Addiction*, 24(1), 19–28.

Quinones-Jenab, V., Perrotti, L. I., Fabian, S. J., Chin, J., Russo, S. J., & Jenab, S. (2001). Endocrinological basis of sex differences in cocaine-induced behavioral responses. *Annals of the New York Academy of Sciences*, 937, 140–171.

Roberts, D. C., Morgan, D., & Liu, Y. (2007). How to make a rat addicted to cocaine. *Progress in Neuropsychopharmacology and Biological Psychiatry*, 31(8), 1614–1624.

Roth, M. E., & Carroll, M. E. (2004). Sex differences in the escalation of intravenous cocaine intake following long- or short-access to cocaine self-administration. *Pharmacology, Biochemistry, and Behavior*, 78(2), 199–207.

Scharf, D., & Shiffman, S. (2004). Are there gender differences in smoking cessation, with and without bupropion? Pooled and meta-analyses of clinical trials of Bupropion SR. *Addiction*, 99(11), 1462–1469.

Shiffman, S., Sweeney, C. T., & Dresler, C. M. (2005). Nicotine patch and lozenge are effective for women. *Nicotine and Tobacco Research*, 7(1), 119–127.

Sofuoglu, M., Mitchell, E., & Kosten, T. R. (2004). Effects of progesterone treatment on cocaine responses in male and female cocaine users. *Pharmacology, Biochemistry, and Behavior*, 78(4), 699–705.

Stevens, S. J., Estrada, B., Murphy, B. S., McKnight, K. M., & Tims, F. (2004). Gender differences in substance use, mental health, and criminal justice involvement of adolescents at treatment entry and at three, six, twelve and thirty month follow-up. *Journal of Psychoactive Drugs*, *36*(1), 13–25.

Substance Abuse and Mental Health Services Administration. (2007). *National Survey on Drug Use and Health, 2006.* Research Triangle Park, NC: Research Triangle Institute.

Swan, G. E., Jack, L. M., Curry, S., Chorost, M., Javitz, H., McAfee, T., et al. (2003). Bupropion SR and counseling for smoking cessation in actual practice: Predictors of outcome. *Nicotine and Tobacco Research*, *5*(6), 911–921.

Tavares, H., Martins, S. S., Lobo, D. S., Silveira, C. M., Gentil, V., & Hodgins, D. C. (2003). Factors at play in faster progression for female pathological gamblers: An exploratory analysis. *Journal of Clinical Psychiatry*, *64*(4), 433–438.

Terner, J. M., & de Wit, H. (2006). Menstrual cycle phase and responses to drugs of abuse in humans. *Drug and Alcohol Dependence*, *84*(1), 1–13. (*)

Tucker, K., Browndyke, J., Gottschalk, P., Cofrancesco, A., & Kosten, T. (2004). Gender-specific vulnerability for rCBF abnormalities among cocaine abusers. *NeuroReport*, *15*, 797–801.

Walitzer, K. S., & Dearing, R. L. (2006). Gender differences in alcohol and substance use relapse. *Clinical Psychology Review*, *26*(2), 128–148. (*)

Walker, Q. D., Rooney, M. B., Wightman, R. M., & Kuhn, C. (2000). Dopamine release and uptake are greater in female than male rat striatum as measured by fast cyclic voltammetry. *Neuroscience*, *95*(4), 1061–1070.

Weiss, R. D., Martinez-Raga, J., Griffin, M. L., Greenfield, S. F., & Hufford, C. (1997). Gender differences in cocaine dependent patients: A 6-month follow-up study. *Drug and Alcohol Dependence*, *44*(1), 35–40.

Westhuis, D. J., Gwaltney, L., & Hayashi, R. (2001). Outpatient cocaine abuse treatment: Predictors of success. *Journal of Drug Education*, *31*(2), 171–183.

Wetherington, C. L. (2007). Sex-gender differences in drug abuse: A shift in the burden of proof? *Experimental and Clinical Psychopharmacology*, *15*(5), 411–417. (*)

Wetter, D. W., Kenford, S. L., Smith, S. S., Fiore, M. C., Jorenby, D. E., & Baker, T. B. (1999). Gender differences in smoking cessation. *Journal of Consulting and Clinical Psychology*, *67*(4), 555–562.

Wong, C. J., Badger, G. J., Sigmon, S. C., & Higgins, S. T. (2002). Examining possible gender differences among cocaine-dependent outpatients. *Experimental and Clinical Psychopharmacology*, *10*(3), 316–323.

Zweben, J. E., Cohen, J. B., Christian, D., Galloway, G. P., Salinardi, M., Parent, D., et al. (2004). Methamphetamine treatment project: Psychiatric symptoms in methamphetamine users. *American Journal of Addiction*, *13*(2), 181–190.

PART VI

SPECIAL POPULATIONS

CHAPTER 25

Adolescent Substance Use and the Role of Gender

Himanshu P. Upadhyaya, MBBS
Kevin M. Gray, MD

Adolescence is a period of rapid physical, cognitive, emotional, social, and behavioral changes. Goals of adolescence include development of trusting relationships with peers, a sense of identity, a path in the world, and independence from parents. In pursuit of these goals, adolescents are often susceptible to peer influence, trying to "find themselves," attempting new things, and challenging parental influence. In both female and male adolescents, these factors may predispose to risk-taking behavior, including substance use. A significant minority of adolescents (8.1% of females and 8.0% of males) progress to substance abuse or dependence.

This chapter provides an overview of substance use disorders (SUDs) in adolescence, highlighting specific areas pertinent to adolescent girls. Prevalence and frequency, as well as potential neurobiological mechanisms underlying heightened risk for SUDs, are reviewed. Psychiatric comorbidity, risk factors, and potential adverse consequences associated with adolescent SUDs are discussed. Finally, a brief overview of evidence-based treatment modalities is provided.

PREVALENCE/EPIDEMIOLOGY

Since 1975, the Monitoring the Future study has surveyed attitudes about, and rates of, substance use among adolescents (Johnston, O'Malley, Bachman, & Schulenberg, 2007). The survey is administered to 8th graders, 10th graders, 12th graders, college students, and young adults. The National Survey on Drug Use and Health provides additional information on substance use in adolescents, including rates of substance abuse and dependence (Substance Abuse and Mental Health Services Administration [SAMHSA], 2007). Table 25.1 provides an overview of adolescent substance use rates by gender. As described below, overall, substance use rates are comparable in female and male adolescents, as opposed to adults, among whom males have a higher rate of substance use (SAMHSA, 2007).

TABLE 25.1. Current Substance Use by 12- to 17-Year-Old Females and Males

	Females	Males
Alcohol	27.4%	29.2%
Alcohol (binge use)[a]	16.5%	21.3%
Alcohol (heavy drinking)[b]	4.3%	7.9%
Cigarettes	10.7%	10.0%
Any illicit drugs	9.7%	9.8%
Marijuana	6.4%	6.8%
Prescription drugs (nonmedical use)	3.5%	3.1%
Substance abuse or dependence	8.1%	8.0%

Note. Data from SAMHSA (2007).

[a]Binge use—five or more drinks on the same occasion (i.e., at the same time or within a couple of hours of each other) on at least 1 day in the past 30 days (includes heavy use).

[b]Heavy use—five or more drinks on the same occasion on each of 5 or more days in the past 30 days.

Illicit Substances

Nearly 10% of adolescents ages 12–17 years are current illicit substance users (SAMHSA, 2007). Notably, 6.7% use marijuana, 3.3% use prescription drugs nonmedically, 1.3% use inhalants, 0.7% use hallucinogens, and 0.4% use cocaine. Eight percent of both female and male adolescents meet criteria for substance abuse or dependence (SAMHSA, 2007).

Overall, gender differences in adolescent current illicit substance use are small, with 9.7% of females and 9.8% of males using any illicit substance, 6.4% of females and 6.8% of males using marijuana, and 3.5% of females and 3.1% of males using prescription psychotropic medications nonmedically (SAMHSA, 2007). However, in most cases, when illicit substance use is tracked by age, gender differences become more pronounced with increasing age. Among younger adolescents (8th–10th graders), only slight gender differences are noted (Johnston et al., 2007). The rate of prior-year marijuana use is slightly higher for males, whereas the rate for use of any illicit drug other than marijuana is slightly higher for females. Among 12th graders and beyond, though, gender differences are notable. Daily marijuana use rates among 12th graders are 3.2% for females versus 6.3% for males. Similar gender differences in daily marijuana use are noted among college students (3.6% females vs. 5.5% males) and young adults (3.4% females vs. 6.5% males; Johnston et al., 2007). Of note, rates of abuse or dependence among females ages 12–17 exceed those among males for prescription psychotherapeutic medications and (1.8% females vs. 1.1% males) pain relievers (1.4% females vs. 0.8% males) (SAMHSA, 2006). However, for young adults ages 18–25, males were more likely than females to meet the criteria for past year pain reliever dependence or abuse (1.1% females vs. 1.4% males; SAMHSA, 2006). In general, there seem to be similar rates of illicit drug use in younger adolescents, but higher prevalence in males in older adolescents and young adults.

Alcohol

The overall rate of current alcohol use in adolescents is 16.6% (SAMHSA, 2007). Alcohol use rates increase gradually through adolescence into adulthood. The most recent data indicate that 3.9% of 12- to 13-year-olds, 15.6% of 14- to 15-year-olds, 29.7% of 16- to 17-year-olds, 51.6% of 18- to 20-year-olds, and 68.6% of 21- to 25-year-olds are current alcohol users. The rates of binge alcohol use in these age groups are 1.5%, 8.9%, 20.0%,

36.2%, and 46.1%, respectively. Alcohol abuse or dependence criteria are met by 5.4% of adolescents (SAMHSA, 2007).

Male adolescents generally report higher rates of alcohol use than females, but the gender difference has been diminishing over time (Johnston et al., 2007). In 2006, among 12th graders, 23% of females versus 30% of males reported having five or more drinks in a row in the last 2 weeks. Since 1975, females have reported rates generally between 20 and 30%, whereas males reported rates as high as 50% around 1980. Thus, among 12th graders, the reduction in gender difference appears mostly attributable to a decline in the rate of heavy episodic drinking among males. In 2006, among college students, the rate of having five or more drinks in a row in the past 2 weeks was 37% in females and 45% in males. A more modest reduction in gender difference for this measure appears attributable to small increases in rates among females and small decreases in rates among males (Johnston et al., 2007).

Female college students and young adults report daily drinking at lower rates than males. In 2006, 3.2% of female and 7.3% of male college students and 4.3% of female and 7.5% of male young adults reported daily drinking (SAMHSA, 2007).

Cigarettes

Cigarette smoking is the leading preventable cause of death in the United States (Centers for Disease Control, 2007). Adults who smoke generally began smoking in adolescence. Adolescents who smoke cigarettes are at significantly higher risk of using illicit substances, with rates of illicit substance use nearly nine times higher than in those who do not smoke cigarettes (SAMHSA, 2007).

Recent trends indicate a gradual decline in overall adolescent cigarette use. Over the past three decades, there has been little gender difference in cigarette smoking rates among adolescents and young adults (Johnston et al., 2007). Since the 1970s, subtle shifts in patterns of cigarette smoking have resulted in periods of greater use by either gender, but overall rates of use have gradually declined among females and males. In 2006, 19.1% of 12th graders smoked cigarettes daily, and 11.3% smoked at least half a pack daily (Johnston et al., 2007).

NEUROBIOLOGY

Adolescence is a period of substantial brain development. Rapid neurobiological changes may underpin the high risk for, and potential lasting effects of, substance abuse during adolescence.

Adult neuroimaging indicates that disturbed dopamine circuitry in the prefrontal cortex and limbic system may adversely affect motivation, drive, and self-control, thereby potentiating the addiction process (Volkow, Fowler, Wang, & Goldstein, 2002). Evidence exists for adolescent developmental changes in dopamine activity in these regions (Chambers, Taylor, & Potenza, 2003; Crews, He, & Hodge, 2007; Spear, 2000). Decreased perception of reward from familiar sources may lead to increased novelty-seeking and risk-taking behavior, including substance use. Additionally, adolescents may be relatively insensitive to negatively reinforcing effects of intoxication, resulting in increased quantities of episodic use (Spear, 2000). The increased propensity to start using and to use larger quantities places adolescents at particular risk of becoming habitual users.

Given the rapid neuronal transitions occurring during adolescence, including cleaving and adjustment in connections of neurons, there may be an enhanced risk of long-term adverse consequences of substance use during this age (Spear, 2002). Although emerging evidence suggests gender differences in some aspects of adolescent brain development (De Bellis et al., 2001), correlation of these differences with substance use has not been established.

COMORBIDITY

Psychiatric disorders are often noted to be comorbid with SUDs in adolescents. Although gender differences in prevalence of various psychiatric disorders exist, data on gender as an independent mediator of these disorders' association with SUDs are limited. Disruptive behavior disorders (including conduct disorder), attention-deficit/hyperactivity disorder (ADHD), mood disorders, and anxiety disorders have been cited frequently as significant risk factors for substance abuse (Bukstein, Brent, & Kaminer, 1989). Among these disorders, conduct disorder, which is more common among adolescent males, has been most closely associated with substance initiation and SUDs, with general agreement that early-onset conduct disorder predicts problematic substance use (Fergusson, Horwood, & Ridder, 2007).

The role of ADHD, which is also more common among adolescent males (female-to-male ratio 1:2.45; Polanczyk, de Lima, Horta, Biederman, & Rhode, 2007), has been debated as an independent risk factor. Researchers have argued that the association is mediated by comorbid conduct disorder (e.g., Fergusson et al., 2007) and may be most applicable to males (Whitmore et al., 1997). However, when the symptom clusters of ADHD are divided, hyperactive/impulsive symptoms strongly correlate with substance initiation and SUDs in females and males, even when controlling for comorbid conduct disorder (Elkins, McGue, & Iacono, 2007). Similarly, there is growing evidence that ADHD is associated with nicotine use, even after controlling for conduct disorder (e.g., Kollins, McClernon, & Fuemmeler, 2005; Upadhyaya, Rose, et al., 2005).

Mood and anxiety disorders, which are more common among adolescent females (e.g., lifetime major depression prevalence female-to-male ratio is 2.1:1; Kuehner, 2003), have been inconsistently associated with adolescent SUDs across studies. The strongest associations have involved cannabis use disorders (Fergusson, Horwood, & Swain-Campbell, 2002; Roberts, Roberts, & Xing, 2007; Wittchen et al., 2007; Zvolensky et al., 2007). Cannabis use in female adolescents ($n = 859$) predicted later onset of depression and anxiety in an Australian prospective study (Patton et al., 2002). Weekly cannabis use among females doubled the risk of depression and anxiety, and daily use quintupled the risk (Patton et al., 2002). Major depressive disorders in adolescents have also been associated with nicotine (Upadhyaya, Deas, Brady, & Kruesi, 2002) and alcohol use disorders (Mason et al., 2008). Whereas adolescent substance use generally precedes the onset of mood and anxiety disorders, social anxiety disorder, which is more common among females (female-to-male ratio 1.8:1; Furmark et al., 1999), may be an exception. Adolescent social anxiety disorder is associated with 4.5-fold and 6.5-fold increased risk of developing alcohol and cannabis dependence, respectively, regardless of gender (Buckner et al., 2008).

Emerging data suggest association of other psychiatric conditions with adolescent SUDs. For example, the presence of Cluster B personality disorders (i.e., borderline and histrionic personality disorders) in adolescence is associated with subsequent development of SUDs, even when controlling for conduct disorder (Cohen, Chen, Crawford, Brook, & Gordon, 2007). Posttraumatic stress disorder (PTSD), which is more common among females (female-to-male ratio 2:1; Kessler, Sonnega, Bromet, Hughes, & Nelson, 1995) during adolescence may predict illicit SUDs (Kilpatrick et al., 2000). Finally, cannabis use during adolescence may be associated with an increased risk for later development of a psychotic illness (Moore et al., 2007).

RISK FACTORS AND PATHWAYS TO SUBSTANCE USE

Adolescent substance abuse does not occur at random or in isolation. Swadi (1999) proposed dividing risk factors into *constitutional predisposition, environmental factors,* and *life events*. Table 25.2 provides an overview of these factors.

Novelty-seeking, risk-taking, and low-harm-avoidant adolescents, regardless of gender, are at increased risk for substance initiation and SUDs (Cloninger, Sigvardsson, & Bohman, 1988; Tarter et al., 2003; Wills, Vaccaro, & McNamara, 1994). Independent of familial risk, exposure to parental SUDs during adolescence was predictive of development of SUDs among a sample of 260 adolescents (Biederman, Faraone, Monuteaux, & Feighner, 2000). Additionally, inadequate or inappropriate parental discipline and supervision, as well as association with deviant peers, substantially increases the risk of antisocial behavior as well as substance abuse (Hawkins, Catalano, & Miller, 1992). Increased perceived risk of using a substance, increased perceived parental disapproval of using a substance, increased parental involvement in daily activities, and increased participation in religious activities are associated with decreased rates of substance use, whereas involvement with fighting and delinquent behaviors is associated with increased rates of substance use (SAMHSA, 2007). Exposure to stressful life events, childhood abuse, violence, or victimization by physical or sexual assault increases the risk for alcohol consumption, cigarette smoking, and SUDs (Kilpatrick et al., 2000; Simantov, Schoen, & Klein, 2000).

Some factors appear unique to female adolescents. Those who eat family dinner at home every day are significantly less likely to initiate drinking than those who inconsistently or never eat family dinner at home (Fisher, Miles, Austin, Camargo, & Colditz, 2007). High social self-esteem is associated with alcohol initiation among females (Fisher et al., 2007). Finally, females are more likely than males to report drinking or smoking to relieve stress (Simantov et al., 2000).

CONSEQUENCES OF SUBSTANCE USE

Of particular concern for females, substance use in adolescence is associated with high-risk sexual behavior that may result in date rape, sexually transmitted diseases, or unintended pregnancy (Dunn, Bartee, & Perko, 2003). Adolescent substance abuse is also significantly correlated with short- and long-term health problems (Aarons et al., 1999), academic failure (Ellickson, Tucker, Klein, & Saner, 2004), motor vehicle accidents (Mayhew, Donelson, Beirness, & Simpson, 1986), homicide (McLaughlin, Daniel, & Joost, 2000), and suicide (Brent, 1995).

TABLE 25.2. Risk Factors for Adolescent Substance Abuse in Females and Males

Constitutional predisposition	Environmental factors	Life events
Genetic risk	Parental substance use	School/academic failure
Novelty seeking and risk taking	Lack of parental monitoring or involvement	Abuse or neglect
Aggression	Peer substance use	Exposure to violence
Psychiatric problems	Deviant peer group	Victimization by assault

Note. Data from Swadi (1999).

TREATMENT

To date, there has been minimal research on gender-specific prevention and treatment interventions for adolescent substance abuse. A review of effective substance abuse prevention programs revealed 10 common elements (Winters, Fawkes, Fahnhorst, Botzet, & August, 2007). These elements are summarized in Table 25.3.

The level of care indicated for adolescent substance abuse varies widely, generally in regard to the acuity of the situation at the time of assessment. If there is potential for medically serious withdrawal, if the continued use of the substance may result in acute serious harm, or if comorbid psychiatric disturbance renders the patient at risk of harm to self or others, then hospitalization is generally warranted. If none of these factors applies, a broad range of outpatient treatment options may be considered, depending on the severity of impairment, the unique characteristics of the situation, and the available treatment options in the community.

A review of controlled treatment studies for adolescent substance abuse revealed the most promising evidence for cognitive-behavioral therapy and family-based/multisystemic therapy (Deas & Thomas, 2001). Other modalities, including contingency management, are gaining increasing attention and validity (Cavallo et al., 2007; Corby, Ledgerwood, & Schuster, 2000; Kamon, Budney, & Stanger, 2005; Krishnan-Sarin et al., 2006; Roll, 2005). In many treatment programs, components of multiple treatment modalities are effectively combined.

The Cannabis Youth Treatment (CYT) study revealed modest treatment success across a range of modalities in adolescents with marijuana use disorders (Dennis et al., 2004). The most cost-effective interventions included a five-session combination of motivational enhancement therapy plus cognitive-behavioral therapy intervention and an adolescent community reinforcement approach. It is possible that shared factors among a variety of approaches may mediate a therapeutic effect in this population.

Evidence indicates that nicotine replacement therapy (Moolchan et al., 2005) and bupropion (Muramoto, Leischow, Sherrill, Matthews, & Stayer, 2007; Upadhyaya, Brady, & Wang, 2004) may be useful options in treating adolescents with nicotine dependence. During treatment, ongoing smoking may be monitored using patient diaries, carbon monoxide breathalyzer readings, and cotinine (nicotine metabolite) levels (Upadhyaya, Deas, et al.,

TABLE 25.3. Elements of Effective Adolescent Substance Abuse Prevention Programs

1. Focuses on altering psychosocial risk factors believed to initiate or maintain substance use.

2. Focuses primarily on alcohol and/or tobacco prevention.

3. Multiple influences and settings are targeted.

4. Program curriculum spans multiple grades and several developmental periods.

5. Activities and curricula are developmentally and socioculturally sensitive.

6. Programs expend a meaningful degree of resources in engaging the target population.

7. Youth component focuses on social skills.

8. Parent component focuses on discipline and support.

9. The structure and philosophy of the programs encourage broad-based involvement in decision making related to their organizational structure.

10. Several aspects of the programs are infused with features that promote their sustainability.

Note. Data from Winters, Fawkes, Fahnhorst, Botzet, and August (2007).

2005). Little is known about differential gender response to smoking cessation treatment in adolescents; limited data suggest similar quit rates among male and female adolescents who smoke (Zhu, Sun, Billings, Choi, & Malarcher, 1999).

Preliminary evidence suggests that buprenorphine may be efficacious for treatment of opiate dependence in adolescents (Marsch et al., 2005). There is also evidence for naltrexone (Deas, May, Randall, Johnson, & Anton, 2005) and acamprosate (Niederhofer & Staffen, 2003) in the treatment of alcohol dependence in adolescents.

Given the high rate of comorbidity between adolescent substance abuse and psychopathology (Bukstein et al., 1989), and the potential for reducing substance abuse risk with successful treatment of psychiatric symptom pathology (Wilens, Faraone, Biederman, & Gunawardene, 2003), it is imperative that any comorbid psychiatric condition be treated in parallel with the SUD (Riggs et al., 2007). Recently, integrated treatment of major depression (with fluoxetine) and SUD (with cognitive-behavioral therapy) was shown to be efficacious for comorbid major depression and SUD (Riggs et al., 2007). Ideally, all aspects of psychiatric and substance abuse treatment should occur in the same setting, but in many cases such combined treatment may not be available.

CONCLUSIONS

The confluence of physical, cognitive, emotional, social, behavioral, and neurobiological changes during adolescence may predispose adolescents to initiate use of, and experience adverse consequences from substances. Whereas significant gender disparities in substance use rates exist among adults, relatively few significant differences are seen in adolescents. Nonetheless, gender may play a role in psychiatric comorbidity and adverse consequences of adolescent substance abuse. Emerging evidence indicates that some prevention and treatment strategies may be successful, but the role of gender in the development of, and response to, these strategies has not been adequately explored.

FUTURE DIRECTIONS

Despite the significant public health implications of substance abuse in adolescence, this topic remains generally understudied. Since many adults with SUDs began using as adolescents, effective prevention and treatment strategies aimed at children and adolescents are crucial. The role of gender in adolescent substance abuse must be further elucidated, as this information may inform the development of individualized prevention and treatment approaches.

KEY POINTS

- Substance use is common in adolescent females and males.
- Gender differences in substance use and SUDs are generally small in early adolescence, but may expand from late adolescence into early adulthood.
- In females and males, significant neurobiological development during adolescence may underlie elevated risk for substance initiation and abuse.
- Psychiatric comorbidity is common in adolescents with SUDs, with conduct disorder and ADHD more common in males, and depression and anxiety more common in females.

- Risk factors for adolescent substance abuse span biological, psychological, and social elements.
- Potential consequences of substance abuse in adolescence are significant. Female adolescents are at particular risk for adverse outcomes from high-risk sexual behavior.
- A variety of adolescent substance abuse prevention and treatment modalities are available, and some have demonstrated efficacy. To date, no studies on gender-specific SUD treatment for adolescents have been conducted.

REFERENCES

Asterisks denote recommended readings.

Aarons, G. A., Brown, S. A., Coe, M. T., Myers, M. G., Garland, A. F., Ezzet-Lofstram, R., al et. (1999). Adolescent alcohol and drug abuse and health. *Journal of Adolescent Health, 24,* 412–421.

Biederman, J., Faraone, S. V., Monuteaux, M. C., & Feighner, J. A. (2000). Patterns of alcohol and drug use in adolescents can be predicted by parental substance use disorders. *Pediatrics, 106,* 792–797.

Brent, D. A. (1995). Risk factors for adolescent suicide and suicidal behavior: Mental and substance abuse disorders, family environmental factors, and life stress. *Suicide and Life Threatening Behavior, 25,* 52–63.

Buckner, J. D., Schmidt, N. B., Lang, A. R., Small, J. W., Schlauch, R. C., & Lewinsohn, P. M. (2008). Specificity of social anxiety disorder as a risk factor for alcohol and cannabis dependence. *Journal of Psychiatric Research, 42,* 230–239.

Bukstein, O. G., Brent, D. A., & Kaminer, Y. (1989). Comorbidity of substance abuse and other psychiatric disorders in adolescents. *American Journal of Psychiatry, 146,* 1131–1141.

Cavallo, D. A., Cooney, J. L., Duhig, A. M., Smith, A. E., Liss, T. B., McFetridge, A. K., et al. (2007). Combining cognitive behavioral therapy with contingency management for smoking cessation in adolescent smokers: A preliminary comparison of two different CBT formats. *American Journal on Addictions, 16,* 468–474.

Centers for Disease Control and Prevention. (2007). Targeting tobacco use: The nation's leading cause of preventable death 2007. Available online at *www.cdc.gov/nccdphp/publications/aag/pdf/osh.pdf.*

Chambers, R. A., Taylor, J. R., & Potenza, M. N. (2003). Developmental neurocircuitry of motivation in adolescence: A critical period of addiction vulnerability. *American Journal of Psychiatry, 160,* 1041–1052.

Cloninger, C. R., Sigvardsson, S., & Bohman, M. (1988). Childhood personality predicts alcohol use in young adults. *Alcoholism, 12,* 494–505.

Cohen, P., Chen, H., Crawford, T. N., Brook, J. S., & Gordon, K. (2007). Personality disorders in early adolescence and the development of later substance use disorders in the general population. *Drug and Alcohol Dependence, 88*(Suppl.), S71–S84.

Corby, E. A., Roll, J. M., Ledgerwood, D. M., & Schuster, C. R. (2000). Contingency management interventions for treating the substance abuse of adolescents: A feasibility study. *Experimental and Clinical Psychopharmacology, 8,* 371–376.

Crews, F., He, J., & Hodge, C. (2007). Adolescent cortical development: A critical period of vulnerability for addiction. *Pharmacology, Biochemistry, and Behavior, 86,* 189–199.

Deas, D., May, M. P., Randall, C., Johnson, N., & Anton, R. (2005). Naltrexone treatment of adolescent alcoholics: An open-label pilot study. *Journal of Child and Adolescent Psychopharmacology, 15,* 723–728.

Deas, D., & Thomas, S. E. (2001). An overview of controlled studies of adolescent substance abuse treatment. *American Journal on Addictions, 10,* 1781–1789.

De Bellis, M. D., Keshavan, M. S., Beers, S. R., Hall, J., Frustaci, K., Masalehdan, A., et al. (2001).

Sex differences in brain maturation during childhood and adolescence. *Cerebral Cortex*, *11*, 552–557.

Dennis, M., Godley, S. H., Diamond, G., Tims, F. M., Babor, T., Donaldson, J., et al. (2004). The Cannabis Youth Treatment (CYT) study: Main findings from two randomized trials. *Journal of Substance Abuse Treatment*, *27*, 197–213. (*)

Dunn, M. S., Bartee, R. T., & Perko, M. A. (2003). Self-reported alcohol use and sexual behaviors of adolescents. *Psychological Reports*, *92*, 339–348.

Elkins, I. J., McGue, M., & Iacono, W. G. (2007). Prospective effects of attention-deficit/hyperactivity disorder, conduct disorder, and sex on adolescent substance use and abuse. *Archives of General Psychiatry*, *64*, 1145–1152.

Ellickson, P. L., Tucker, J. S., Klein, D. J., & Saner, H. (2004). Antecedents and outcomes of marijuana use initiation during adolescence. *Preventive Medicine*, *39*, 976–984.

Fergusson, D. M., Horwood, L. J., & Ridder, E. M. (2007). Conduct and attentional problems in childhood and adolescence and later substance use, abuse, and dependence: Results of a 25-year longitudinal study. *Drug and Alcohol Dependence*, *88*(Suppl.), S14–S26.

Fergusson, D. M., Horwood, L. J., & Swain-Campbell, N. (2002). Cannabis use and psychosocial adjustment in adolescence and young adulthood. *Addiction*, *97*, 1123–1135.

Fisher, L. B., Miles, I. W., Austin, S. B., Camargo, C. A., & Colditz, G. A. (2007). Predictors of initiation of alcohol use among US adolescents: Findings from a prospective cohort study. *Archives of Pediatrics and Adolescent Medicine*, *161*, 959–966.

Furmark, T., Tillfors, M., Everz, P. O., Marteinsdottir, I., Gefvert, O., & Fredrikson, M. (1999). Social phobia in the general population: Prevalence and sociodemographic profile. *Social Psychiatry and Psychiatric Epidemiology*, *34*, 416–424.

Hawkins, J. D., Catalano, R. F., & Miller, J. Y. (1992). Risk and protective factors for alcohol and other drug problems in adolescence and early adulthood: Implications for substance abuse prevention. *Psychological Bulletin*, *112*, 64–105.

Johnston, L. D., O'Malley, P. M., Bachman, J. G., & Schulenberg, J. E. (2007). *Monitoring the Future national survey results on drug use, 1975–2006. Volume I: Secondary school students* (NIH Publication No. 07-6205). Bethesda, MD: National Institute on Drug Abuse. Available at *monitoringthefuture.org/pubs/monographs/vol1_2006.pdf*. (*)

Kamon, J., Budney, A., & Stanger, C. (2005). A contingency management intervention for adolescent marijuana abuse and conduct problems. *Journal of the American Academy of Child and Adolescent Psychiatry*, *44*, 513–521.

Kessler, R. C., Sonnega, A., Bromet, E., Hughes, M., & Nelson, C. B. (1995). Posttraumatic stress disorder in the National Comorbidity Study. *Archives of General Psychiatry*, *52*, 1048–1060.

Kilpatrick, D. G., Acierno, R., Saunders, B., Resnick, H. S., Best, C. L., & Schnurr, P. P. (2000). Risk factors for adolescent substance abuse and dependence: Data from a national sample. *Journal of Consulting and Clinical Psychology*, *68*, 19–30.

Kollins, S. H., McClernon, F. J., & Fuemmeler, B. F. (2005). Association between smoking and attention-deficit/hyperactivity disorder symptoms in a population-based sample of young adults. *Archives of General Psychiatry*, *62*, 1142–1147.

Krishnan-Sarin, S., Duhig, A. M., McKee, S. A., McMahon, T. J., Liss, T., McFetridge, A., et al. (2006). Contingency management for smoking cessation in adolescent smokers. *Experimental and Clinical Psychopharmacology*, *14*, 306–310.

Kuehner, C. (2003). Gender differences in unipolar depression: An update of epidemiological findings and possible explanations. *Acta Psychiatrica Scandinavica*, *108*, 163–174.

Marsch, L. A., Bickel, W. K., Badger, G. J., Stothart, M. E., Quesnel, K. J., Stanger, C., et al. (2005). Comparison of pharmacological treatments for opioid-dependent adolescents: A randomized controlled trial. *Archives of General Psychiatry*, *62*, 1157–1164.

Mason, W. A., Kosterman, R., Haggerty, K. P., Hawkins, J. D., Redmond, C., Spoth, R. L., et al. (2008). Dimensions of adolescent alcohol involvement as predictors of young-adult major depression. *Journal of Studies on Alcohol and Drugs*, *69*, 275–285.

Mayhew, D. R., Donelson, A. C., Beirness, D. J., & Simpson, H. M. (1986). Youth, alcohol, and relative risk of crash involvement. *Accident Analysis and Prevention*, *18*, 273–287.

McLaughlin, C. R., Daniel, J., & Joost, T. F. (2000). The relationship between substance use, drug selling, and lethal violence in 25 juvenile murderers. *Journal of Forensic Sciences, 45*, 349–353.

Moolchan, E. T., Robinson, M. L., Ernst, M., Cadet, J. L., Pickworth, W. B., Heishman, S. J., et al. (2005). Safety and efficacy of the nicotine patch and gum for adolescent tobacco addiction. *Pediatrics, 115*, e407–e414.

Moore, T. H., Zammit, S., Lingford-Hughes, A., Barnes, T. R., Jones, P. B., Burke, M., et al. (2007). Cannabis use and risk of psychotic or affective mental health outcomes: A systematic review. *Lancet, 370*, 319–328.

Muramoto, M. L., Leischow, S. J., Sherrill, D., Matthews, E., & Strayer, L. J. (2007). Randomized, double-blind, placebo-controlled trial of 2 dosages of sustained-release bupropion for adolescent smoking cessation. *Archives of Pediatrics and Adolescent Medicine, 161*, 1068–1074. (*)

Niederhofer, H., & Staffen, W. (2003). Acamprosate and its efficacy in treating alcohol dependent adolescents. *European Child and Adolescent Psychiatry, 12*, 144–148.

Patton, G. C., Coffey, C., Carlin, J. B., Degenhardt, L., Lynskey, M., & Hall, W. (2002). Cannabis use and mental health in young people: Cohort study. *British Medical Journal, 325*, 1195–1198.

Polanczyk, G., de Lima, M. S., Horta, B. L., Biederman, J., & Rohde, L. A. (2007). The worldwide prevalence of ADHD: A systematic review and metaregression analysis. *American Journal of Psychiatry, 164*, 942–948.

Riggs, P. D., Mikulich-Gilbertson, S. K., Davies, R. D., Lohman, M., Klein, C., & Stover, S. K. (2007). A randomized controlled trial of fluoxetine and cognitive behavioral therapy in adolescents with major depression, behavior problems, and substance use disorders. *Archives of Pediatrics and Adolescent Medicine, 161*, 1026–1034. (*)

Roberts, R. E., Roberts, C. R., & Xing, Y. (2007). Comorbidity of substance use disorders and other psychiatric disorders among adolescents: Evidence from an epidemiologic survey. *Drug and Alcohol Dependence, 88*(Suppl.), S4–S13.

Roll, J. M. (2005). Assessing the feasibility of using contingency management to modify cigarette smoking by adolescents. *Journal of Applied Behavioral Analysis, 38*, 463–467.

Simantov, E., Schoen, C., & Klein, J. D. (2000). Health-compromising behaviors: Why do adolescents smoke or drink?: Identifying underlying risk and protective factors. *Archives of Pediatrics and Adolescent Medicine, 154*, 1025–1033.

Spear, L. P. (2000). The adolescent brain and age-related behavioral manifestations. *Neuroscience and Biobehavioral Reviews, 24*, 417–463. (*)

Spear, L. P. (2002). Alcohol's effects on adolescents. *Alcohol Research and Health, 26*, 287–293.

Substance Abuse and Mental Health Services Administration (SAMHSA). (2006). *Office of Applied Studies website.* Available at *www.oas.samhsa.gov/prescription/Ch6.htm.*

Substance Abuse and Mental Health Services Administration (SAMHSA). (2007). *Results from the 2006 National Survey on Drug Use and Health: National findings* (Office of Applied Studies, NSDUH Series H-32, DHHS Publication No. SMA 07-4293). Rockville, MD: Author. (*)

Swadi, H. (1999). Individual risk factors for adolescent substance use. *Drug and Alcohol Dependence, 55*, 209–224.

Tarter, R. E., Kirisci, L., Mezzich, A., Cornelius, J. R., Pajer, K., Vanyukov, M., et al. (2003). Neurobehavioral disinhibition in childhood predicts early age at onset of substance use disorder. *American Journal of Psychiatry, 160*, 1078–1085.

Upadhyaya, H. P., Brady, K. T., & Wang, W. (2004). Bupropion SR in adolescents with comorbid ADHD and nicotine dependence: A pilot study. *Journal of the American Academy of Child and Adolescent Psychiatry, 43*, 199–205.

Upadhyaya, H. P., Deas, D., & Brady, K. T. (2005). A practical clinical approach to the treatment of nicotine dependence in adolescents. *Journal of the American Academy of Child and Adolescent Psychiatry, 44*, 942–946.

Upadhyaya, H. P., Deas, D., Brady, K. T., & Kruesi, M. (2002). Cigarette smoking and psychiatric comorbidity in children and adolescents. *Journal of the Academy of Child and Adolescent Psychiatry, 41*, 1294–1305.

Upadhyaya, H. P., Rose, K., Wang, W., O'Rourke, K., Sullivan, B., Deas, D., et al. (2005). Attention-deficit/hyperactivity disorder, medication treatment, and substance use patterns among adolescents and young adults. *Journal of Child and Adolescent Psychopharmacology, 15,* 799–809.

Whitmore, E. A., Mikulich, S. K., Thompson, L. L., Riggs, P. D., Aarons, G. A., & Crowley, T. J. (1997). Influences on adolescent substance dependence: Conduct disorder, depression, attention deficit hyperactivity disorder, and gender. *Drug and Alcohol Dependence, 47*(2), 87–97.

Wills, T. A., Vaccaro, D., & McNamara, G. (1994). Novelty seeking, risk taking, and related constructs as predictors of adolescent substance use: An application of Cloninger's theory. *Journal of Substance Abuse, 6,* 1–20.

Volkow, N. D., Fowler, J. S., Wang, G. J., & Goldstein, R. Z. (2002). Role of dopamine, the frontal cortex, and memory circuits in drug addiction: Insight from imaging studies. *Neurobiology of Learning and Memory, 78,* 610–624.

Wilens, T., Faraone, S. V., Biederman, J., & Gunawardene, S. (2003). Does stimulant therapy of attention-deficit/hyperactivity disorder beget later substance abuse? A meta-analytic review of the literature. *Pediatrics, 111,* 179–185.

Winters, K. C., Fawkes, T., Fahnhorst, T., Botzet, A., & August, G. (2007). A synthesis review of exemplary drug abuse prevention programs in the United States. *Journal of Substance Abuse Treatment, 32,* 371–380.

Wittchen, H., Fröhlich, C., Behrendt, S., Günther, A., Rehm, J., Zimmermann, P., et al. (2007). Cannabis use and cannabis use disorders and their relationship to mental disorders: A 10-year prospective-longitudinal community study in adolescents. *Drug and Alcohol Dependence, 88*(Suppl.), S60–S70.

Zhu, S. H., Sun, J., Billings, S. C., Choi, W. S., & Malarcher, A. (1999). Predictors of smoking cessation in U.S. adolescents. *American Journal of Preventive Medicine, 16,* 202–207.

Zvolensky, M. J., Lewinsohn, P., Bernstein, A., Schmidt, N. B., Buckner, J. D., Seeley, J., & Bonn-Miller, M. O. (2007). Prospective associations between cannabis use, abuse, and dependence and panic attacks and disorder. *Journal of Psychiatric Research, 42*(12), 1017–1023.

CHAPTER 26

Substance Use in Pregnancy

Chaya Bhuvaneswar, MD, MA, MPH
Grace Chang, MD, MPH

The problem of substance use in pregnancy remains a major public health challenge. The use of any substances of abuse during pregnancy correlates with increased rates of medical complications for both the mother and fetus (Berenson, Wilkinson, & Lopez, 1995). This chapter reviews the epidemiology of substance use in pregnancy, consequences of prenatal exposure (see Table 26.1), and clinical approaches to treating substance use during pregnancy. We cover the most commonly used substances during pregnancy: alcohol, nicotine, marijuana, opioids, and cocaine.

ALCOHOL USE IN PREGNANCY

Epidemiology

In the Substance Abuse and Mental Health Services Administration (SAMHSA) National Survey on Drug Use and Health, a cross-sectional survey of households using telephone interviews prior to 2001, up to 20% of all women ($n = 35,000$) admitted to using some alcohol during pregnancy (U.S. Department of Health and Human Services, 1994). In contrast, between 2002 and 2003, 9.3% of pregnant women reported use of some alcohol, with 4% reporting binge drinking (SAMHSA, 2003). In 2005, 12.1% of pregnant women reported use of some alcohol, with 3–4% reporting binge drinking during pregnancy (SAMHSA, 2005).

Preconception alcohol consumption has been shown to be the strongest predictor of continued alcohol use during pregnancy (Caetano, Ramisetty-Mikler, & Floyd, 2006). Other risk factors include substance use by one's partner, lack of stable housing, and psychiatric illness, including mood and anxiety disorders (Hans, 1999). In one 16-year longitudinal study, depressive symptoms during pregnancy were as predictive of heavy postnatal alcohol consumption as were episodes of binge drinking during pregnancy. Race has also been found to be associated with alcohol use during pregnancy. In one population-based obstetrics study ($n = 903$), European Americans were more likely to report alcohol, nicotine, and illicit substance use during pregnancy than were African Americans or Mexican Americans, though African Americans and Native Americans have historically been considered the highest risk groups (Wiemann, Berenson, & San Miguel, 1994). The 2002 National Epidemiologic Survey

TABLE 26.1. Potential Consequences of Prenatal Substance Exposure

Alcohol

Fetal alcohol syndrome (FAS)
- Craniofacial: smooth philtrum, thinned vermilion of upper lip, short palpebral fissures, midface hypoplasia, microphthalmia, strabismus, ptosis
- Neurological: microcephaly, mild-to-moderate mental retardation, developmental delay, irritability, hyperactivity, seizures
- Skeletal: radioulnar synostosis, contractures, scoliosis, hemivertebrae

Features of fetal alcohol spectrum disorders (FASD)
ADHD; MCI; cardiac, renal, and visual defects (including lens abnormalities, reduced orbital size); higher prevalence of substance and behavioral disorders

Tobacco
Pre-eclampsia, placental abruption, low birth weight, IUGR, neurocognitive deficits

Marijuana
Organophosphate poisoning and other pesticide complications for mother; neonatal jitteriness, increased malignancy risk, motor delays

Opioids
Opioid overdose complications (e.g., decreased fetal heart rate variability, respiratory depression), opioid withdrawal complications (including neonatal abstinence syndrome), altered HPA axis reactivity and analgesia threshold

Cocaine
Cardiovascular (e.g., fetal/maternal cerebrovascular and cardiac events), placental abruption, migraine headaches, coagulopathy (maternal)

ADHD, attention-deficit/hyperactive disorder; HPA, hypothalamic–pituitary axis; IUGR, intrauterine growth restriction; MCI, myocardial infarction.

ADHD, attention-deficit/hyperactive disorder; HPA, hyopthalamic–pituitary axis; IUGR, intrauterine growth restriction; MCI, myocardial infarction.

on Alcohol and Related Conditions (NESARC; n = 43,093) found that binge drinking during pregnancy was highest among European Americans between the ages of 18 and 44 (25%; n = 653) as compared to matched African American women (9%, n = 303). Other factors associated with binge drinking during pregnancy were younger age (21–29 years of age), being single (without a spouse or significant other), and an annual income greater than $40,000 (Caetano et al., 2006). These findings are similar to the 2000–2001 National Pregnancy Risk Assessment Monitoring System (PRAMS; n = 16,000), which identified two cohorts of prenatal drinkers: (1) below age 30, single, with nicotine and polysubstance dependence (with marijuana the most common comorbid drug); or (2) above age 35, high socioeconomic status and level of education, nonuser of any illicit drugs, married, and European American. The prevalence of alcohol use during pregnancy was found to be 1–3% for the first cohort and 6–15% for the second (Phares et al., 2004).

Consequences of Prenatal Exposure to Alcohol

Prenatal alcohol exposure affects the physiology of pregnancy, the neonatal period, childhood and adolescent development, and adult behavior. It has been estimated that, for the 2.6 million infants who experience intrauterine alcohol exposure each year in the United States, treatment and services for mental retardation and other neurocognitive sequelae incur a national cost of over $700 million per year (Office of National Drug Policy, 2002).

One factor mediating the negative consequences is that women have more rapid and severe end-organ effects from alcohol than men (Meschke, Holl, & Messelt, 2003). Women's decreased "first-pass" metabolism is linked to the presence of less alcohol dehydrogenase (AD) enzyme in their gastric mucosa, resulting in a slower metabolizing of alcohol in women than men. In general, the fetus has less AD than the mother and is therefore exposed longer to the same amount of alcohol (Little, Gilstrap, & Cunningham, 1990). Pregnancy-related complications from alcohol use may include preterm labor, decreased production of breast milk, and increased risk of spontaneous abortion by as much as four times (Mennella, Pepino, & Teff, 2005; Rasch, 2003). It is not clear whether the teratogenic effects of alcohol (see Table 26.1) are dose dependent, with some studies implicating binge drinking, and many determining significant effects from even a very low level of consumption. In addition, genetic factors are increasingly being explored, adding to what is already known about polymorphisms in the aldehyde dehydrogenase (ADH) gene among Native Americans and Asians that may increase susceptibility to developmental consequences of exposure (Mulligan, Robin, Osier, et al., 2003). Possible protective alleles have been identified, including maternal *ADH1B*3* allele among African Americans and Afro-Caribbeans (Scott & Taylor, 2007).

Since its first description in a 1973 *Lancet* article by the American pediatricians Kenneth Lyon Jones and David L. Smith, fetal alcohol syndrome (FAS) has been the focus of public health interventions against the long-term consequences of prenatal alcohol exposure (Jones & Smith, 1973). The overall incidence of FAS is estimated at 1 in 300 to 1 in 1,000 live births per year in the United States. Since 1996, the syndrome has been designated fetal alcohol spectrum disorders (FASD), in recognition of clinical heterogeneity and a higher prevalence of subtle developmental abnormalities that may occur. This new term, FASD, broadened the scope of congenital anomalies originally described, some of which may emerge as late as young adulthood (Calhoun, et al., 2006). FASD reflects the way in which alcohol affects central nervous system (CNS) development, as well as the growth of the heart, eyes, legs, arms, teeth, ears, palate, and external genitalia, and can be a consequence of alcohol exposure at any point in pregnancy rather than simply during the first trimester (Floyd, Davis, Martin, Hungerford, & Hymbaugh, 1994).

Key features of FASD include (1) neonatal dysmorphology, (2) cognitive and behavioral changes, (3) and increased vulnerability to substance use and other psychiatric disorders. Neonatal dysmorphic features were initially characterized as microcephaly with a head circumference below the fifth percentile on the growth chart, small palpebral fissures, a flat nasal bridge, a smooth or indistinct philtrum, a thin upper lip, and flattening of the midface. Minor criteria include epicanthal folds as well as low-set or mildly malformed ears (Chudley, Kilgour, Cranston, & Edwards, 2007).

Cognitive and behavioral changes associated with FASD include higher rates of attention-deficit/hyperactivity disorder (ADHD; with up to 73% prevalence in one FASD cohort) and a spectrum of cognitive impairments under the rubric of alcohol-related neurodevelopmental deficit, which include learning disabilities, self-injury, anger and impulse control problems (Manning & Eugene Hoyme, 2007). Delays in early literacy skills have also been associated with FASD. Attempts have been made to use intensive classroom interventions to improve deficits in reading and computational skills, though their effectiveness is unclear given the diversity in the neurobehavioral phenotypes of FASD (Adnams et al., 2007). Specific brain regions appear to be more vulnerable to alcohol exposure, with neuroimaging of FASD children showing a narrowing in the parietal region, decreased growth of the frontal lobe, and deficits in cerebellar vermis, corpus callosum, and caudate nucleus (Spadoni, McGeer, Fryer,

& Riley, 2007). Imaging studies have not yet correlated sex of the fetus with nature or severity of any specific abnormality (Bookstein et al., 2007).

Prenatal alcohol exposure may also be a risk factor for psychiatric disorders in young adulthood and beyond, including substance use disorders (SUDs) and other Axes I and II psychopathologies. One longitudinal study attempting to establish this link through 21-year follow-up (n = 500) found that binge drinking during pregnancy carried increased risk for problem drinking at age 21, even after controlling for ongoing environmental factors and family history (Barr et al., 2006). The interaction of parental psychiatric illness, maternal alcohol consumption during pregnancy, and genetic risk and environmental factors as contributors to psychiatric disorders among offspring continues to be investigated, with one adoption study (n = 95) describing different genetic pathways for increased risk of alcohol abuse by offspring (Cadoret, Yates, Troughton, Woodworth, & Stewart, 1995); another finding genetic alcohol diathesis (with maternal alcohol consumption) predictive of mood disorders (n = 197) (Cadoret et al., 1996); and a third attributing conduct and behavioral disorders in adolescence to prenatal alcohol exposure (Langbehn & Cadoret, 2001).

Identification of Prenatal Alcohol Use

Screening represents the first step of primary and secondary prevention. Screening alone has been associated with reduced alcohol intake among pregnant women (Bradley, Boyd-Wickizer, Powell, & Burman, 1998). Specific considerations about screening may be gleaned from guidelines on problem drinking for women of reproductive age released by the American College of Obstetrics and Gynecology (ACOG) in 2006 (Sokol, Floyd, Dang, & Ceperich, 2006). "Problem drinking" for reproductive-age women who are not pregnant is defined by the National Institute on Alcohol Abuse and Alcoholism (NIAAA) as greater than seven drinks per week and greater than three drinks at any one sitting (Saunders, Aasland, Babor, de al Fuente, & Grant, 1993). Many women meeting these criteria for problem drinking may fail to recognize themselves as being "at risk" because of the absence of appreciable negative consequences. Targeting at-risk women for interventions such as education and referral has been identified as a priority for the prevention of FASD. The T-ACE and the TWEAK (tolerance, worried, eye-opener, amnesia/black-outs, cut-down) have been shown to have greater sensitivity than the CAGE or MAST among pregnant women and may be useful screening tools (Chang, Wilkins-Haug, & Berman, 1999).

Treatment of Alcohol Use

Treatment interventions can be classified into the following types: (1) primary care clinician counseling of reproductive-age women who meet criteria for problem drinking; (2) brief interventions delivered by primary care doctors, obstetricians, gynecologists, or other health professionals for pregnant women who are at risk but not dependent; (3) detoxification and referral services for pregnant women with alcohol dependence; and (4) follow-up services for women known to have consumed alcohol during pregnancy.

Brief interventions have been studied among pregnant women who drink to excess but who may not be alcohol dependent. For example, one study found that a brief motivational intervention in a community sample (n = 800) involving five sessions (four using motivational interviewing to determine stage of change; the fifth dealing with contraception and basic prenatal care) reduced the risk of alcohol use during pregnancy by twofold (Floyd et al., 2007). Delivery of another intervention (involving manualized motivational interviewing) by a nutritionist over a few sessions appeared to decrease alcohol consumption by fivefold in another cohort of women (n = 255) (O'Connor & Whaley, 2006).

For pregnant woman who are physiologically dependent, specialized inpatient detoxification treatment is required. Because the rate of benzodiazepine elimination may be faster in pregnancy, a tailored short-acting benzodiazepine protocol, often dosed hourly, may be useful. Referral to detoxification services should be accompanied by ongoing, coordinated follow-up by the primary care physician, obstetrician, and addictions specialist. Concurrent participation in Alcoholics Anonymous meetings, specialized support groups for pregnant women attempting medically monitored sobriety, and individualized social work services are recommended for pregnant women undergoing alcohol treatment to ensure that, in the immediate postpartum and longer-term period after delivery, the patient will have the support required to maintain sobriety and to care for a child who may have special needs. With close clinical supervision, psychopharmacological treatments (e.g., acamprosate, naltrexone, disulfiram) may play a role in helping women maintain sobriety; however, at the current time, none of these, nor any other psychopharmacological treatment for alcohol, is Federal Drug Administration (FDA)-approved for use in pregnant or breastfeeding women (Lamberg, 2005).

NICOTINE USE IN PREGNANCY

Epidemiology

Nicotine is one of the most commonly used substances by pregnant women. Annually, an estimated 2 million infants are thought to be exposed to cigarette smoke *in utero* (Orleans, Barker, Kaufman, & Marx, 2000). In the past few decades, however, the rate of cigarette smoking has declined among pregnant women. Data from the 2006 National Survey on Drug Use and Health (NSDUH; n = 35,000) found that cigarette smoking among pregnant women ages 15–44 in the 1 month preceding data collection was 16.5%, significantly lower than for women who were not pregnant (29%). For pregnant adolescents, this does not hold: for females ages 15–17, rates of cigarette smoking are higher for pregnant (23%) than for nonpregnant females (17%) (SAMHSA, 2007).

Risk factors for nicotine use during pregnancy include partner and family nicotine use, living alone (Mueller, Munk, & Thomsen, 2007), high caffeine consumption (Spinillo et al., 1994; Strinic, Bukovic, & Sumilin, 2005), use of any illicit substances (Phares et al., 2004), and an unplanned pregnancy (Than, Honein, & Watkins, 2005). Women with occupations where alcohol is served or where secondhand smoke is routine in the workplace (e.g., bars or nightclubs) are also more likely to smoke cigarettes during pregnancy (Mueller et al., 2007). Furthermore, an estimated 45% of women who use nicotine during pregnancy meet criteria for at least one psychiatric disorder, such as an anxiety disorder, bipolar I disorder, oppositional defiant disorder, or ADHD (Flick et al., 2006; Goodwin, Keyes, & Simuro, 2007). Significant comorbidities of cigarette smoking during pregnancy include binge drinking and depressive symptoms (Blalock, Robinson, Wetter, & Cinciripini, 2006).

Consequences of Prenatal Exposure to Nicotine

Pregnancy complications associated with nicotine use that have been studied, to date include pregnancy-induced hypertension or pre-eclampsia (for which there have been ambiguous findings and no clear establishment of causality by smoking); arterial thrombotic events, including cerebrovascular accidents (CVAs), particularly in women with antiphospholipid antibody syndrome who smoke during pregnancy or who were taking oral contraceptives prior to conceiving; acute myocardial infarction in pregnancy, a rare event (1 in 35,000) mediated by coronary vasospasm in connection with smoking; and placental abruption (James, Jamison, & Biswas, 2006; Salihu & Wilson, 2007; Walker, 2003; Yang et al., 2006). Another possible pregnancy-related complication of smoking cigarettes is induction of vitamin and mineral deficiencies (i.e., vitamin A and zinc) that are thought to be caused by antioxidant depletion. (Bolisetty, Naidoo, & Lui, 2002).

In general, cigarette smoking has been thought to interfere with maternal–fetal circulation during pregnancy, increasing vascular resistance on the fetal side and thereby inducing fetal hypoxia (Cnattingius & Nordstrom, 1996). Among those women with pre-eclampsia from any cause, smoking during pregnancy may disrupt maternal–fetal circulation and cause poorer neonatal outcomes. For example, one study among African American women at a university hospital demonstrated higher rates of low birth weight and placental abruption among women with pre-eclampsia who smoked (n = 1,862) as compared to the nonsmoking group (n = 16,508) (Newman, Lindsay, & Graves, 2001). In a meta-analysis of outcomes among 1,358,083 pregnant women, maternal cigarette smoking was associated with up to a 90% increase in placental abruption, across both case–control and prospective studies (Ananth, Smulian, & Vintzileos, 1999). Finally, a prospective cohort study of 30,681 pregnant women who smoked found a twofold increase in rate of placental abruption as compared to matched nonsmokers, with the risk of abruption rising in a dose-dependent manner with cigarette exposure, and each pack of cigarettes smoked per day increasing the risk of abruption by 40% (Raymond & Mills, 1993). A higher fetal mortality rate with abruption occurred among pregnant women who smoked at least one pack per day.

Neonatal complications of nicotine exposure reported in the literature include low birth weight (with attendant increased risks for cardiovascular disease in later life); prematurity; intrauterine growth restriction (IUGR); and increased congenital malformations, such as polydactyly, syndactyly, cleft palate, hypospadias, cryptorchidism, gastroschisis, and craniosyntosis (Alderman, Bradley, Greene, Fernbach, & Barón, 1994; Andres & Day, 2000; Berghella, 2007; Carmichael, Shaw, & Laurent, 2005; Hampton, 2006; Jensen, Toft, Thulstrup, Bonder, & Olsen, 2007; Meyer, Williams, Hernandez-Diaz, & Cnattingius, 2004; Raatkainen, Huurinainen, & Heinonen, 2000; Torfs, Christianson, & Iovannisci, 2006). Other complications include decreased neonatal respiratory function (as well as increased risk of pulmonary hypertension from disruption of fetal circulation); sudden infant death syndrome (SIDS); dysregulated immunity and increased infections; and dysregulation of fetal hypothalamic–pituitary–adrenal axis (HPA) with increased adrenocorticotropin hormone (ACTH) and circulating cortisol reflective of abnormal stress physiology (McDonald et al., 2006; Shah, Sullivan, & Carter, 2006; Van Marter, Leviton, & Allred, 1996). Nicotine withdrawal has also been observed in the neonatal period. The metabolite cotinine in cord blood has been correlated with reduced neurological scores and increased Finnegan scale withdrawal ratings (Godding, Bonnier, & Fiasse, 2006). In addition, maternal cigarette smoking has been linked to longer length of stay in neonatal intensive care (NICU) in a dose-dependent manner (by number of cigarettes smoked per day) while controlling for other substance exposures (Miles, Lanni, Jansson, & Svikis, 2006).

Longer-term consequences of prenatal exposure to nicotine may include cognitive and language deficits, particularly during the first 4 years of life, with at least a mild to moderate effect remaining after controlling for maternal education and other environmental factors; and increased prevalence of smoking as adults (Batty, Der, & Deary, 2006; Buka, Shenassa, & Niaura, 2006). The cognitive deficits, which include deficits in verbal learning, appear to persist with time and also to have a dose–response relationship with amount of nicotine used (Mortensen, Michaelsen, Sanders, & Reinisch, 2005).

Identification of Prenatal Cigarette Smoking

Approximately 25% women who smoke cigarettes in the United States attempt to quit smoking upon learning that they are pregnant (Orleans, Barker, Kaufman, & Marx, 2000). It appears that a significant proportion (10–25%) of women who stop smoking during pregnancy do so early on and without formal intervention (Ershoff, Quinn, & Mullen, 1995). Although as many as 33% of these women relapse sometime before delivery, one large study found that up to 96% of women maintained smoking cessation in the final 3 months of pregnancy (Suellentrop, Morrow, Williams, D'Angelo, & CDC, 2006). Thus the desire to quit has been observed among many pregnant women at multiple points in pregnancy, and having a nonsmoking partner appears to increase the likelihood of reaching abstinence (Ockene, Ma, & Zapka, 2002).

Clinical history is the mainstay for detection of smoking during pregnancy; in addition, the Fagerstrom test for nicotine dependence can be useful. The Fagerstrom test is a six-item questionnaire that evaluates the intensity of physical dependence on nicotine. Questions, such as, "How soon after you wake up do you smoke your first cigarette?" and "Do you still smoke if you are so sick that you are in bed or are having trouble breathing?," help clinicians and patients determine the extent of the intervention that will be required (Rustin, 2000). Other useful screening methods may include assays for the nicotine metabolite cotinine, which may be present in maternal urine for up to 30 days (Chan, Caprara, Blanchette, Klein, & Koren, 2004).

Treatment of Cigarette Smoking

Interventions for cigarette smoking cessation include both pharmacological and nonpharmacological approaches. Bupropion has been shown to have efficacy in pregnant women who smoke (n = 10), without demonstrated teratogenic effects during the first trimester (Chan, Einarson, & Koren, 2005). In one open-label, randomized trial in which pregnant women were offered the choice between gum, patch, or lozenges, although the combination of nicotine replacement therapy with cognitive-behavioral therapy did increase abstinence rates, the study was suspended because nicotine replacement therapy appeared to carry a 20% greater risk of negative birth outcomes such as preterm birth, NICU admissions, small-for-gestational-age birth, placenta abruption, and fetal demise (Pollak, Oncken, & Lipkus, 2007). Therefore, clinicians are advised to have risk–benefit discussions with the patient before initiating nicotine replacement therapy, to consider bupropion as an alternative, and to prioritize the use of psychosocial or behavioral interventions, as described below.

Behavioral interventions for smoking cessation in pregnancy have shown promising results. Setting quit dates and being contacted by phone by a midwife at multiple points during pregnancy produce quit rates of over 30%, as verified by breath carbon monoxide tests (Hajek, West, & Lee, 2001). Interventions promoting life skills (such as stress management and assertiveness) and self-efficacy in quitting also appear to have an impact on cessation (Kilby, 1998). Nontraditional therapies are still being investigated, with one randomized trial of hypnosis (n = 158) achieving a 43% quit rate (compared with a 31% quit rate for the pregnant women in the control group who smoked and received cessation counseling only) (Valbo & Eide, 1996).

MARIJUANA USE IN PREGNANCY

Epidemiology

Marijuana is thought to be the most commonly used illicit drug in both the general population and among pregnant women. In one public hospital cross-sectional study (n = 1,000) using hair analysis, a 4% rate of marijuana use in the third trimester among pregnant adolescents was detected (Mitsuhiro, Chalem, Barros, Guinsburg, & Laranjeira, 2007). However, data from the 2001 multisite Maternal Lifestyle Study (MLS; n = 8,527) using meconium testing found a marijuana prenatal exposure rate of 11.1% (Lester et al., 2001; SAMHSA, 2007). Marijuana and other cannabis formulations have been also used by women outside of hospital settings for normal nausea and vomiting in pregnancy, as well as for hyperemesis gravidarum, despite the potential toxic exposure of pesticides and possible teratogenic effects of cannabis (Westfall, Janssen, & Lucas, 2006).

Consequences of Prenatal Exposure to Marijuana

Data on pregnancy-related complications of marijuana use are limited. However, its psychoactive component, exocannabinoid delta-9-tetrahydrocannabinol (THC), is hypothesized to have negative effects on ovulation, spermatogenesis, implantation, and duration of pregnancy. (Taylor, Ang, & Bell, 2007). In contrast, complications for the neonate and child have been more extensively characterized (see Table 26.1). Findings in the neonate include increased jitteriness (possibly as part of a withdrawal syndrome of autonomic disruption); a twofold risk of ventricular septal defect; higher pitched infant cry; possible decreases in birth weight and length via intrauterine growth retardation; and increases in the incidence of malignancies ranging from acute myeloblastic leukemia (AML) to rhabdomyosarcoma (Parker et al., 1990; Wilson, Loffredo, Correa-Villasenor, & Ferencz, 1998).

Longer-term effects of maternal marijuana use have also been investigated, with a particular emphasis on cognitive and motor development. Marijuana exposure during lactation (as measured by positive urine screens) was associated with decreased motor development measured at age 1 in a cohort study (n = 68) (Astley & Little, 1990). In addition, at 3-year follow-up in the National Maternal and Infant Health Survey (n = 13,417), increased fearfulness and shorter length of play were related to prenatal marijuana exposure (Faden & Graubard, 2000). Depressive symptoms in early adolescence, as well as disturbed nocturnal sleep in early childhood, may also be long-term sequelae of prenatal marijuana exposure (Dahl, Scher, Williamson, Robles, & Day, 1995; Grey, Day, & Leech, 2005).

Identification of Prenatal Marijuana Use

Urine toxicology and clinical history are used to screen for marijuana use during pregnancy. Injected sclerae, dilated pupils, or inappropriate laughter or apathy may be warning signs of marijuana use. Consent is required for urine testing but may be routinely included in a discussion of medically indicated tests for baseline and serial prenatal assessments. The primary metabolite detectable in urine for up to 30 days after initial use is 9-carboxy-THC. In obtaining the clinical history for marijuana use during pregnancy, standardized instruments such as the Severity of Dependence Scale (SDS), which consists of five questions focusing on the impact of continued use despite occupational and social dysfunction, may be helpful as a starting point (Gossop et al., 1995).

Treatment of Marijuana Use

General interventions for substance treatment and outreach, rather than specific marijuana cessation programs, have been studied among pregnant women. Targeted interventions have taken the form of public service announcements as well as written brochures created by the American Pregnancy Association, ACOG, and pharmaceutical companies promoting prenatal care and safety (American Pregnancy Association, 2000). The impact of such interventions remains to be studied further, though analogous programs relying primarily on written brochures for cigarette smoking cessation have not been proven effective (Acharya, Jauniaux, & Sathia, 2002).

OPIOID USE IN PREGNANCY

Epidemiology

It is estimated that approximately 7,000 births of babies exposed to opiates occur annually in the United States (Luty, Nikolau, & Beam, 2003). The most common opioids abused during pregnancy include heroin and fentanyl (Little et al., 1990). The use of prescription opioids as illicit drugs may also be masked by peripartum analgesics, making detection challenging, despite the need for maintenance in pregnancy and monitoring after delivery to manage neonatal abstinence syndrome from oxycodone and fentanyl abuse (Ludlow, Christmas, Paech, & Orr, 2007). Prescription opioid use may also be commonly accompanied by benzodiazepine use, with implications for detoxification protocol as well as a wider range of teratogenic effects attributable to both illicit substances (Sander & Hays, 2005).

Consequences of Prenatal Exposure to Opioids

Opioid use carries serious consequences for both maternal and fetal physiology (see Table 26.1). Although the exact prevalence of opioid overdose in pregnancy is unknown, the same signs and symptoms (e.g., coma, circulatory collapse, pinpoint pupils, bradycardia, hypothermia, and severe respiratory depression) are present for opioid overdose in nonpregnant women and carry risks for both mother and fetus; cautious use of naloxone for reversal without causing withdrawal is the treatment of choice (Center for Substance Abuse Treatment, 2005; LoVecchio, Pizon, Riley, Sami, & D'Incognito, 2007). Early signs of pregnancy, such as fatigue or abdominal discomfort, may be mistaken for opioid withdrawal and may lead women to initially increase their use (Center for Substance Abuse Treatment, 2005). Opioid exposure during pregnancy (including methadone exposure) may reduce fetal heart rate, meriting regular monitoring at serial follow-up visits, along with initial screening tests for hepatitis serologies, human immunodeficiency virus (HIV), and toxicology, along with other routine chemistries (Navaneethakrishnan, Tutty, Sinha, & Lindow, 2006).

Long-term effects of prenatal opiate exposure on the fetus have not been extensively characterized. However, the comorbidities associated with the relatively high-risk and low-prevalence behavior of injection opiate use during pregnancy have both short-term and long-term effects on the fetus. These include *in utero* exposure to HIV, hepatitis B and C, and bacterial endocarditis. During pregnancy bacterial endocarditis can carry up to a 30% fetal mortality rate (and similar rates of maternal mortality) (Montoya, Karnath, & Ahmad, 2003). Hepatitis carries up to a 75% maternal–fetal transmission among women with active infection, and infection rates among pregnant women who use opioid have been estimated at 41% in one recent hospital-based study ($n = 108$) (Fajemirokun-Odudeyi et al., 2006). HIV prevalence among pregnant women who inject opioids was 59% in one study, with HIV prevalence among individuals who inject drugs, in general, more recently estimated at 13–15% (DesJarlais et al., 2007; European Collaborative Study, 2001).

Opioid withdrawal may be difficult to distinguish from other more commonly observed syndromes, such as upper respiratory infections. Opioids have a rapid transplacental passage (less than 60 minutes), and withdrawal is likely to begin 6–48 hours after last usage

(Farrell, 1994). The maternal opioid withdrawal syndrome is characterized by influenza-like symptoms (e.g., myalgias) and signs (e.g., rhinorrhea and lacrimation), as well as anorexia, which can result in impaired fetal growth (Little et al., 1990). The stress state that characterizes withdrawal may also have a negative impact on the fetus; some studies show increased epinephrine in amniotic fluid (Zuspan, Gumpel, Mejia-Zelaya, Madden, & Davis, 1975).

Neonatal abstinence syndrome (NAS) from opioids has been well characterized. NAS involves wakefulness, irritability, tremulousness, temperature dysregulation, as well as disorganized suck, failure to thrive, and, more rarely, seizures (Kuschel, 2007). Enduring for up to 10 weeks following delivery, NAS may require management in an intensive care unit (Ebner et al., 2007). The incidence of NAS among opioid-exposed neonates may be as high as 90%, though not all of these infants will require pharmacological treatment. Treatment is most often with tincture of opium, available as "Neonatal Opiate Solution" (Burns & Mattick, 2007; Rementeria & Nunag, 1973). Naloxone may also play a role in the treatment of NAS-related respiratory depression (McGuire & Fowlie, 2003). Measuring the level of methadone in neonatal cord blood may also assist in identifying the most severe cases and initial dosing of treatment (Kuschel, Austerberry, Cornwell, Couch, & Rowley, 2004). One study found that only half of 27 hospitals surveyed used standardized procedures for evaluation and treatment and guidelines for maternal toxicology screening, determination of length-of-stay criteria, and infant monitoring based on established safe protocols such as the Neonatal Abstinence Syndrome Scale (Crocetti, Amin, & Jansson, 2007).

Identification of Prenatal Opioid Use

Confirmation of opioid use during pregnancy relies on urine toxicology screening. After findings on the physical examination (such as track marks) or patient self-report, urine screening is efficient and often the most rapid tool available. Methadone can be detected in the urine up to 2 weeks after use, although a specific "drugs of abuse" urine toxicology may be required that is not available at all facilities. Heroin remains detectable in the urine for up to 72 hours after use. Fentanyl, like methadone, may not be revealed in conventional urine toxicology screens and may require a specific screening request (Haley, Roy, Leclerc, Boudreau, & Boivin, 2004). Neonatal meconium, while shown to have equivalent or greater sensitivity for maternal opioid use compared with urine toxicology, is not yet widely available and represents screening at a later stage during pregnancy. For screening in the office, the Drug Abuse Screen Test (DAST) can be useful (Luty et al., 2003).

Treatment of Opioid Use

Since the early 1970s, the standard of care for management of prenatal opiate use has been methadone maintenance (Wang, 1999). A still-investigational alternative involves the use of buprenorphine or naltrexone, as is described below. A third treatment option is opioid detoxification (particularly during the second trimester), which is not currently recognized as standard care (Luty et al., 2003).

The metabolism of methadone is increased during pregnancy via the effect of increased progesterone on liver cytochrome P450 enzymes. In addition to the decreased plasma protein-binding of methadone, increased metabolism results in a shortened half-life of methadone during the third trimester in particular (somewhat less than the standard 24- to 36-hour half-life of the drug) (Burns, Mattick, Lim, & Wallace, 2007; Wolff, Boys, Rostami-Hodjegan, Hay, & Raistrick, 2005). Hence, pregnant women may report withdrawal symptoms on their maintenance dose, thereby requiring dosage adjustment.

To begin the maintenance regimen, patients already on outpatient methadone maintenance should be continued on their outpatient dose (after it has been verified, preferably via a written record, with their outpatient provider or licensed clinic). Women who use heroin, fentanyl, or codeine should be converted to using methadone during pregnancy so that there will be fewer withdrawal cycles, fewer spontaneous abortions associated with oral substitution than with injection drug use, and a reduced risk of infectious diseases, compared with intravenous usage (Kashiwagi et al., 2005). In making the conversion to methadone, the starting dose often ranges from 1 mg to 20 mg (Hulse, Milne, English, & Holman, 1998). Patients are then dosed on an as-needed basis for signs and symptoms of opiate withdrawal (including subjective cravings) every 6 hours, with most patients reaching a stable dose after 48–72 hours (McCarthy, Leamon, Stenson, & Biles, 2007).

Potential cultural and psychological barriers to methadone treatment should be addressed. Women in early recovery may be resistant to being "on drugs" again. Incarcerated pregnant women may have difficulties gaining access to the medication or be the target of disapproval from prison authorities for receiving it under federal mandate (Rich et al., 2005). Discussion of taboos against methadone should be balanced with a fact-based discussion of benefits of avoiding withdrawal in pregnancy versus the risk of methadone-induced cardiac arrhythmias (such as torsades de pointes, which, if unchecked, may lead to ventricular fibrillation and cardiac arrest) in pregnant women and possible induction of fetal arrhythmias by methadone exposure (which has been reported in case reports among methadone-exposed neonates) (Hunt, Lipton, Goldsmith, Strug, & Spunt, 1985; Hussain & Ewer, 2007).

It is unclear whether specialized multiservice programs for pregnant women, versus receiving methadone from an outpatient methadone clinic, carry greater physiological, psychosocial, and medical benefits. An early study ($n = 6$) by Chang and colleagues showed that enhanced prenatal care and comprehensive services may achieve better neonatal outcomes (measured by birth weight and decreased rates of prematurity) than traditional methadone programs, despite equivalent dose ranges for maintenance (Chang, Carroll, Behr, & Kosten, 1992). This finding has been duplicated in a recent prospective multicenter study ($n = 259$) in France (Lejeune, Simmat-Durand, & Gourier, 2006). There is also some debate about whether higher or lower doses at delivery are of particular benefit. Lower doses are associated with less neonatal withdrawal, but higher doses during the pregnancy and at delivery are associated with better patient compliance, reduced relapse risk, and higher neonatal birth weights (McCarthy, Leamon, Parr, & Anania, 2005). Split-dosing trials (in which the total daily dose is given in two parts) of methadone have also been associated with preliminary favorable results and may also reduce concomitant cocaine cravings for women who use several substances (DePetrillo & Rice, 1995). Analgesia during delivery for women maintained on methadone may also require adaptation, with one clinical trial showing a 70% increase in opiate analgesic dose for cesarean deliveries among this group (Meyer, Wagner, Benvenuto, Plante, & Howard, 2007).

As an alternative to methadone during pregnancy, buprenorphine has been validated by several naturalistic studies in France, where outpatient physicians can use buprenorphine without specialized training, so that up to 70,000 patients annually receive the medication on an outpatient basis (Lacroix et al., 2004). Though several French and some American studies have reported that buprenorphine, when started in the second trimester of pregnancy, is safe and well tolerated (Auriacombe et al., 1999), greater severity of the NAS and higher rates of SIDs have been described in one prospective study ($n = 67$) (Kahila, Saisto, Kivitie-Kallio, Haukkamaa, & Halmesmäki, 2007).

Naltrexone may also play a role in relapse prevention, and has been used for maintenance after initial taper with buprenorphine. In one Australian pilot study ($n = 8$), naltrexone was used for detoxification in pregnancy with the positive outcome measure of abstinence from heroin throughout the pregnancy; subjects reported a preference for the implant rather than daily dosing (Hulse & O'Neill, 2004). However, the use of an opiate antagonist during pregnancy is not yet FDA approved.

Opioid detoxification is typically avoided in the first trimester due to an association of spontaneous abortion with withdrawal (Luty et al., 2003). Major drawbacks of this approach (which make it unlikely to attain status of standard of care) include high risk of relapse and the complications of opioid withdrawal in pregnancy, as detailed above.

Studies are underway on achieving harm reduction, in conjunction with methadone maintenance, among pregnant women who are using opioids. Cognitive-behavioral therapy, for example, has been found to reduce HIV risk behaviors in this population, including decreased use of contaminated needles for injection drug use and greater participation in needle exchange programs (O'Neill, Baker, Cooke, Haukkamaa, & Halmesmäki, 1996).

COCAINE USE IN PREGNANCY

Epidemiology

Data from the 1996–1998 National Household Survey on Drug Abuse found that, among pregnant women (n = 1,249), 10% of those who used illicit drugs also used cocaine (Ebrahim & Gfroerer). Other studies, such as a multisite study of university hospitals, have found prevalence to be as high as 10% in a general antenatal population (n = 1,185 pregnant women using cocaine, out of a total participating 11,181); most authors describe higher prevalence in urban versus rural areas (Bauer et al., 2002).

Consequences of Prenatal Exposure to Cocaine

Placental abruption, caused by vasospasm and hypoxia to the placental bed, is a well-established effect of cocaine use during pregnancy (see Table 26.1) (Little et al., 1990). It is typically associated with cocaine bingeing as opposed to sporadic cocaine use (Burkett, Yasin, Palow, LaVoie, & Martinez, 1995). Premature rupture of membranes, preterm labor, preterm delivery, and maternal seizures are also possible side effects of maternal cocaine use (Plessinger & Woods, 1998).

Migraine headaches, which may become more prevalent during pregnancy due to increased production of estrogen, are more common among those who use cocaine, further contributing to the irritability that may characterize intermittent withdrawal (Dhopesh, Maany, & Herrig, 1991). Among pregnant women who use cocaine, both hemorrhagic and ischemic CVAs may occur as a result of cocaine-induced hypertension. Dyspnea during pregnancy, which is due to a decreased tidal volume from the compression of the lower lung fields by the expanding uterus, may be indicative of "crack lung" or pneumonitis in a woman who uses cocaine—characterized by fevers, pulmonary infiltrates, and leukocytosis. Pneumonitis is treated with oral steroids but can be severe enough to cause acute respiratory failure and make patients ventilator dependent (O'Donnell, Mappin, Sebo, & Tazelaar, 1991). Hyperthermia mediated by vasoconstriction and/or the hypermetabolic state of cocaine use may also be observed and should be considered during pregnancy as an effect that might counteract the expected physiological vasodilation (and normal lowering of blood pressure seen in pregnancy) from increased levels of progesterone. Cocaine-induced hyperthermia may also cause an altered mental status, including an excited delirium and other cocaine-induced states of delirium resulting from cardiac or respiratory failure, stroke, the intoxication syndrome, or infections more common among pregnant women who use cocaine (including endocarditis, sepsis, and hepatitis for those who inject crack cocaine, as for those who inject opioid) (Blaho, Winbery, & Park, 2000). Cocaine-induced psychosis or delirium should be managed with intensive care that includes cardiac monitoring; unopposed beta blockade should be avoided for the risk of exacerbating hypertension, and the use of antipsychotics, while often warranted for an excited delirium with risks of injury or death, should be measured carefully against the risk of neuroleptic malignant syndrome (which may be increased among those who use cocaine) (Akpaffiong & Ruiz, 1991; Kuczowski, 2005).

In addition to jeopardizing the fetal–placental circulation, cocaine may cause longer-term complications for the fetus, the neonate, and the developing child. There is an increased risk of infection with HIV and other infectious agents via vertical transmission from mother to fetus, due to cocaine-induced vasculopathy (Storen, Wijdicks, Crum, & Schultz, 2000).

Identification of Prenatal Cocaine Use

Urine toxicology is used for screening and detects the metabolite benzoylecogine up to 72 hours after use (Cone & Dickerson, 1992). Some authors have noted that metabolites may show up in urine as long as 2 weeks after use, depending on the screening sensitivity (Osterloh & Lee, 1989). Benzoylecogine can also be detected in a serum toxicology screen for up to 8 hours after cocaine use (Kraemer & Paul, 2007).

Treatment of Cocaine Use

The syndrome of cocaine withdrawal is not life-threatening for the mother or for the fetus, and the associated mood symptoms (and potential effect on noncompliance) may be treated with a variety of medications, among them serotonin selective reuptake inhibitors (SSRIs), methylphenidate, atypical antipsychotics, and tricyclic antidepressants for depression and irritability (Gardner & Kosten, 2007). Standard care does not currently include the use of anti-craving medications for pregnant women, though several agents that are FDA-approved for other uses (e.g., disulfiram, modafinil, propanolol, topiramate, pramipexole, and vigabatrin) have been shown to reduce cocaine cravings among study subjects who were not pregnant (Kampman, 2005). Of these, all are designated as "Category C" (i.e., not established as safe in pregnancy through human randomized clinical trials, but not contraindicated). Therefore, the risks and benefits must be weighed for each individual pregnant woman before treatment is initiated.

FUTURE DIRECTIONS

Clinical challenges yet to be addressed by services and other research include designing substance treatments that are tailored to pregnant women; integrating counseling about problem drinking into routine care for reproductive-age women to reduce the risk of exposure during pregnancy; and increasing access to and availability of pharmacological and psychosocial treatments for pregnant women who are substance using, abusing, or dependent. Further research should also address the needs of special populations, including treatment priorities for culturally diverse women who use substances during pregnancy, adolescents, women with posttraumatic stress disorder and other Axis I diagnoses, rural women, and women who are coping with intimate partner violence (Velez et al., 2006).

KEY POINTS

- During pregnancy, 15% of women use alcohol, 16–20% use nicotine, and 4% use illicit substances (e.g., marijuana, cocaine, opioids, amphetamines).
- The most commonly used substance of abuse during pregnancy is alcohol, and this is also the most well-established teratogen.
- Risk factors for substance use during pregnancy vary by substance but include preconception use of the substance, continued use by a partner, lack of social support, and unplanned pregnancy.
- Substance use screening early during pregnancy is critical.
- Currently, there are no FDA-approved psychopharmacological treatments for alcohol, nicotine, marijuana, or amphetamine dependence among pregnant women. Methadone maintenance is FDA approved for pregnant women who have opioid dependence.
- All women, and all pregnant women, should be routinely screened for intimate partner violence at primary care and prenatal visits, and the American College of Obstetrics and Gynecology also recommends screening all reproductive-age women for problem drinking well in advance of conception.

REFERENCES

Asterisks denote recommended readings.

Acharya, G., Jauniaux, E., & Sathia, L. (2002). Evaluation of the impact of current anti-smoking advice in the UK on women with planned pregnancies. *Journal of Obstetrics and Gynaecology*, 22(5), 498–500.

Adnams, C. M., Sorour, P., Kalberg, W. O., Kodituwakku, P., Perold, M. D., Kotze, A., et al. (2007). Language and literacy outcomes from a pilot intervention study for children with fetal alcohol spectrum disorders in South Africa. *Alcohol*, 41(6), 403–414.

Akpaffiong, M. J., & Ruiz, P. (1991). Neuroleptic malignant syndrome: A complication of neuroleptics and cocaine abuse. *Psychiatric Quarterly*, 62(4), 299–309.

Alderman, B. W., Bradley, C. M., Greene, C., Fernbach, S. K., & Barón, A. E. (1994). Increased risk of craniosynostosis with maternal cigarette smoking during pregnancy. *Teratology*, 50(1), 13–18.

American Pregnancy Association. (2000). *Using illegal street drugs during pregnancy*. Irving, TX: Author. Retrieved March 30, 2008, from *www.americanpregnancy.org/pregnancy health/illegaldrugs.html*.

Ananth, C. V., Smulian, J. C., & Vintzileos, A. M. (1999). Incidence of placental abruption in relation to cigarette smoking and hypertensive disorders during pregnancy: A meta-analysis of observational studies. *Obstetrics and Gynecology*, 93(4), 622–628.

Andres, R. L., & Day, M. C. (2000). Perinatal complications associated with maternal tobacco use. *Seminars in Neonatology*, 5(3), 231–241.

Astley, S. J., & Little, R. E. (1990). Maternal marijuana use during lactation and infant development at one year. *Neurotoxicology and Teratology*, 12(2), 161–168.

Auriacombe, M., Affelou, S., Lavignasse, P., Lafitte, C., Roux, D., Daulouède, J. P., et al. (1999). Pregnancy, abortion and delivery in a cohort of heroin dependent patients treated with drug substitution (methadone and buprenorphine) in Aquitaine. *Presse Medicale*, 28(4), 177.

Barr, H. M., Bookstein, F. L., O'Malley, K. D., Connor, P. D., Huggins, J. E., & Streissguth, A. P. (2006). Binge drinking during pregnancy as a predictor of psychiatric disorders on the Structured Clinical Interview for DSM-IV in young adult offspring. *American Journal of Psychiatry*, 163(6), 1061–1065. (*)

Batty, G. D., Der, G., & Deary, I. J. (2006). Effects of maternal smoking during pregnancy on offspring's cognitive ability: Empirical evidence for complete confounding in the U.S. national longitudinal survey of youth. *Pediatrics, 118*(3), 943–950.

Bauer, C. R., Shankaran, S., Bada, H. S., Lester, B., Wright, L. L., Krause-Steinrauf, H., et al. (2002). The Maternal Lifestyle Study: Drug exposure during pregnancy and short term maternal outcomes. *American Journal of Obstetrics and Gynecology, 186*(3), 487–495.

Berenson, A. B., Wilkinson, G. S., & Lopez, L. A. (1995). Substance use during pregnancy and peripartum complications in a triethnic population. *International Journal of the Addictions, 30*(2), 135–145.

Berghella, V. (2007). Prevention of recurrent fetal growth restriction. *Obstetrics and Gynecology, 110*(4), 904–912.

Blaho, K., Winbery, S., & Park, L. (2000). Cocaine metabolism in hyperthermic patients with excited delirium. *Journal of Clinical Forensic Medicine, 7*(2), 71–76.

Blalock, J. A., Robinson, J. D., Wetter, D. W., & Cinciripini, P. M. (2006). Relationship of DSM-IV-based depressive disorders to smoking cessation and smoking reduction in pregnant smokers. *American Journal on Addictions, 15*(4), 268–277.

Bolisetty, S., Naidoo, D., & Lui, K. (2002). Postnatal changes in maternal and neonatal plasma antioxidant vitamins and the influence of smoking. *Archives of Disease in Childhood: Fetal and Neonatal Edition, 86*(1), F36–40.

Bookstein, F. L., Connor, P. D., Huggins, J. E., Barr, H. M., Pimentel, K D., & Streissguth, A. P. (2007). Many infants prenatally exposed to high levels of alcohol show one particular anomaly of the corpus callosum. *Alcoholism: Clinical and Experimental Research, 31*(5), 868–879.

Bradley, K. A., Boyd-Wickizer, J., Powell, S. H., & Burman, M. L. (1998). Alcohol screening instruments in women: A critical review. *Journal of the American Medical Association, 280*(2), 166–171. (*)

Buka, S. L., Shenassa, E. D., & Niaura, R. (2003). Elevated risk of tobacco dependence among offspring of mothers who smoked during pregnancy: A 30-year prospective study. *American Journal of Psychiatry, 160*(11), 1978–1984. (*)

Burkett, G., Yasin, S. Y., Palow, D., LaVoie, L., & Martinez, M. (1995). Patterns of cocaine binging: Effect on pregnancy. *American Journal of Obstetrics and Gynecology, 172*(2), 372–378.

Burns, L., & Mattick, R. P. (2007). Using population data to examine the prevalence and correlates of neonatal abstinence syndrome. *Drug and Alcohol Review, 26*(5), 487–492.

Burns, L., Mattick, R. P., Lim, K., & Wallace, C. (2007). Methadone in pregnancy: Treatment retention and neonatal outcomes. *Addiction, 102*(2), 264–270. (*)

Cadoret, R. J., Winokur, G., Langbehn, D., Troughton, E., Yates, W. R., & Stewart, M. A. (1996). Depression spectrum disease: I. The role of gene–environment interaction. *American Journal of Psychiatry, 153*(7), 892–899.

Cadoret, R. J., Yates, W. R., Troughton, E., Woodworth, G., & Stewart, M. A. (1995). Adoption study demonstrating two genetic pathways to drug abuse. *Archives of General Psychiatry, 52*(1), 42–52.

Caetano, R., Ramisetty-Mikler, S., & Floyd, L. R. (2006). The epidemiology of drinking among women of child-bearing age. *Alcoholism: Clinical and Experimental Research, 30*(6), 1023–1030.

Calhoun, F., Attilia, M. L., Spagnolo, P. A., Rotondo, C., Mancinelli, R., & Ceccanti, M. (2006). National Institute on Alcohol Abuse and Alcoholism and the study of fetal alcohol spectrum disorders. *International Consortium [Annali dell'Instituto Superior di Sanita], 42*(1), 4–7.

Carmichael, S. L., Shaw, G. M., & Laurent, C. (2005) Hypospadias and maternal exposures to cigarette smoke. *Paediatric and Perinatal Epidemiology, 19*(6), 406–412.

Center for Substance Abuse Treatment. (2005). *Medication-assisted treatment for opioid addiction in pregnancy*. Treatment Improvement Protocol (TIP) Series 43. DHHS Publication No. (SMA) 05-4048. Rockville, MD: Substance Abuse and Mental Health Services Administration. 2005. Accessed March 30, 2008, *www.ncbi.nlm.nih.gov/books/bv.fcgi?rid=hstat5.section.83488*. (*)

Chan, B., Einarson, A., & Koren, G. (2005). Effectiveness of bupropion for smoking cessation during pregnancy. *Journal of Addictive Diseases, 24*(2), 19–23.

Chan, D., Caprara, D., Blanchette, P., Klein, J., & Koren, G. (2004). Recent developments in meconium and hair testing methods for the confirmation of gestational exposures to alcohol and tobacco smoke. *Clinical Biochemistry, 37*(6), 429–438.

Chang, G. (2001). Alcohol-screening instruments for pregnant women. *Alcohol Research and Health, 25*(3), 204–209.

Chang, G., Carroll, K. M., Behr, H. M., & Kosten, T. R. (1992). Improving treatment outcome in pregnant opiate-dependent women. *Journal of Substance Abuse Treatment, 9*(4), 327–330.

Chang, G., Wilkins-Haug, L., Berman, S., & Goetz, M. A. (1999). The TWEAK: Application in a prenatal setting. *Journal of Studies on Alcohol, 60*(3), 306–309.

Chudley, A. E., Kilgour, A. R., Cranston, M., & Edwards, M. (2007). Challenges of diagnosis in fetal alcohol syndrome and fetal alcohol spectrum disorder in the adult. *American Journal of Medical Genetics Part C: Seminars in Medical Genetics, 145*(3), 261–272.

Cnattingius, S., & Nordstrom, M. L. (1996). Maternal smoking and feto-infant mortality: Biological pathways and public health significance. *Acta Paediatrica, 85*(12), 1400–1402.

Cone, E. J., & Dickerson, S. L. (1992). Efficacy of urinalysis in monitoring heroin and cocaine abuse patterns: Implications in clinical trials for treatment of drug dependence. *NIDA Research Monograph, 128*, 46–58.

Crocetti, M. T., Amin, D. D., & Jansson, L. M. (2007). Variability in the evaluation and management of opiate-exposed newborns. *Clinical Pediatrics (Phila), 46*(7), 632–635.

Dahl, R. E., Scher, M. S., Williamson, D. E., Robles, N., & Day, N. (1995). A longitudinal study of prenatal marijuana use: Effects on sleep and arousal at age 3 years. *Archives of Pediatric and Adolescent Medicine, 149*(2), 145–150.

DePetrillo, P. B., & Rice, J. M. (1995). Methadone dosing and pregnancy: Impact on program compliance. *International Journal of the Addictions, 30*(2), 207–217.

DesJarlais, D. C., Arasteh, K., Perlis, T., Hagan, H., Abdul-Quader, A., Heckathorn, D. D., et al. (2007). Convergence of HIV seroprevalence among injecting and non-injecting drug users in New York City. *AIDS, 21*(2), 231–235.

Dhopesh, V., Maany, I., & Herrig, C. (1991). The relationship of cocaine to headache in polysubstance abusers. *Headach, 31*(1), 17–19.

Ebner, N., Rohrmeister, K., Winklbaur, B., Baewert, A., Jagsch, R., Peternell, A., et al. (2007). Management of neonatal abstinence syndrome in neonates born to opioid maintained women. *Drug and Alcohol Dependence, 87*(2–3), 131–138.

Ebrahim, S. H., & Gfroerer, J. (2003). Pregnancy-related substance use in the United States during 1996–1998. *Obstetrics and Gynecology, 101*(2), 374–379.

Emory Maternal Substance Abuse and Child Development Program. (2008). *Facts about drug use in pregnancy.* Retrieved March 31, 2008, from *www.psychiatry.emory.edu/PROGRAMS/GADrug/ Factsheets/Drugs%20Fact%20Sheet.pdf.*

Ershoff, D H., Quinn, V. P., & Mullen, P. D. (1995). Relapse prevention among women who stop smoking early in pregnancy: A randomized clinical trial of a self-help intervention. *American Journal of Preventive Medicine, 11*(3), 178–184.

European Collaborative Study. (2001). HIV-infected pregnant women and vertical transmission in Europe since 1986 European collaborative study. *AIDS, 15*(6), 761–770.

Faden, V. B., & Graubard, B. I. (2000). Maternal substance use during pregnancy and developmental outcome at age three. *Journal of Substance Abuse, 12*(4), 329–340.

Fajemirokun-Odudeyi, O., Sinha, C., Tutty, S., Pairaudeau, P., Armstrong, D., Phillips, T., et al. (2006). Pregnancy outcome in women who use opiates. *European Journal of Obstetrics, Gynecology, and Reproductive Biology, 126*(2), 170–175.

Farrell, M. (1994). Opiate withdrawal. *Addiction, 89*(11), 1471–1475.

Flick, L. H., Cook, C. A., Homan, S. M., McSweeney, M., Campbell, C., & Parnell, L. (2006). Persistent tobacco use during pregnancy and the likelihood of psychiatric disorders. *American Journal of Public Health, 96*(10), 1799–1807.

Floyd, R. L., Davis, M. K., Martin, M. L., Hungerford, D., & Hymbaugh, K. J. (1994). *From data to action: CDC's Public Health Surveillance for Women, Infants and Children.* Department of Health and Human Services: Centers for Disease Control and Prevention, Atlanta, GA. Retrieved March 29, 2008, from *www.cdc.gov/reproductivehealth/Products&Pubs/DatatoAction/pdf/Chlt8.pdf.*

Floyd, R. L., Sobell, M., Velasquez, M. M., Ingersoll, K., Nettleman, M., Sobell, L., et al. (2007). Project CHOICES Efficacy Study Group. *American Journal of Preventive Medicine, 32*(1), 1–10.

Gardner, T. J., & Kosten, T. R. (2007). Therapeutic options and challenges for substances of abuse. *Dialogues in Clinical Neuroscience, 9*(4), 431–445. (*)

Godding, V., Bonnier, C., & Fiasse, L. (2004). Does in utero exposure to heavy maternal smoking induce nicotine withdrawal symptoms in neonates? *Pediatric Research, 55*(4), 645–651.

Goodwin, R. D., Keyes, K., & Simuro, N. (2007). Mental disorders and nicotine dependence among pregnant women in the United States. *Obstetrics and Gynecology, 109*(4), 875–883. (*)

Gossop, M., Darke, S., Griffiths, P., Hando, J., Powis, B., Hall, W., et al. (1995). The Severity of Dependence Scale (SDS): Psychometric properties of the SDS in English and Australian samples of heroin, cocaine, and amphetamine users. *Addiction, 90*(5), 607–614.

Grey, K. A., Day, N. L., & Leech, S. (2005). Prenatal marijuana exposure: Effect on child depressive symptoms at ten years of age. *Neurotoxicology and Teratology, 27*(3), 439–448.

Hajek, P., West, R., & Lee, A. (2001). Randomized controlled trial of a midwife-delivered brief smoking cessation intervention in pregnancy. *Addiction, 96*(3), 485–494.

Haley, N., Roy, R., Leclerc, P., Boudreau, J. F., & Boivin, J. F. (2004). Characteristics of adolescent street youth with a history of pregnancy. *Journal of Pediatric and Adolescent Gynecology, 17*(5), 313–320. (*)

Hampton, T. (2006). Prenatal smoking linked to digit defects. *Journal of the American Medical Association, 295*(8), 879.

Hans, S. L. (1999). Demographic and social characteristics of substance-abusing pregnant women. *Clinical Perinatology, 26* (1), 55–74.

Hulse, G. K., Milne, E., English, D. R., & Holman, C. D. (1998). Assessing the relationship between maternal opiate use and neonatal mortality. *Addiction, 93*(10), 1553–1558.

Hulse, G. K., & O'Neill, G. (2002). Using naltrexone implants in the management of the pregnant heroin user. *Australia and New Zealand Journal of Obstetrics and Gynaecology, 42*(5), 569–573.

Hunt, D. E., Lipton, L. S., Goldsmith, D. S., Strug, D. L., & Spunt, B. (1985). It takes your heart: The image of methadone maintenance in the addict world and its effect on recruitment into treatment. *International Journal of the Addictions, 20*(11–12), 1751–1771.

Hussain, T., & Ewer, A. K. (2007). Maternal methadone may cause arrhythmias in neonates. *Acta Paediatrica, 96*(5), 768–769.

James, A. H., Jamison, M. G., & Biswas, M. S. (2006). Acute myocardial infarction in pregnancy: A United States population-based study. *Circulation, 113*(12), 1564–1571.

Jensen, M. S., Toft, G., Thulstrup, A. M., Bonde, J. P., & Olsen, J. (2007). Cryptorchidism according to maternal gestational smoking. *Epidemiology, 18*(2), 220–225.

Jones, K. L., & Smith, D. W. (1973). Recognition of the fetal alcohol syndrome in early infancy. *Lancet, 2*(7836), 999–1001. (*)

Kahila, H., Saisto, T., Kivitie-Kallio, S., Haukkamaa, M., & Halmesmäki, E. (2007). A prospective study on buprenorphine use during pregnancy: Effects on maternal and neonatal outcome. *Acta Obstetrica Gynecologica Scandinavic, 86*(2), 185–190. (*)

Kampman, K. M. (2005). Medications for cocaine abuse. *Psychiatric Times, 22*(2), 38–46.

Kashiwagi, M., Arlettaz, R., Lauper, U., Lauper, U., Zimmermann, R., & Hebisch, G. (2005). Methadone maintenance program in a Swiss perinatal center: Management and outcome of 89 pregnancies. *Acta Obstetetrica Gynecologica Scandinavica, 84*(2), 145–150.

Kilby, J. W. (1998). A smoking cessation plan for pregnant women. *Journal of Obstetric, Gynecologic, and Neonatal Nursing, 26*(4), 397–402.

Kraemer, T., & Paul, L. D. (2007). Bioanalytical procedures for determination of drugs of abuse in blood. *Analytical and Bioanalytical Chemistry, 388*(7), 1415–1435.

Kuczowski, K. M. (2005). Peripartum care of the cocaine-abusing parturient: Are we ready? *Acta Obstetrica Gynecologica Scandinavica, 84*(2), 108–116.

Kuschel, C. A. (2007). Managing drug withdrawal in the newborn infant. *Seminars on Fetal and Neonatal Medicine, 12*(2), 127–133. (*)

Kuschel, C. A., Austerberry, L., Cornwell, M., Couch, R., & Rowley, R. S. (2004). Can methadone concentrations predict the severity of withdrawal in infants at risk of neonatal abstinence syndrome? *Archives of Disease in Childhood: Fetal and Neonatal Edition, 89*(5), F390–F393.

Lacroix, I., Berrebi, A., Chaumerliac, C., Lapeyre-Mestre, M., Montastruc, J. L., & Damase-Michel, C. (2004). Buprenorphine in pregnant opioid-dependent women: First results of a prospective study. *Addiction, 99*(2), 209–214.

Lamberg, L. (2005). Risks and benefits key to psychotropic use during pregnancy and postpartum period. *Journal of the American Medical Association, 294*(13), 1604–1608. (*)

Langbehn, D. R., & Cadoret, R. J. (2001). The adult antisocial syndrome with and without antecedent conduct disorder: Comparisons from an adoption study. *Comprehensive Psychiatry, 42*(4), 272–282.

Lejeune, C., Simmat-Durand, L., Gourier, L., Aubisson, S., & Groupe d'Etudes Grossesse et Addictions (GEGA). (2006). Prospective multicenter observational study of 260 infants born to 259 opiate-dependent mothers on methadone or high-dose buprenorphine substitution. *Drug and Alcohol Dependence, 82*(3), 250–257.

Lester, B. M., ElSohly, M., Wright, L. L., Smeriglio, V. L., Verter, J., Bauer, C. R., et al. (2001). The Maternal Lifestyle Study: Drug use by meconium toxicology and maternal self-report. *Pediatrics, 107*(2), 309–317.

Little, B. B., Gilstrap, L. C., Cunningham, F. G., McDonald, P. C., & Gant, N. F. (1990). Social and illicit substance use during pregnancy. In Cunningham, McDonald, & Gant (Eds.), *Williams obstetrics* (18th ed.). Norwalk, CT: Appleton & Lange.

LoVecchio, F., Pizon, A., Riley, B., Sami, A., & D'Incognito, C. (2007). Onset of symptoms after methadone overdose. *American Journal of Emergency Medicine, 25*(1), 57–59.

Ludlow, J., Christmas, T., Paech, M. J., & Orr, B. (2007). Drug abuse and dependency during pregnancy: Anaesthetic issues. *Anaesthesia and Intensive Care, 35*(6), 881–893.

Luty, J., Nikolau, V., & Beam, J. (2003). Is opiate detoxification unsafe in pregnancy? *Journal of Substance Abuse Treatment, 24*(4), 363–367.

Manning, M. A., & Eugene Hoyme, H. (2007). Fetal alcohol spectrum disorders: A practical clinical approach to diagnosis. *Neuroscience and Biobehavioral Review, 31*(2), 230–238.

McCarthy, J. J., Leamon, H., Stenson, G., & Biles, L. A. (2008). Outcomes of neonates conceived on methadone maintenance therapy. *Journal of Substance Abuse Treatment, 35*(2), 202–206.

McCarthy, J. J., Leamon, M. H., Parr, M. S., & Anania, B. (2005). High-dose methadone maintenance in pregnancy: Maternal and neonatal outcomes. *American Journal of Obstetrics and Gynecology, 193*(3, Pt. 1), 606–610.

McDonald, S. D., Walker, M., Perkins, S. L., Beyene, J., Murphy, K., Gibb, W., et al. (2006). The effect of tobacco exposure on the fetal hypothalamic–pituitary–adrenal axis. *British Journal of Obstetrics and Gynecology, 113*(11), 1289–1295.

McGuire, W., & Fowlie, P. W. (2003). Naloxone for narcotic exposed newborn infants: Systematic review. *Archives of Disease in Childhood: Fetal and Neonatal Edition, 88*(4), F308–F311.

Mennella, J. A., Pepino, M. Y., & Teff, K. L. (2005). Acute alcohol consumption disrupts the hormonal milieu of lactating women. *Journal of Clinical Endocrinology and Metabolism, 90*(4), 1979–1985.

Meschke, L. C., Holl, J. A., & Messelt, S. (2003). Assessing the risk of fetal alcohol syndrome: Understanding substance use among pregnant women. *Neurotoxicology and Teratology, 25*(6), 667–674.

Meyer, K. A., Williams, P., Hernandez-Diaz, S., & Cnattingius, S. (2004). Smoking and the risk of oral clefts: Exploring the impact of study designs. *Epidemiology, 15*(6), 671–678.

Meyer, M., Wagner, K., Benvenuto, A., Plante, D., & Howard, D. (2007). Intrapartum and postpartum analgesia for women maintained on methadone during pregnancy. *Obstetrics and Gynecology, 110*(2, Pt.1), 261–266.

Miles, D. R., Lanni, S., Jansson, L., & Svikis, D. (2006). Smoking and illicit drug use during pregnancy: Impact on neonatal outcome. *Journal of Reproductive Medicine, 51*(7), 567–572.

Mitsuhiro, S. S., Chalem, E., Barros, M. C., Guinsburg, R., & Laranjeira, R. (2007). Prevalence of cocaine and marijuana use in the last trimester of adolescent pregnancy: Socio-demographic, psychosocial, and behavioral characteristics. *Addictive Behaviors, 32*(2), 392–397.

Montoya, M. E., Karnath, B. M., & Ahmad, M. (2003). Endocarditis during pregnancy. *Southern Medical Journal, 96*(11), 1156–1157.

Mortensen, E. L., Michaelsen, K. F., Sanders, S. A., & Reinisch, J. M. (2005). A dose–response relationship between maternal smoking during late pregnancy and adult intelligence in male offspring. *Paediatric and Perinatal Epidemiology, 19*(1), 4–11.

Mueller, L. L., Munk, C., & Thomsen, B. L. (2007). The influence of parity and smoking in the social environment on tobacco consumption among daily smoking women in Denmark. *European Addiction Research, 13*(3), 177–184.

Mulligan, C. J., Robin, R. W., Osier, M. V., Sambuughin, N., Goldfarb, L. G., Kittles, R. A., et al. (2003). Allelic variation at alcohol metabolism genes (ADH1B,ADH1C,ALDH2) and alcohol dependence in an American Indian population. *Human Genetics, 113*(4), 325–326.

Navaneethakrishnan, R., Tutty, S., Sinha, C., & Lindow, S. W. (2006). The effect of maternal methadone use on the fetal heart pattern: A computerized CTG analysis. *British Journal of Obstetrics and Gynecology, 113*(8), 948–950.

Newman, M. G., Lindsay, M. K., & Graves, W. (2001). Cigarette smoking and pre-eclampsia: Their association and effects on clinical outcomes. *Journal of Maternal and Fetal Medicine, 10*(3), 166–170.

Ockene, J., Ma, Y., & Zapka, J. (2002). Spontaneous cessation of smoking and alcohol use among low-income pregnant women. *American Journal of Preventive Medicine, 23*(3), 150–159.

O'Connor, M. J., & Whaley, S. E. (2006). Brief intervention for alcohol use by pregnant women. *American Journal of Public Health, 97*(2), 252–258.

O'Donnell, A. E., Mappin, F. G., Sebo, T. J., & Tazelaar, H. (1991). Interstitial pneumonitis associated with crack cocaine abuse. *Chest, 100*(4), 1155–1157.

Office of National Drug Policy. (2002). *The economic costs of drug abuse in the United States*. Washington, DC: Office of National Drug Policy. Retrieved March 30, 2008, from *www.whitehousedrugpolicy.gov/publications/economic_costs/e_summary.pdf*.

Oncken, C. A., & Kranzler, H. R. (2003). Pharmacotherapies to enhance smoking cessation during pregnancy. *Drug and Alcohol Reviews, 22*(2), 191–202.

O'Neill, K., Baker, A., Cooke, M., Haukkamaa, M., & Halmesmäki, E. (1996). Evaluation of a cognitive-behavioral intervention for pregnant injecting drug users at risk of HIV infection. *Addiction, 91*(8), 1115–1125. (*)

Orleans, C. T., Barker, D. C., Kaufman, N. J., & Marx, J. F. (2000). Helping pregnant smokers quit: Meeting the challenge in the next decade. *Tobacco Control, 174*(4), 276–281.

Osterloh, J. D., & Lee, B. L. (1989). Urine drug screening in mothers and newborns. *American Journal of Disease in Childhood, 143*(7), 791–793.

Parker, S., Zuckerman, B., Bauchner, H., Frank, D., Vinci, R., & Cabral, H. (1990). Jitteriness in full-term neonates: Prevalence and correlates. *Pediatrics, 85*(10), 17–23.

Phares, T. M., Morrow, B., Lansky, A., Barfield, W. D., Prince, C. B., & Marchi, K. S. (2004). Surveillance for disparities in maternal health related behaviors: Selected states. Pregnancy Risk Assessment Monitoring System (PRAMS), 2000–2001. *MMWR Surveillance Summary, 53*(4), 1–13. (*)

Plessinger, M. A., & Woods, J. R., Jr. (1998). Cocaine in pregnancy: Recent data on maternal and fetal risks. *Obstetric and Gynecology Clinics of North America, 25*(1), 99–118. (*)

Pollak, K. I., Oncken, C. A., & Lipkus, I. M. (2007). Nicotine replacement and behavioral therapy for smoking cessation in pregnancy. *American Journal of Preventive Medicine, 33*(4), 297–305. (*)

Raatkainen, K., Huurinainen, P., & Heinonen, S. (2007). Smoking in early gestation or through pregnancy: A decision crucial to pregnancy outcome. *Preventive Medicine, 44*(1), 59–63.

Rasch, V. (2003). Cigarette, alcohol, and caffeine consumption: Risk factors for spontaneous abortion. *Acta Obstetrica et Gynecologica Scandinavica, 82*(2), 182–188.

Raymond, E. G., & Mills, J. L. (1993). Placental abruption: Maternal risk factors and associated fetal conditions. *Acta Obstetrica et Gynecologica Scandinavica, 72*(8), 633–639.

Rementeria, J. L., & Nunag, N. N. (1973). Narcotic withdrawal in pregnancy: Stillbirth incidence with a case report. *American Journal of Obstetrics and Gynecology, 116*(8), 1152–1156.

Rich, J. D., Boutwell, A. E., Shield, D. C., Key, R. G., McKenzie, M., Clarke, J. G., et al. (2005). Attitudes and practices regarding the use of methadone in U.S. state and federal prisons. *Journal of Urban Health, 82*(3), 411–419.

Rustin, T. A. (2000). Assessing nicotine dependence. *American Family Physician, 62*(3), 579–584. (*)

Sander, S. C., & Hays, L. R. (2005). Prescription opioid dependence and treatment with methadone in pregnancy. *Journal of Opioid Management, 1*(2), 91–97.

Salihu, H. M., & Wilson, R. E. (2007). Epidemiology of pre-natal smoking and perinatal outcomes. *Early Human Development, 83*(11), 713–720.

Saunders, J. B., Aasland, O. G., Babor, T. F., de al Fuente, J. R., & Grant, M. (1993). Development of the Alcohol Use Disorders Identification Test (AUDIT): WHO collaborative project on early detection of persons with harmful alcohol consumption: II. *Addiction, 88*(6), 791–804.

Scott, D. M., & Taylor, R. E. (2007). Health-related effects of genetic variations of alcohol-metabolizing enzymes in African Americans. *Alcohol Research and Health, 30*(1), 18–21.

Shah, T., Sullivan, K., & Carter, J. (2006). Sudden infant death syndrome and reported maternal smoking during pregnancy. *American Journal of Public Health, 96*(10), 1757–1759.

Sokol, R., Floyd L., Dang, E. P., & Ceperich, S. D. (2006). Drinking and reproductive health: A fetal alcohol spectrum disorders toolkit. Detroit, MI: American College of Obstetrics and Gynecology. Retrieved March 30, 2008, from *www.acog.org/departments/healthIssues/FASDToolKit.pdf*. (*)

Spadoni, A. D., McGee, C. L., Fryer, S. L., & Riley, E. P. (2007). Neuroimaging and fetal alcohol spectrum disorders. *Neuroscience and Biobehavioral Reviews, 31*(2), 239–245.

Spinillo, A., Capuzzo, E., Nicola, S. E., Spinillo, A., Capuzzo, E., Nicola, S. E., et al. (1994). Factors potentiating the smoking-related risk of fetal growth retardation. *British Journal of Obstetrics and Gynaecology, 101*(11), 954–958.

Storen, E. C., Wijdicks, E. F., Crum, B. A., & Schultz, G. (2000) Moyamoya-like vasculopathy from cocaine dependency. *American Journal of Neuroradiology, 21*(6), 1008–1010.

Strinic, T., Bukovic, D., & Sumilin, L. (2005). Sociodemographic characteristics and lifestyle habits of pregnant women smokers. *Collegium Antropologicum, 29*(2), 611–614.

Substance Abuse and Mental Health Services Administration. (2003). *Overview of findings from the 2002 National Survey on Drug Use and Health* (Office of Applied Studies, NHSDA Series H-21, DHHS Publication No. SMA 03-3774). Rockville, MD: Author.

Substance Abuse and Mental Health Services Administration. (2006). *Results from the 2005 National Survey on Drug Use and Health: National findings* (Office of Applied Studies, NSDUH Series H-30, DHHS Publication No. SMA 06-4194). Rockville, MD: Author.

Substance Abuse and Mental Health Services Administration. (2007). *Results from the 2006 National Survey on Drug Use and Health: National findings* (Office of Applied Studies, NSDUH Series H-32, DHHS Publication No. SMA 07-4293). Rockville, MD: Author.

Suellentrop, K., Morrow, B., Williams, L., D'Angelo, D., & Centers for Disease Control and Prevention (CDC). (2006). *Monitoring progress toward achieving Maternal and Infant Healthy People 2010 Objectives: 19 states*. Pregnancy Risk Assessment Monitoring System (PRAMS), 2000–2003. *MMWR Surveillance Summary, 55*(9), 1–11. (*)

Taylor, A. H., Ang, C., & Bell, S. C. (2007). The role of the endocannabinoid system in gametogenesis: Implantation and early pregnancy. *Human Reproduction Update, 13*(5), 501–513.

Than, L. C., Honein, M. A., & Watkins, M. L. (2005). Intent to become pregnant as a predictor of exposures during pregnancy: Is there a relation? *Journal of Reproductive Medicine, 50*(6), 389–396.

Torfs, C. P., Christianson, R. E., & Iovannisci, D. M. (2006). Selected gene polymorphisms and their interaction with maternal smoking, as risk factors for gastroschisis. *Birth Defects Research: Part A. Clinical and Molecular Teratology, 76*(10), 723–730.

U.S. Department of Health and Human Services. (1994). *National Household Survey on Drug Abuse*. Rockville, MD: Substance Abuse and Mental Health Services Administration, Office of Applied Sciences.

Valbo, A., & Eide, T. (1996). Smoking cessation in pregnancy: The effect of hypnosis in a randomized study. *Addictive Behaviors, 21*(1), 29–35.

Van Marter, L. J., Leviton, A., & Allred, E. N. (1996). Persistent pulmonary hypertension of the newborn and smoking and aspirin and nonsteroidal anti-inflammatory drug consumption during pregnancy. *Pediatrics, 97*(5), 658–663.

Velez, M. L., Montoya, I. D., Jansson, L. M., Walters, V., Svikis, D., Jones, H. E., et al. (2006). Exposure to violence among substance-dependent pregnant women and their children. *Journal of Substance Abuse Treatment, 30*(1), 31–38.

Walker, I. D. (2003). Venous and arterial thrombosis during pregnancy: Epidemiology. *Seminars on Vascular Medicine, 3*(1), 25–32.

Wang, E. C. (1999). Methadone treatment during pregnancy. *Journal of Obstetric, Gynecological, and Neonatal Nursing, 28*(6), 615–622.

Westfall, R. E., Janssen, P. A., & Lucas, P. (2006). Survey of medicinal cannabis use among childbearing women: Patterns of its use in pregnancy and retroactive self-assessment of its efficacy against "morning sickness." *Complementary Therapies in Clinical Practice, 12*(1), 27–33.

Wiemann, C. M., Berenson, A. B., & San Miguel, V. V. (1994) Tobacco, alcohol, and illicit drug use among pregnant women: Age and racial/ethnic differences. *Journal of Reproductive Medicine, 39*(10), 769–776.

Wilson, P. D., Loffredo, C. A., Correa-Villasenor, A., & Ferencz, C. (1998). Attributable fraction for cardiac malformations. *American Journal of Epidemiology, 148*(5), 414–423.

Wolff, K., Boys, A., Rostami-Hodjegan, A., Hay, A., & Raistrick, D. (2005). Changes to methadone clearance during pregnancy. *European Journal of Clinical Pharmacology, 61*(10), 763–768.

Yang, Q., Wen, S. W., Smith, G. N., Chen, Y., Krewski, D., Chen, X. K., et al. (2006). Maternal cigarette smoking and the risk of pregnancy-induced hypertension and eclampsia. *International Journal of Epidemiology, 35*(2), 288–293.

Zuspan, F. P., Gumpel, J. A., Mejia-Zelaya, A., Madden, J., & Davis, R. (1975). Fetal stress from methadone withdrawal. *American Journal of Obstetrics and Gynecology, 122*(1), 43–46.

CHAPTER 27

Ethnic and Cultural Correlates of Addiction among Diverse Women

Latoya C. Conner, PhD
Charlene E. Le Fauve, PhD
Barbara C. Wallace, PhD

A bodily disease, which we look upon as whole and entire within itself, may, after all, be but a symptom of some ailment in the spiritual past.

—Nathaniel Hawthorne

Substance abuse is inextricably connected to historical, social, ethnic, and cultural experiences of the diverse women (i.e., members of racial/ethnic groups) affected. Integrating ethnicity and culture into the framework of women and addictions is imperative to understanding the intricate behavioral, psychological, and medical outcomes that occur among diverse women. Such an understanding also enhances cross-cultural awareness by examining how cultural dynamics inform psychological functioning and sequelae, clinical practice, empirical research, and evidence-based addiction treatment for diverse women.

The purpose of this chapter is to provide a cultural and contextual framework for understanding addictions among women of diverse backgrounds. The chapter (1) introduces the ethnic and cultural correlates of addictions; (2) presents epidemiological data on the prevalence of substance use and treatment among African American, Native American/Alaska Native, Latino, and Asian American women; (3) provides the historical contexts that give rise to the culture of addiction among women from diverse ethnic groups; and (4) summarizes current empirical research, evidence-based prevention, and culturally specific clinical treatment geared toward addiction recovery.

DEFINITION OF ETHNICITY AND CULTURE

Definitions of ethnicity and culture have been used interchangeably in other texts (Boyd-Franklin, 2000); however, we believe that although they inform each other, there are distinct differences between the two. In this chapter we refer to "ethnicity" as encompassing both (1) *subjective factors*, such as social norms, cultural values, attitudes, behaviors, and an individual's identification with an ethnic group; and (2) *objective factors*, including the ways in which individuals or a group of people are viewed based on ancestry, nationality, religion, shared experiences, including but not limited to economic, social, and political injustices, discrimination, or oppression (Alba, 1990; Juby & Concepción, 2005; Phinney, 1996). Pinderhughes (1989) asserts that societal definitions, values, and other factors determine whether ethnic meaning becomes positive, ambivalent, or negative, which then has great significance for an individual's behavior and psychological functioning. She also recommends that "all helping professionals … understand the dynamics of ethnicity as these affect themselves as well as their clients, in order to ensure effectiveness" in their treatment (p. 39).

In this chapter we refer to the term "culture" as the "transmission of knowledge, skills, attitudes, [learned] behaviors, and language from one generation to the next, usually within the confines of a physical environment" (Carter, 1995, p. 12). Although the positive influence of culture on drug and alcohol use may be indirect (Saylors, 2003), the social influences significantly compound the experiences, needs, and clinical presentations of diverse women (Comas-Diaz & Greene, 1994). Underlying mood and anxiety disorders have been found among women across cultures, with current substance use problems being predictive of mental health service use (Alvidrez, 1999). Patterns of substance use, beliefs about the cause of mental illness and addiction, and subsequent service utilization vary by ethnicity and culture. In the next section we review diagnostic criteria for the psychological sequelae of substance abuse and the prevalence of substance abuse in ethnically diverse women, followed by key findings of epidemiological and treatment admissions data.

DSM-IV SUBSTANCE-RELATED AND SUBSTANCE-INDUCED DISORDERS AND CULTURAL CONTEXT

According to the text revision of the fourth edition of the *Diagnostic and Statistical Manual of Mental Disorders* (DSM-IV-TR), alcohol, amphetamines, inhalants, prescription medications that may be abused (e.g., sedatives), opioids (morphine, heroin), marijuana (cannabis), cocaine, hallucinogens, and phencyclidine (PCP) are classified into two types of disorders: (1) substance-related disorders, which are disorders of intoxication, dependence, abuse, and withdrawal caused by various substances, both legal and illegal; and (2) substance-induced disorders, including intoxication, withdrawal, and various mental states (e.g., dementia, psychosis, anxiety, mood disorders) (American Psychiatric Association, 2000). Diagnostic criteria for either substance-related or substance-induced disorders must be evaluated in the context of the impact of the individual's cultural context and in a manner that includes an awareness of the culture-bound syndromes described in Appendix I of the DSM-IV-TR. A cultural formulation, designed to supplement the multiaxial assessment paradigm, facilitates the careful and systematic examination of background, context, symptoms, apparent dysfunction, and the clinical presentation, while mindful of unique cultural factors. Key issues that are highly relevant to women of diverse backgrounds include cultural identity and ethnic reference group, language and customs, cultural explanations of presenting symptoms, the individuals' (and their significant others') interpretation of the meaning and severity of those symptoms, and cultural attributions or explanations for the etiology of the symptoms. Women from various cultures have historically maintained diverse roles in society, which necessitated methods of coping and behavioral adaptations for survival that have influenced mental health and associated substance use and abuse across generations. Accordingly, methods of communication, issues of trust, social support structures, and culturally sanctioned norms must be considered when conducting a comprehensive diagnostic assessment and case formulation.

When conducting a diagnostic interview about substances of abuse, it is paramount that the service provider be familiar with street names of drugs, have an awareness of the current patterns of distribution and use of substances in the local community and region, and that he or she demonstrate both sensitivity to the perspective of the individual seeking care as well as credibility and a self-assured empathic, nonjudgmental disposition. Clinical knowledge and judgment are invaluable tools in creating a safe environment in which the individual can disclose information about illegal activities, such as illicit drug use (or other behaviors that are often highly associated with drug use, such as theft, prostitution, distribution, or other illegal acts). Further, women of diverse ethnic groups are faced with daily stressors associated with holding membership in a minority group in a predominantly European American society. As such, inherent frustrations associated with oppression, racism, perceived and real discrimination, and other general aspects of daily living become compounded by clinical syndromes such as trauma, spousal abuse, multigenerational trauma, abandonment, mood and anxiety disorders, greater prevalence of high blood pressure, greater risk for stroke, various forms of cancer, diabetes, other medical conditions, and substance use and abuse.

EPIDEMIOLOGY

Prevalence of Substance Use among Ethnically Diverse Women

In May, 2006 the United States Census Bureau (United States Bureau of the Census, 2007) announced that nearly one in every three U.S. residents was part of a group other than single-race non-Hispanic White. The collective group "other" than European American is a highly heterogeneous group of people who represent a growing number of citizens who have diverse contextual and cultural origins that influence health outcomes. This announcement was based on national estimates by race, Hispanic origin, and age. As of 2005, the nation's minority population totaled 98 million, or 33%, of the country's total of 296.4 million. Such data support what many scientists, policymakers, health care providers, and private citizens observe in activities of daily living, and underscore the necessity of recognizing that diversity and a culturally informed substance abuse treatment and services approach should be the rule rather than the exception (Bourgois et al., 2006; Fleck, Keck, Corey, & Strakowski, 2005; Heinz, Epstein, & Preston, 2007; Westermeyer, 1995). Hispanics are the largest minority group at 42.7 million and the fastest-growing group, followed by African Americans (39.7 million), Asians (14.4 million), Native Americans/Alaska Natives (4.5 million), and Native Hawaiians and other Pacific Islanders (990,000). In addition, there are 104 males per every 100 females under age 18. As the population ages, there are 72 men for every 100 women age 65 and over, and 46 men per every 100 women age 85 and over. Racially and ethnically diverse women outlive their male counterparts (Hoyert, Kung, & Smith, 2005: Agency for Healthcare Research and Quality, 2008), and data on patterns of alcohol and substance use prevalence show an inverse pattern, such that males in general tend to use alcohol and illicit substance at higher rates than women (Substance Abuse and Mental Health Services Administration, 2008).

This section describes factors that influence national policy and practice, with particular focus on the implications of epidemiological survey data concerning women of color. As providers strive to develop effective strategies to engage, treat, and maintain positive treatment outcomes, their understanding of the issues diverse women face must be informed by epidemiological knowledge of the population and research on effective practices. Learning to better understand these clients will help clinicians remove the barriers that keep ethnically diverse women from seeking treatment and deter their recovery. What follows is a review of key findings among Hispanic, African American, Native American/Alaska Native, and Asian American women that emerge from recent surveys. This review also highlights relevant historical contexts and adaptive strengths that may be clinically important to understand the data.

Key Findings of Epidemiological and Treatment Admissions Data

Three sources provide much of the data available on adult women who use or abuse alcohol or other substances: the National Survey on Drug Use and Health (SAMHSA, 2007), the National Epidemiologic Survey on Alcohol and Related Conditions (Grant et al., 2004), and the Treatment Episode Data Set (SAMHSA, 2006), among other sources. The epidemiology of women and addiction is reviewed elsewhere in this text. However, pertinent findings regarding race/ethnicity, which inform this discussion, are highlighted here.

Data from NSDUH in 2006 showed that past-month illicit drug use varied by race/ethnicity. Among persons ages 12 and older, the rate was lowest among Asian Americans (3.6%), followed by 6.9% for Hispanics, 7.5% for Native Hawaiians or other Pacific Islanders, 8.5% for European Americans, 8.9% for persons reporting two or more races, 9.8% for African Americans, and 13.7% for Native Americans or Alaska Natives. Male past-month illicit drug use among persons ages 12 and older was 10.5%, which is higher than that of females (6.2%). Male substance use tends to be higher than female use in general and therefore is expected to be higher within race/ethnicity as well. Among youth ages 12–17 in 2006, the rate of current illicit drug use among Native Americans or Alaska Natives was about twice the overall rate among youths in general (18.7% vs. 9.8%, respectively). The rates were 11.8% among youths reporting two or more races, 10.2% among African Americans, 10.0% among European Americans, 8.9% among Hispanics, and 6.7% among Asian Americans. Illicit drug use by youths ages 12–17 for European American females in this cohort is higher than that of males, with a rate of 10.3% for past-month use (vs. 9.7% for males). African American and Hispanic female rates are 9.5 and 8.6% respectively, and are lower than that of males (10.8% for African American males and 9.1% for European American males).

Alcohol

Of all persons sampled in the NSDUH (ages 12 and older), European Americans in 2006 were more likely than other racial/ethnic groups to report current use of alcohol (55.8%), followed by 47.1% for persons reporting two or more races, 41.8% for Hispanics, 40.0% for African Americans, 37.2% for Native Americans or Alaska Natives, 36.7% for Native Hawaiians or other Pacific Islanders, and 35.4% for Asian Americans. In addition, the NSDUH (2006) reports that among persons ages 12–20, current alcohol use rates are highest among European Americans again, followed by Native Americans or Alaska Natives. Specifically, rates were 18.6% among African Americans, 19.7% among Asian Americans, 25.3% among Hispanics, 27.5% among those reporting two or more races, 31.3% among Native Americans or Alaska Natives, and 32.3% among European Americans. Rates for Native Americans or Alaska Natives increased since the 2005 rate, which was 21.7%.

Substance Dependence

In 2006, among persons ages 12 and older, the rate of substance dependence or abuse was the lowest among Asian Americans (4.3%). Racial/ethnic groups reporting similar rates included Native Hawaiians or other Pacific Islanders (12.0%), persons reporting two or more races (12.0%), Hispanics (10.0%), European Americans (9.2%), and African Americans (9.0%).

The rate among Native Americans or Alaska Natives (19.0%) was higher than the rates among Hispanics, European Americans, and African Americans. These rates were all similar to the rates reported in 2005.

HISTORICAL CONTEXTS AND SALIENT ISSUES FOR DIVERSE WOMEN

The heterogeneity of women of color—their historical realities and current psychological experiences—must be explored in the context of their addictive behaviors. Women's substance use and addictions are influenced by the cultural norms and practices of the ethnic groups to which they belong, in addition to other environmental and biological factors (Collins & McNair, 2002). Clinically, it is imperative for counselors to understand the cultural expectations that influence the lives of women, and to ask culturally informed questions to be effective with women with addictions (Mora, 2002). For example, Mora (2002) suggests that counselors ask the following questions: What are the historical contributions to the shaming and destructive behaviors of diverse women? Does exploring the impact of ethnic, cultural, and family histories on their current addictive behavior create risks or resilience among these women? What are the culturally appropriate guidelines for prevention and treatment? In this section, we turn to salient issues present in the experiences of diverse women, including African American, Native American/Alaska Native, Hispanic, and Asian American women. The link between ethnic and cultural experiences, expectations, and substance use is highlighted.

African American Women

The cultural history of African American women in the United States is wrought with institutional racism and multiple oppressions, including sexism, economic poverty, and health disparities (Greene, 1994). African American women are descendents of Native Americans and Africans who were transplanted from West Africa to the Caribbean, parts of South America, and the United States during the trans-Atlantic slave trade. "No other group entered the [American] society as involuntary immigrants, and no other group was subsequently victimized by two centuries of slavery," rendering the African American history unique (Marger, 1997, p. 227). African American women were stripped of many personal, familial, social, and sexual rights that compromised their psychological health (Wyatt, 1997). Given the contextual history of loss and oppression, African American women are faced with a range of challenges that impact their psychological realities, adaptive functioning, and overall sexual, emotional, and medical health. The empirical literature has much to offer in highlighting culturally and ethnically informed health behavior.

Substance abuse in the context of such painful life experiences has been described as "escapism alcohol," for example (Battle, 1990, as cited in Ehrmin, 2002, p. 787). In a qualitative study by Ehrmin (2002), African American women revealed that substance abuse was a way to numb the painful feelings associated with loss of a loved one, especially parents during their youth; overt and covert forms of racism and prejudice; societal, cultural, and familial rejection; physical abuse; incest, sexual abuse, and rape; and unresolved feelings of shame and guilt for the impact their active substance use had on their mothering. Ehrmin suggests that a *culture care* model for African American women would include providing support to help them resolve past pains, anger, guilt, and comorbid depression by creating meaning in social, religious, and cultural ways, thus thwarting of potential substance relapse.

In another study Alvidrez (1999), found that African American women reported greater alcohol and drug problems, compared to other Latin American and European American women. They also endorsed religious or supernatural factors to account for their substance abuse, as a form of mental illness. In addition to the role of religion and spirituality in the etiology of mental illness, spiritual faith, religious practice, and help-seeking support from family and community impact the coping strategies used among women with substance use disorders (SUDs). The transcendent role of spirituality is well documented in the literature on African Americans (Akbar, 1996; Ani, 1997; Brome, Owens, Allen, & Vevaina, 2000; Constantine, Lewis, Conner, & Sanchez, 2000; Frame & Williams, 1996; Mattis, 2002). Research reveals that African-centered principles (i.e., spiritual faith and interconnectedness) serve as protective factors against anxiety, depression, hostility, interpersonal sensitivity, and somatization (Conner, 2003; Ferraro & Koch, 1994), all of which are psychological challenges that may trigger substance use or relapse. Among African American women in recovery from substance abuse, those who coped in spiritual ways also reported a greater quality of life and more positive attitudes about self and others (Brome et al., 2000, as cited in Witherspoon & Richardson, 2006).

Furthermore, ethnic identity and cultural worldview may also serve as protective factors against substance abuse or relapse in the face of life challenges. A woman's internalized belief about her ethnic group or her ethnic identity affects her self-esteem and mood, which also affects her chances of using substances or relapsing. Perceptions of discrimination or internalized racism have been linked to higher levels of psychological distress, lower life satisfaction, and poorer health outcomes (Witherspoon & Richardson, 2006).

Native American and Alaska Native Women

The mental health landscape for Native American women includes the struggle with the loss of cultural values, generational ties, and the disintegration of indigenous ways of being—which also impacts the mental health and subsequent substance use or abuse among them (Napholz, 2000). The loss of ethnic identity and cultural knowledge, in general, leads to loss of a sense of self (LaFramboise, 1994, as cited in Napholz, 2000). Napholz (2000) found that successful "retraditionalism"—going forward by going backward—in the form of bicultural resynthesis was an effective means to assist Native American women achieve a healthy self-identity and positive coping skills to overcome emotional and behavioral problems. Bicultural resynthesis is a hierarchical model that illustrates how a person experiences bicultural stress, guilt, anger, shame, and isolation, to which he or she acculturates or adapts to survive in mainstream culture. Next, the process of deculturation—releasing attachment to mainstream values—is necessary in order to engage in ethnic switching—an embracing of indigenous ways of being—whereby the individual develops an authentic connection with self, ethnic identity, and ancestry. It is only when a person reaches this stage of historical enlightenment and bicultural identity that he or she successfully achieves a bicultural resynthesis (Napholz, 2000).

The process of coming full circle in the process of bicultural resynthesis is reflective of the perspective that Native American culture is circular and interdependent (Lowery, 1998). Several of the treatment and recovery models for Native American women with substance abuse problems include the use of overlapping concentric circles that share the same axis and include an integration of physical, emotional, and spiritual healing support (Lowery, 1998). For instance, women's circles have been effective in addressing the needs of Native American women in ways that link spiritual and physical wellness to the community, the culture, and the natural world (Saylors, 2003).

The predominant health problems for Native American women are often referred to as a triad that includes substance abuse, violence, and depression (Saylors, 2003). In one study on Native American women living in a coed residential substance abuse treatment center, 85% of the women reported that they had been abused (emotionally, physically, and/or sexually) in their lifetime (Saylors, 2003). Following the culturally congruent treatment of a women's circle, Saylors found that substance use had decreased significantly at 6-month follow-up, the number of women legally employed had doubled, and self-reported health status had increased.

Treatment for Native American populations must be integrative, empowering, culturally unique, and include traditional indigenous healing practices, such as tribal groups, medicine men, relatives, and community members (LaFramboise, Trimble, & Mohatt, 1995; Lowery, 1998). Mental health professionals must be competent in treating women in culturally and contextually appropriate ways. It is at this intersection that the treatment of health problems (e.g., substance abuse) for Native American women will both empower and heal.

Hispanic or Latina Women

The diversity within Hispanic or Latino populations requires both an ethnic and cultural approach to explore the specific influences on health behaviors. Although the term "Hispanic" suggests a homogeneous group united by similarities, this is not the case (Vasquez, 1994). The term refers to an ethnic group who may share common cultural values and the Spanish language (Trepper, Nelson, McCollum, & McAvoy, 1997), and who may be first-, second-, or third-generation U.S.-born citizens or more recent immigrants. We will use the term Hispanic to include all Spanish-speaking groups regardless of country of origin. Others use the term "Latino" to refer to individuals who were born in Latin America with the exclusion of those born in other countries. Included in the Hispanic or Latino ethnic group are diverse individuals with familial origins from a variety of countries in Latin America, the Caribbean, and Europe. The major groups identified by the U.S. Census are Mexican Americans, Puerto Ricans, and Cuban Americans (Paz, 2004). Migration and cultural adaptation experiences are heterogeneous among Hispanic women and impact their socioeconomic and socio-demographic profiles. In addition, Hispanics can be of any race (Borrell & Hatch, 2005); thus, the population ranges from dark-skinned to light-skinned individuals and includes a plethora of shades in between who also may have admixtures with Native Americans, Mexican or South American Indians, African Americans, Afro-Caribbeans, European Americans, and Asians or Asian Americans. This is true for all of the women described in this chapter. As such, a clinician who observes a woman and makes an attribution that she holds membership within a particular racial group based only on phenotypic presentation may be grossly mistaken, and might therefore behave in a manner that could create a barrier for relationship building before rapport is established.

Many Hispanic family households in the United States are headed by females (National Institutes of Health [NIH], 2006). Although many of these women work outside the home (Mora, 2002), their households have incomes below the poverty level more often than other types of households (United States Bureau of Census, 2007); more than 43% of poor Hispanic families are female-headed and are likely to have no health insurance, have little or no health care for themselves or their children, and have no support network. Poverty combines with these multiple barriers to receiving adequate health services and increases the likelihood that mental illness and alcohol and SUDs will occur. Migration experiences and consequences associated with a lack of citizenship create a strong reluctance to enter the public health service systems in the United States. Real and perceived fear of detection, deportation, or separation of the mother from her children obstructs pursuit and receipt of mental health and/or substance abuse services for recent immigrants.

Other issues related to age, level of acculturation, and cultural and ethnic identity are the most salient for first-, second-, or third-generation Hispanic women (Mora, 2002). Acculturation was found to be predictive of substance abuse, especially among Cuban, Puerto Rican American, and Mexican women compared to their male counterparts (Black & Markides, 1993). That is the more educated, employed, and/or acculturated a women was, the greater her chances of using/abusing alcohol and drugs. Another aspect of acculturation is encountering discrimination, prejudice, and exclusion based on language or complexion. Racial identity among Hispanic women can be influenced by personal reactions to differential treatment between racial hierarchies (Borrell & Hatch, 2005). The extent to which cultural heritage and religion in the family, or "familism," govern family mores also determines the degree which an individual pursues "help," and from whom, when in need. For example, the family norm might be to first speak to trusted members of the family (Alvidrez, 1999), then a pastoral counselor or folk healer, rather than a health professional about a problem. Although religiosity and the family are deemed protective factors against alcohol and substance use, conversely, both factors might deter women from seeking professional care.

Asian American Women

The presence of Asians in the United States dates back to the 1800s, beginning with the first wave of Chinese immigrants, followed by the Japanese (Marger, 1997). The term "Asian American" refers to a culturally heterogeneous group of people, including those from Japan, Korea, India, Southeast Asia, Micronesia, Melanesia, Polynesia, and the Hawaiian Islands (Bradshaw, 1994), representing even greater diversity in language, culture, and ethnic origins. Though Asian Americans represent dozens of ethnic groups, with the exception of the model minority label attached to their successful assimilation to American society (Marger, 1997), Asian women are often regarded in such a way that their diversity is overlooked (Kitano & Louie, 2002; Joe, 1996).

Asian men were the first to migrate to the United States, in part due to cultural roles, but by the mid 1900s, following the 1965 Immigration Act, the number of Asian women among the immigrant population had reached approximately 50% (Bradshaw, 1994; Joe, 1996). Many myths about Asian/Asian American women "ranged from the erotic Oriental beauty to the evil dragon lady to the obedient wife and mother" (Joe, 1996, p. 199). Asian women are faced with the task of challenging the ethnic stereotypes, gendered myths, and discrimination or exploitation based on those myths. As a result of such ethnic stereotypes and their own cultural ways of being, there are relatively low numbers of Asian Americans seek mental health treatment, including substance abuse treatment. From a treatment perspective, there are also structural, financial and cultural barriers resulting from such stereotypes that further complicate the mental health picture for Asian Americans (Kitano & Louie, 2002).

It is important to understand specific ethnic and cultural issues that go beyond race-based stereotypes (Bradshaw, 1994). Although the overall prevalence of substance use among Asians is reportedly lower than other ethnic groups, researchers (e.g., Chi, Lubben, & Kitano, 1989; D'Avanzo, Frye, & Froman, 1994; Joe, 1996) report on the within-race variance, which is important to understanding the diversity of behaviors, circumstances, cultural styles, and assimilation/acculturation levels as they relate to substance use. Chi et al. (1989) assert that Asian Americans' substance use practices, especially alcohol, are related to their degree of assimilation. They hypothesize that the more Asians assimilate, the more their substance use behavior may reflect the dominant group. The authors acknowledge that the opposite may also be true: More recent immigrants may have had preexisting substance abuse behaviors prior to their migration.

Asians vary tremendously in their cultural values, beliefs, and practices (Bradshaw, 1994); however, traditional Asian cultural values include several common components, such as interdependence, collective self-esteem, fatalism, "saving face," and shame aversion (Kitano & Louie, 2002). In an ethnographic study, Joe (1996) uncovered "unstoried" histories of Asian/Pacific American women found that their drug use was a way to deal with family chaos, violence, abuse, poverty, gender and cultural norms, marginalization. She found that the most common pattern of drug use, which started as early as preadolescent years with peers and family members in some cases, began with alcohol, followed by tobacco, marijuana, and cocaine, then "ice" or crystal methamphetamine.

An exploration of Cambodian refugee women and their families living on the East and West coasts of the United States (D'Avanzo et al., 1994) found that in those families where alcohol was perceived as a problem, the majority of problem drinkers were husbands. About 45% of the women, however, said that they used alcohol for nervousness, stress, headaches, insomnia, and pain. In addition, about 15% of the East Coast women reported that a family member used street drugs and was having dependency problems. Whereas use of alcohol or street drugs was not perceived as problematic by West Coast Cambodian women, over 58% of the women and their families reported using prescription drugs for self-treatment of illnesses other than those targeted by the prescription. When prescription drugs were misused by the women in this study, it was most frequently to effect an altered state or street-drug "high" (D'Avanzo et al., 1994).

The effects of historical lineage and ethnic stereotypes on health behavior must be addressed in order to provide culturally informed assessment and evidence-based addiction treatment. More empirical data are needed to identify the drinking and drug use behaviors among Asian subgroups by context, including refugees, immigrants (Bradshaw, 1994), and first-, second-, or third-generation U.S.-born Asian American women, who may present a slightly different picture from more recent immigrants. The differences may exist in terms of the extent to which their experiences with assimilation, acculturation, pluralism, and cultural values impact their substance use.

Collectively, the women highlighted in this section share a common experience as members of visible ethnic groups in the United States. Their drinking and drug behaviors are influenced by factors related to migration from their countries of origin; community or family practices with substances (Collins & McNair, 2002); racial microaggressions or daily hassles, or challenges; racism and oppression; as well as intrapsychic pain (see Sue et al., 2007). The psychological sequelae from historical traumas, powerlessness, marginalization, gender socialization, violence, and victimization contribute to the development of addiction among these diverse women. For many, their substance use is the most pervasive, stigmatizing, and telling of all addictions among women both within and across ethnic groups (Straussner & Attia, 2002). Therefore, it is imperative that successful addiction treatment address social, psychological, cultural, ethnic, economic, physical, and political variables (Shoultz, Tanner, & Harrigan, 2000). In the next section we review the correlates of addictions among diverse women, followed by implications for integrating and adapting evidence-based addiction treatment.

TOWARD THE DELIVERY OF EVIDENCE-BASED ADDICTION TREATMENT TO WOMEN OF DIVERSE CULTURES

The Need for Evidence-Based Interventions

A wide range of addiction correlates can be found in the population of women from various ethnic and cultural groups seeking community-based addiction treatment. These correlates suggest both the necessity and challenge of deploying evidence-based interventions. It may be necessary to integrate, adapt, and tailor evidence-based interventions in order to meet the needs of individual diverse female clients. However, evidence-based addiction treatments often emerge as a result of trials with homogenous samples, where those included met rigorous inclusion and exclusion criteria (e.g., mostly European American males using only alcohol, no current arrest/legal case, never suicidal/homicidal, no comorbidity, and excellent contact information for long-term follow-up—as in the case of Project MATCH); as a result, the generalization of findings to treatment in the real world with diverse clients ends up being limited (Marlatt, 1999). The use of rigorous inclusion and exclusion criteria for the selection of research participants typically results in the following: as the number of inclusion and exclusion criteria increases, the generalizability of the findings from treatment efficacy research decreases (Goldfried & Wolfe, 1996).

In response to this reality, Moos (2002) discusses the issues of fidelity versus flexibility. Practitioners are urged to exercise fidelity in deploying empirically supported treatments disseminated via expert consensus guidelines and manuals. However, in the real-world treatment context practitioners may also need to exercise flexibility. Flexibility may mean using the results of naturalistic observation to inform steps to be taken (Moos, 2002). Or, flexibility may mean using assessment findings and adapting and integrating evidence-based approaches in relation to client characteristics (e.g., their ethnic and cultural characteristics) and the emergent correlates of addiction (Wallace, 2005). There is also the contemporary principle and outcry of consumers advocating for themselves—"Nothing about us without us"—necessitating the question: How can we implement evidence-based practices and yet fully incorporate clients' preferences into clinical decision making (Moos, 2003)? Others have used extensive case histories to illustrate how to conduct the kind of thorough, individualized assessment that will bring to light client characteristics and preferences, then to select from a menu of evidence-based options while exercising flexibility in integrating, adapting, and tailoring interventions in light of assessment findings (Wallace, 2005).

The Variety of Contemporary Client Characteristics and Correlates of Addiction

Common correlates of addiction are readily encompassed in descriptions of contemporary client characteristics. These correlates or characteristics are numerous. Some of these are common correlates of addiction, regardless of client demographics. Others are correlates common to ethnic/minority women entering addiction treatment.

Multiproblem Clients

First, individuals may have multiple addictions and related problem behaviors (Wallace, 2005). For example, there may be the presence of more than one SUD (e.g., alcohol, crack, and marijuana) and more than one problem behavior (e.g., experiencing domestic violence, engaging in violence, and high-risk/unprotected sex), creating complex combinations and subsequent treatment challenges. This has led to the assertion that contemporary clients entering community-based addiction treatment can be aptly described as multiproblem clients (Wallace, 2005).

Mental, Behavioral, and Physical Health Correlates

Clinicians may be faced with the challenge of patients who have multiple co-occurring DSM-IV-TR Axis I and Axis II mental disorders, including those commonly rooted in experiences of trauma across the lifespan (Handmaker, Packard, & Conforti, 2002; Landsberg, Rock, Berg, & Smiley, 2002; Ouimette & Brown, 2003); the presence of varied health, disability, and medical conditions; and a risk for conditions such as HIV/AIDS, sexually transmitted diseases, and hepatitis B and C viruses. Also possible are reproductive or gynecological problems among women, as well as smoking-related disease (asthma, coronary heart disease, cancer), chronic disease (e.g., diabetes, hypertension), obesity, and lifelong learning disabilities (Haller, Miles, & Cropsey, 2004; National Institute on Drug Abuse, 2003; Palepu et al., 2003; Strathdee, 2003; Timpson, Williams, Bowen, & Keel, 2003; Wallace, 2005).

A mental health, behavioral health, and physical health nexus has been described (Wallace, 2005) wherein the following occurs: Mental health problems compromise behavioral health, and compromised behavioral health may lead to serious physical health problems. Examples include the possible etiology of conditions such as HIV/AIDS, sexually transmitted diseases, or serious physical disabilities from exposure to violence.

Other pertinent findings suggest a connection between mental health and physical health indices. Cochran, Mays, Alegria, Ortega, and Takeuchi (2007) indicate that when diversity includes sexual orientation, those who are lesbian, bisexual, or homosexually experienced heterosexuals may be subject to a greater variety of health conditions relative to heterosexual women. Meanwhile, levels of psychological distress for all subjects emerge as key variables in determining health.

Implications for practitioners and researchers include paying attention to the additional sources of stress that may attend the experience of engaging in a nonheterosexual lifestyle. The call to attain cultural competence includes acquiring the sensitivity to empathically engage with lesbian and bisexually active women, while conveying respect and acceptance (Wallace, 2005).

Trauma and Multiple Traumas as Common Correlates

Women from diverse ethnic/racial groups may also present with traumatic histories (Ouimette & Brown, 2003), whether of childhood neglect and/or abuse (emotional, physical, sexual), parental domestic violence, adolescent and adult rapes, battering/domestic violence, drug culture violence, or from varied patterns of both victimization from, and perpetration of, violence (Acierno, Coffey, & Resnick, 2003; Locke & Newcomb, 2003; Parrott, Drobes, Saladin, Coffey, & Dansky, 2003; Riggs, Rukstalis, Volpicelli, Kalmanson, & Foa, 2003; Stuart, Moore, Ramsey, & Kahler, 2003).

One source of trauma involves loss of children due to the disruption and dysfunction chronic addiction typically causes in women's lives. Indeed, any substance use currently renders women vulnerable to loss of child custody. The majority of women who have lost child custody experience this as quite traumatic, often developing anxiety and depression which complicates their recovery process and ability to adhere to treatment. One result is difficulty maintaining stable abstinence; another result is the subsequent experience of graduated negative sanctions, including the ultimate sanction of termination of parental rights. Unresolved guilt over the loss of children can lead to more severe mental health problems, including evolution of psychotic depression (Wallace, 2005). The result of unresolved guilt can be a chronic pattern of relapse or inability to terminate drug use, which contributes to the additional risk of recidivism or being charged with a criminal offense (Wallace, 2005).

Additional sources of trauma are being reported by contemporary clinicians observing the most recent effects of the ongoing Iraq war upon ethnically and culturally diverse female armed service personnel. Clinicians are reporting that these women are increasingly presenting histories of trauma. Negative outcomes for this vulnerable population include PTSD, addiction, and homelessness, and returning female armed services personnel are presenting with all three conditions in historically high numbers. Etiology of these conditions is found in their high level of exposure to combat operations in the Iraq war, relative to prior wars (Gamache, Rosenheck, & Tessler, 2003; Holmstedt, 2007; Schnurr et al., 2008), including heretofore unprecedented high rates of exposure to rape/sexual abuse by fellow U.S. soldiers, along with exposure to roadside bombs and other classic sources of overstimulation that characterize a war zone (e.g., seeing dead bodies, witnessing the death of colleagues in uniform, fearing one's own death).

Given all of these possible sources of trauma and resultant comorbid SUD and PTSD, there is a need for integrated treatment that simultaneously addresses both disorders (Najavits et al., 2003). Ideally, such treatment emphasizes stabilizing clients, teaching them to cope in safe ways, reducing their most destructive symptoms, while explicitly avoiding any actual processing of the trauma. This integrated model differs from widespread policies and practices that require clients to become abstinent before working on their PTSD (Najavits et al., 2003). This recommended simultaneous treatment of the comorbid SUD and PTSD constitutes an evidence-based approach (Brown, Read, & Kahler, 2003, p. 186); however, the evidence does not indicate what constitutes the most effective focus and timing of the trauma/PTSD treatment, suggesting an area of much-needed research. The diverse women presenting comorbidity must be treated in light of these recommendations. Meanwhile, the current challenge will only be exacerbated with the rise in diverse women being exposed to war in Iraq.

Functional Problems as a Common Correlate

Co-occurring functional problems create additional difficulties in the daily lives of these women of diverse backgrounds. Problems encompass a greater risk of unemployment, low income, and a risk for premature termination from treatment. Such functional difficulties may mean a tendency to arrive late for appointments, necessitating flexibility on the part of those clinicians, or clinical systems, treating such women (Riggs et al., 2003).

Women may also arrive late or tend to cancel at the last minute due to child care responsibilities or sick children. Access to transportation can be a challenge, given a lack of funds or inconsistent funds associated with unemployment and poverty. In light of functional difficulties, common adaptations recommended in service delivery involve still working with/ seeing late arrivals, operating with a walk-in policy, and the double-booking of appointment slots to accommodate the high frequency of "no shows" or late arrivals. In our own work we have witnessed the double-booking of appointment slots to accommodate the high frequency of "no shows" or late arrivals. New clients are informed of this policy and asked to be somewhat flexible and patient in waiting to be seen when double-booked clients both show up. Such policies are not without controversy, yet they do respond to practical realities in outpatient settings where a significant portion of clients are plagued with such functional difficulties.

Other adaptations recommended include taking a harm reduction approach, given how functional difficulties, comorbidity, and a multitude of problems combine such that women have difficulty attaining and maintaining abstinence. Women who are still using substances as well as those who arrive intoxicated/high to appointments can be accepted and engaged in treatment in a pragmatic harm reduction approach (Marlatt, 1998; Tatarsky, 2003). Such an approach can help women stabilize as well as gradually minimize and eliminate the impact of functional difficulties, even as they are supported over time in exploring abstinence options.

Incarceration Histories as a Common Correlate

Women who end up involved with illegal substances are quite vulnerable to arrest and incarceration, often partly due to romantic/intimate/sexual involvement with men who are dealing drugs. The risk of unemployment is even greater for those who also end up with an arrest history; indeed, incarceration can bar one from employment and even housing, destabilizing families (and communities), making them even more vulnerable to crime (Drucker, 2006). Any women using drugs in our current era, during which policies of mass incarceration and overincarceration have prevailed for the past 30 years (Chesney-Lind & Pasko, 2004; Drucker, 2006; Haney, 2006), is most unfortunate, given that the practice of readily incarcerating women is highly prevalent.

Indeed, many data support how women have been well represented for nearly two decades among those involved with the criminal justice system. As of 2003, 40–60% of all those entering addiction treatment programs in the United States come from the courts, probation, parole, or the correctional systems (McLellan, 2003, p. 187). Others have suggested that the numbers of those who are court mandated for criminal offenses are even higher in outpatient addiction treatment programs located in poorer communities, urban communities, or communities with large numbers of African American clients (Howard, 2003).

Current drug sentencing policies have had a disproportionate negative impact upon the most vulnerable in our society—women and communities of color; and, within the group of women, women of color are being incarcerated at higher rates. Bearing this out, from 1980 to 1999 there was a more than sixfold increase in the number of women incarcerated (i.e., from 12,000 in 1980 to 90,000 in 1999), which is ten times greater than the number of women incarcerated in all of Western Europe (Chesney-Lind, 2002, pp. 80–81). Also, from 1995 to 2002, the average annual rate of increase for female inmates was 5.25%, exceeding the 3.5% annual rate increase for male inmates (Harrison & Beck, 2003). Within this societal trend, there were also racial and ethnic disparities in female incarceration rates; a 191 per 100,000 incarceration for African American females, an 80 per 100,000 rate for Hispanic females, and a mere 35 for 100,000 rate for European American females, by year end 2002 (Harrison & Beck, 2003).

Mandates to Treatment as Common Correlates

As a result of incarceration histories, clients are typically mandated to community-based addiction treatment as a condition of parole. Also, those seeking to regain child custody are typically coerced into drug treatment by child welfare and foster care agencies. The possibility of regaining child custody is made contingent on engagement in substance abuse treatment. Welfare applicants are also being screened for addiction problems; the receipt and maintenance of benefits are contingent on engagement in treatment. Clients experiencing all such mandates/coercion are subject to drug testing and may face graduated negative sanctions for testing positive.

Another consequence of these treatment mandates is that initial motivation to enter treatment may be largely extrinsically based, in contrast with motivation that is internally based, arising from personal self-perceptions or desires (De Leon, Melnick, & Tims, 2001). A resultant clinical challenge involves the task of assisting clients in shifting their motivation from an external to an internal, while drawing on motivational interviewing techniques (Miller & Rollnick, 2002; Wallace, 2005), so as to maximize the potential positive impact of participation in treatment.

Experiences of Racism as Common Correlates

Other potential correlates of addiction may include exposure to the racism that operates in the contemporary social-environmental context. Evidence of this racism can be seen in the previously noted mass incarceration policies and practices in the United States, which are a modern-day heir to those historical state mechanisms long utilized to perpetuate social and racial injustice in the tradition of slavery, segregation, and discriminatory immigration; moreover, these are all policies that effectively serve to isolate, stigmatize, and marginalize the most economically disadvantaged, such as racial and ethnic minorities (Drucker, 2006).

Other evidence can be found in reports from female members of racial/ethnic groups of having had experiences—often daily—of being attacked, disrespected, or merely feeling that something is not right, suggesting the experience of "racial microaggressions" in everyday life, as described by Sue et al. (2007). These racial microaggressions are brief and commonplace verbal, behavioral, and environmental indignities (whether intentional or unintentional) that serve to communicate hostile, derogatory, or negative racial slights and insults. Typically, they are invisible to the perpetrator, and often invisible to the recipient, even as recipients tend to be left with vague unpleasant feelings. The potential damage done to the identity of those who have accumulated a lifetime of such experiences, or have had such encounters since immigrating to this country, may also emerge as a factor to be addressed in treatment (Sue & Sue, 2003; Wallace, Carter, Nanin, Keller, & Alleyne, 2003).

Experiences of racial microaggressions serve to sensitize clients to any instances of being disrespected. This sensitization necessitates that practitioners address their own social conditioning for stigmatizing women and any related negative countertransference; a recommended solution is to acquire adaptive affective, behavioral, and cognitive responses to those who come from diverse ethnic/cultural backgrounds (Wallace, 2005). Examples of adaptive affective responses are empathy (a key nonspecific factor identified in research on treatment outcome), respect, and acceptance. All those who work with diverse women need to strive to replace any maladaptive responses (e.g., stigma, prejudice, racism, sexism, heterosexism, homophobia) with these adaptive affective responses (Wallace, 2005). Thus, training in multicultural counseling competencies (Sue et al., 1998) emerges as essential, ideally as a condition of delivering addiction treatment to diverse women.

Implications for Varied Stages of Change

Complex findings may emerge from a thorough individualized assessment. This complexity can also be conveyed via the concept of stages of change. Diverse female clients may be in different states of readiness to change for any given problem behavior. Indeed, a client may be in different stages of change (Prochaska & DiClemente, 1983; Velasquez, Maurer, Crouch, & DiClemente, 2001) for a number of problem behaviors.

For example, consider how "Mrs. Z" could be in the following multiple stages of change at the same time: in a stage of precontemplation (not thinking about it) for taking psychiatric medication and terminating marijuana smoking; in a stage of contemplation (thinking about it) for using condoms; an action stage (having taken action to change) for crack cocaine smoking; and in a maintenance stage (maintaining change for over 6 months) for taking HIV medication. Of note, that Mrs. Z is still smoking marijuana means that she is testing positive for drug use and receiving ongoing negative sanctions from drug court, parole, and a child welfare agency. Both the drug use and the sanctions increase her risk of reincarceration and termination of her parental rights.

IMPLICATIONS FOR INTEGRATING AND ADAPTING EVIDENCE-BASED APPROACHES FOR DIVERSE WOMEN

The correlates of addiction among racially, ethnically, and culturally diverse women have implications for the engagement of these women in treatment and for their receipt of interventions tailored to their specific needs, given individualized assessment findings. This review of the addiction correlates of addiction commonly found among contemporary diverse female clients immediately begins to suggest the need for interventions that will accomplish the following: recognize that women arriving for addiction treatment will be in various stages of change regarding their behavior, making the transtheoretical model of Prochaska and DiClemente (1983) highly pertinent; address comorbidity, such as that which follows from PTSD, by utilizing an integrated treatment approach that simultaneously addresses both the addiction and trauma (Brown et al., 2003; Najavits et al., 2003); provide individual and group interventions that can enhance coping skills; shift clients' motivation from extrinsic (given an external mandate or coercion) to an intrinsic, possibly be applying motivational interviewing techniques (Miller & Rollnick, 2002); reduce the risk of relapse and recidivism by providing a relapse prevention program (Marlatt & Donovan, 2005; Marlatt & Gordon, 1985); and include a harm reduction policy and approach when clients refuse the goal of abstinence or are not yet ready to terminate all substance use (Marlatt, 1998; McLellan, 2003; Tatarsky, 2003). The following is a more complete presentation of the range of evidence-based approaches appropriate for diverse women.

An Array of Evidence-Based Alternatives

Several summaries of evidence-based addiction treatment approaches for use with adults are available in the literature; these approach share substantial overlap and point toward a contemporary standard of care. For example, the National Institute on Drug Abuse (NIDA, 1999) recommended relapse prevention, supportive–expressive psychotherapy, individualized drug counseling, motivational enhancement therapy, the community reinforcement approach plus vouchers, day treatment with abstinence contingencies and vouchers, and the MATRIX model. As effective psychosocial modalities, Moos (2003) recommended cognitive-behavioral interventions, social skills training, stress management and relapse prevention training, a community reinforcement approach, motivational interviewing, behavioral contracting, and behavioral marital therapy.

Wallace (2005) recommended a menu of seven evidence-based approaches, as follows: (1) special focus on building a strong therapeutic alliance/social support (TASS) network; (2) motivational interviewing/motivational enhancement therapy/brief interventions; (3) cognitive-behavioral therapy (CBT)/relapse prevention (RP)/social skills training; (4) 12-step facilitation/guidance using Alcoholics and/or Narcotics Anonymous; (5) individual drug counseling (IDC) and/or supportive–expressive psychotherapy; (6) community reinforcement approach/vouchers: contingency management; or (7) the MATRIX model or a day treatment approach or "IEC" outpatient model—that is, "I" (intensive, 4–5 days per week), "E" (extensive, 6–12 months), and "C" (comprehensive, combining multiple elements, such as TASS, CBT/RP, IDC, group drug counseling, drug testing, etc.). Also recommended were a number of state-of-the-art practices, with selected examples, as follows: the integration of motivational interviewing and stages of change; integration of harm reduction, moderation approaches, and abstinence models; and incorporating contemporary trends in psychology, such as multiculturalism, positive psychology, the strengths-based approach, and optimistic thinking/learned optimism.

These three summaries of evidence-based approaches (i.e., NIDA, 1999; Moos, 2003; Wallace, 2005) underscore a point made by Miller and Hester (2003, p. 1) that contemporary practitioners have "an array of alternatives with reasonable empirical support, offering a choice among promising options." Such options may be essential, given the assertion of Blume and Garcia de la Cruz (2005) that one size does *not* fit all, within the context of delivering treatment. Blume and Garcia de la Cruz (2005) go on to suggest how it is possible that we do not know, as yet, what works with people of color, because they have not been adequately represented in research studies.

Following the Standard of Care: Avoiding Discrimination and Disparities in Service Delivery

It has been asserted that evidence-based approaches should be viewed as a recommended standard of care (Wallace, 2005). As such, it is important that we extend contemporary standards of care arising from evidence-based approaches to ethnic minorities. Certainly it is important that more efficacy and effectiveness research be conducted with diverse samples (e.g., Blume et al., 2005). However, until those studies are done, it is a valid approach to endorse the prevailing standards of care embodied in evidence-based approaches (Wallace, 2005). Deviation from contemporary standards of care or recommended evidence-based protocols may constitute discrimination in the context of treating racial/ethnic minorities. Furthermore, to deviate from the contemporary evidence-based standards of care could contribute to disparities in service delivery and exacerbate substance-related disparities in health—such as those that disproportionately impact ethnic minorities. Such discrimination, as embodied in any deviations from contemporary standards of care or recommended protocols, may also be seen as constituting a maladaptive response to diversity. An adaptive behavioral coping response to client diversity would include, at a minimum, adherence to evidence-based standards of care (Wallace, 2005).

Making Treatment Work

Given the many correlates of addiction to be found among diverse women, as reviewed earlier, practitioners may need to, metaphorically, hold the menu of evidence-based addiction treatment options in hand. A next step may involve selecting from the menu of options in light of individual assessment findings, while going on to integrate, adapt, and tailor treatment to the complex characteristics and preferences of multiproblem clients (Wallace, 2005). What does the resultant treatment approach look like?

Consider integrating treatment for Mrs. Z, mentioned earlier. For her treatment, the practitioner would need to consider her stage of change for a number of problem behaviors (precontemplation stage for taking psychiatric medication and terminating marijuana smoking; contemplation stage for using condoms) and select the use of motivational interviewing to enhance her intrinsic motivation to change. Also indicated is the use of a number of interventions from the menu of options reviewed earlier: some form of evidence-based individual and group work to address trauma, simultaneously conducted with addiction treatment; behavioral marital therapy for the woman and her husband (or partner); CBT, relapse prevention, and social skills training; participation in 12-step groups (e.g., Narcotics Anonymous); and, as the need arises, interventions to address issues of identity and coping with the stress of racism, drawing on work from the field of multiculturalism. These all constitute very practical steps in making treatment work, given Mrs. Z's characteristics and preferences as a consumer.

In sum, such correlates of addiction need to be addressed, along with the addiction, while drawing upon contemporary evidence-based approaches. The goal is to ensure clinician adherence to a contemporary standard of care embodied in evidence-based approaches, while avoiding discrimination and disparities in service delivery. Ultimately, the goal is to move toward equity in service delivery (Wallace, 2008) so as to maximize positive treatment outcomes with diverse women.

FUTURE DIRECTIONS

Addressing addictions among women of diverse backgrounds requires participation by public health sectors and individual communities. We recommend that future discussions build on the literature reviewed in this chapter so that the historical realities and current psychological experiences of diverse women are explored in the context of addiction, its etiology and outcomes. One way to begin this process is by understanding the role of cumulative stressors, multiple oppressions, and health disparities in the lives of women from diverse backgrounds. Research should also explore the biopsychosociocultural determinants of substance use and addiction among women, particularly the relationships between genetic predisposition to addictions, family and community exposure, and trauma and health sequelae. The treatment of trauma and mental health disorders, including substance use/abuse disorders, must be contextualized within social, political, and systemic domains. Integrated assessments of patient racial and ethnic identity, including religiosity and clinician perspectives in understanding historical correlates of addictions among diverse women must be presented in culturally and linguistically appropriate language. Culturally congruent and contextual treatment models (e.g., urban, suburban, rural) are needed.

KEY POINTS

- Substance abuse in the United States is inextricably connected to historical, social, ethnic and cultural experiences of the diverse women affected by it.
- Integrating ethnicity and culture into the framework of women and addictions is imperative to understand the intricate behavioral, psychological, and medical outcomes of diverse women. Such an understanding also enhances cross-cultural awareness by examining how cultural dynamics inform psychological functioning and sequelae, clinical practice, empirical research, and evidence-based addiction treatment for diverse women.
- Diagnostic criteria for either substance-related or substance-induced disorders must be evaluated in the context of the impact of the individual's culture, and in a manner that includes an awareness of the culture-bound syndromes described in Appendix I of the DSM-IV-TR.
- Key issues that are highly relevant to women of diverse backgrounds include the cultural identity and ethnic reference group, language and customs, cultural explanations of presenting symptoms, individuals' (and their significant others') interpretation of the meaning and severity of those symptoms, and cultural attributions or explanations for the etiology of the symptoms.
- Clinically, it is imperative to understand the cultural expectations that influence the lives of women and for clinicians to ask culturally informed questions of themselves. For example, Mora (2002) suggests the following: What are the historical contributions to the shaming and destructive behaviors of diverse women? Does exploring the impact of ethnic, cultural, and family histories on their current addictive personality or behavior create risks or resilience

among these women? What are the culturally appropriate guidelines for prevention and treatment?

• The correlates of addiction among racially, ethnically, and culturally diverse women have implications for their engagement in treatment and for their receipt of interventions tailored to their characteristics, given individualized assessment findings.

• The diverse correlates of addiction need to be addressed, along with the addiction, while drawing upon contemporary evidence-based approaches. The goal is to ensure clinician adherence to a contemporary standard of care embodied in evidence-based approaches, while avoiding discrimination and disparities in service delivery. Ultimately, the goal is to move toward equity in service delivery (Wallace, 2008) so as to maximize positive treatment outcomes with diverse women.

REFERENCES

Asterisks denote recommended readings.

Acierno, R., Coffey, S. F., & Resnick, H. S. (2003). Introduction to the special issue: Interpersonal violence and substance use problems. *Addictive Behaviors*, *28*(9), 1529–1532.

Agency for Healthcare Research and Quality (2008). *2007 National Healthcare Quality Report*. AHRQ Pub. No. 08-0040. Rockville, MD: U.S. Department of Health and Human Services, Agency for Healthcare Research and Quality.

Akbar, N. (1996). African metapsychology of human personality. In D. A. Azibo (Ed.), *African psychology in historical perspective and related commentary* (pp. 29–45). Trenton, NJ: Africa World Press.

Alba, R. (1990). *Ethnic identity: The transformation of White America*. New Haven, CT: Yale University Press.

Alvidrez, J. (1999). Ethnic variations in mental health attitudes and service use among low-income African American, Latina, and European American young women. *Community Mental Health Journal*, *35*(6), 515–530.

American Psychiatric Association. (2000). *Diagnostic and statistical manual of mental disorders* (4th ed., text rev.). Washington, DC: Author.

Ani, M. (1997). *Let the circle be unbroken: The implication of African spirituality in the diaspora* (4th ed.). Trenton, NJ: Red Sea Press.

Black, S. A., & Markides, K. S. (1993). Acculturation and alcohol consumption in Puerto Rican, Cuban-American, and Mexican-American women in the United States. *American Journal of Public Health*, *83*(6), 890–893.

Blume, A. W.., & de la Cruz, B. G. (2005). Relapse prevention among diverse populations. In A. G. Marlatt & D. M. Donovan (Eds.), *Relapse prevention: Maintenance strategies in the treatment of addictive behaviors* (pp. 45–64). New York: Guilford Press.

Borrell, L. N., & Hatch, S. L. (2005). Racial/ethnic minority and health: The role of the urban environment. In S. Galeo & D. Vlahov (Eds.), *Handbook of urban health: Populations, methods, and practice* (pp. 63–78). New York: Springer.

Bourgois, P., Martinez, A., Kral, A., Edlin, B. R., Schonberg, J., & Ciccarone, D. (2006). Reinterpreting ethnic patterns among white and African American men who inject heroin: A social science of medicine approach. *PLoS Medicine*, *3*(10), e452.

Boyd-Franklin, N. (2000). Families in their cultural and multisystemic contexts. In R. T. Carter (Ed.), *Addressing cultural issues in organizations: Beyond the corporate context* (pp. 89–100). Thousand Oaks, CA: Sage.

Bradshaw, C. K. (1994). Asian and Asian American women: Historical and political considerations in psychotherapy. In L. Comas-Diaz & B. Greene (Eds.), *Women of color: Integrating ethnic and Gender identities in psychotherapy* (pp. 72–113). New York: Guilford Press.

Brome, D. R., Owens, M. D., Allen, K., & Vevaina, T. (2000). An examination of spirituality among

African American women in recovery from substance abuse. *Journal of Black Psychology*, 26(4), 470–486.

Brown, P. J., Read, J. P., & Kahler, C. W. (2003). Comorbid posttraumatic stress disorder and substance use disorders: Treatment outcomes and the role of coping. In P. Ouimette & P. Brown (Eds.), *Trauma and substance abuse: Causes, consequences, and treatment of comorbid disorders* (pp. 171–188). Washington, DC: American Psychological Association.

Carter, R. T. (1995). *The influence of race and racial identity in psychotherapy: Toward a racially inclusive model.* New York: Wiley.

Chesney-Lind, M. (2002). Imprisoning women: The unintended victims of mass imprisonment. In M. Mauer & M. Chesney-Lind (Eds.), *Invisible punishment: The collateral consequences of mass imprisonment.* New York: The New Press.

Chesney-Lind, M., & Pasko, L. (2004). *The female offender: Girls, women and crime* (2nd ed.). Thousand Oaks, CA: Sage.

Chi, I., Lubben, J. E., & Kitano, H. H. L. (1989). Differences in drinking behavior among three Asian-American groups. *Journal of Studies on Alcohol*, 50(1), 15–23.

Cochran, S. D., Mays, V. M., Alegria, M., Ortega, A. N., & Takeuchi, D. (2007). Mental health and substance use disorders among Latino and Asian American lesbian, gay, and bisexual adults. *Journal of Consulting and Clinical Psychology*, 75(5), 785–794.

Collins, R., & McNair, L. D. (2002). Minority women and alcohol use. *Alcohol Research and Health*, 26(4), 251–256.

Comas-Diaz, L., & Greene, B. (Eds.). (1994). *Women of color: Integrating ethnic and gender identities in psychotherapy.* New York: Guilford Press. (*)

Conner, L. C. (2003). *Spiritual, collective and creative coping among black urban youth: The impact of an African-centered worldview* (doctoral dissertation, Columbia University, Teacher's College). *Dissertation Abstracts International*, 64(6-B), 2981.

Constantine, M. G., Lewis, E. L., Conner, L. C., & Sanchez, D. (2000). Addressing spiritual and religious issues in counseling African Americans: Implications for counselor training and practice. *Counseling and Values*, 45, 28–38.

D'Avanzo, C. E., Frye, B., & Froman, R. (1994). Culture, stress and substance use in Cambodian refugee women. *Journal of Studies on Alcohol*, 55(4), 420–426.

De Leon, G., Melnick, G., & Tims, F. M. (2001). The role of motivation and readiness in treatment and recovery. In F. M. Tims, C. G. Leukefeld, & J. J. Platt (Eds.), *Relapse and recovery in addictions* (pp. 143–171). New Haven, CT: Yale University Press.

Drunker, E. M. (2006). Incarcerated people. In B. S. Levy & V. W. Sidel (Eds.), *Social injustice and public health.* New York: Oxford University Press.

Ehrmin, J. T. (2002). "That feeling of not feeling": Numbing the pain for substance-dependent African American women. *Qualitative Health Research*, 2(6), 780–791.

Ferraro, K. K., & Koch, J. R. (1994). Religion and health among Black and White adults: Examining social support and consolation. *Journal for the Scientific Study of Religion*, 33(4), 362–375.

Fleck, D. E., Keck, P. E., Jr., Corey, K. B., & Strakowski, S. M. (2005). Factors associated with medication adherence in African American and white patients with bipolar disorder. *Journal of Clinical Psychiatry*, 66(5), 646–652.

Frame, M. W., & Williams, C. B. (1996). Counseling African Americans: Integrating spirituality in therapy. *Counseling and Values*, 41(1), 16–28.

Gamache, G., Rosenheck, R., & Tessler, R. (2003). Overrepresentation of women veterans among homeless women. *American Journal of Public Health*, 93(7), 1132–1136.

Goldfried, M. R., & Wolfe, B. E. (1996). Psychotherapy practice and research: Repairing a strained relationship. *American Psychologist*, 51(10), 1007–1016.

Grant, B. F., Stinson, F. S., Dawson, D. A., Chou, S. P., Dufour, M. C., Compton, W., et al. (2004). Prevalence and co-occurrence of substance use disorders and independent mood and anxiety disorders: Results from the National Epidemiologic Survey on Alcohol and Related Conditions. *Archives of General Psychiatry*, 61(8), 807–816.

Greene, B. (1994). African American women. In L. Comas-Diaz & B. Greene, (Eds.). *Women of color: Integrating ethnic and gender identities in psychotherapy* (pp. 10–29). New York: Guilford Press.

Haller, D. L., Miles, D. R., & Cropsey, K. L. (2004). Smoking stage of change is associated with retention in a smoke-free residential drug treatment program for women. *Addictive Behaviors, 29*(6), 1265–1270.

Handmaker, N., Packard, M., & Conforti, K. (2002). Motivational interviewing in the treatment of dual disorders. In W. R. Miller & S. Rollnick, *Motivational interviewing: Preparing people for change* (2nd ed., pp. 362–376). New York: Guilford Press.

Haney, C. (2006). *Reforming punishment: Psychological limits to the pains of imprisonment*. Washington, DC: American Psychological Association.

Harrison, P. M., & Beck, A. J. (2003). *Prisoners in 2002*. Bureau of Justice Statistics, Washington, DC: U.S. Department of Justice.

Heinz, A., Epstein, D. H., & Preston, K. L. (2007). Spiritual/religious experiences and in-treatment outcome in an inner-city program for heroin and cocaine dependence. *Journal of Psychoactive Drugs, 39*(1), 41–49.

Holmstedt, K. (2007). *Band of sisters: American women at war in Iraq*. Mechanicsburg, PA: Stackpole Books.

Howard, D. L. (2003). Culturally competent treatment of African American clients among a national sample of outpatient substance abuse treatment units. *Journal of Substance Abuse Treatment, 24*, 89–102.

Hoyert, D. L., Kung, H. C., & Smith, B. L. (2005). Deaths: Preliminary data for 2003. *National Vital Statistics Report, 53*(15), 1–48. Available at *http://www.cdc.gov/nchs/pressroom/05facts/lifeexpectancy.htm*.

Joe, K. A. (1996). The lives and times of Asian-Pacific American women drug users: An ethnographic study of their methamphetamine use. *Journal of Drug Issues, 26*(1), 199–218.

Juby, H., & Concepción, W. (2005). Ethnicity: The term and its meaning. In R. T. Carter (Eds.), *The handbook for racial–cultural psychology and counseling: Theory and research* (pp. 26–40). Hoboken, NJ: Wiley.

Kitano, K. J., & Louie, L. J. (2002). Asian and Pacific Islander women and addiction. In S. L. A. Straussner & S. Brown (Eds.), *The handbook of addiction treatment for women: Theory and practice* (pp. 348–374). San Francisco: Jossey-Bass.

LaFramboise, T. D., Trimble, J. E., & Mohatt, G. V. (1995). Counseling intervention and American Indian tradition: An integrative approach. In R. Hornby (Ed.), *Alcohol and Native Americans* (pp. 149–169). Mission, SD: Sinte Gleska University Press.

Landsberg, G., Rock, M., Berg, L. K. W., & Smiley, A. (Eds.). (2002). *Serving mentally ill offenders: Challenges and opportunities for mental health professionals*. New York: Springer.

Locke, T. F., & Newcomb, M. D. (2003). Childhood maltreatment, parental alcohol/drug-related problems, and global parental dysfunction. *Professional Psychology: Research and Practice, 34*(1), 73–79.

Lowery, C. T. (1998). American Indian perspective on addiction and recovery. *Health and Social Work, 23*(2), 127–135.

McLellan, A. (2003). What's the harm in discussing harm reduction: An introduction to a three-paper series. *Journal of Substance Abuse Treatment, 25*(4), 239–240.

Marger, M. N. (1997). *Race and ethnic relations: American and global perspectives*. Belmont, CA: Wadsworth.

Marlatt, G. A. (1985). Abstinence and controlled drinking: Alternative treatment goals for alcoholism and problem drinking? *Bulletin of the Society of Psychologists in Addictive Behaviors, 4*(3), 123–150.

Marlatt, G. A. (1998). *Harm reduction: Pragmatic strategies for managing high-risk behaviors*. New York: Guilford Press.

Marlatt, G. A. (1999). From hindsight to foresight: A commentary on Project MATCH. In J. A. Tucker, D. M. Donovan, & G. A. Marlatt (Eds.), *Changing addictive behavior: Bridging clinical and public health strategies* (pp. 45–66). New York: Guilford Press.

Marlatt, G. A., & Donovan, D. M. (Eds.). (2005). *Relapse prevention: Maintenance strategies in the treatment of addictive behaviors* (2nd ed.). New York: Guilford Press.

Marlatt, G. A., & Gordon, J. R. (1985). *Relapse prevention: Maintenance strategies in the treatment of addictive behaviors*. New York: Guilford Press.

Mattis, J. S. (2002). Religion and spirituality in the meaning-making and coping experiences of African American women: A qualitative analysis. *Psychology of Women Quarterly*, 26(4), 309–321.

McLellan, A. T. (2003). Crime and punishment and treatment: Latest findings in the treatment of drug-related offenders. *Journal of Substance Abuse Treatment*, 25, 187–188.

Miller, W. R., & Hester, R. K. (2003). Treating alcohol problems: Toward an informed eclecticism. In R. K. Hester & W. R. Miller (Eds.), *Handbook of alcoholism treatment approaches: Effective alternatives* (3rd ed., pp. 1–12). Boston: Allyn & Bacon.

Miller, W. R., & Rollnick, S. (2002). *Motivational interviewing: Preparing people for change.* New York: Guilford Press.

Moos, R. (2002, August). Addictive disorders in context: Principles and puzzles of effective treatment and recovery. An invited address at the 110th convention of the American Psychological Association, Chicago, IL.

Moos, R. (2003). Addictive disorders in context: Principles and puzzles of effective treatment and recovery. *Psychology of Addictive Behaviors*, 17(1), 3–12.

Mora, J. (2002). Latinas in cultural transition: Addiction, treatment, and recovery. In S. L. A. Straussner & S. Brown (Eds.), *The handbook of addiction treatment for women* (pp. 323–347). San Francisco: Jossey-Bass.

Najavits, L. M., Runkel, R., Neuner, C., Frank, A. F., Thase, M. E., Crits-Christoph, P., et al. (2003). Rates and symptoms of PTSD among cocaine-dependent patients. *Journal of Studies on Alcohol*, 64(5), 601–606.

Napholz, L. (2000). Balancing multiple roles among a group of urban midlife American Indian working women. *Health Care for Women International*, 21(4), 255–266.

National Institute on Drug Abuse. (1999). *Principles of drug addiction treatment: A research-based guide*, U.S. Department of Health and Human Services, NIH Publication No. 99-4180. Bethesda, MD: National Institute on Drug Abuse.

National Institute on Drug Abuse. (2003). *Drug use among racial/ethnic minorities.* National Institutes of Health, Publication No. 03-3888. Available at *www.drugabuse.gov/pdf/minorities03.pdf.* (*)

Office of Research on Women's Health. (2006). *Women of color health data book* (3rd ed.). National Institutes of Health, Publication No. 06-4247. *orwh.od.nih.gov/pubs/WomenofColor2006.pdf.* (*)

Ouimette, P., & Brown, P. J. (Eds.). (2003). *Trauma and substance abuse: Causes, consequences, and treatment of comorbid disorders.* Washington, DC: American Psychological Association.

Palepu, A., Horton, N. J., Tibbetts, N., Dukes, K., Meli, S., & Samet, J. H. (2003). Substance abuse treatment and emergency department utilization among a cohort of HIV-infected persons with alcohol problems. *Journal of Substance Abuse Treatment*, 25(1), 37–42.

Parrott, D. J., Drobes, D. J., Saladin, M. E., Coffey, S. F., & Dansky, B. S. (2003). Perpetration of partner violence: Effects of cocaine and alcohol dependence and posttraumatic stress disorder. *Addictive Behaviors*, 28(9), 1587–1602.

Paz, J. (2002). Culturally competent substance abuse treatment with Latinas. *Journal of Human Behavior in the Social Environment*, 5(3–4), 123–126.

Phinney, J. S. (1996). When we talk about American ethnic groups, what do we mean? *American Psychologist*, 51(9), 918–927.

Pinderhughes, E. (1989). *Understanding race, ethnicity, and power: The key to efficacy in clinical practice.* New York: Free Press.

Prochaska, J. O., & DiClemente, C. C. (1983). Stages and processes of self-change of smoking: Toward an integrative model of change. *Journal of Consulting and Clinical Psychology*, 51(3), 390–395.

Riggs, D. S., Rukstalis, M., Volpicelli, J. R., Kalmanson, D., & Foa, E. B. (2003). Demographic and social adjustment characteristics of patients with comorbid posttraumatic stress disorder and alcohol dependence: Potential pitfalls to PTSD treatment. *Addictive Behaviors*, 28(9), 1717–1730.

Saylors, K. (2003). The Women's Circle comes full circle. *Journal of Psychoactive Drugs*, 35(1), 59–62.

Schnurr, P. P., Friedman, M. J., Engel, C. C., Foa, E. B., Shea, M. T., Chow, B. K., et al. (2008). Cognitive behavioral therapy for posttraumatic stress disorder in women: A randomized controlled trial. *Journal of the American Medical Association*, 297(8), 820–830.

Shoultz, J., Tanner, B., & Harrigan, R. (2000). Culturally appropriate guidelines for alcohol and drug abuse prevention. *Nurse Practitioner*, 25(11), 50–56.

Strathdee, S. A. (2003). Sexual HIV transmission in the context of injection drug use: Implications for interventions. *International Journal of Drug Policy*, *14*(1), 79–81.

Straussner, S. L. A., & Attia, P. R. (2002). Women's addiction and treatment through a historical lens. In S. L. A. Straussner & S. Brown (Eds.), *The handbook of addiction treatment for women: Theory and practice* (pp. 3–25). San Francisco: Jossey-Bass.

Straussner, S. L. A., & Brown, S. (Eds.). (2002). *The handbook of addiction treatment for women: Theory and practice*. San Francisco, CA: Jossey-Bass. (*)

Stuart, G. L., Moore, T. M., Ramsey, S. E., & Kahler, C. W. (2003). Relationship aggression and substance use among women court-referred to domestic violence intervention programs. *Addictive Behaviors*, *28*(9), 1603–1610.

Substance Abuse and Mental Health Services Administration. (2008). Results from the 2007 National Survey on Drug Use and Health: National Findings. Rockville, MD: Office of Applied Studies, NSDUH Series H-34, DHHS Publication No. SMA 08-4343.

Substance Abuse and Mental Health Services Administration. (2006). *Treatment Episode Data Set (TEDS). Highlights—2005. National Admissions to Substance Abuse Treatment Services.* Rockville, MD: Office of Applied Studies, DASIS Series: S-36, DHHS Publication No. (SMA) 07-4229.

Substance Abuse and Mental Health Services Administration. (2007). *Results from the 2006 National Survey on Drug Use and Health: National Findings.* Rockville, MD: Office of Applied Studies, NSDUH Series H-32, DHHS Publication No. SMA 07-4293.

Sue, D. W., Capodilupo, C. M., Torino, G. C., Bucceri, J. M., Holder, A. M., Nadal, K. L., et al. (2007). Racial microaggressions in everyday life: Implications for clinical practice. *American Psychologist*, *62*(4), 271–286.

Sue, D. W., Carter, R. T., Casas, J., Fouad, N. A., Ivey, A. E., Jensen, M., et al. (1998). *Multicultural counseling competencies: Individual and organizational development*. Thousand Oaks, CA: Sage.

Sue, D. W., & Sue, D. (2003). *Counseling the culturally diverse: Theory and practice* (4th ed.). New York: Wiley.

Tatarsky, A. (2003). Harm reduction by psychotherapy: Extending the reach of traditional substance use treatment. *Journal of Substance Abuse Treatment*, *25*, 249–256.

Timpson, S. C., Williams, M. L., Bowen, A. M., & Keel, K. (2003). Condom use behaviors in HIV-infected African American crack cocaine users. *Substance Abuse*, *24*(4), 211–220.

Trepper, T. S., Nelson, T. S., McCollum, E. E., & McAvoy, P. A. (1997). Improving substance abuse service delivery to Hispanic women through increased cultural competencies. *Journal of Substance Abuse Treatment*, *14*(3), 225–234.

Vasquez, M. J. (1994). Latinas. In L. Comas-Diaz & B. Greene (Eds.), *Women of color: Integrating ethnic and gender identities in psychotherapy* (pp. 114–138). New York: Guilford Press.

Velasquez, M. M., Maurer, G. G., Crouch, C., & DiClemente, C. C. (2001). *Group treatment for substance abuse: A stages-of-change therapy manual.* New York: Guilford Press.

Wallace, B. C. (2005). *Making mandated treatment work.* New York: Jason Aronson.

Wallace, B. C. (Ed.). (2008). *Toward equity in health: A new global approach to health disparities.* New York: Springer.

Wallace, B. C., Carter, R. T., Nanin, J. E., Keller, R., & Alleyne, V. (2003). Identity development for "diverse and different others": Integrating stages of change, motivational interviewing, and identity theories for race, people of color, sexual orientation, and disability. In B. C. Wallace & R. T. Carter (Eds.), *Understanding and dealing with violence: A multicultural approach* (pp. 41–92). Thousand Oaks, CA: Sage.

Westermeyer, J. (1995). Cultural aspects of substance abuse and alcoholism: Assessment and management. *Psychiatric Clinics of North America*, *18*(3), 589–605.

Witherspoon, K. M., & Richardson, A. W. (2006). Sisters in support together against substances (SISTAS): An alcohol abuse prevention group for black women. *Journal of Ethnicity in Substance Abuse*, *5*(3), 49–60.

Wyatt, G. E. (1997). *Stolen women: Reclaiming our sexuality, taking back our lives.* New York: Wiley.

CHAPTER 28

Substance Use Disorders among Sexual-Minority Women

Thomas W. Irwin, PhD

Until the mid-1990s, the addiction treatment literature focused almost exclusively on men, and differences in etiology, course, and treatment went uninvestigated. During the past 15 years, there has been an increased effort to better understand substance use disorders (SUDs) and addiction treatment among women and how it may differ in comparison to men (Greenfield et al., 2007). A similar disparity, if not more extreme, exists in the addiction treatment literature focused on SUDs among sexual minorities. Since the early 1990s, there has been a significant amount of research investigating the relationship between SUDs and HIV risk taking among gay men (Stall, Hays, Waldo, Ekstrand, & McFarland, 2000). By comparison, there have been very few studies that have investigated substance use and SUDs among sexual-minority women exclusively.

The primary goal of this chapter is to provide an overview of the literature on addiction among sexual-minority women. The factors that are unique to this population are presented in terms of etiology, epidemiology, and best practices for the treatment of addiction. While this remains an understudied population, during the past decade, researchers and clinicians have gained a somewhat better understanding of substance use and misuse and SUDs among lesbians and bisexual women and how to best meet the treatment needs of this group.

SOCIAL IDENTITY AND SEXUAL BEHAVIOR

Researchers use a variety of terms to define sexual minorities. Depending on the nature of the research, studies may include participants across the spectrum of sexual minorities: lesbian women, gay men, and bisexual men and women, and individuals identifying as transgendered (LGBT). The collective LGBT population is extraordinarily heterogeneous, however, and recognizing this diversity is an important starting point in any review of how substance use, abuse, and dependence impact this population. This chapter focuses primarily on lesbian and bisexual women, with comparisons made to heterosexual women and, at times, gay and bisexual men. Although those who identify as transgendered are referenced within the context of the larger community in this chapter, it is worth noting that there is an extremely limited amount of research regarding addiction within this specific group. Therefore, at present, there is insufficient information to address SUDs within the transgendered population in this chapter.

The addiction treatment literature, as in all areas of behavioral heath, is inconsistent in how sexual-minority women are defined, and, depending on the study, the definition of the sample may include either sexual behavior or sexual identity but usually not both. Unfortunately, the lack of specificity, usually in defining differences between behavior and identity, is one of the largest problems in addiction research and behavioral health studies with this population. One of the challenges of interpreting existing research findings involves the lack of consistency across studies in terms of how samples are defined and the extent to which results and the interpretation of those results generalize to the larger population of sexual-minority women.

"Sexual orientation" generally refers to the target of one's desire for sexual, physical, and emotional intimacy, which may be toward women, men, or both. Although an individual's sexual orientation may fluctuate over time, it is generally believed that one cannot choose his or her orientation. How these desires are expressed through behavior is yet another construct that may or may not be congruent with sexual orientation. Although an individual may be oriented toward same-sex relationships, because of the burden of stigma and discrimination, he or she may choose to pursue opposite-sex relationships. Similarly, if he or she is oriented toward opposite-sex relationships and there are no outlets for expressing these desires, the individual may engage in same-sex relationships.

Sexual identity is a more complicated, multidimensional construct which includes how individuals incorporate sexual orientation and sexual experience into their perceptions of self and how they integrate these elements with other aspects of their social identity. To identify as a lesbian or gay person suggests some acculturation into the lesbian/gay community and some awareness of its culture and history. If a large sample were taken of women who have had or intend to have sex with women, there would be a wide range in how those individuals group identified themselves. These could include lesbian, "gay woman," bisexual, or "queer." It would also include women who identify as heterosexual.

In defining their identity, sexual minorities face numerous struggles. Sexual minorities are required to cope with discrimination that continues to be socially sanctioned and vindicated through legislation from federal, state, and local governments (Herek, 1989). Unlike racial and ethnic minorities, sexual minorities do not generally mature in an environment where there are models for coping with discrimination based on sexual orientation. Unfortunately, the process of "coming out" also has negative consequences and is associated with increased levels of discrimination (Craw, Fok, & Hartman, 1998).

The process of sexual identity development is referred to as "coming out" and is most often characterized as a process that unfolds through stages (Cass, 1979; Coleman, 1982). Generally, the process involves recognizing same-sex sexual orientation, increasing acceptance of the orientation, disclosing to others, and increasing association with, and integration into, LGBT culture. Through the process, individuals must cope with and manage homophobia, both their own and from external sources, including family and the larger society. Ultimately, the sexual orientation is integrated into the individual's sense of self along with other aspects of identity. It is important to consider, too, that LGBT individuals may not "come out" in all environments (e.g., professional, academic, family). They may instead choose not to disclose in situations when criticism or discrimination might be expected. Because of this lack of disclosure, LGBT individuals are generally underrepresented in most settings, which is one reason why it is a difficult population to study. LGBT individuals are more "hidden" or "invisible" compared to ethnic and racial minority groups.

EPIDEMIOLOGY

Survey Methods and External Validity

Another challenge to researchers is to develop methodologies that will allow for investigating differences in SUDs among sexual-minority women based on both identity and sexual behavior. To understand the factors that impact the etiology, epidemiology, and treatment of SUDs among sexual-minority women, it is important to recognize that assessing both sexual behaviors and sexual identity is critical (Young & Meyer, 2003). One of the difficulties of interpreting existing research findings involves the lack of consistency across studies in terms of how samples are defined and the extent to which results and the interpretation of those results generalize to larger populations. To the extent possible, the research question should be considered carefully and should inform assessment decisions. For example, if hypotheses relate to sexual behaviors specifically, excluding women who have sex with women but do not identify as lesbian might alter important findings. However, if the research question focuses on effects of discrimination, creating groups based on identity may be the most relevant choice, regardless of sexual activity.

The difficulty of this challenge is underscored by the results of a recent study. A population-based probability sample was used to compare sexual-minority women with heterosexual women (Drabble & Trocki, 2005). The number of research participants who identified as heterosexual and had same-sex partners (1.8%) in the past 5 years outnumbered lesbian-identified women (0.9%) by almost 2 to 1. Bisexual-identified women (1.3%) outnumbered lesbians in this sample as well. This study found important differences between groups that would have been overlooked if all sexual-minority participants were combined and compared to "exclusively heterosexual women."

Alcohol Use

There has been a slow but positive progression toward a better understanding of the nature and significance of alcohol use disorders (AUDs) among lesbians and bisexual women. To a great extent, this progress is due to increased methodological rigor during the past decade. As Cochran (2001) points out, questions that assess sexual behavior or identity have only recently been included in large-scale surveys used for estimating prevalence of mental health morbidity, including AUDs, and because of this several studies have been published during the past decade that have included probability sampling methodology.

Early studies tended to rely on recruiting samples from the community taken from venues where LGBT individuals gathered or socialized. Often referred to as "convenience sampling," these studies were nonprobability surveys that were likely very biased toward sexual minorities that identified as lesbian or gay and who had high levels of community involvement and higher levels of substance use. Although now over a decade old, the most comprehensive review of problem drinking among lesbian and gay men was completed by Bux (1996), and it provided a very thorough review of study findings and a good summary of the methodological problems of these studies. Stressed in this review is the concern that early research likely overestimated alcohol use among LGBT individuals because of sampling bias.

In summarizing the patterns of alcohol use and prevalence of AUDs among LGBT individuals, Bux found that lesbians and gay men were less likely than heterosexual men and women to abstain from drinking. Whereas lesbians were more likely to be heavy drinkers compared to heterosexual women, this was not found for gay men in comparison to heterosexual men. Bux also suggested that drinking among gay men had declined during the previous decade, perhaps due to a community response to HIV.

The results of the population-based survey studies on alcohol use among sexual-minority women have been generally consistent in supporting earlier findings indicating that this population has a significantly higher risk of problem drinking than heterosexual women. Using data from a national survey, Cochran and Mays (2000a) found that women who reported having sex with women (WSW) reported using alcohol more frequently and in greater amounts and also experienced greater alcohol-related morbidity than exclusively heterosexually active women. In that same year, Valanis et al. (2000) reported on a study involving a national population-based sampling strategy that included more than 90,000 women 50–79 years. Results indicated that sexual minority women were more likely to drink alcohol. Diamant, Wold, Spritzer, and Gelberg (2000) found similar results using data ($n =$ 4,697) gathered in California. In this study, lesbians and bisexual women were more likely than heterosexual women to report any alcohol consumption. Lesbians, but not bisexual women, were more likely than heterosexual women to drink heavily.

In another study using data from California ($n = 11,204$), Burgard, Cochran, and Mays (2005) found that WSW were higher than heterosexual women on a variety of alcohol use indices. WSW were more likely to consume alcohol at least weekly, drink on more days per month, drink more drinks per drinking day, experience more binge-drinking days per month, and report more binge-drinking behavior.

It has been a rare instance when sexual identity and sexual behaviors are included in epidemiological studies of SUDs in sexual minorities. Drabble and Trocki (2005) categorized women into four groups: lesbian identified, bisexual identified, exclusively heterosexual, and heterosexual-identified women who had sex with women. The demographic variables of age, ethnicity, relationship status (partnered or not partnered), median income, and educational level were controlled for in these analyses. Comparing across groups, results indicated that heterosexual women who reported no same-sex sexual partners were less likely to be heavy drinkers compared to the other three groups. In analyzing mean number of drinks per year, the only significant difference between groups was that exclusively heterosexual women drank less as compared to heterosexual-identified women who reported some same-sex sexual experiences. Lesbian- and bisexual-identified women were more likely than heterosexual-identified women to have experienced negative consequences related to drinking, to endorse alcohol dependence criteria, and to have participated in alcohol treatment.

One of the few population-based studies that did not find differences between sexual-minority women and heterosexual women was one of the first published (Bloomfield, 1993). In a household sample ($n = 395$) from San Francisco, no significant differences were found in levels of drinking between lesbian/bisexual women and heterosexual women. The study was not without its limitations, however, as behavioral anchors were not used to define differences between light, moderate, and heavy drinking. The study also had limited power to detect differences due to small sample size.

Drug Use

Estimates of the extent of drug use, abuse, and dependence among lesbians and bisexual women have been rarer than for drinking. Skinner (1994) conducted one of the first studies of drug use among lesbian and gay men from two metropolitan areas of a Southern state. In comparing lesbians and gay men, results of the study showed that lesbians were more likely to use marijuana, stimulants, sedatives, and tranquilizers than gay men, and were more likely to report lifetime, illicit-drug use. Few comparisons were made to the general population in this study, but prevalence rates across most drugs were higher for both lesbians and gay men. Cochran and Mays (2000a) found that WSW were more likely to show evidence of drug dependency than women who reported having sex only with men, although data on specific drugs were not analyzed. In another national survey, WSW were more likely to report marijuana and analgesic use compared to exclusively heterosexual women. Differences were greater between groups for lifetime drug use than when comparing recent use (Cochran, Ackerman, Mays, & Ross, 2004).

Scheer et al. (2002) investigated drug use among younger women (ages 18–29; n = 2,547) in low-income neighborhoods in Northern California. Findings indicated that women who reported having sex with women, compared to women who had sex only with men, were more likely to report past and recent injection drug use. In a survey of sexual-minority women in California (n = 2,011), drug use was very common, with one-third of the sample using marijuana during the past year (Corliss, Grella, Mays, & Cochran, 2006). Although this study did not compare lesbians to heterosexual women, the rates of drug use were elevated and were estimated to be five times higher than the women in the general population. In surveying psychiatric disorders, two studies found that responders who had same-sex sexual experiences had a higher 12-month prevalence of SUDs (Gilman et al., 2001; Sandfort, de Graaf, Bijl, & Schnabel, 2001). Drabble and Trocki (2005) compared heterosexual-identified women who had sex only with men to lesbian, bisexual, and heterosexual-identified women who had sex with women. Compared to exclusively heterosexual women, all other groups were more likely to report marijuana use, with lesbians reporting the highest rates. There were no differences between groups on rates of other drug use.

Nicotine Use

Although there are limited data on nicotine use among LGBT individuals, research in the area points to higher levels of tobacco use. A review of the smoking literature among this population (Ryan, Wortley, Easton, Pederson, & Greenwood, 2001) included eight studies, most of which included sexual-minority women, and found that the prevalence of smoking among lesbians and bisexual women ranged from 11 to 50%, and in gay and bisexual men from 25 to 50%. With only one exception, each study reviewed showed an increased rate of smoking above comparison groups of heterosexuals or compared to the general population for both gay men and lesbians. An important point that the authors make is that the LGBT samples in these studies can largely be characterized as demographically different in favor of reduced smoking compared to the general population. In particular, education level, which has a strong inverse relationship with smoking, was higher, on average, among LGBT samples. This review found that although LGBT individuals were, in general, college educated, smoking rates were found to be comparable to high school graduates in the general population.

Additional studies across both population-based samples (Burgard et al., 2005; Diamant & Wold, 2003; Gruskin, Hart, Gordon, & Ackerson, 2001) and community-based samples (Aaron et al., 2001; Cochran et al., 2001; Mays, Yancey, Cochran, Weber, & Fielding, 2002; Sanchez, Meacher, & Beil, 2005) have shown consistent and significantly elevated rates of smoking for lesbians and bisexual women, as compared to heterosexual women in the general population.

Summary

The evidence for increased rates of substance use and SUDs among sexual-minority women is clear. Although more research is needed to draw firm conclusions, it appears that sexual-minority women are at higher risk for drinking, drug use, and smoking across the lifespan.

Research among adolescents suggests that problems with alcohol and drugs may be more prominent for adolescent lesbians (Remafedi, 1987; Rotheram-Borus, Hunter, & Rosario, 1994). High school students who identify as gay, lesbian, or bisexual were more likely to smoke, drink alcohol, and use drugs than those who identified as heterosexual (Garofalo, Wolf, Kessel, Palfrey, & DuRant, 1998). In a study investigating a wide range of age groups, Burgard et al. (2005) found the greatest difference in levels of drinking between WSW and women who reported having sex only with men were in the age group of 26–35. In testing differences between sexual-minority women and heterosexual women, significant differences have been found in midlife and for those 50–79 (Mays & Cochran, 2001; Valanis et al., 2000).

While sexual minority women may have a higher prevalence of SUDs, data also indicate that they are more likely than heterosexual women to seek professional help for addictions, use mental health services, and seek professional services when experiencing psychiatric syndromes (Cochran & Mays, 2000a; Cochran, Sullivan, & Mays, 2003). Although Bloomfield (1993) did not find differences when comparing drinking patterns between lesbians and heterosexual women, a higher number of lesbians identified as being in recovery. This was a significant finding, in spite of little statistical power to detect differences.

Although these studies have provided very important contributions, there is still much to explore. A summary of the results do not conclude with certainty which subgroups, particularly in regard to sexual identity, might have the most severe problems with SUDs. It is unfortunate indeed that, in general, studies that have utilized the best methodology for both probability sampling techniques and assessment of alcohol and drug use measures have also suffered from a lack of specificity regarding sexual identity and have relied almost exclusively on sexual behavior as the basis of creating comparison groups. In doing so, there is a significant loss in the ability to understand how the use of tobacco, alcohol, and drugs differs depending on the cultural and social context in which it occurs in this very diverse group of women.

RISK FACTORS

Numerous factors have been hypothesized to increase vulnerability to SUDs among lesbian and bisexual women relative to women generally. While some of these factors are also associated with elevated drinking in heterosexual women, this chapter focuses primarily on influences specific to intrapersonal, interpersonal, and sociocultural factors that are unique to minority status and which are likely to increase vulnerability to SUDs. Increasingly, data point to sexual-minority stress as a powerful mechanism in the development of both psychological distress and psychiatric and substance use problems (Meyer, 2003).

There is a growing body of evidence that suggests that discrimination, victimization, and sexual-minority stress may have very large consequences for the subsequent development of both SUDs and other mental health problems, and the evidence is clear that sexual minorities endure traumatic events at significantly higher rates compared to heterosexual counterparts (Meyer, 1995). For many, these experiences begin at a young age. Children and adolescents who express, or are interpreted by peers to have, a sexual-minority orientation and those who exhibit gender-role nonconformity have dramatically higher rates of trauma in both home and school environments (Balsam, Beauchaine, Mickey, & Rothblum, 2005). Research indicates that LGBT youths are often the victim of attacks, from verbal harassment to physical assault (D'Augelli & Dark, 1994; Dean, Wu, & Martin, 1992; Rivers & D'Augelli, 2001). Disclosure of sexual orientation or coming out in the high school context and gender atypical dress and behaviors are associated with increased frequency of victimization within the school environment. School avoidance is higher among LGBT youths. Garofalo et al. (1998) found in one study that 25% of LGBT students in high school reported missing school because of fear of victimization in the past month, compared to 5% of heterosexual students.

LGBT individuals are more likely to report psychological and physical victimization in childhood and in adulthood. Further, gay men, in particular, are more likely to experience sexual assaults than heterosexual men. Balsam et al. (2005) investigated lifetime victimization by comparing LGBT with heterosexual siblings. Results indicated that LBGT siblings were more likely to be victimized at home by parents (psychological and physical abuse), experience childhood sexual abuse, and experience more psychological and physical victimization by partners as adults.

Research suggests that lesbians are more likely to be victimized by a partner than gay men. Compared to heterosexual women, lesbians may be just as likely to be in abusive relationships, although differences may exist in the nature of abuse between lesbians and heterosexuals (Waldner-Haugrud, Gratch, & Magruder, 1997). Psychological and verbal abuse may be more prevalent among lesbians than among heterosexual women, with estimates of 70–90% reporting psychological abuse in their relationships (Lockhart, White, Causby, & Isaac, 1994; Renzetti, 1989). Lie and Gentlewarrier (1991) found that both psychological and physical abuse were more commonly seen together in lesbian relationships than psychological abuse alone or physical abuse alone.

Although causal links from overt discrimination and experiences of discrimination and victimization are difficult to attribute to the development of SUDs, several studies have found strong associations between the two. Mays and Cochran (2001) found that LGBT individuals were more likely to experience discrimination (both lifetime and day to day). Forty-two percent of LGBT individuals who experience discrimination attribute this discrimination to sexual orientation. Perceived discrimination was positively associated with reduced quality of life and with indicators of psychiatric morbidity (Kessler, Mickelson, & Williams, 1999).

Adversity and stress are strongly associated with increased levels of distress and psychological functioning as well as exacerbating psychiatric disorders within minorities generally (Dohrenwend, 2000) and sexual minorities specifically (Gilman et al., 2001; Mays & Cochran, 2001). As has been demonstrated, lesbians and bisexual women have a significantly higher rate of substance use and dependence. Sexual minorities also have higher elevations of mood and anxiety disorders (Gilman et al., 2001; Sandfort et al., 2001), levels of psychological distress (Warner et al., 2004), and rates of suicidality (Cochran & Mays, 2000b; Gilman et al., 2001; Paul et al., 2002).

A variety of social structures may not cause but may perpetuate heavy substance use among lesbians and bisexual women. Social outlets have traditionally been very limited. Gay and lesbian bars have been settings where LGBT individuals are able to socialize with others without fear of scrutiny or ostracism. It has often been suggested that reliance on bars as social outlets increases the risk of heavy drinking and the development of SUDs. While an association between bar going and heavy drinking for lesbians exists (Heffernan, 1998), a causal relationship is difficult to demonstrate without prospective studies, and these have not been conducted.

The past 20 years have witnessed the emergence of a growing number of alcohol-free social outlets (coffee shops and restaurants), outside of bar environments, for LGBT individuals in large urban areas. During this same period, however, alcohol, tobacco, and pharmaceutical companies, recognizing a potentially very profitable market in the LGBT community, have developed very aggressive strategies in promoting use of their products. In 2001 a document was revealed to the media that had been developed by R. J. Reynolds as a project to increase market share of Camel cigarettes among both the LGBT community in the Castro section of San Francisco and the homeless population in the Tenderloin. The "Sub Culture Urban Marketing Project," also known by the acronym Project SCUM, was discovered by Anne Landman of the American Lung Association of Colorado and the story published by the *San Francisco Weekly* (Smith & Malone, 2003). During the past 10 years, it has become common for LGBT events to be sponsored by alcohol companies, including fund raising and gay pride events. This turn of events is particularly troubling, given the difficulty of finding LGBT social venues that are alcohol free. The heightened visibility of these companies in the LGBT community has raised the concern of community leaders about the ethics of marketing these products to an already vulnerable population (Drabble, 2001).

While causal links between these environmental factors and the development of SUDs have not been demonstrated among LGBT populations, minority stress and the challenge of maintaining an identity that is highly stigmatized have been shown to have a negative impact on psychological functioning and quality of life. In addition to the challenge that these may pose to LGBT individuals, it may also be that there are fewer social structures that provide protective factors for these individuals.

It is generally thought that lesbians and gay men have few social structures that provide support for "maturing out" of heavy drinking (Bux, 1995). While change is occurring in small areas of the country, same-sex relationships are not a socially sanctioned institution, and same-sex couples have considerably more challenges, in some cases impossible legal or financial barriers, for having children through adoption or surrogacy. Klaas-Jan and Knibble (1998) note that marriage and parental roles serve as stabilizing factors. These authors point out that there is a complex relationship among social, family, and career roles/obligations and the impact these have on drinking for women generally, and research has not been conducted to illuminate how these factors may impact levels of drinking among lesbians and bisexual women.

TREATMENT

During the past 30 years, there has been a dramatic change in how lesbians and gay men are perceived by mental health service providers. In 1973 Robert Spitzer led the effort within the American Psychiatric Association to remove homosexuality as a clinical disorder from the *Diagnostic and Statistical Manual of Mental Disorders* (Spitzer, 1981). The American Psychological Association followed 2 years later with a resolution supporting the decision. Professional organizations across disciplines, including the National Association of Social Workers and the American Association for Marriage and Family Therapy, have embraced the need for culturally appropriate treatment for LGBT patients.

In spite of these changes, there are still considerable barriers that need to be addressed. The reality of these barriers might be best emphasized by the fact that there continues to be a debate over the ethics of "reparative" or "conversion" therapy (Wainberg, 2004). In spite of a lack of a theoretical basis or evidence of effectiveness, proponents of conversion therapy suggest that treatment for homosexuality is appropriate and effective in converting sexual orientation and identity toward heterosexuality (Rosik, 2003; Spitzer, 2004). There remain professionals across all disciplines who actively treat homosexuality as a pathological condition that can and should be changed (Nicolosi, 1994).

The slow change in attitudes by mental health professionals is demonstrated by a study investigating attitudes among psychologists (Garnets, Hancock, Cochran, Goodchilds, & Peplau, 1991). This study identified numerous harmful practices used by psychologists that were incongruent with the ethical principles identified by the American Psychological Association ethical guidelines. Fifty-eight percent of psychologists surveyed were aware of negative incidents involving colleagues that defined lesbians and gay men as pathological, including instances when the focus on sexuality interfered with treating the individual for the primary presenting problem. A study of psychoanalysts (Lilling & Friedman, 1995) identified a negative bias toward homosexual patients, particularly those with serious psychopathology.

There are relatively few published data specific to addiction treatment in terms of the progress toward culturally competent services. What little there is does not suggest that much progress has been made. In an early study, Weathers (1980) found that most addiction treatment programs had negative attitudes about lesbians and did not provide adequate services; these programs either limited or refused services altogether or provided treatment focused on changing sexuality and ignoring the addiction. In conducting a survey of government-funded addiction treatment programs, Hellman (1989) found that drug and alcohol counselors had a very limited understanding of how to assess and treat gay and lesbian clients with alcohol and drug problems. Further, the amount of training and supervision providers received in treating sexual minorities was virtually nonexistent. These results were replicated in a more recent study. Eliason (2000) found that counselors had very little formal education on working with LGBT clients, and they lacked knowledge about legal issues and family issues specific to this population. Almost half had negative or ambivalent attitudes about gays and lesbians.

In a study comparing counselors from urban versus rural settings, Eliason and Hughes (2004) found that although urban counselors had more contact with LGBT clients and had more training about LGBT issues, they did not have more positive attitudes or report more knowledge about LBG issues. Counselors had negative or ambivalent attitudes about LGBT clients in this study as well.

Similar findings come from another study that attempted to identify factors that predict affirmative treatment among addiction counselors. Interestingly, level of education was not a significant predictor of affirmative treatment practices—which likely indicates that if there is formal training for providing affirmative or culturally sensitive LGBT treatment for graduate-level therapists, effects of such training were not demonstrated in this study. Women counselors were more affirmative about LGBT issues than male counselors, and more experience as a counselor predicted higher levels of affirmative treatment (Eliason, 2000). One of the strongest predictors of affirmative therapy was at the organizational level, indicating that the environment in which the counselor works may have a greater positive effect on the client than counselor-specific attributes.

It is clear from the evidence that addiction treatment programs are ill-equipped to provide appropriate treatment for sexual-minority women and often assume that women (and men) entering treatment are heterosexual. As a general rule, sexuality is not assessed or addressed in addiction treatment. Very little research has been conducted on "special populations" generally in addiction treatment. Research does indicate that treatment specifically designed and implemented for women are more effective (Greenfield et al., 2007). However, efficacy studies have not been conducted to determine whether LGBT-specific treatments are more effective for sexual-minority women. Research has been able to demonstrate that LGBT clients are more likely to participate in a program that includes LGBT-specific material (Colcher, 1982; Driscoll, 1982). Also, minority clients generally have the expectation that a counselor who belongs to a similar minority as they do will be more accepting of them (Brooks, 1981; Goz, 1973).

Treatment Recommendations

Sexual orientation/identity should not be ignored in treatment, and counselors should never assume that clients are heterosexual. In order to create an environment that is culturally appropriate for LBGT clients, literature or signage should be visible in waiting or treatment areas that include statements regarding nondiscrimination of sexual orientation. Literature on resources for treatment and recovery in the LGBT community should be visible and available to patients. Intake forms and questionnaires should be designed in such a way as to be inclusive of same-sex relationships and family structures, and staff should be trained to use language that is consistent with these goals. If heterosexuality is assumed, it is likely to lead to reduced disclosure by LGBT clients.

Training and supervision related to the improvement in providing culturally sensitive treatment for LGBT clients and patients are very much needed. Organizational leadership in modeling appropriate behavior and language toward LBGT issues is critical. Staff should be encouraged to explore their own attitudes about LGBT individuals. If staff members are unwilling or unable to manage their own negativity, they should be encouraged to find a more appropriate setting or population with which to work. Consistency across the treatment team regarding these issues is critical as well. If one staff member expresses homonegativity or has a heterocentric bias, a treatment team that primarily holds an LGBT-positive clinical style may not be sufficient to make a patient feel comfortable enough to disclose important information.

In providing referrals for additional care, staff should be informed of LGBT-specific resources and be knowledgeable about the appropriateness of placements, with an awareness that placements that may provide poor or even harmful services to their LGBT clients. In large urban areas, community centers may provide addiction treatment and/or referral services, and gay and lesbian Alcoholics Anonymous (AA) meetings are available in almost all large metropolitan areas.

It is very important that counselors understand the cultural context in which SUDs develop and are maintained in the LGBT population. This is not an easy task. Even within the LGBT umbrella there are many subcultures, each with different norms and alcohol and drug use patterns. Part of this understanding includes knowledge of the environments to which clients return and the environmental cues that will challenge them. Understanding the social context and pressures that clients face and what it will take to cope with those pressures are critical in any good addiction treatment program. It is also important that staff have an adequate understanding of the perceived or expected positive and negative consequences of alcohol and drug use that are unique to LGBT clients.

The question of how to address sexuality specifically is a complex one. The first rule should be to respect the client's identity as he or she defines it. As discussed previously, making assumptions about sexual orientation or sexual identity based on sexual behavior alone is a mistake. Ideally, these components of sexuality are assessed in a mindful and respectful way during the intake process. Another highly sensitive area is related to where clients are "at" in the coming-out process. Earlier stages of coming out tend to be more intrapsychic, and individuals may not be able or willing to discuss the conflict they are experiencing. They also may not be wholly comfortable interacting with other LGBT patients. During the middle stages, in contrast, acknowledging that clients may have strong needs to identify with other LGBT individuals and culture is important. At this point it may be difficult or uncomfortable for these individuals to interact with heterosexuals. Clinicians who work with LGBT patients should be trained and supervised to help them develop skill in obtaining culturally sensitive psychosocial histories, including sexual histories, when relevant, in a nonjudgmental style.

The primary psychosocial treatment modality for SUDs is group, not individual, therapy.

One important consideration is how to manage other patients' reactions to LGBT patients. It is critical that the institution take responsibility for creating an environment that is intolerant of homonegativity. This goal can be accomplished in different ways. As discussed previously, the physical environment is critical. At intake, having all patients read policies that identify the clinic/institution as being nondiscriminatory to sexual diversity will reduce the likelihood that negativity will be expressed and provide a mechanism for managing it when it is expressed. Second, staff members serve as behavioral models for patient groups and, generally, if the staff have an LGBT-affirmative perspective, the patients/clients are much more likely to adopt this stance.

FUTURE DIRECTIONS

Given the disparity between the high rates of SUDs among sexual-minority women compared to women generally and the relatively limited literature, there is a critical need for more research on addiction among this population. Compared to gay men and women generally, lesbians and bisexual women are underserved by the research community. Much needs to be done to better understand the etiological and maintenance factors that underlie SUDs in this population. Studies have indicated that sexual minorities face challenges in childhood and adolescence that have potential for seriously impacting mental health and well-being across the lifespan, including the development of SUDs. Increased efforts are needed to develop prevention and treatment services for addictive disorders specifically among sexual-minority women. In the past decade, a comparable wealth of federal funding has gone toward understanding and treating alcohol and drug use among gay and bisexual men. Similar resources need to open up, particularly from the National Institutes of Health (NIH) and the Substance Abuse and Mental Health Services Administration (SAMHSA), specifically directed toward SUDs among lesbians and bisexual women.

KEY POINTS

- One of the greatest challenges in the area of addiction among sexual-minority women is the inherent diversity that exists within this population.
- Studies have consistently shown that sexual-minority women are more likely to drink and use drugs more heavily, and are more likely to experience problems related to their use, than heterosexual women. Tobacco use is also much higher in sexual-minority women compared to heterosexual women.
- Although sexual-minority women may have a higher prevalence of SUDs, data also indicate that they may seek treatment services for addiction and mental health services at higher rates than heterosexual women.
- Discrimination, victimization, and stress among LGBT individuals may have very large consequences for the subsequent development of SUDs and other mental health problems. Adversity and stress are strongly associated with increased levels of distress and psychological functioning among sexual minorities.
- Other risk factors include social structures that may influence SUDs among sexual-minority women, including social outlets where alcohol and drug use are common, marketing strategies by alcohol and tobacco companies targeting GLBT individuals, and probably most importantly, the lack of support or validation of same-sex relationships and family structures.
- Although there has been a positive shift toward mental health services that are more accepting of LGBT individuals, few efforts have been made to develop treatment services that are

fully accommodating or specifically designed for sexual-minority women. There remains considerable negativity toward those who express sexual diversity in treatment programs and individual providers.

• Sexual orientation/identity should not be ignored in treatment, and counselors should never assume that clients are heterosexual.

• Training and supervision related to the improvement in providing culturally sensitive treatment for LGBT clients and patients are greatly needed.

REFERENCES

Asterisks denote recommended readings.

Aaron, D. J., Markovic, N., Danielson, M. E., Honnold, J. A., Janosky, J. E., & Schmidt, N. J. (2001). Behavioral risk factors for disease and preventive health practices among lesbians. *American Journal of Public Health*, 91(6), 972–975.

Balsam, K. F., Beauchaine, T. P., Mickey, R. M., & Rothblum, E. D. (2005). Mental health of lesbian, gay, bisexual, and heterosexual siblings: Effects of gender, sexual orientation, and family. *Journal of Abnormal Psychology*, 114(3), 471–476.

Bloomfield, K. (1993). A comparison of alcohol consumption between lesbians and heterosexual women in an urban population. *Drug Alcohol Dependency*, 33(3), 257–269.

Brooks, V. R. (1981). Sex and sexual orientation as variables in therapists' biases and therapy outcomes. *Clinical Social Work Journal*, 9(3), 198–210.

Burgard, S. A., Cochran, S. D., & Mays, V. M. (2005). Alcohol and tobacco use patterns among heterosexually and homosexually experienced California women. *Drug Alcohol Dependency*, 77(1), 61–70.

Bux, D. A. (1996). The epidemiology of problem drinking in gay men and lesbians: A critical review. *Clinical Psychology Review*, 16, 277–298.

Cass, V. C. (1979). Homosexual identity formation: A theoretical model. *Journal of Homosexuality*, 4(3), 219–235.

Cochran, S. D. (2001). Emerging issues in research on lesbians' and gay men's mental health: Does sexual orientation really matter? *American Psychologist*, 56, 931–947. (*)

Cochran, S. D., Ackerman, D., Mays, V. M., & Ross, M. W. (2004). Prevalence of non-medical drug use and dependence among homosexually active men and women in the U.S. population. *Addiction*, 99, 989–998.

Cochran, S. D., & Mays, V. M. (2000a). Relation between psychiatric syndromes and behaviorally defined sexual orientation in a sample of the U.S. population. *American Journal of Epidemiology*, 151, 516–523.

Cochran, S. D., & Mays, V. M. (2000b). Lifetime prevalence of suicide symptoms and affective disorders among men reporting same-sex sexual partners: Results from NHANES. *American Journal of Public Health*, 90(4), 573–578.

Cochran, S. D., Mays, V. M., Bowen, D., Gage, S., Bybee, D., Roberts, S. J., et al. (2001). Cancer-related risk indicators and preventive screening behaviors among lesbians and bisexual women. *American Journal of Public Health*, 91(4), 591–597.

Cochran, S. D., Sullivan, J. G., & Mays, V. M. (2003). Prevalence of mental disorders, psychological distress, and mental health services use among lesbian, gay, and bisexual adults in the United States. *Journal of Consulting and Clinical Psychology*, 71, 53–61. (*)

Colcher, R. W. (1982). Counseling the homosexual alcoholic. *Journal of Homosexuality*, 7(4), 43–52.

Coleman, E. (1982). Developmental stages of the coming out process. *Journal of Homosexuality*, 7(2–3), 31–43.

Corliss, H. L., Grella, C. E., Mays, V. M., & Cochran, S. D. (2006). Drug use, drug severity, and help seeking behaviors of lesbian and bisexual women. *Journal of Women's Health*, 15(5), 556–568.

Craw, S. M., Fok, L. Y., & Hartman, S. J. (1998). Who is at greatest risk of work-related discrimination—women, blacks, or homosexuals? *Employee Responsibilities and Rights Journal*, 11(1), 1998.

D'Augelli, A. R., & Dark, L. J. (1994). Lesbian, gay, and bisexual youths. In L. D. Eron, J. H. Gentry, & P. Schlegel (Ed.), *Reason to hope: A psychosocial perspective on violence and youth* (pp. 177–196). Washington, DC: American Psychological Association.

Dean, L., Wu, S., & Martin, J. L. (1992). Trends in violence and discrimination against gay men in New York City: 1984 to 1990. In G. M. Herek & K. T. Berrill (Eds.), *Hate crimes: Confronting violence against lesbians and gay men* (pp. 46–64). Thousand Oaks, CA: Sage.

Diamant, A. L., & Wold, C. (2003). Sexual orientation and variation in physical and mental health status among women. *Journal of Women's Health*, 12(1), 41–49.

Diamant, A. L., Wold, C., Spritzer, K., & Gelberg, L. (2000). Health behaviors, health status, and access to and use of health care: A population-based study of lesbian, bisexual, and heterosexual women. *Archives of Family Medicine*, 9(10), 1043–1051.

Drabble, L. (2001). *The ethics of tobacco, alcohol, and pharmaceutical funding: A practical guide for LGBT organizations*. San Francisco: Coalition of Lavender Americans on Smoking and Health and Progressive Research and Training for Action.

Drabble, L., & Trocki, K. (2005). Alcohol consumption, alcohol-related problems, and other substance use among lesbian and bisexual women. *Journal of Lesbian Studies*, 9(3), 19–30.

Eliason, M. J. (2000). Substance abuse counselors' attitudes about lesbian, gay, bisexual, and transgender clients. *Journal of Substance Abuse*, 12, 311–328.

Eliason, M. J., & Hughes, T. (2004). Treatment counselor's attitudes about lesbian, gay, bisexual, and transgendered clients: Urban vs. rural settings. *Substance Use and Misuse*, 39(4), 625–644.

Garnets, L., Hancock, K. A., Cochran, S. D., Goodchilds, J., & Peplau, L. A. (1991). Issues in psychotherapy with lesbian and gay men: A survey of psychologists. *American Psychologist*, 46(9), 964–972.

Garofalo, R., Wolf, R. C., Kessel, S., Palfrey, J., & DuRant, R. H. (1998). The association between health risk behaviors and sexual orientation among a school-based sample of adolescents. *Pediatrics*, 101, 895–902. (*)

Gilman, S. E., Cochran, S. D., Mays, V. M., Hughes, M., Ostrow, D., & Kessler, R. C. (2001). Risk of psychiatric disorders among individuals reporting same-sex sexual partners in the National Comorbidity Survey. *American Journal of Public Health*, 91(6), 933–939.

Goz, R. (1973). Women patients and women therapists: Some issues that come up in psychotherapy. *International Journal of Psychoanalytic Psychotherapy*, 2(3), 298–319.

Greenfield, S. F., Brooks, A. J., Gordon, S. M., Green, C. A., Kropp, F., McHugh, R. K., et al. (2007). Substance abuse treatment entry, retention, and outcome in women: A review of the literature. *Drug and Alcohol Dependence*, 86, 1–21.

Gruskin, E. P., Hart, S., Gordon, N., & Ackerson, L. (2001). Patterns of cigarette smoking and alcohol use among lesbians and bisexual women enrolled in a large health maintenance organization. *American Journal of Public Health*, 91(6), 976–979.

Heffernan, K. (1998). The nature and predictors of substance use among lesbians. *Addictive Behaviors*, 23, 517–528.

Hellman, R. E., Stanton, M., Lee, J., et al. (1989). Treatment of homosexual alcoholics, in government funded agencies: Provider training and attitudes. *Hospital Community Psychiatry*, 40, 1163–1168.

Kessler, R. C., Mickelson, K. D., & Williams, D. R. (1999). The prevalence, distribution, and mental health correlates of perceived discrimination in the United States. *Journal of Health and Social Behavior*, 40(3), 208–230.

Klaas-Jan, H., & Knibbe, R. A. (1998). Changes in social roles as predictors of changes in drinking behaviour. *Addiction*, 93(11), 1717–1727.

Lie, G.-Y., & Gentlewarrier, S. (1991). Intimate violence in lesbian relationships: Discussion of survey findings and practice implications. *Journal of Social Service Research*, 15, 41–59.

Lilling, A. H., & Friedman, R. C. (1995). Bias towards gay patients by psychoanalytic clinicians: An empirical investigation. *Archives of Sexual Behavior*, 24(5), 563–570.

Lockhart, L. L., White, B. W., Causby, V., & Isaac, A. (1994). Letting out the secret: Violence in lesbian relationships. *Journal of Interpersonal Violence, 9,* 469–492.

Mays, V. M., & Cochran, S. D. (2001). Mental health correlates of perceived discrimination among lesbian, gay, and bisexual adults in the United States. *American Journal of Public Health, 91*(11), 1869–1876.

Mays, V. M., Yancey, A. K., Cochran, S. D., Weber, M., & Fielding, J. E. (2002). Heterogeneity of health disparities among African American, Hispanic, and Asian American women: Unrecognized influences of sexual orientation. *American Journal of Public Health, 92*(4), 632–639.

Meyer, I. H. (1995). Minority stress and mental health in gay men. *Journal of Health and Social Behavior, 36*(1), 38–56.

Meyer, I. H. (2003). Prejudice, social stress, and mental health in lesbian, gay, and bisexual populations: Conceptual issues and research evidence. *Psychological Bulletin, 129,* 674–697. (*)

Nicolosi, J. (1994). Objections to AAP statement on homosexuality and adolescence. *Pediatrics, 93*(4), 696.

Paul, J. P., Catania, J., Pollack, L., Moskowitz J., Canchola, J., Mills, T., et al. (2002). Suicide attempts among gay and bisexual men: Lifetime prevalence and antecedents. *American Journal of Public Health, 92*(8), 1338–1345.

Remafedi, G. (1987). Adolescent homosexuality: Psychosocial and medical implications. *Pediatrics, 79,* 331–337.

Renzetti, C. M. (1989). A second closet: Third-party responses to victims of lesbian partner abuse. *Family Relations, 38*(2), 157–163.

Rivers, I., & D'Augelli, A. R. (2001). The victimization of lesbian, gay, and bisexual youths: Implications for intervention. In A. R. D'Augelli & C. J. Patterson (Eds.), *Lesbian, gay, bisexual identities and youths: Psychological perspectives* (pp. 199–223). New York: Oxford University Press.

Rosik, C. H. (2003). Motivational, ethical, and epistemological foundations in the treatment of unwanted homoerotic attraction. *Journal of Marital and Family Therapy, 29*(1), 13–28.

Rotheram-Borus, M. J., Hunter, J., & Rosario, M. (1994). Suicidal behavior and gay related stress among gay and bisexual male adolescents. *Journal of Adolescent Research, 9*(4), 498–508.

Sanchez, J. P., Meacher, P., & Beil, R. (2005). Cigarette smoking and lesbian and bisexual women in the Bronx. *Journal of Community Health, 30*(1), 23–37.

Sandfort, T. G., de Graaf, R., Bijl, R. V., & Schnabel, P. (2001). Same-sex sexual behavior and psychiatric disorders: Findings from the Netherlands Mental Health Survey and Incidence Study (NEMESIS). *Archives of General Psychiatry, 58*(1), 85–91.

Scheer, S., Peterson, I., Page-Shafer, K., Delgado, V., Gleghorn, A., Ruiz, J., et al. (2002). Sexual and drug use behavior among women who have sex with both women and men: Results of a population-based survey. *American Journal of Public Health, 92,* 1110–1112.

Skinner, W. F. (1994). The prevalence and demographic predictors of illicit and licit drug use among lesbians and gay men. *American Journal of Public Health, 84,* 1307–1310.

Smith, E. A., & Malone, R. E. (2003). The outing of Philip Morris: Advertising tobacco to gay men. *American Journal of Public Health, 93,* 988–993.

Spitzer, R. L. (1981). The diagnostic status of homosexuality in DSM-III: A reformulation of the issues. *American Journal of Psychiatry, 138,* 210–215.

Spitzer, R. L. (2004). 200 participants reporting a change from homosexual to heterosexual orientation. *Archives of Sexual Behavior, 32*(5), 2004.

Stall, R. D., Hays, R. B., Waldo, C. R., Ekstrand, M., & McFarland, W. (2000). The gay '90s: A review of research in the 1990s on sexual behavior and HIV risk among men who have sex with men. *AIDS, 14*(Suppl. 3), 14.

Valanis, B. G., Bowen, D. J., Bassford, T., Whitlock, E., Charney, P., & Carter, R. A. (2000). Sexual orientation and health: Comparisons in the women's health initiative sample. *Archives of Family Medicine, 9*(9), 843–853.

Wainberg, M. L. (2004). Reply to Spitzer's (2003) reply. *Archives of Sexual Behavior, 33*(2), 83–85.

Waldner-Haugrud, L. K., Gratch, L. V., & Magruder, B. (1997). Victimization and perpetration rates of violence in gay and lesbian relationships: Gender issues explored. *Violence and Victims, 12,* 173–184.

Warner, J., McKeown, E., Griffin, M., Johnson, K., Ramsay, A., Cort, C., et al. (2004). Rates and predictors of mental illness in gay men, lesbians, and bisexual men and women: Results from a survey based in England and Wales. *British Journal of Psychiatry, 185,* 479–485.

Weathers, B. (1980). Alcoholism and the lesbian community. In M. C. Eddy & J. ford (Eds.), *Alcoholism and women* (pp. xx–xx). Dubuque, IA: Kendall/Hunt.

Young, R. M., & Meyer, I. H. (2005). The trouble with MSM and WSW: Erasure of the sexual-minority person in public health discourse. *American Journal of Public Health, 95*(7), 1144–1149.

PART VII

SOCIAL AND POLICY ISSUES

CHAPTER 29

Violence and Victimization among Women with Substance Use Disorders

Angela E. Waldrop, PhD

The relationship between violence and substance use disorders (SUDs) is complex and often reciprocal in nature. As this chapter describes, addiction places women at risk for violent victimization. It also enhances their likelihood of engaging in violent behavior. The experience of victimization, furthermore, places women at risk for SUDs, particularly when they use substances to self-medicate symptoms of anxiety and depression. This chapter reviews the epidemiology of the co-occurrence of violence, victimization, and addiction and the functional relationships among these factors.

EPIDEMIOLOGY

Although violent crime appears to be on the decline in the United States, the National Crime Victimization Survey (NCVS) reported that in 2006, 6.1 million violent crimes were committed, including sexual assault, robbery, and aggravated and simple assault (Rand & Catalano, 2007). The most recent results of the NCVS (from 2006) indicate that, among every 1,000 females age 12 and older, 22.9 experienced some form of violent victimization (excluding homicide) in the prior 12 months.

The National Violence Against Women Survey (NVAWS) (Tjaden & Thoennes, 2000) sampled men and women (n = 8,000 for each sex) and assessed physical assault, forcible rape, and stalking. Over half of the women (51.9%) reported having experienced a physical assault in their lives. Lifetime completed or attempted rape was reported by 17.6% and being the victim of stalking at some time in the past was reported by 8.1% of women. The National Women's Study (NWS; n = 4,008; Resnick, Kilpatrick, Dansky, Saunders, & Best, 1993) found that 13% of women had experienced a completed rape in their lifetimes.

In a recent large epidemiological study, the California Women's Health Survey, community women were assessed for exposure to physical and sexual violence and repeat victimization (Kimerling, Alvarez, Pavao, Kaminski, & Baumrind, 2007). About one-fourth (24.3%) of women reported an experience of physical and/or sexual violence from childhood and almost as many (22.9%) reported at least one such experience in adulthood (Kimerling et al., 2007). The authors of the study highlighted the fact that multiple victimization occurred for 12% of their sample and was associated with worse outcomes on measures of anxiety, depression, and posttraumatic stress disorder (PTSD; Kimerling et al., 2007).

WOMEN'S SUDs ASSOCIATED WITH GREATER EXPOSURE TO VIOLENCE/VICTIMIZATION

Violence Exposure → SUDs

Although Hien (Chapter 14, this volume) addresses the link between PTSD and addiction, it is worth noting here that substance use often develops as part of a chain of reactions to violence exposure. A typical pattern commences with an individual witnessing or experiencing a physical or sexual assault; followed by posttraumatic stress symptoms, including depression, PTSD, and other anxiety disorders; culminating in the use of alcohol, drugs, or over-the-counter medications to manage distress. This model of the violence–addiction equation attributes their link to the mediating role of psychological distress. Often, these factors interact in a reciprocal nature, through a cycle of substance use and violence exposure (Kilpatrick, Acierno, Resnick, Saunders, & Best, 1997). The following sections review the co-occurrence of substance use and violence from clinical and population-based studies.

Sexual and Physical Abuse

Among a sample of women (*n* = 105) presenting to a substance use clinic, 22% reported a history of adult physical assault by an intimate partner, and 14% had experienced child abuse (Easton, Swan, & Sinha, 2000). In another study of women (*n* = 369) recruited from community domestic violence agencies, participants with recent incidents of intimate partner violence were more likely to report drinking to cope (Kaysen et al., 2007). This choice of coping strategies also mediated the relationship of alcohol use to trauma symptom severity (Kaysen et al., 2007). In a sample of women who had applied for an order of protection from a district attorney's domestic violence specialty unit, researchers found that women who experienced more than one, as compared to one, sexual assault from a partner were 3.5 times more likely to start or escalate substance use (McFarlane et al., 2005). In the NVAWS study, minority women, in particular, were at increased risk for problematic alcohol use and illicit drug use if they had experienced sexual violence in adulthood (Kaukinen & Demaris, 2005).

In a carefully conducted analysis of twin data (combining monozygotic and dizygotic female–female pairs) from a population-based sample (*n* = 1,411), Kendler and colleagues (2000) found that child sexual abuse put women at increased risk for SUDs in adulthood. Twins discordant for sexual abuse were examined, with confounding factors controlled in the analyses; the abused twin was at much greater risk for psychopathology, including drug and alcohol use disorders (odds ratios = 2.8–3.1). Similarly, in a study using both retrospective and prospective methods, women with abuse and neglect histories were more likely to have lifetime and current SUDs, particularly cocaine and stimulant use (Widom, 1999).

These studies highlight the role that substances of abuse can play in the lives of many women who have experienced violent assault. The use of intentional strategies to avoid trauma-related distress has been termed "effortful avoidance" (Feuer, Nishith, & Resick, 2005). Use of substances may reduce distressing symptoms in the short term, but like other forms of avoidance, it serves to maintain chronic symptoms of anxiety and posttraumatic stress associated with traumatic experiences.

SUDs → Violence Exposure

Compared to the literature that seeks to understand victimization as a risk factor for substance use, the work on understanding substance use preceding victimization is much sparser. This is probably due, in part, to the delicate balance between attempting to understand risk factors for victimization without resorting to victim blaming. A question that is often overlooked is the possibility that a third factor is increasing the risk for both substance use and victimization. Unfortunately, because most research in this area is cross-sectional, this question is difficult to address. Proposed models for understanding addiction preceding violence exposure have focused on potential deficits in detection of danger cues that might have decreased the risk of victimization and engagement in high-risk activities, such as drug use (cf. Chilcoat & Breslau, 1998; Hien, Cohen, & Campbell, 2005).

In one of the few longitudinal studies to assess the temporal order of violence exposure and substance use problems, an analysis of the NWS data found that Wave I illicit drug use, but not alcohol abuse, predicted an increased risk for a new assault in the 2-year follow-up period (Kilpatrick et al., 1997). In a subset of this nationally representative sample, drug use and assaults were part of a cycle in which each increased the risk of the other. Wave III data from the NWS indicated that women who had used illicit drugs on four or more occasions were at greater risk for experiencing a physical assault, although this relationship declined with the inclusion of major depression in the model (Acierno, Resnick, Kilpatrick, Saunders, & Best, 1999), highlighting the importance of examining other possible explanatory factors.

In the National Study of Couples, a broad sample of married and cohabiting couples was assessed for intimate partner violence (Caetano, Schafer, & Cunradi, 2001). In the European American and African American segments of the sample, women with alcohol-related problems (endorsed from a list of 29 items, e.g., belligerence, accidents) were more likely to be both the victim and the perpetrator of intimate partner violence. This relationship did not hold among Hispanic participants. Couples in which the male partners had alcohol problems were also more likely to report violence perpetrated by either partner. In a study of women who presented to emergency departments for treatment, those who were physically assaulted by a partner were more likely to engage in heavy alcohol use, meet criteria for alcohol abuse or dependence, and use illicit drugs (Lipsky, Caetano, Field, & Larkin, 2005). Male partners who engaged in partner abuse were more likely to have been using alcohol during the assault, whether or not the woman was drinking at the time. The authors review proposed explanations for these relationships, including proximal factors, such as disinhibiting effects of alcohol on partners' behavior, and deleterious effects on reasoning that may also serve the role of rationalizing the abuse (Lipsky et al., 2005).

These findings extend to sexual aggression by partners, as well. In the National Study of Couples, sexual aggression from male partners toward female partners was associated with binge drinking among European American and Hispanic men (Ramisetty-Mikler, Caetano, & McGrath, 2007). Among African American men, sexual aggression toward female partners was about equally likely whether or not binge drinking occurred. In this sample, sexual aggression was characterized primarily by insisting on sex, without the use of physical force.

A small literature examines the role of environmental context for increased risk of victimization. These studies have assessed women from targeted populations of high alcohol use, including college women and women who frequent bars. In a 6-week study of college women, the risk of experiencing a physical or sexual assault was strongly associated with the quantity of alcohol use on the day of the assault (Parks & Fals-Stewart, 2004). On days with heavy alcohol use (five or more standard drinks), risk of experiencing sexual aggression was 9 times higher than on nondrinking days. On days with less-than-heavy use (one to four standard drinks), the risk was 3 times higher than on nondrinking days. Similarly, the risk for physical assault was 7 times higher on heavy drinking days and about 3 times higher on less-than-heavy drinking days, when compared to nondrinking days (Parks & Fals-Stewart, 2004). Abbey (2002) reviewed the literature and concluded that, among other factors, heavy alcohol use likely reduces a woman's ability to defend herself, influences a perpetrator's perception of the woman as a target, and increases disinhibition in a potential perpetrator.

Women with SUDs as Violent Offenders

The literature on women as perpetrators is limited, perhaps in part because women are less likely than men to commit violent acts. Research in the area of family violence, however, has assessed women as perpetrators against partners and children. Other investigators have examined violent offending in women who are substance users.

In a clinic-based study, women with cocaine or alcohol dependence reported a greater frequency of physical and psychological aggression toward their partners, when compared with controls (Parrott, Drobes, Saladin, Coffey, & Dansky, 2003). This pattern was even stronger among women with comorbid PTSD. In another study of women seeking substance abuse treatment, 18% reported having committed an act of physical violence toward a spouse or partner (Easton et al., 2000). In a sample of young adults who used methamphetamine, a significant proportion of young women (30%) reported engaging in violence while under the influence of the drug at rates relatively similar to young men (38%) (Sommers, Baskin, & Baskin-Sommers, 2006).

Caregivers with substance use problems are more likely to engage in child abuse and neglect. Several reviews have highlighted this issue (e.g., Arellano, 1996; Johnson & Leff, 1999), but the explanations for this link continue to be investigated, particularly given that some children of substance users fare better than others (Nair, Schuler, Black, Kettinger, & Harrington, 2003). In a study of women who abuse substances and were enrolled in a home-based intervention, the results indicated that the cumulative stress from a number of risk factors helped to determine the risk for child abuse (Nair et al., 2003). Women were assessed for 10 categories of environmental risk (e.g., ongoing violence exposure, family size, homelessness, absence of children's father[s]). The presence of any five or more of these risk factors discriminated between women at high and low risk for abuse and neglect of their infants. This study highlights the complex life circumstances of women with SUDs and the multiple stressors that may contribute to the violence they may experience and perpetrate.

In a study that highlights the relationship between addiction and violent behavior, researchers measured criminal convictions before and after substance use treatment. In a large sample of adults ($n = 1,075$), recidivism to criminal activities was reduced from baseline to multiple posttreatment follow-up points over 5 years (Gossop, Trakada, Stewart, & Witton, 2005). Although the sample was only about one-fourth female, no sex differences were found in these outcomes.

The findings of these studies point to addiction interventions as a means of indirectly reducing other harmful negative behaviors, including violence. The benefits associated with substance use treatment include improved family relationships, safety for children, and reduced criminal behavior. These facts highlight the need for agencies that interact with women offenders to provide effective addiction treatment services as an investment in the prevention of other problematic behaviors.

SAFETY PLANS AND TREATMENT NEEDS

Given the frequent co-occurrence of violence and substance use in women, both factors should be assessed in patients presenting for substance use treatment, victimization, or violent offenses. In cases in which women are involved in an ongoing risk for violence exposure, a safety plan may assist in preparation for the move to a safer environment. Safety plans typically include steps to prepare for leaving an acutely violent situation, such as keeping important documents (e.g., birth certificate), change of clothes, and cash in an easily accessible location. They typically also involve information on individuals and agencies that can be contacted in case crisis housing or other resources are needed. When children are involved, mothers may need to prepare them for a quick escape when violence erupts (see the American Bar Association Commission on Domestic Violence's *www.abanet.org/tips/dvsafety.html#safetips* for more information on safety plans). In cases in which the presenting problem is violence exposure, it is important to assess whether a woman is using substances as a coping strategy and the extent to which use with a partner is contributing to the problematic behavior. SUDs triggered by victimization can have effects that last long after the danger of further victimization is gone. Women who have been identified as violent offenders in cases such as child abuse stand to benefit from substance use treatment when substance use is a contributing factor.

In many cases, when women receive treatment for SUDs, their active efforts to reduce risk for use will include removing themselves from triggering situations such as a social situations that emphasize substance use (e.g., bars) or a relationship with a partner who uses. Comprehensive treatment will also include the development of alternative strategies for managing interpersonal conflict, setting boundaries, and deescalating strong affective states. Some programs have integrated parenting skills training, as well (Killeen & Brady, 2000; Magura & Laudet, 1996).

FUTURE DIRECTIONS

Research on the relationships between substance abuse and violent victimization and perpetration still requires the implementation of prospective studies that can address issues of causation. Integrated treatments that address the symptom interplay of SUDs and PTSD may aid in the prevention of chronic emotional distress, substance use, and revictimization. The program Seeking Safety (Hien, Cohen, Miele, Litt, & Capstick, 2004; Najavits, Weiss, Shaw, & Muenz, 1998) and at least one exposure-based treatment (Brady, Dansky, Back, Foa, & Carroll, 2001; Back, Dansky, Carroll, Foa, & Brady, 2001) for comorbid substance use and PTSD have shown promising results. Perhaps further development of interventions in the cycle of violence and substance use at the family level may also prevent intergenerational transmission of both problems.

KEY POINTS

- Violence and substance use are intimately connected, often in a reciprocal fashion.
- When women present for substance use treatment, they should also be evaluated for potential violence exposure and its associated effects, such as depression, anxiety, and PTSD.
- For women who have been perpetrators in the context of substance use, services (e.g., intensive parenting skills training) should be made available to enhance alternative forms of coping.
- Addressing violence issues is important to maintaining abstinence and improving additional outcomes, such as adequate parenting skills and occupational functioning.

REFERENCES

Asterisks denote recommended readings.

Abbey, A. (2002). Alcohol-related sexual assault: a common problem among college students. *Journal of Studies on Alcohol Supplement*, *14*, 118–128.

Acierno, R., Resnick, H., Kilpatrick, D. G., Saunders, B., & Best, C. L. (1999). Risk factors for rape, physical assault, and posttraumatic stress disorder in women: Examination of differential multivariate relationships. *Journal of Anxiety Disorders*, *13*(6), 541–563.

Arellano, C. M. (1996). Child maltreatment and substance use: A review of the literature. *Substance Use and Misuse*, *31*(7), 927–935.

Back, S. E., Dansky, B. S., Carroll, K. M., Foa, E. B., & Brady, K. T. (2001). Exposure therapy in the treatment of PTSD among cocaine-dependent individuals: Description of procedures. *Journal of Substance Abuse Treatment*, *21*(1), 35–45.

Brady, K. T., Dansky, B. S., Back, S. E., Foa, E. B., & Carroll, K. M. (2001). Exposure therapy in the treatment of PTSD among cocaine-dependent individuals: Preliminary findings. *Journal of Substance Abuse Treatment*, *21*(1), 47–54.

Caetano, R., Schafer, J., & Cunradi, C. B. (2001). Alcohol-related intimate partner violence among white, black, and Hispanic couples in the United States. *Alcohol Research and Health*, *25*(1), 58–65.

Chilcoat, H. D., & Breslau, N. (1998). Posttraumatic stress disorder and drug disorders: Testing causal pathways. *Archives of General Psychiatry*, *55*, 913–917. (*)

Easton, C. J., Swan, S., & Sinha, R. (2000). Prevalence of family violence in clients entering substance abuse treatment. *Journal of Substance Abuse Treatment*, *18*(1), 23–28.

Feuer, C. A., Nishith, P., & Resick, P. (2005). Prediction of numbing and effortful avoidance in female rape survivors with chronic PTSD. *Journal of Traumatic Stress*, *18*(2), 165–170.

Gossop, M., Trakada, K., Stewart, D., & Witton, J. (2005). Reductions in criminal convictions after addiction treatment: 5-year follow-up. *Drug and Alcohol Dependence*, *79*(3), 295–302.

Hien, D., Cohen, L., & Campbell, A. (2005). Is traumatic stress a vulnerability factor for women with substance use disorders? *Clinical Psychology Review*, *25*(6), 813–823. (*)

Hien, D. A., Cohen, L. R., Miele, G. M., Litt, L. C., & Capstick, C. (2004). Promising treatments for women with comorbid PTSD and substance use disorders. *American Journal of Psychiatry*, *161*(8), 1426–1432.

Johnson, J. L., & Leff, M. (1999). Children of substance abusers: Overview of research findings. *Pediatrics*, *103*(5, Pt. 2), 1085–1099.

Kaukinen, C., & Demaris, A. (2005). Age at first sexual assault and current substance use and depression. *Journal of Interpersonal Violence*, *20*(10), 1244–1270.

Kaysen, D., Dillworth, T. M., Simpson, T., Waldrop, A., Larimer, M. E., & Resick, P. A. (2007). Domestic violence and alcohol use: Trauma-related symptoms and motives for drinking. *Addictive Behaviors*, *32*(6), 1272–1283.

Kendler, K. S., Bulik, C. M., Silberg, J., Hettema, J. M., Myers, J., & Prescott, C. A. (2000). Childhood sexual abuse and adult psychiatric and substance use disorders in women: An epidemiological and cotwin control analysis. *Archives of General Psychiatry*, *57*(10), 953–959.

Killeen, T., & Brady, K. T. (2000). Parental stress and child behavioral outcomes following substance abuse residential treatment. Follow-up at 6 and 12 months. *Journal of Substance Abuse Treatment*, *19*(1), 23–29.

Kilpatrick, D. G., Acierno, R., Resnick, H. S., Saunders, B. E., & Best, C. L. (1997). A 2-year longitudinal analysis of the relationships between violent assault and substance use in women. *Journal of Consulting and Clinical Psychology*, *65*(5), 834–847.

Kimerling, R., Alvarez, J., Pavao, J., Kaminski, A., & Baumrind, N. (2007). Epidemiology and consequences of women's revictimization. *Women's Health Issues*, *17*(2), 101–106. (*)

Lipsky, S., Caetano, R., Field, C. A., & Larkin, G. L. (2005). Is there a relationship between victim and partner alcohol use during an intimate partner violence event? Findings from an urban emergency department study of abused women. *Journal of Studies on Alcohol*, *66*(3), 407–412.

Magura, S., & Laudet, A. B. (1996). Parental substance abuse and child maltreatment: Review and implications for intervention. *Children and Youth Services Review, 18*(3), 193–220.

McFarlane, J., Malecha, A., Gist, J., Watson, K., Batten, E., Hall, I., et al. (2005). Intimate partner sexual assault against women and associated victim substance use, suicidality, and risk factors for femicide. *Issues in Mental Health Nursing, 26*(9), 953–967.

Nair, P., Schuler, M. E., Black, M. M., Kettinger, L., & Harrington, D. (2003). Cumulative environmental risk in substance abusing women: Early intervention, parenting stress, child abuse potential and child development. *Child Abuse and Neglect, 27*(9), 997–1017.

Najavits, L. M., Weiss, R. D., Shaw, S. R., & Muenz, L. R. (1998). "Seeking safety": Outcome of a new cognitive-behavioral psychotherapy for women with posttraumatic stress disorder and substance dependence. *Journal of Traumatic Stress, 11*(3), 437–456.

Parks, K. A., & Fals-Stewart, W. (2004). The temporal relationship between college women's alcohol consumption and victimization experiences. *Alcoholism: Clinical and Experimental Research, 28*(4), 625–629.

Parrott, D. J., Drobes, D. J., Saladin, M. E., Coffey, S. F., & Dansky, B. S. (2003). Perpetration of partner violence: Effects of cocaine and alcohol dependence and posttraumatic stress disorder. *Addictive Behaviors, 28*(9), 1587–1602.

Ramisetty-Mikler, S., Caetano, R., & McGrath, C. (2007). Sexual aggression among [sic] white, [sic] black, and Hispanic couples in the U.S.: Alcohol use, physical assault, and psychological aggression as its correlates. *American Journal of Drug and Alcohol Abuse, 33*(1), 31–43.

Rand, M., & Catalano, S. (2007). *Criminal victimization, 2006.* Washington, DC: U.S. Department of Justice.

Resnick, H. S., Kilpatrick, D. G., Dansky, B. S., Saunders, B. E., & Best, C. L. (1993). Prevalence of civilian trauma and posttraumatic stress disorder in a representative national sample of women. *Journal of Consulting and Clinical Psychology, 61,* 984–991.

Sommers, I., Baskin, D., & Baskin-Sommers, A. (2006). Methamphetamine use among young adults: Health and social consequences. *Addictive Behaviors, 31*(8), 1469–1476.

Tjaden, P., & Thoennes, N. (2000). *Full report of the prevalence, incidence, and consequences of violence against women: Findings from the National Violence Against Women Survey.* Washington, DC: U.S. Department of Justice, Office of Justice Programs, National Institute of Justice.

Widom, C. S. (1999). Posttraumatic stress disorder in abused and neglected children grown up. *American Journal of Psychiatry, 156,* 1223–1229.

CHAPTER 30

Legal Issues, Addiction, and Gender

Rebecca W. Brendel, MD, JD
Matthew F. Soulier, MD

Individuals with substance use disorders (SUDs) frequently come into contact with the legal system. For the forensic mental health practitioner, any evaluation involves a thorough assessment of substance use, and substance use may be relevant in almost any civil or criminal context. Examples of types of evaluations in which substance use may be forensically relevant in civil contexts include commitment proceedings, determinations of capacity or competence to make medical or legal decisions, disability evaluations, tort claims, and child custody evaluations (Gendel, 2006). In the criminal context, substance use may be relevant to determinations of competency and criminal responsibility evaluations (Schouten & Brendel, 2008) as well as to sentencing evaluations. Although it is unconstitutional to criminally prosecute an individual with substance dependence for the crime of addiction or substance use (*Powell v. Texas*, 1968; *Robinson v. California*, 1962), substance use is inextricably linked with the criminal justice system in this country through drug-related crimes of possession and distribution, crimes committed to obtain drugs, illegal activity that occurs under the influence of substances, and the relationship of substance use to domestic violence (U.S. Department of Justice [USDOJ], 2007a). In addition, because of the connection between addiction and crime, correctional institutions are challenged with a population that has significant treatment needs (USDOJ, 2007a).

Although substance abuse is relevant to a wide range of civil and criminal legal settings, several legal issues are particularly relevant, and even unique, to women. This chapter focuses on a subset of civil and criminal legal issues with particular relevance to women. Specifically, in the civil arena, the topics of civil commitment for substance use, including laws related to involuntary treatment of pregnant women, and the relationship between addiction and child custody are explored. In the context of criminal law, the role of substance use in crime, characteristics of jail and prison inmates, differences between male and female offenders, and treatment programs and outcomes in correctional settings are discussed.

500

ISSUES IN CIVIL LAW

Pregnant Women with Substance Use Disorders:
Prevalence, Clinical Characteristics, and Legal Issues

Large numbers of children are affected by parental substance abuse, with estimates ranging from 8.3 million to 17.5 million (Gregoire & Schultz, 2001). A developing child can be exposed to maternal substance use at the earliest stages of prenatal development, causing treatment providers to struggle with how to manage and take care of mothers who abuse substances during their pregnancies. Parental substance abuse may also continue to have a significant impact throughout childhood. An estimated 5.5% of women ages 18–49 who have one or more children living with them are dependent on alcohol or illicit drugs, and 70% of women entering substance use treatment report having children (Brady & Ashley, 2005). Because so many children are affected by parental substance abuse, it has become a key area of concern in child welfare law due to states' *parens patriae* role in protecting children.

Nearly 4% of pregnant women use illicit drugs according to a 2005 government survey (March of Dimes, 2006). It is estimated that 2–3% of newborns have been exposed to cocaine, and 3–12% are exposed to marijuana *in utero*. Twenty-seven percent of pregnant women smoke cigarettes, and as many as 73% of pregnant women may have used alcohol at some time during their pregnancy (Gomby & Shiono, 1991). All of these substances cross the placenta and may have a direct effect on the developing brain and nervous system (Zuckerman, 1991). Prenatal exposure to a variety of substances can potentially have long-reaching consequences for children, involving abilities related to attention, behavioral control, and emotional regulation.

The care of pregnant women with SUDs requires sensitivity to the unique conditions of these women, including other co-occurring psychiatric disorders, the need for prenatal care, and the needs of their already existing children (Lester & Twomey, 2008). A variety of approaches to pregnant women with SUDs has developed, ranging from treatment-based approaches to criminal prosecution. In general, physicians have largely disapproved of criminal prosecution of women with SUDs. However, most physicians have agreed that existing child abuse and neglect laws need to be redefined to include alcohol and drug abuse during pregnancy, and also have highly favored the compulsory treatment of substance-abusing pregnant women in the criminal justice system (Abel & Kruger, 2002).

Over the last two decades, stimulated by the crack cocaine epidemic in the 1980s, states have attempted to address the treatment of pregnant women who use substances (Linder, 2005). Specifically nationwide coverage of crack cocaine abuse highlighted the associated social and economic consequences of drug abuse. States have sought to protect the unborn child from the effects of prenatal substance abuse through the passage of legislation and the attempted criminal prosecution of over 200 women, based on the theory that drug dependency is a crime against the fetus (Minkoff & Paltrow, 2004). Pregnant women have been prosecuted, civilly committed and jailed for drug use, and new mothers have lost custody of their children (Paltrow, 1991). Proponents of these punitive approaches to maternal substance use have argued that children need to be protected; they also cite the heavy financial burden to society of children born to mothers with SUDs, including the increased use of child welfare services (Lester, Andreozzi, & Appiah, 2004; Paltrow, 1991).

Punitive approaches may in effect, create two separate and adversarial individuals: the "innocent" fetus and the "bad" woman who does not care if she hurts the fetus. The problems of the pregnant woman may be minimized, and her privacy rights may be compromised, as the fetus becomes the focus of attention (Paltrow, 1991). Traditional principles of medical ethics and treatment rely on a patient's knowing, voluntary, and competent consent. Substituting this approach with the criminal enforcement of medical treatment may undermine a woman's right to determine her fate and that of the fetus (Minkoff & Paltrow, 2004). Criminal enforcement, however, may be considered ethical in scenarios where pregnant women are seen as having the same moral obligation to a not-yet-born child as to a born child (Murray, 1991). This ethical analysis has contributed to the legal debate regarding the constitutional rights of the unborn child. Specifically, although federal constitutional jurisprudence in the United States has historically held that the unborn child is not entitled to constitutional protection because the fetus is not a separate legal entity from the mother (Linder, 2005), state laws that punish pregnant women for behavior hazardous to their fetuses have been based on claims of fetal rights. Prosecutors have attempted to consider a fetus a child, and in this vein have argued that maternal substance abuse is a form of abuse against this separate "person." For example, as of 2007, there were 18 states with provisions pertaining to child abuse and neglect in the context of a pregnant woman's abuse of alcohol (National Institute on Alcohol Abuse and Alcoholism [NIAAA], 2007), though the constitutionality of these laws is controversial (Larson, 1991). Women have been charged with child endangerment/abuse, illegal drug delivery to a minor, and manslaughter for drug use during pregnancy. All courts, however, with the exception of those in the jurisdiction of South Carolina, have rejected the expansion of existing state laws to punish pregnant woman based on claims of fetal rights (Harris & Paltrow, 2003).

South Carolina has had the most attempted prosecutions of pregnant women who use substances (Linder, 2005). In 1996 it became the first state to uphold a conviction based on a child endangerment statute against a pregnant, drug-using woman in the case of Cornelia Whitner, a 28-year-old woman with little education who abused crack cocaine during her pregnancy. After Ms. Whitner gave birth, her child tested positive for cocaine, and she was charged with criminal child abuse. She received an 8-year sentence after she pled guilty, and the South Carolina Supreme Court upheld the decision (Gendel, 2004). South Carolina continued its application of child abuse and neglect laws to the unborn child in the 1999 homicide conviction of Regina McKnight. Ms. McKnight was sentenced to 20 years in prison after her stillborn child's toxicology was positive for cocaine. This decision was again upheld by the South Carolina Supreme Court, and the U.S. Supreme Court declined to review the case. With assistance from organizations such as the American Civil Liberties Union (ACLU) and National Advocates for Pregnant Women (NAPW), Ms. McKnight's conviction was reversed on May 12, 2008 after the South Carolina Supreme Court unanimously ruled that the research linking cocaine use to stillbirths was inaccurate and "outdated" (National Advocates for Pregnant Women, 2008).

The reversal of Ms. McKnight's conviction and others (e.g., *Cruz v. State of Maryland*, 2006) illustrate some of the limitations of, and flaws in, the punitive approach to pregnant women with SUDs. First, the majority of the women prosecuted have been low-income women of color, even though the rates of drug abuse among pregnant women is highest for whites (Lester et al., 2004; Paltrow, 1991). Second, the use of cocaine has been especially targeted criminally, but the rates of alcohol and nicotine use among pregnant females are much higher (Gomby & Shiono, 1991). Further, while the results of studies examining the effects of prenatal cocaine use on later child development have been mixed to inconclusive, the negative effects of in utero alcohol and nicotine exposure are more clearly demonstrated. For example, children born to nicotine-abusing and/or alcohol-abusing mothers are smaller and are delivered at an earlier gestational age (Lester et al., 2004; Sood et al., 2001) than unexposed children.

However, the consumption of alcohol and nicotine is legal for pregnant women, and numerous other legal hazards, such as poor nutrition, advanced maternal age, and poor prenatal care, also pose potential risks to a developing fetus or postnatal child. Several courts have stated that the application of child abuse laws to the unborn fetus would make them unconstitutionally vague, holding pregnant women criminally liable for an unlimited number of behaviors. Under such an expansion, women could not know what behavior would be deemed criminal (Harris & Paltrow, 2003). Some courts have also recognized that extension of the law to cover unborn fetuses could unintentionally encourage women to have abortions or prevent detection of substance use by avoiding medical care. These decisions would jeopardize the safety of the mother and child, while never addressing the root problems of addiction (Linder, 2005) that would be better served in treatment programs (ACLU, 2006). In addition, the application of child abuse statutes during pregnancy ignores the shortage of treatment programs and specialized services for those women who would seek them if they were more available (Paltrow, 1991). In addition, these programs targeting prenatal drug exposure may be extremely cost-effective, given the overall burden of this problem (Phibbs, 1991).

States' approaches to substance abuse during pregnancy vary widely from a strictly criminal perspective to one that emphasizes mothers' treatment (Lester et al., 2004). Some state legislation may emphasize early identification and the allocation of treatment resources (Steven & Ahlstrom, 1991), whereas other states have commitment statutes designed to protect the fetus through the involuntary restriction of substance abuse for a pregnant woman (NIAAA, 2007). Such commitment could include the holding of a pregnant woman in a noncriminal setting, such as a hospital, until she delivers the baby, but it does not necessarily mandate substance abuse treatment.

The first state began civil commitment of women in these circumstances in 1999. Specific legal protections may attach in the course of these proceedings. For example, in Wisconsin, if commitment is sought for a prolonged period of time, the pregnant woman is entitled to legal representation and a judicial hearing (NIAAA, 2007a). As of January 1, 2007, four states had statutes providing for the involuntary civil commitment of women who abuse alcohol during pregnancy: North Dakota, South Dakota, Oklahoma, and Wisconsin (NIAAA, 2007b). In order for a pregnant substance-using woman to be committed under these commitment statutes, it must be demonstrated that the woman presents a danger to herself or the fetus by reason of mental illness. Because the rate of drug-exposed infant cases is escalating, judges have limited time to consider each one (Boland, 1991).

States have also struggled with how to identify pregnant women who abuse substances, and with the reporting of toxicology results of a child after birth (Lester et al., 2004). Pregnant women are not obligated to participate in nonconsensual drug testing for the purpose of criminal prosecution (Harris & Paltrow, 2003). Minnesota and Virginia are the only states to mandate prenatal screening for substance use, and Minnesota is the only state to mandate neonatal testing for drugs (Lester et al., 2004). Concern about the implications of mandatory drug screening and reporting of positive toxicology results has emerged among health care providers, who worry that these measures will deter pregnant women with SUDs from seeking prenatal care due to their fear of prosecution or loss of child custody.

Substance Abuse, Parenting, and Implications for Child Welfare and Child Custody Laws

A mother or father's ability to parent and attend to the emotional and developmental needs of the child may be significantly affected by ongoing substance use. Women are often the primary caregivers for young children; therefore, substance abuse among women who are the primary caretakers of children is important for overall child safety and development (Kronstadt, 1991). The child's environment is of central concern in child custody cases, in which determinations must be made regarding the safety of a home environment, the removal of children from parental custody, and the best interest of the child.

In addition to affecting the quality of the caregiving environment, parental substance abuse is frequently reported to coexist with child maltreatment. Children born to mothers who used illicit drugs during pregnancy, as determined by neonatal toxicology screens and maternal records, have been shown to be at a higher risk of subsequent abuse or neglect compared to children from a general population. In one study, 155 (30.2%) of the 513 children exposed to drugs during pregnancy were reported as abused or neglected, and 102 (19.9%) of the reports were substantiated. This proportion was 2–3 times that of other children living in the same geographic area (i.e., the south side of Chicago). Toddlers were the most susceptible to this abuse, and neglect was most often reported (72.6% of cases) (Jaudes, Ekwo, & Van Voorhis, 1995). Associations between alcohol abuse and physical maltreatment and between cocaine abuse and sexual maltreatment have also been identified (Famularo, Kinscherff, & Fenton, 1992). Substance abuse has contributed to child mistreatment in one-third to two-thirds of families served by child welfare agencies (Semidei, Radel, & Nolan, 2001).

Maternal substance abuse can also destabilize and compromise the safety and nurturing consistency that children need for healthy development. For example, studies have demonstrated that children raised with a parent who abuses substances show more adjustment, behavior, conduct, and attention-deficit problems than other children (Semidei et al., 2001). Childhood behavioral problems increase proportionally in the setting of mothers who continue to abuse substances, experience domestic violence, or have mental health problems (Whitaker, Orzol, & Kahn, 2006). Youths living with a mother who abused substances were more likely to report illicit drug use than youths of non-drug-using mothers (National Survey of Drug Use and Health [NSDUH], 2005). Even more, if the influence of serious maternal mental illness and illicit drug use were both considered, the odds of offspring illicit drug use increased 93% over that of offspring of mothers not abusing drugs (NSDUH, 2005).

Women who abuse substances during or after their pregnancies are more likely to have out-of-home placement of their child (Sarkola, Kahila, Gissler, & Halmesmaki, 2007). Drug-exposed infants are increasingly referred to child protective services, which in turn increases the need for out-of-home care (McCullough, 1991). Overall, women who abuse drugs have higher rates of perinatal complications, psychiatric symptoms, and early reported childhood trauma. These women are at a high risk of experiencing an interruption in the continuity of their caregiving, and their exposed children are less likely to remain in their care. In the first 3 years of life, 20–46% of children from cocaine-affected pregnancies have been shown to be in nonparental care (Eiden, Foote, & Schuetze, 2007). Approximately 19% of mothers with cocaine abuse or dependence lost custody of their infants by 1 month of age, compared to 0.02% of noncocaine using mothers (Eiden et al., 2007). Mothers with SUDs were unable to provide care to 44% of their infants during the first 18 months of life, with younger mothers with heroin dependence and reported depressive symptoms the least likely to maintain care (Nair et al., 1997).

Lack of prenatal services, heavier substance abuse, an early childhood history of trauma, and greater psychiatric impairment are all factors that have been associated with loss of custody of an infant (Minnes, Singer, Humphrey-Wall, & Satayathum, 2008). The likelihood of loss is associated with substance abuse treatment after delivery and having a partner who abuses substances (Sarkola et al., 2007). These women may also struggle with limited employment, education, housing, and have previous children who are already in custody outside of their home—all of which increase the risk of early childhood out-of-home care (Sarkola et al., 2007). Should such cumulative risk factors not be addressed, the likelihood that mothers who lose custody will reunite with their children is decreased (Larrieu, Heller, & Smyke, 2008).

Child placement significantly affects the mother with SUDs. Women with cocaine dependence who retain custody of their children have been shown to have different characteristics and risk factors than women who use cocaine but do not maintain custody of their children. For instance, poor urban women who used cocaine prenatally and lost custody of their infant reported greater psychological and functional impairment postpartum than women who maintained custody of their infant. Such women who lost custody reported more somatization, anxiety, psychosis, and distress. They had higher rates of childhood trauma, including neglect and physical abuse, than women who did not lose custody of their infant (Minnes et al., 2008).

Among parents who initiate outpatient treatment for cocaine dependence, Lewis and Petry (2005) compared characteristics of those who retained custody versus those who did not. Noncustodial parents demonstrated more psychological distress, more prior history of alcohol problems, and greater current employment and legal problems than custodial parents. Other studies have confirmed that noncustodial parents have reported higher frequencies of drug use, homelessness, risky sex practices, psychological distress, and victimization experiences (Lam, Wechsberg, & Zule, 2004).

However, retaining custody of an infant could make it more difficult for a mother with an SUD to continue drug treatment if child care is not provided as part of treatment. Mothers who maintain custody of their children need to arrange child care for such treatment. Whereas custodial parents have been shown to have less psychiatric and functional impairment than noncustodial parents, they are also less likely to complete substance abuse treatment. The risk of dropping out of treatment was greatest for younger than 21, African American pregnant mothers, who had custody of minor children (Scott-Lennox, Rose, Bohlig, & Lennox, 2000). Even though custodial mothers have been shown to be more likely to have health insurance, they are less likely than noncustodial parents to have received drug treatment (Lam et al., 2004). Importantly, drug treatment compliance is associated with faster reunification between children who have been removed from the home and their parents, even when accounting for ongoing drug use (Smith, 2003).

Given the significant implications of maternal substance abuse on the mother, the child, and their relationship, the standard of practice for child custody evaluations includes a careful and systematic assessment of substance abuse. (For more detail see the American Academy of Child and Adolescent Psychiatry practice parameters for child custody evaluation, 1997, and the Association of Family and Conciliation Courts Model Standards of Practice for Child Custody Evaluation, 2006.) Allegations of abuse raised in mediations and custody investigations in California most frequently concern domestic violence and substance abuse (39% and 38%, respectively) (Johnston, Lee, Olesen, & Walters, 2005). The purpose of the evaluation should not be to determine that a parent is abusing substances. Rather, the clinician must assess the impact of possible parental substance abuse on the developmental needs of the child. Each potential drug of abuse should be investigated in a structured manner, and physical tests (e.g., urine toxicology) may be necessary (Schleuderer & Campagna, 2004). It should not be assumed that prenatal substance abuse reflects intentional maltreatment of a fetus or indifference to the health of the child, especially given the numerous barriers to receiving treatment. Additionally, a single drug test should not substitute for a thorough evaluation of parenting ability in the context of the child's best interest (Paltrow, 1991).

Although one study (Sorensen et al., 1995) showed that judges considering primary physical residence were more influenced by allegations of maltreatment than substance abuse, custody evaluators should nevertheless craft parenting plans that will benefit a child living with or having contact with a parent with an SUD. Parenting plans should consider the needs of each child relative to the problems created by the parental pattern of substance use. Supervised or therapeutic visitation may be recommended. Refusal of postdivorce visits with the noncustodial parent by a child is associated with having at least one parent with psychopathology, especially substance abuse (Racusin, Copans, & Mills, 1994). Given the potential dangers to children who reside with or visit a parent who is actively abusing substances, the risks and benefits should be considered in a way that favors the developmental interests of the child.

Judges will also be aided by an assessment of a parent's insight into the drug use, past substance treatment, and prognosis for future treatment. The substance abuse treatment system has increasingly recognized and sought to address the need for programming specifically designed for women. Motivation has been repeatedly shown to be an important predictor of whether a woman enters and completes a substance treatment program (Pelissier, 2004). Motivation can be difficult to sustain when women who abuse substances encounter barriers to treatment, including child care responsibilities, stigmatization, and lack of resources to pay for treatment if it is available. It is estimated that 30% of the treatment programs in the United States offer special programs or services for women, and that 14% offer programs for pregnant women; 13% of substance abuse treatment facilities surveyed offered child care services, and 12% offered prenatal services (Brady & Ashley, 2005). Two-thirds of major hospitals in 15 cities reported in 1989 that they had no place to refer pregnant women with SUDs (Kumpfer, 1991). With such a limited supply of drug treatment programs for pregnant women, 25 states have funded, and given priority access to, substance treatment programs for pregnant women (Lester et al., 2004).

Notwithstanding the limited availability of programs for women with SUDs, women who received treatment at women-only facilities or facilities offering child care services stayed in treatment longer than women who received treatment in mixed-gender facilities or facilities not offering child care services (Substance Abuse and Mental Health Services Administration [SAMHSA], 2007). One study of residential substance abuse programs for pregnant and parenting women found that a majority of former clients (61%) reported being completely drug- and alcohol free throughout the 6-month follow-up (Porowski, Burgdorf, & Herrell, 2004). Positive outcomes at such programs include reduced substance use, improvement in mental health symptoms, better perinatal/birth outcomes, better employment, improved self-reported health status, and HIV risk reduction (Orwin, Francisco, & Bernichon, 2001). Research also shows the importance of engaging families in services. More than three-quarters of women participating in the Residential Women's and Children's Program and the Pregnant and Parenting Women's Program (RWC/PPW) reported that their families were involved in alcohol- or drug-related activities. Almost half of them (42.9%) reported having fewer than two friends who did not use drugs. Having a support network greatly increases treatment retention and reductions in drug use for women (SAMHSA, 2007).

Family Drug Courts and Rehabilitative Approaches to the Treatment of Parents with Substance Use Disorders

Emerging findings indicate that there may be a role for family treatment drug courts that combine long-term substance abuse treatment and judicial supervision to support individual recovery. Participation in most drug courts is voluntary, but once enrolled, participation in treatment is required. These programs have the potential to strengthen families and improve child health because they are integrated with the public child welfare system. Drug courts have been shown to improve employment status, earned income, and social functioning (Bryan

& Havens, 2008). The presence of parental substance abuse necessitates the coordination of multiple social services, including the child welfare agency, court, and other community providers. Drug courts can facilitate communication among these services and mandate the treatment that a parent needs, with regular scrutiny and accountability by the court, while maintaining a family-based perspective (Semidei et al., 2001).

Such rehabilitative approaches that shift the focus from parental substance abuse to a whole-family context, including significant others, appear to be promising. When entire families are treated, the abilities of parents to support one another and their children increase (SAMHSA, 2007). For example, nine months after referral to a substance treatment program, clients who maintained sobriety were more likely to have significant-other support, child custody, and parental rights. These outcomes were not associated with court-ordered treatment (Gregoire & Schultz, 2001). Improving the existing support systems can maximize the potential for ongoing recovery while maintaining the safety of the child. More treatment programs designed for women are needed, and more research is required to assess their treatment effectiveness (Kumpfer, 1991).

ISSUES IN THE CRIMINAL JUSTICE SYSTEM

Overview of Drug Use and Arrest and Prosecution

Drug use is inextricably interwoven into the criminal justice system in the United States through a number of nexuses; including drug offenses, drug-related crime, crime that occurred when the perpetrator was under the influence of drugs or alcohol, and treatment of drug- and alcohol-addicted inmates in local, state, and federal correctional institutions (USDOJ, 2007a). The most obvious nexus between drug use and the criminal justice system is entry as a result of a drug offense. According to the Federal Bureau of Investigation, drug abuse violations are defined as offenses "relating to the unlawful possession, sale, use, growing, manufacturing, and making of narcotic drugs including opium, cocaine and their derivatives, marijuana, synthetic narcotics, and dangerous nonnarcotic drugs such as barbiturates" (Federal Bureau of Investigation (FBI), 2005b; USDOJ, 2007a).

Federal, state, and local authorities make between 1.8 and 1.9 million arrests per year for drug abuse violations (FBI, 2005b, 2007) out of approximately 14 million total arrests per year, not including traffic violations. This arrest rate makes drug abuse violations the most common category of arrests in the United States. Within the category of drug violations, approximately 80% are for substance possession (FBI, 2006; USDOJ, 2007a). Of substance possession arrests nationwide, the most common substance is marijuana (37–39%), with some regional variation (FBI, 2007; USDOJ, 2007a). Overall, women represent approximately 24% of annual arrests and 19% of drug abuse violations (FBI, 2006).

The connection between addiction and entry into the criminal justice system goes beyond arrests for drug use violations. Studies of postconviction correctional institution inmates have shown that between 16 and 18% of crimes are committed to obtain drug money (USDOJ, 2007a). In local and state facilities, between 25 and 33% of property offenses were committed to obtain money for drugs, approximately 25% of drug offenses were committed to obtain money for drugs, and less than 10% of violent offenses were committed to support a drug habit (USDOJ, 2007a). Within the federal correctional system, the distribution of offenses to obtain drugs has been somewhat different from that in state and local facilities: 25% of drug crimes, nearly 15% of violent crime, and less than 11% of property crimes reportedly were committed to obtain drug money (USDOJ, 2007a).

A third connection between drug use and entry into the criminal justice system is through offenses committed while under the influence of an addictive substance. In a 2004 survey, approximately 25% of federal inmates and nearly 33% of state inmates reported that they had committed the offense for which they were incarcerated while under the influence of drugs (USDOJ, 2007a). Individuals incarcerated for drug offenses had the highest reported rate of crimes committed under the influence of drugs: 44% in state and 32% in federal custody (USDOJ, 2007a). In state facilities, 39% of property offenders said they were under the influence of drugs at the time of their instant offense (the offense for which they were arrested), making these offenses the second most likely to be committed under the influence of drugs (USDOJ, 2007a). Second among federal offenses committed under the influence of drugs were violent crimes, with nearly 25% of offenders reported under the influence of drugs at the time of the crime (USDOJ, 2007a). Similarly, a 2005 survey of victims of violent crime showed that more than 25% of victims reported that the perpetrator of the crime against them was under the use of alcohol, drugs, or both (USDOJ, 2007a).

Gender Differences in Offender Populations

Gender differences clearly exist in the proportion of correctional system inmates incarcerated for drug, property, and other nonviolent offenses. Specifically, women are less likely than men to be confined for violent offenses and more likely to be confined for drug or property crimes; government data from 2005 showed that nearly 60% of women in state prison facilities were confined due to property or drug crimes, compared to 40% of men (FBI, 2006; Sentencing Project, 2007). The number of female prisoners has risen steadily since 1980 and is increasing at a rate greater than the male prison population (Centers for Disease Control [CDC], 2001; Messina, Burdon, Hagopian, & Prendergast, 2006; USDOJ, 2007b, 2007c, 2007d, 2007e). Historically, female inmates have had higher rates of drug use than male inmates; in some samples approximately 80% of incarcerated women reported using drugs and/or alcohol in the past, with more than half using in the month prior to their instant offense, 25% under the influence at the time of the crime, and 25% committing a crime to obtain money for drugs (CDC, 2001). More recent data from 2004 found that 60% of women in state prison had a history of drug dependence (Sentencing Project, 2007).

Retrospective data analysis has suggested that, over time, women have been disproportionately incarcerated for drug-related activity. For example, between 1986 and 1996, rates of incarceration for nondrug offences of women slightly more than doubled (130%), and the number of women in correctional custody for drug-related offenses rose nearly ninefold (888%) (ACLU, 2006; Sentencing Project, 2007). Half of the increase in the state female inmate population from 1986 to 1996 was due to drug offenses, compared to one-third of the increase for men during the same time period (ACLU, 2006). Overall, women are more likely than men to serve time for drug offenses (Sentencing Project, 2007).

The proportion of female juvenile drug arrests also appears to be increasing, relative to male juvenile offenders. Even though more than 80% of juvenile drug arrests were of males in 2003, the proportion of female juvenile arrests for drug-related offenses increased steadily between 1994 and 2003 by approximately 5.5% (FBI, 2005a). In addition, an increasing proportion of juvenile females appear to be arrested for drug offenses at younger ages compared to male juveniles. Specifically, a 9-year retrospective analysis of trends in juvenile drug arrests from 1994 to 2003 showed that a higher proportion of female juveniles were arrested at a younger age (15 and under) than were male juveniles (FBI, 2005a).

Women may also be negatively affected by changes in drug laws, leading to their incarceration at a higher rate than men for less serious and less or nonviolent offenses than men. For example, although historical data have suggested that women are less likely than men to play a central role in the drug trade, a broadening sphere of criminal liability, including accomplices, conspiracy, and mandatory sentences, has apparently affected women disproportionately (ACLU, 2006; Rathbone, 2005). In addition, analysis of men and women seeking entry into drug treatment in the California prison system showed that men had more serious criminal justice involvement than women prior to incarceration (Messina, Burdon & Prendergast, 2006). Finally, according to the ACLU, these changes in drug laws have allowed criminal liability for drug crimes to attach to "partners, relatives, and bystanders" of drug-offense perpetrators (ACLU, 2006).

Given the association between substance use and entry into the criminal justice system, it is no surprise that addiction is widespread in individuals under the supervision of the criminal justice system. What is not entirely clear is how these individuals should be treated by society. Specifically, are individuals with SUDs criminals who should be punished, or do these individuals become offenders as a result of their addiction and other associated factors (Gendel, 2004, 2006)? How society views the nature of addiction has important repercussions for how drug use behaviors are treated within the criminal justice system. If drug use should be punished criminally, then offenders should be punished, but if criminal acts are the result of addiction-related behavior, then treatment should be more effective than punishment (Gendel, 2006). In fact, the criminal justice system appears to use a hybrid approach, combining incarceration with or without treatment for addiction (as evidenced by the growth in prison populations), with some diversion programs through mechanisms such as drug courts, which are generally limited to nonviolent offenders (Gendel, 2004, 2006)

Treatment for Substance Abuse within Correctional Facilities: Implications for Women

Within correctional facilities, substance abuse treatment includes detoxification, counseling, residential programs such as therapeutic communities, maintenance programs, 12-step and self-help groups, and education/awareness programs. Although the proportion of inmates with alcohol and drug addiction in local, state, and federal facilities is high, treatment resources have historically been inadequate to meet this need. A 2002 study indicated that only 18% of local jail inmates who met the criteria for drug abuse or dependence and only 17% who met the criteria for alcohol abuse or dependence had participated in treatment programs since incarceration (USDOJ, 2007a).

Treatment rates in state and federal facilities were higher, according to 2004 data that showed that 39% of state and 45% of federal inmates who had used drugs in the month before their offense had received some drug treatment or participated in a drug program (USDOJ, 2007a). Both of these percentages represented approximately a 5% increase since 1997 and were attributed to increased participation in self-help groups, peer counseling, and drug abuse education programs (USDOJ, 2007a). It should also be noted, however, that notwithstanding only a small percentage increase in participation in drug-related programs in federal and state facilities, due to the increase in the state and federal prison populations during the period from 1997 to 2004, the actual number of inmates receiving substance abuse treatment grew by 33% in state facilities and by 90% in federal prisons (USDOJ, 2007a)

But even with these increases in the actual number of inmates receiving treatment, the availability of treatment falls significantly short of guidelines promulgated by the National Commission on Correctional Health Care (NCCHC; 1992); the American Psychiatric Association, which contends that correctional mental health care should be required to meet the prevailing community care standards (Gendel, 2006); and principles endorsed by the

National Institute on Drug Abuse (NIDA), which include integration of treatment planning for substance abuse with criminal justice supervision (NIDA, 2006).

The limitations in the provision of mental health and substance abuse treatment services in correctional facilities are especially problematic for women. Once women with addiction come to the attention of the criminal justice system, regardless of the setting in which treatment is provided, their treatment needs are substantially different from, and generally much greater than, those of their male cohort. Specifically, research focused on women offenders entering correctionally based treatment has shown inmate characteristics such as consistently high numbers of trauma and abuse histories, interpersonal violence, and chronic mental and physical health problems, compared with men (Messina, Burdon, & Prendergast, 2006; UDDOJ, 2007a). Approximately half of incarcerated women have been the victim of physical or sexual abuse, and women are also more likely than men to be victims of domestic violence (NIDA, 2006), for which substance abuse is a risk factor (Beck, 2004). Female offenders are also more likely to have mental illness and to have used more drugs more frequently prior to incarceration than male offenders (NIDA, 2006). The presence of psychiatric disorders among women in prison has been documented over time and in the United Kingdom as well as the United States (NIDA, 2006; Turner & Tofler, 1986).

Although these gender-associated differences have been well established, outcomes of correctional treatment programs for women have been poorly studied and understood. Treatment programs serving both men and women may provide effective treatment for women, but gender-specific programs may be more effective within the female correctional population, especially for women with trauma and abuse histories (NIDA, 2006). In one study based at a California women's facility that implemented a traditional therapeutic community (TC) program, for example, findings showed that there were no differences between the TC treatment group and the no-treatment control population in 6- and 12-month return-to-custody rates, in contrast to evidence that the TC model is effective in men (Messina, Burdon, & Prendergast, 2006). In the same study the only significant difference in return-to-custody rates occurred between treatment only and treatment plus community-based aftercare populations, suggesting an important role for postrelease aftercare (Messina, Burdon, & Prendergast, 2006). The authors suggested that the lack of effect from a TC treatment program for women may be an indication that gender-specific and responsive treatment is required for female offenders with drug dependence. This conclusion mirrors data about gender differences in treatment needs in noncorrectional studies, which have shown that specialized, gender-specific services are required to treat women with SUDs, and that programs that are effective for men may fall short for women (Pelissier, Camp, Gaes, Saylor, & Rhodes, 2003)

Another analysis of male and female inmates entering prison-based TC treatment in California similarly showed that success in avoiding return to custody was associated with participation in aftercare, and that mental illness was associated with an increased likelihood of reincarceration (Messina, Burdon, Hagopian, et al., 2006). A third multisite study of substance abuse treatment outcomes for male and female federal prison programs showed that implementation of a cognitive-behavioral treatment model could result in comparable outcomes across programs, but that specific program implementation factors could affect outcomes (Pelissier, Motivans, & Rounds-Bryant, 2005). In this study, however, whereas there was no difference in treatment outcomes for 16 male programs studied, in the four female programs studied, one had significantly higher drug use rates and one had significantly lower recidivism rates that could not be statistically accounted for based on the data characteristics (Pelissier et al., 2005). Furthermore, for both men and women, motivation to change appears to be an important predictor of treatment entry and completion (Pelissier, 2004).

FUTURE DIRECTIONS

Based on the available research, continued study of effective treatment modalities for incarcerated women is needed to elucidate what interventions are effective for SUDs. What is clear at this point, however, is that any effective treatment is likely to include postrelease aftercare, address the significant psychiatric comorbidity of women with SUDs in correctional custody, and target the psychosocial factors such as trauma and abuse that have been well documented to occur among women offenders. Other factors that will also likely need to be addressed include the relatively low academic achievement of female prison inmates and familial factors such as parenting, maintenance of familial integrity, and child custody (Sentencing Project, 2007).

KEY POINTS

- Different jurisdictions have developed varying approaches toward women who use drugs or alcohol during pregnancy, ranging from treatment-based approaches to criminal sanctions.
- Provision of substance abuse treatment to pregnant women is associated with positive outcomes, including reduced substance use, improvement in mental health symptoms, better perinatal/ birth outcomes, better employment, improved self-reported health status, and HIV risk reduction.
- Because it often affects the nature and quality of parenting, a thorough assessment of substance use is standard practice in child custody evaluations.
- Women are more likely than men to be incarcerated for drug and property crimes and less likely than men to be incarcerated for violent crime.
- Among individuals involved in the criminal justice system, women are more likely than men to have a history of trauma or abuse, mental illness, and a longer and more extensive substance abuse history.
- The availability of substance abuse treatment for women in correctional institutions is limited, and there are few outcome data regarding the efficacy of these treatment programs.

REFERENCES

Asterisks denote recommended readings.

Abel, E. L., & Kruger, M. (2002). Physician attitudes concerning legal coercion of pregnant alcohol and drug abusers. *American Journal of Obstetrics and Gynecology, 186*(4), 768–772.
American Academy of Child and Adolescent Psychiatry. (1997). Practice parameters for child custody evaluation. *Journal of the American Academy of Child and Adolescent Psychiatry, 36*(10, Suppl.), 57S–68S.
American Civil Liberties Union. (2006). *Women in prison: An overview.* Retrieved May 31, 2008, from *www.aclu.org/womensrights/violence/25829res20060612.html.*
Association of Family and Conciliation Courts. (2006). *Model standards of practice for child custody evaluation.* Madison, WI.
Boland, P. (1991). Perspective of a juvenile court judge. *The Future of Children, 1*(1), 100–104.
Brady, T. M., & Ashley, O. S. (2005). *Women in substance abuse treatment: Results from the Alcohol and Drug Services Study (ADSS).* Substance Abuse and Mental Health Services Administration Office of Applied Studies. Retrieved June 6, 2008, from *www.drugabusestatistics.samhsa.gov/womenTX/womenTX.htm.*
Bryan, V., & Havens, J. (2008). Key linkages between child welfare and substance abuse treatment:

Social functioning improvements and client satisfaction in a family drug treatment court. *Family Court Review*, 46(1), 151–162. (*)

Centers for Disease Control. (2001). *Women, injection drug use, and the criminal justice system.* Retrieved on May 21, 2008, from *www.cdc.gov/idu/facts/cj-women.pdf.*

Eiden, R. D., Foote, A., & Schuetze, P. (2007). Maternal cocaine use caregiving status: Group differences in caregiver and infant risk variables. *Addictive Behaviors*, 32(3), 465–476.

Famularo, R., Kinscherff, R., & Fenton, T. (1992). Parental substance abuse and the nature of child maltreatment. *Child Abuse and Neglect*, 16(4), 475–483.

Federal Bureau of Investigation. (2005a). *Uniform crime report: Crime in the United States 2004, Special Report: Arrest of juveniles for drug abuse violations 1994–2003.* Washington, DC: U.S. Department of Justice. Retrieved May 30, 2008, from *www.fbi.gov/ucr/cius_04/special_reports/arrest_juveniles.html.*

Federal Bureau of Investigation. (2005b). *Uniform crime report: Crime in the United States 2004, Appendix II: Offenses in uniform crime reporting.* Washington, DC: U.S. Department of Justice. Retrieved May 30, 2008, from *www.fbi.gov/ucr/cius_04/appendices/appendix_02.html.*

Federal Bureau of Investigation. (2006). *Uniform crime report: Crime in the United States 2005, persons arrested.* Retrieved May 30, 2008, from *www.fbi.gov/ucr/05cius/arrests/index.html.*

Gendel, M. H. (2004). Forensic and medical legal issues in addiction psychiatry. *Psychiatric Clinics of North America*, 27, 611–626.

Gendel, M. H. (2006). Substance misuse and substance-related disorders in forensic psychiatry. *Psychiatric Clinics of North America*, 29, 649–673. (*)

Gomby, D. S., & Shiono, P. H. (1991). Estimating the number of substance-exposed infants. *The Future of Children*, 1(1), 17–25.

Gregoire, K. A., & Schultz, D. J. (2001). Substance-abusing child welfare parents: Treatment and child placement outcomes. *Child Welfare Journal*, 80(4), 433–452.

Harris, L. H., & Paltrow, L. (2003). The status of pregnant women and fetuses in U.S. criminal law. *Journal of the American Medical Association*, 289(13), 1697–1699.

Jaudes, P. K., Ekwo, E., & Van Voorhis, J. (1995). Association of drug abuse and child abuse. *Child Abuse and Neglect*, 19(9), 1065–1075.

Johnston, J. R., Lee, S., Olesen, N. W., & Walters, M. G. (2005). *Family Court Review*, 43(2), 283–294.

Kronstadt, D. (1991). Complex developmental issues of prenatal drug exposure. *The Future of Children*, 1(1), 36–49.

Kumpfer, K. L. (1991). Treatment programs for drug-abusing women. *The Future of Children*, 1 (1), 50–60.

Lam, W. K. K., Wechsberg, W., & Zule, W. (2004). African-American women who use crack cocaine: A comparison of mothers who live with and have been separated from their children. *Child Abuse and Neglect*, 28(11), 1229–1247.

Larrieu, J. A., Heller, S. S., & Smyke, A. T. (2008). Predictors of permanent loss of custody for mothers of infants and toddlers in foster care. *Infant Mental Health Journal*, 29(1), 48–60.

Larson, C. S. (1991). Overview of state legislative and judicial responses. *The Future of Children*, 1(1), 72–84.

Lester, B. M., Andreozzi, L., & Appiah, L. (2004). Substance use during pregnancy: Time for policy to catch up with research. *Harm Reduction Journal*, 1(5), 5.

Lester, B. M., & Twomey, J. E. (2008). Treatment of substance abuse during pregnancy. *Women's Health*, 4(1), 67–77.

Lewis, M. W., & Petry, N. M. (2005). Relationship between custodial status and psychosocial problems among cocaine-abusing parents initiating substance abuse treatment. *American Journal of Addiction*, 14(5), 403–415.

Linder, E. N. (2005). Punishing prenatal alcohol abuse: The problems inherent in utilizing civil commitment to address addiction. *University of Illinois Law Review*, 3, 873–902.

March of Dimes. (2006). Quick reference fact sheets: Illicit drug use during pregnancy. Retrieved May 27, 2008, from *www.marchofdimes.com/professionals.*

McCullough, C. B. (1991). The child welfare response. *The Future of Children*, 1(1), 61–71.

Messina, N., Burdon, W., Hagopian, G., & Prendergast, M. (2006). Predictors of prison-based treatment outcomes: A comparison of men and women participants. *American Journal of Drug and Alcohol Abuse, 32*, 7–28.

Messina, N., Burdon, W., & Prendergast, M. (2006). Prison-based treatment for drug-dependent women offenders: Treatment versus no treatment. *Journal of Psychoactive Drugs*, SARC Suppl. 3, 333–343.

Minkoff, H., & Paltrow, L. M. (2004). Melissa Rowland and the rights of pregnant women. *Obstetrics and Gynecology, 104*(6), 1234–1236.

Minnes, S., Singer, L. T., Humphrey-Wall, R., & Satayathum, S. (2008). Psychosocial and behavioral factors related to the post-partum placements of infants born to cocaine-using women. *Child Abuse and Neglect, 32*(3), 353–366.

Murray, T. H. (1991). Prenatal drug exposure: Ethical issues. *The Future of Children, 1*(1), 105–112.

Nair, P., Black, M. M., Schuler, M., Keane, V., Snow, L., et al. (1997). Risk factors for disruption in primary caregiving among infants of substance abusing women. *Child Abuse and Neglect, 21*(11), 1039–1051.

National Advocates for Pregnant Women. (2008). *Regina McKnight: Victory at long last.* Retrieved June 9, 2008, from *www.advocatesfor pregnantwomen.org.*

National Commission on Correctional Health Care Position Statements. (1992). *Mental health services in correctional settings.* National Commission on Correctional Health Care 1992. Retrieved May 28, 2008, from *www.ncchc.org/resources/statements/mentalhealth.html.*

National Institute on Alcohol Abuse and Alcoholism. (2007a). Alcohol and pregnancy: Civil commitment. Alcohol Policy Information System. Retrieved May 27, 2008, from *www.alcoholpolicy. niaaa.nih.gov.*

National Institute on Alcohol Abuse and Alcoholism. (2007b). *Alcohol and pregnancy: Number of states with provisions authorizing civil commitment, January 1, 1998 through January 1, 2007.* Alcohol Policy Information System. Retrieved May 27, 2008, from *www.alcoholpolicy.niaaa.nih. gov.*

National Institute on Alcohol Abuse and Alcoholism. (2007c). *Alcohol and pregnancy: Number of states with provisions pertaining to child abuse/child neglect, January 1, 2003 through January 1, 2007.* Alcohol Policy Information System. Retrieved May 27, 2008, from *www.alcoholpolicy. niaaa.nih.gov.*

National Institute on Drug Abuse. (2006). *Principles of drug abuse treatment for criminal justice populations* (Publication No. 06-5316). National Institutes of Health 2006. Retrieved on May 27, 2008, from *www.drugabuse.gov/PDF/PODAT_CJ/PODAT_CJ.pdf.* (*)

National Survey on Drug Use and Health Report. (2005). *Mothers' serious mental illness and substance use among youths.* Department of Health and Human Services 2005. Retrieved May 27, 2008, from *www.oas.samhsa.gov.*

Orwin, R. G., Francisco, L., & Bernichon, T. (2001). *Effectiveness for women's substance abuse treatment programs: A Meta-Analysis Center for Substance Abuse Treatment.* Arlington, VA: SAMHSA.

Paltrow, L. M. (1991). Perspective of a reproductive rights attorney. *The Future of Children, 1*(1), 85–92.

Paltrow, L. M. (1998). Punishing women for their behavior during pregnancy: An approach that undermines the health of women and children. *Drug Addiction Research and the Health of Women.* Rockville, MD: National Institute on Drug Abuse.

Pelissier, B. (2004). Gender differences in substance use treatment entry and retention among prisoners with substance use histories. *American Journal of Public Health, 94*(8), 1418–1424.

Pelissier, B., Camp, S. D., Gaes, G. G., Saylor, W. G., & Rhodes, W. (2003). Gender differences in outcomes from prison-based residential treatment. *Journal of Substance Abuse Treatment, 24*, 149–160.

Pelissier, B., Motivans, M., & Rounds-Bryant, J. L. (2005). Substance abuse treatment outcomes: A multi-site study of male and female prison programs. *Journal of Offender Rehabilitation, 41*(2), 57–80.

Phibbs, C. S. (1991). The economic implications of prenatal substance exposure. *The Future of Children, 1*(1), 113–120.

Porowski, A. W., Burgdorf, K., & Herrell, J. M. (2004). Effectiveness and sustainability of residential substance abuse treatment programs for pregnant and parenting women. *Evaluation and Program Planning, 27,* 191–198.

Powell v. Texas, 392 U.S. 514 (1968).

Racusin, R. J., Copans, S. A., & Mills, P. (1994). Characteristics of families of children who refuse post-divorce visits. *Journal of Clinical Psychology, 50*(5), 792–801.

Rathbone, C. (2005). *A world apart: Women, prison, and life behind bars.* New York: Random House.

Robinson v. California, 370 U.S. 660 (1962).

Sabol, W. J., Minton, T. D., & Harrison, P. M. (2007). *Bureau of justice statistics bulletin: Prison and jail inmates at midyear 2006.* Report NCJ 217675, U.S. Department of Justice 2007. Retrieved on May 30, 2008, from *www.ojp.usdoj.gov/bjs/pub/pdf/pjim06.pdf.*

Sarkola, T., Kahila, H., Gissler, M., & Halmesmaki, E. (2007). Risk factors for out-of-home custody child care among families with alcohol and substance abuse problems. *Acta Paediatrica, 96*(11), 1571–1576.

Schleuderer, C., & Campagna, V. (2004). Assessing substance abuse questions in child custody evaluations. *Family Court Review, 42*(2), 375–383.

Schouten, R., & Brendel, R. W. (2008). The role of psychiatrists in the criminal justice system. In T. A. Stern, J. F. Rosenbaum, M. Fava, J. Biederman, & S. L. Rauch (Eds.), *Comprehensive clinical psychiatry* (pp. 1155–1164). Philadelphia: Mosby.

Scott-Lennox, J., Rose, R., Bohlig, A., & Lennox, R. (2000). The impact of women's family status on completion of substance abuse treatment. *Journal of Behavioral Health Services and Research, 27*(4), 366–379.

Semidei, J., Radel, L. F., & Nolan, C. (2001). Substance abuse and child welfare: Clear linkages and promising responses. *Child Welfare, 80*(4), 109–128.

Sentencing Project, The. (2007). *Women in the criminal justice system* (briefing sheets). Washington, DC: Author.

Smith, B. D. (2003). How parental drug use and drug treatment compliance relate to family reunification. *Child Welfare, 82*(3), 335–365.

Sood, B., Delaney-Black, V., Covington, C., Nordstrom-Klee, B., Ager, J., Templin, T., et al. (2001). Prenatal alcohol exposure and childhood behavior at age 6 to 7 years: I. Dose–response effect. *Pediatrics, 108*(2), E34.

Sorensen, E., Goldman, J., Ward, M., Albanese, I., Graves, L., & Chamberlain, C. (1995). Judicial decision-making in contested custody cases: The influence to reported child abuse, spouse abuse, and parental substance abuse. *Child Abuse and Neglect, 19* (2), 251–260.

Steven, S., & Ahlstrom, A. S. (1991). Perspective from a Minnesota county attorney's office. *The Future of Children, 1*(1), 93–99.

Substance Abuse and Mental Health Services Administration. (2007). *Family-centered treatment for women with substance use disorders: History, key elements, and challenges.* Retrieved June 7, 2008, from *womenandchildren.treatment.org/Family_Treatment_Paper.pdf.*

Turner, T. H., & Tofler, D. S. (1986). Indicators of psychiatric disorder among women admitted to prison. *British Medical Journal, 292,* 651–653.

U.S. Department of Justice Bureau of Justice Statistics. (2007a). *Drugs and crime facts* (Report NCJ 165148). Retrieved May 21, 2008, from *www.ojp.usdoj.gov/bjs/dcf/contents.htm.* (*)

U.S. Department of Justice Bureau of Justice Statistics. (2007b). *Jail statistics.* Retrieved May 21, 2008, from *www.ojp.usdoj.gov/bjs/jails.htm.*

U.S. Department of Justice Bureau of Justice Statistics. (2007c). *Prison statistics.* Retrieved May 21, 2008, from *www.ojp.usdoj.gov/bjs/prisons.htm.*

U.S. Department of Justice Bureau of Justice Statistics. (2007d). *Prison and jail inmates at midyear 2006* (Report NCJ 217675). Retrieved May 21, 2008, from *www.ojp.usdoj.gov/bjs/pub/pdf/pjim06.pdf.*

U.S. Department of Justice Bureau of Justice Statistics. (2007e). *Prisoners in 2006* (Report NCJ 219416). Retrieved May 21, 2008, from *www.ojp.usdoj.gov/bjs/abstract/p06.htm.*

Wetherington, C. L., & Roman, A. B. (Eds.). (1998). *Drug addiction research and the health of women.* Rockville, MD: National Institute on Drug Abuse.

Whitaker, R. C., Orzol, S. M., & Kahn, R. S. (2006). Maternal mental health, substance use, and domestic violence in the year after delivery and subsequent behavior problems in children at age 3 years. *Archives of General Psychiatry, 63,* 551–560.

Zuckerman, B. (1991). Drug-exposed infants: Understanding the medical risk. *The Future of Children, 1*(1), 26–35.

Index